Cognitive Therapy across the Lifespan

In this balanced and critical overview, an international team of experts examines systematically the evidence in support of the effectiveness of cognitive-behavioral approaches to treating clinical problems across the lifespan. They analyze the cognitive models of psychopathology on which these treatments are based, and identify the clinical and conceptual problems, giving specific recommendations for addressing them. The range of disorders covered includes depression, anxiety, panic disorder, schizophrenia, obsessive-compulsive disorder, personality disorders, eating disorders, posttraumatic stress disorder, conduct problems, and addiction.

Mark A. Reinecke is Chief of the Division of Psychology at the Northwestern University Medical School.

David A. Clark is Professor of Psychology at the University of New Brunswick. Both have published widely in the area of cognitive behavior therapy.

Cognitive Therapy across the Lifespan

Edited by

Mark A. Reinecke
Northwestern University Medical School

David A. Clark
University of New Brunswick

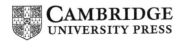
CAMBRIDGE
UNIVERSITY PRESS

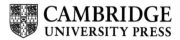

CAMBRIDGE
UNIVERSITY PRESS

Shaftesbury Road, Cambridge CB2 8EA, United Kingdom

One Liberty Plaza, 20th Floor, New York, NY 10006, USA

477 Williamstown Road, Port Melbourne, VIC 3207, Australia

314–321, 3rd Floor, Plot 3, Splendor Forum, Jasola District Centre, New Delhi – 110025, India

103 Penang Road, #05–06/07, Visioncrest Commercial, Singapore 238467

Cambridge University Press is part of Cambridge University Press & Assessment,
a department of the University of Cambridge.

We share the University's mission to contribute to society through the pursuit of
education, learning and research at the highest international levels of excellence.

www.cambridge.org
Information on this title: www.cambridge.org/9780521533775

© Cambridge University Press & Assessment 2004

First published 2003
Reprinted 2009

A catalogue record for this publication is available from the British Library

ISBN   978-0-521-65109-7   Hardback
ISBN   978-0-521-53377-5   Paperback

Contents

Contributors

Julie Wargo Aikins, PhD
Department of Psychology
Yale University
2 Hillhouse Avenue
New Haven CT 06520
USA

Arthur D. Anastopoulos, PhD
Department of Psychology
University of North Carolina at Greensboro
Box 26164
Greensboro NC 27402-6164
USA

R. Lindsey Bergman, PhD
UCLA Child OCD, Anxiety, & Tourette
   Disorders Program
Division of Child and Adolescent Psychiatry
UCLA Neuropsychiatric Institute, Room
   68-251
UCLA School of Medicine
760 Westwood Plaza
Los Angeles CA 90024
USA

Joseph D. Calabrese
Center for Psychiatric Rehabilitation
Department of Psychiatry
University of Chicago School of Medicine
7230 Arbor Drive
Tinley Part IL 60477
USA

Cheryl N. Carmin, PhD
Stress & Anxiety Disorders Clinic
Department of Psychiatry (M/C913)
University of Illinois-Chicago
913 South Wood Street
Chicago IL 60612-7327
USA

Nicola M. Chung, BA
Center for Alcohol Studies
Rutgers, the State University of
   New Jersey
607 Allison Rd
Piscataway NJ 08854-8001
USA

David A. Clark, PhD
Department of Psychology
University of New Brunswick
Bag Service # 45444
Fredericton
Canada NB E3B 6E4

Patrick W. Corrigan, PsyD
Center for Psychiatric Rehabilitation
Department of Psychiatry
University of Chicago School of
   Medicine
7230 Arbor Drive
Tinley Park IL 60477
USA

Sona Dimidjian, PhD
Center for Clinical Research
Department of Psychology
University of Washington
1107 NE 45th Street, #310
Seattle WA 98105
USA

Keith S. Dobson, PhD
Department of Psychology
University of Calgary
2500 University Drive NW
Calgary T2N 1N4
Alberta
Canada

David L. DuBois, PhD
Department of Psychology
University of Missouri
210 McAllester Hall
Columbia MO 65211
USA

Edna B. Foa, PhD
Center for the Study & Treatment of
    Anxiety
Department of Psychiatry
University of Pennsylvania School of
    Medicine
3535 Market Street, Suite 600N
Philadelphia PA 19104
USA

David A. F. Haaga, PhD
Department of Psychology
American University
Washington DC 20016-8062
USA

Richard G. Heimberg, PhD
Adult Anxiety Clinic of Temple University
Department of Psychology
Weiss Hall
Temple University
1701 North 13th Street
Philadelphia PA 19122-6085
USA

Elizabeth A. Hembree, PhD
Center for the Study & Treatment of Anxiety
Department of Psychiatry
University of Pennsylvania School of
    Medicine
3535 Market Street, Suite 600N
Philadelphia PA 19104
USA

Stefan G. Hofmann, PhD
Department of Psychology
Boston University
101 Newburg Street
Boston MA 02131
USA

Daniel le Grange, PhD
Department of Psychiatry
University of Chicago School of Medicine
5841 South Maryland Avenue, MC3077
Chicago IL 60637
USA

John E. Lochman, PhD
Department of Psychology
Box 870348
University of Alabama
Tuscaloosa AL 35487
USA

Christy Lopez
Department of Psychology
University of Missouri
210 McAllester Hall
Columbia MO 65211
USA

Thomas N. Magee
Department of Psychology
Box 870348
University of Alabama
Tuscaloosa AL 35487
USA

Douglas S. Mennin, PhD
Department of Psychology
Yale University
Box 208205
New Haven CT 06520-8205
USA

Thomas J. Morgan, PsyD
Center for Alcohol Studies
Rutgers, the State University of New Jersey
607 Allison Rd
Piscataway NJ 08854-8001
USA

Cory F. Newman, PhD
Center for Cognitive Therapy
Department of Psychiatry
University of Pennsylvania School of
Medicine
3600 Market Street
Philadelphia PA 19104-2649
USA

Dustin A. Pardini
Department of Psychology
Box 870348
University of Alabama
Tuscaloosa AL 35487
USA

Gilbert R. Parra
Department of Psychology
University of Missouri
210 McAllester Hall
Columbia MO 65211
USA

John Piacentini, PhD
UCLA Child OCD, Anxiety, & Tourette
    Disorders Program
Division of Child and Adolescent Psychiatry
UCLA Neuropsychiatric Institute, Room
    68–251
UCLA School of Medicine
760 Westwood Plaza
Los Angeles CA 90024
USA

Christine Purdon, PhD
Department of Psychology
University of Waterloo
200 University Avenue West
Waterloo
Ontario N2L 3G1
Canada

Ronald M. Rapee, PhD
Department of Psychology
Macquarie University
Sydney
NSW 2109
Australia

Christine L. Ratto, PhD
Department of Psychiatry and Behavioral
    Sciences
Albert Einstein College of Medicine
110 East 210th Street
Bronx NY 01467-2490
USA

Helen S. Raytek, PsyD
National Council on Alcoholism and Drug
    Dependence
6th Floor
18 Rector St
Newark NJ 07102
USA

Mark A. Reinecke, PhD
Division of Psychology
Department of Psychiatry & Behavioral
    Sciences
Northwestern University Medical School
Abbott Hall, Suite 1205
710 North Lakeshore Drive
Chicago IL 60610
USA

Paul M. Salkovskis, PhD
Department of Psychology
Institute of Psychiatry
de Crespigny Park
Denmark Hill
London SE5 8AF
UK

Jan Scott, PhD
University Department of Psychological
    Medicine
Gartnavel Royal Hospital
Glasgow University
Glasgow G12 OXH
Scotland
UK

Stephanie D. Shaffer
Department of Psychology
University of North Carolina at Greensboro
Box 26164
Greensboro NC 27402-6164
USA

Ari Solomon, PhD
Department of Psychology
Williams College
Williamstown MA 01267
USA

Susan H. Spence, PhD, MBA
School of Psychology
University of Queensland
Brisbane
QLD 4072
Australia

E. Paige Temple
Department of Psychology
Campus Box 7160
Chapel Hill NC 27599-7160
USA

Cynthia L. Turk, PhD
Department of Psychology
LaSalle University
1900 W. Oleny Avenue
Philadelphia PA 19141
USA

Karina Wahl
Department of Psychiatry
University of Oxford
Warneford Hospital
Oxford OX3 7JX
UK

Judith K. Wilson, BA (Hons)
Department of Psychology
Macquarie University
Sydney
NSW 2109
Australia

Foreword

A. T. Beck, M.D.

The remarkable development of cognitive intervention strategies to ameliorate maladaptive emotional and behavioral responses began in the 1960s with a specific focus on the use of cognitive constructs of depression and anxiety. In those days we relied on rather simple research methodologies and treatment formulations. What began as an attempt to redress oft-cited deficiencies in psychoanalytic and behavioral theory and treatment of emotional disorders has evolved 40 years later into a genuine paradigmatic shift in our approach to a broad range of psychological problems in children, adolescents, and adults.

Cognitive theory, therapy, and research have shown remarkable progress in a number of ways over the last few decades. Cognitive and cognitive-behavioral perspectives have been applied in very creative ways to a much broader range of clinical phenomena than originally imagined. New and innovative treatment approaches are continually under development and refinement. There is a greater understanding of therapeutic issues involved in the immediate effectiveness and long-term efficacy of cognitive therapy, and in the processes of change. Research into the cognitive basis of psychological disorders has attained a much higher standard as a result of contributions from experimental cognitive, developmental, and social psychology. Newer theoretical models that recognize the multidimensional, interactive, and dynamic nature of the human condition have been proposed. Cognitive theory and research have been enriched by the ongoing contributions of a large number of researchers and practitioners from diverse backgrounds in experimental, social, and developmental psychology as well as psychiatry and the neurosciences. It has now become daunting to keep abreast of developments that are occurring on so many fronts.

This book is the latest edited volume on cognitive and cognitive-behavior therapy. What makes it different from many of the previous publications is evident even from a perusal of the table of contents. The editors have succeeded in bringing together the leading researchers within the field of cognitive-clinical psychology to deal with a wide range of clinical disorders. In fact, this is one of the few edited books to cover such a broad range of psychological disorders. For the most part, each of the chapters discusses research on cognitive theory and treatment with an effort show how each informs the other. This emphasis on both theory and therapy is very much in keeping with the strong empirical basis of the cognitive and cognitive-behavioral perspectives. As well, the contributors raise many interesting and perplexing issues that will continue to drive much of the research and development in cognitive-clinical theory and therapy for the next few years. A final strength of the current volume is its lifespan perspective. By bringing together experts in child and adolescent mental health, the present volume has much to offer the mental health professional. For students and professionals wanting an introduction to cognitive-clinical theory and treatment, this volume provides an excellent introduction to the field. For the advanced cognitive-clinical researcher or practitioner, this book will be a valuable resource for updating your knowledge base on a wide range of clinical disorders.

Perhaps the most important contribution of this volume, however, is found in the discerning, critical stance taken by the contributors. More than a review of the current literature, this volume critiques both the clinical literature on the effectiveness of cognitive therapy and the scientific foundations on which these interventions are based. As C. S. Peirce wrote nearly a century ago, "to reason well ... it is absolutely necessary to possess ... intellectual honesty and sincerity and a real love of truth." The contributors to this volume demonstrate intellectual honesty and sincerity. They recognize that for the field of cognitive therapy to develop it is necessary to maintain a skeptical eye toward our models and treatments. It is only by genuine and critical inquiry that these can be refined and developed, and that they may come to be accepted. This book unflinchingly examines the strengths and weaknesses of cognitive approaches to psychotherapy and the empirical foundations on which they stand, and so provides guidelines for future developments in the field. This is a remarkable and valuable volume.

REFERENCE

Hartshorne, C., Weiss, P., and Burks, A. (eds) (1931–58). *Collected Papers of Charles Sanders Peirce.* Cambridge, MA: Harvard University Press.

Cognitive therapy across the lifespan: conceptual horizons

Mark A. Reinecke[1] and David A. Clark[2]

[1] Northwestern University Medical School, Chicago, IL, USA
[2] University of New Brunswick, Fredericton, Canada

Important advances have been made in the field of cognitive therapy during the past 30 years, and numerous books have been published describing the application of these models to a range of clinical problems and populations. The ascent of cognitive therapy has been rapid and, in many ways, quite remarkable. It has become an integral part of training in psychiatry and clinical psychology, and has emerged as a dominant paradigm for understanding psychopathology and psychosocial intervention. Even a brief perusal of the contents of contemporary journals attests to the strength and breadth of these approaches.

How did this come about? Cognitive therapy emerged during the late 1950s and early 1960s as the result of the convergence of several historical trends (Mahoney, 1991; Clark and Beck, 1999; Dobson and Dozois, 2001). These included: (1) a growing recognition of the importance of information-processing models in linguistics and experimental cognitive psychology; (2) the publication of studies supporting mediational models of human adaptation, and the emergence of social learning theory as a paradigm for understanding the development of psychopathology; (3) a growing dissatisfaction with traditional drive models of human motivation and the dearth of empirical support for the effectiveness of psychodynamic forms of psychotherapy; and (4) a recognition of limits of classical behavioral models for understanding human development. Cognitive therapy emerged, then, in response to social needs, and as a result of a growing recognition of the limitations of existing models. Its development was supported by the availability of social tools or resources – in this case, experimental methodologies for putting models and treatments based on them to the test, philosophical support for the role of linguistic symbols and cognitive constructs as mediators of human behavior, and a need to develop more effective treatments for specific disorders, such as major depression. It is likely that cognitive therapy, as a paradigm for understanding psychopathology and psychotherapy, would not have emerged in its present form had these historical trends, social needs, and empirical resources not converged.

Cognitive therapy, then, is a product of its time. Its evolution during the years ahead will be determined by these same factors – the recognition of the limits of extant models, the press of social needs, and the availability of new tools for addressing these shortcomings. A goal of this volume is to examine critically the shortcomings of current cognitive-behavioral models (both conceptually and in clinical practice), and to clarify the limits or bounds of extant theories – what George Kelly (1955) referred to as their "range of convenience." Related goals are to clarify social needs, and to note what emerging tools and resources might be used in addressing them.

Much of the current appeal of cognitive-behavioral therapy (CBT) stems from three factors – its intuitive simplicity, its reliance upon empirical methods for testing the validity of its models and the effectiveness of its treatments, and its clinical utility. These are not unimportant factors. Parsimony, empiricism, and clinical utility are values that have served the field of cognitive therapy well over the past 30 years – they should not be abandoned as models are developed to address a wider range of social concerns.

Cognitive theories of psychopathology and psychotherapy are founded upon a substantial base of experimental research regarding cognitive concomitants of emotional disorders (Dobson and Kendall, 1993; Clark and Beck, 1999). This reliance upon experimental methods for putting theories to the test and for documenting the efficacy of interventions has contributed to an ongoing process of "creative destruction" by which cognitive-behavioral models are made and remade, tested and refined.

The definition of cognitive-behavioral therapy

CBTs are based upon a simple proposition – that thought processes occur, and that they matter. As William James succinctly noted, "the first fact for us ... is that some form of thinking goes on." This acknowledgment of the central role of cognition in human adaptation, though controversial at the time, was prescient. As research abundantly demonstrates, cognitive processes are implicated in many forms of psychopathology (Dobson and Kendall, 1993), and attempts to modify maladaptive beliefs and attitudes can ameliorate these difficulties. What, however, constitutes a CBT? Is any model that acknowledges the role of cognitive processes in human adaptation a form of cognitive therapy? Are there specific therapeutic strategies and techniques that are shared by alternative forms of CBT? Is cognitive therapy, in essence, defined by its therapeutic strategies and techniques? Are the various forms of CBT that have been developed during recent years similar in practice, and can they be discriminated from other noncognitive forms of psychotherapy? Is cognitive change necessary and/or sufficient for behavioral and emotional improvement to occur? If it is not, then how does CBT exert its effects? These are questions which must be resolved if we are to understand the nature of cognitive-behavioral psychotherapy.

Kendall and Hollon (1979), in defining CBT, proposed that cognitive-behavioral models "attempt to . . . incorporate the cognitive activities of the client in the effort to produce therapeutic change." They are suggesting, as such, that a defining feature of CBT is the explicit focus on promoting cognitive change as a means of bringing about clinical improvement. This is consistent with the view that cognitive processes play a central role in the etiology and treatment of behavioral and emotional disorders. As Dobson (2001) stated, "in order for a treatment to be labeled a cognitive-behavioral therapy, it must be based on the mediational model. A therapist using this model is presumed to make the assumption that cognitive change will mediate or lead to behavioral change. . . . [they] use treatment methods to effect cognitive change in the service of behavioral change"(p. xii).

Dobson and Dozois (2001) proposed that all forms of CBT share three assumptions: (1) that cognitive activity affects behavior; (2) that cognitive contents and processes may be monitored and changed; and (3) that behavioral (and emotional) change may be affected through cognitive change. Other authors have, during recent years, suggested that alternative forms of CBT share additional assumptions as well. Freeman and Reinecke (1995), for example, observed that cognitive-behavioral models implicitly assume that the processing of information is active and adaptive, and that it allows individuals to derive a sense of meaning from their experiences. They noted, as well, that cognitive-behavioral models assume that belief systems are idiosyncratic, and that incoming information is typically assimilated to existing belief systems. Finally, they noted that cognitive-behavioral models assume that clinical disorders can be distinguished on the basis of specific belief (cognitive contents or products) and information-processing strategies (cognitive processes). Additional assumptions of cognitive therapy have been described by Clark and Beck (1999). Whether a model, clinical strategy, or technique may be viewed as a form of CBT depends on whether it is consistent with these assumptions. To the degree that models and techniques diverge from these assumptions, they will be seen as incompatible with cognitive-behavioral theories of psychopathology and change.

CBTs are not, from this perspective, defined by their techniques or by the strategies and technologies of change. Any intervention that brings about cognitive change as a means of facilitating behavioral and emotional change may be considered a form of cognitive therapy. Moreover, any model that explicitly acknowledges the mediating (or moderating) role of cognitive factors in human adaptation may be viewed as a variant of CBT. CBT may be viewed as a family of models, with alternative forms sharing all, many, or few of the fundamental assumptions of the theory. There is, as such, no bright line or critical feature (save the acknowledgment of the central role of cognitive mediation in human adaptation) that discriminates cognitive-behavioral theories and forms of treatment from those that are not. Models may be more or less similar to the exemplar (the Beck standard model of therapy for depression) depending upon how many of the fundamental assumptions of the model they incorporate. Finally, it is worth acknowledging that cognitive models do not assert that the only pathways to psychopathology involve cognitive vulnerability, or that the only mechanisms of change are cognitive in nature. Rather, they acknowledge that human adaptation and psychopathology are multiply determined. Most psychiatric disorders are multifactorial in origin, and risk factors for them often involve dimensional factors that operate within both the normal and abnormal range. Cognitive models are entirely consistent with contemporary research in developmental psychopathology indicating that environmental, biological, social, personality, and cognitive factors interact in contributing to individual patterns of psychopathology and behavioral maladaptation. Understanding the ways in which these factors interact over time stands as a important challenge for the field.

Efficacy of cognitive-behavioral treatments

Controlled-outcome studies suggest that therapies based upon these assumptions can be efficacious in treating a number of behavioral and emotional problems (Chambless et al., 1996; Nathan and Gorman, 1998; Strunk and DeRubeis, 2001). Cognitive-behavioral models have, over the years, been found to be clinically useful. Cognitive-behavioral treatment guidelines are typically presented in the form of manuals specifying procedures and techniques in a fairly prescriptive manner. There have been, to date, over 325 outcome studies completed examining the effectiveness of CBT (Butler and Beck, 2001). Although studies vary with regard to their methodological rigor, and long-term outcome studies are few, trials completed to date suggest that cognitive-behavioral interventions can be quite effective in treating a number of disorders and conditions. They have consistently been found to be more effective than no treatment in treating mood and anxiety disorders, and have been typically found to be as effective as alternative psychosocial and pharmacological interventions. As a consequence, cognitive therapy has been designated as an "empirically supported" or "well-established" treatment for a number of disorders, including major depression, panic, obsessive-compulsive disorder, and social anxiety (Chambless et al., 1996).

To be sure, the recent development of cognitive-behavioral treatment manuals and a literature on empirically supported forms of treatment has proven controversial (Fensterheim and Raw, 1996; Silverman, 1996; Addis, 1997; Nathan, 1998;

Addis et al., 1999). Concerns have been raised that these approaches are conceptually narrow, that they encourage rigid, formulaic treatment which does not attend to the needs of individual patients, that cognitive-behavioral approaches do not recognize the central importance of the therapeutic relationship as a facilitator of clinical improvement, and that methodologies for demonstrating the efficacy of treatments are biased in favor of problem-focused treatments, such as CBT. Many of these concerns are not entirely without merit. It is worth acknowledging, none the less, that the objectives of work on empirically supported treatments – to develop efficacious interventions, to evaluate the relative effectiveness of alternative treatments for specific clinical problems, and to disseminate information on effective interventions to clinicians in the community – are entirely reasonable. We have an obligation, as clinicians and scholars, to be accountable to our communities by attempting to develop effective treatments, by demonstrating their utility, by acknowledging their limitations, and by training our students accordingly. Although discussions of research into empirically supported psychotherapies have been spirited, a number of larger issues have not been addressed. Treatment manuals are typically developed so that the efficacy of standardized forms of treatment can be examined. What other functions do these manuals serve, and why have they become so prevalent at this point in time? Can these manuals assist us in better understanding the nature of the therapeutic relationship, and the ways in which relationship variables and therapeutic techniques affect treatment outcome? Finally, should treatment manuals be seen as guides for formulating cases and developing strategic treatment plans, or as proscriptive lists of techniques to be introduced in a regimented manner? These are important issues. They are issues that form the core of why treatment manuals have proven controversial.

Treatment manuals, assessment-driven treatment protocols, and best-practice guidelines have proven useful in many areas of medicine, including cardiology and oncology. Despite the increasing availability during recent years of manuals, guidelines, and protocols for empirically supported forms of psychotherapy, it is not at all clear that practitioners actually use them, or if they do, that they follow the manual as intended. Many of these programs, though effective, are not regularly used in everyday practice. Many clinicians do not like structured guidelines or protocols. They are seen as too inflexible and too tied to theories they find unacceptable. Why might this be? As Beutler (2000) observed, clinicians tend to give greater weight to their personal opinions and beliefs than to empirical evidence when making clinical decisions. Beliefs and personal experience are given credence and, when supported by others, are taken as evidence for the validity of their clinical approach. Adopting and effectively implementing something as broad and complex as an empirically supported treatment protocol, as such, can be daunting. It requires support, training, an openness to innovation, and an ability to set aside one's beliefs and preexisting clinical opinions. As Beutler (2000) succinctly stated, efforts to encourage the use of empirically supported treatments "ignore the unrealistic assumption that practitioners will willingly and easily forsake their own experience and preferences, that they will efficiently learn many different and contradictory methods . . . and that once these skills and techniques have been learned, they will continue, unaffected, indefinitely." Changing clinicians' behavior, as such, can be as complex and challenging as changing that of our patients. Empirically supported treatments, such as CBT, have true potential. The value of empirically supported treatment protocols for psychiatry and clinical psychology, and the ways in which they will influence clinical practices and the culture of psychotherapy, are only now becoming apparent.

The bounds of cognitive-behavioral theory

Although CBTs were developed as models of psychopathology and psychotherapy, need they be limited to these domains? What, for example, is the relationship of CBT to rational, postrationalist, and poststructuralist models currently used in such diverse fields as economics, political science, literature, history, and cultural anthropology? These are important questions in so far as they direct our attention to identifying the defining features of cognitive-behavioral theories and therapies, and to identifying the limits of our models. They direct our attention, as well, to issues, questions, and problems that are just beyond this boundary.

CBT has traditionally relied on quantitative research methods to put its models to the test and to examine the efficacy of treatments based on them. There is now a strong movement in psychology advocating the value of qualitative research methodologies and questioning the legitimacy of concepts such as objectivism, validity, empiricism, and scientific neutrality. This postrationalist tradition traces its lineage not to the view of psychology and psychiatry as sciences (based on the German experimental laboratory ideal and Lockean or Democritan models), but to the French ideal of *la clinique* in which all interventions had to be demonstrated as effective with individual patients, at the bedside, before they could be accepted as scientifically validated, and to Kantian or Platonic models. Postrationalist models are often associated with postmodern schools of thought, and are most clearly apparent in cognitive-constructivist theories of psychopathology and psychotherapy. How the field of cognitive therapy will evolve as postrationalist understandings are applied to an essentially rationalist model is not yet clear.

Cognitive formulations based upon the assumptions of cognitive therapy – that cognitive activity (broadly conceived) affects behavior, that cognitive contents and processes may be monitored and changed, and that change may be effected through cognitive processes – may usefully be applied to a range of issues and concerns outside clinical psychology, psychiatry, and social work. Cognitive and perceptual processes, many of which appear, at first glance, to be irrational or maladaptive, appear, for example, to play a role in economic and political decision-making. These observed limits on human rationality have profound philosophical and social implications (Gigerenzer and Selten, 2001; Searle, 2001) and are worthy of exploration from a cognitive-behavioral perspective. In a similar manner, shared beliefs, attitudes, expectations, goals, attributions, and values (many of which may be tacit or unstated) may serve as a foundation for cultural identity. This view is consistent with a strong cognitive research tradition in social psychology that looks at culture from a cognitive perspective. Culture may be understood from a cognitive perspective as a set of shared tacit beliefs, attitudes, expectancies, and values that characterize a group, along with cultural "products" derived from these beliefs. These would include the art, music, architecture, and social or political institutions developed by the group. Culture, as a set of stable, shared beliefs, will have an influence on social patterns and adaptation. There may, as such, be links between culture, cognition, and mental health. It would not be implausible to hypothesize that cognitive processes may influence cultural assimilation and the ways in which groups with differing tacit beliefs interact.

Goals of this book

Although CBTs enjoy wide acceptance and are supported by an impressive body of empirical evidence, there are a number of unresolved concerns and issues. One goal in developing this book has been to provide a broad and critical examination of the field of cognitive therapy and the historical context in which the model evolved. Few articles or chapters have attempted systematically to identify weaknesses of the models and obstacles to developing more effective cognitive approaches for understanding and treating clinical disorders (Segal, 1988; Haaga et al., 1991; Segal and Dobson, 1992; Robins and Hayes, 1993; Clark and Steer, 1996). It is unclear, for example, that cognitive factors associated with various forms of emotional distress are specific to the disorder in question, or that they serve as vulnerability factors for the development of the condition. Moreover, it is also not clear whether relationships exist between changes in proposed mechanisms and clinical improvement. The ways in which social, biological, environmental, and cognitive factors interact over time in contributing to vulnerability for psychopathology are not well understood (Rutter, 1996; Ingram and Price, 2001), and the role of emotion in CBT is deserving of additional study (Lazarus, 1991; Safran and Greenberg, 1991; Samoilov and Goldfried, 2000). Cognitive processes are often viewed as static – the depressed individual, for example, may be viewed as possessing a relatively stable set of maladaptive beliefs, attitudes, attributions, and cognitive biases which will be the focus of treatment. More recent clinical and theoretical formulations, however, have focused upon understanding the individual in context. An emphasis is placed on understanding the individual's social environment and the ways in which this intersects with cognitive factors in maintaining and exacerbating his or her distress (Joiner, 2000). Familial influences on adaptation and the ways in which culture and history influence individuals' understanding of themselves, their relationships with others, and their mood represent new arenas for development in CBT. This research will be of both theoretical and practical importance as it may inform the development of cognitive-behavioral primary and secondary prevention programs (Jaycox et al., 1994; Clarke et al., 1995; Hannan et al., 2000).

An explicit goal in developing this volume, then, has been to review the current status of cognitive-behavioral models for understanding and treating clinical problems, to identify weaknesses in the theoretical and empirical literatures surrounding these approaches, and to suggest strategies for resolving these obstacles. We have asked our authors to identify emerging themes and issues in the literature. Although empirical papers and reviews regularly conclude with a call for additional research, these needs are rarely specified. Our authors have been encouraged to recommend specific areas in need of exploration and to suggest novel approaches for addressing intransigent clinical and conceptual issues. We asked each of our contributors to address several specific questions. These included: (1) What are the primary unresolved issues or questions confronting the field? (2) What are the most important trends as you review the recent development of the field? (3) What specific areas, issues or problems are most in need of investigation? and (4) What strategies might be employed to address these issues?

CBT is a rapidly evolving field. Although many writers cite the original Cognitive Therapy of Depression treatment manual (Beck et al., 1979) as a touchstone for understanding cognitive-behavioral interventions, the model and therapy have evolved dramatically since that time in both scope and sophistication. With this in mind, our contributors were encouraged to emphasize research focusing upon more recent models and interventions.

Many principles and techniques of CBT, once considered revolutionary, have now been assimilated into other forms of therapy. Maintaining a trusting collaborative therapeutic relationship, educating patients about their difficulties and providing a rationale for treatment, developing a shared vocabulary for understanding their concerns, therapeutic activity, maintaining a structured and problem-focused therapeutic stance, developing coping skills, providing feedback and support, facilitating the development of feelings of hope and personal efficacy, and conducting a developmental examination of the origins of maladaptive beliefs and interpersonal styles are widely accepted clinical strategies. As Rehm (1995) cogently observed, many forms of effective psychotherapy share these characteristics. Like dynamic concepts of unconscious motivation and person-centered notions of therapeutic rapport before them, cognitive-behavioral procedures are being accepted as an integral part of contemporary clinical practice. As we have seen, however, there are many unanswered questions, and a range of issues which have simply not been addressed.

If there is a difficulty in contemporary scholarship it is not that we think too broadly, but too narrowly. Specialization and hyperspecialization are valuable both for developing academic careers and for refining our conceptual models. They do so, however, in a tedious, incremental manner. Clinical scholars tend, as a group, to crawl along the frontiers of knowledge on all fours, magnifying glass in hand. We rarely lift our heads to see the wide vistas before us. Our subject matter – human development, adaptation, emotion, the making of meaning, and the amelioration of human suffering – is important, engaging, and noble. Too often, however, our discussions are reduced to debates regarding conceptual minutia, the psychometrics of specific instruments, and details of research methodology. To be sure, these are important issues. They are not, in the final analysis, the *most* important ones. They rarely yield paradigmatic shifts or rapid gains in understanding. Our goal, in this book, was to encourage our contributors to lift our eyes to the broad vistas before us. What are the strengths and limitations of our models? What are the strengths and limitations of our clinical approaches? How can we understand our field from historical and cultural perspectives? What are the most important opportunities for interdisciplinary scholarship? Where, looking toward the horizon, should we be heading?

REFERENCES

Addis, M. (1997). Evaluating the treatment manual as a means of disseminating empirically validated psychotherapies. *Clinical Psychology: Science and Practice*, **4**, 1–11.

Addis, M., Wade, W., and Hatgis, C. (1999). Barriers to dissemination of evidence-based practices: addressing practitioners' concerns about manual-based psychotherapies. *Clinical Psychology: Science and Practice*, **6**, 430–41.

Beck, A., Rush, A., Shaw, B., and Emery, G. (1979). *Cognitive Therapy of Depression*. New York: Guilford.

Beutler, L. (2000). Empirically based decision making in clinical practice. *Prevention and Treatment*, **3**, article 27. Available online at http://journals.apa.org/prevention. 1 September 2000.

Butler, A. and Beck, J. (2001). Cognitive therapy outcomes: a review of meta-analyses. *Journal of the Norwegian Psychological Association*, **37**, 1–9.

Chambless, D., Sanderson, W., Shoham, V., et al. (1996). An update on empirically-validated therapies. *Clinical Psychologist*, **49**, 5–18.

Clark, D. and Beck, A. (1999). *Scientific Foundations of Cognitive Theory and Therapy of Depression*. New York: Wiley.

Clark, D. and Steer, R. (1996). Empirical status of the cognitive model of anxiety and depression. In *Frontiers of Cognitive Therapy*, ed. P. Salkovskis, pp. 75–96. New York: Guilford Press.

Clarke, G. N., Hawkins, W., Murphy, M., and Sheeber, L. (1993). School-based primary prevention of depressive symptomatology in adolescents: findings from two studies. *Journal of Adolescent Research*, **8**, 183–204.

Clarke, G., Hawkins, W., Murphy, M., et al. (1995). Targeted prevention of unipolar depressive disorder in an at-risk sample of high school adolescents: a randomized trial of a group cognitive intervention. *Journal of the American Academy of Child and Adolescent Psychiatry*, **34**, 312–21.

Dobson, K. (2001). Preface. In *Handbook of Cognitive-Behavioral Therapies*, 2nd edn, ed. K. Dobson, pp. xi–xiv. New York: Guilford.

Dobson, K. and Dozois, D. (2001). Historical and philosophical bases of cognitive-behavioral therapies. In *Handbook of Cognitive-Behavioral Therapies*, 2nd edn, ed. K. Dobson, pp. 3–39. New York: Guilford.

Dobson, K. and Kendall, P. (eds) (1993). *Psychopathology and Cognition*. San Diego: Academic Press.

Fensterheim, H. and Raw, S. (1996). Psychotherapy research is not psychotherapy practice. *Clinical Psychology: Science and Practice*, **3**, 168–71.

Freeman, A. and Reinecke, M. (1995). Cognitive therapy. In *Essential Psychotherapies: Theory and Practice*, ed. A. Gurman and S. Messer, pp. 182–225. New York: Guilford Press.

Gigerenzer, G. and Selten, R. (eds) (2001). *Bounded Rationality: The Adaptive Toolbox.* Cambridge, MA: MIT Press.

Haaga, D., Dyck, M., and Ernst, D. (1991). Empirical status of cognitive theory of depression. *Psychological Bulletin*, **110**, 215–36.

Hannan, A. P., Rapee, R. M., and Hudson, J. L. (2000). The prevention of depression in children: a pilot study. *Behaviour Change*, **17**, 78–83.

Ingram, R. and Price, J. (eds) (2001). *Vulnerability to Psychopathology: Risk Across the Lifespan.* New York: Guilford.

James, W. (1948). *The Principles of Psychology*. New York: World. (Originally published 1890.)

Jaycox, L. H., Reivich, K. J., Gillham, J., and Seligman, M. E. P. (1994). Prevention of depressive symptoms in school children. *Behaviour Research and Therapy*, **32**, 801–16.

Joiner, T. (2000). Depression's vicious scree: self-propagating and erosive processes in depression chronicity. *Clinical Psychology: Science and Practice*, **7**(2), 203–18.

Kelly, G. (1955). *The Psychology of Personal Constructs*. New York: Norton.

Kendall, P. and Hollon, S. (eds) (1979). *Cognitive-Behavioral Interventions: Theory, Research and Procedures*. New York: Academic Press.

Lazarus, R. (1991). *Emotion and Adaptation*. New York: Oxford University Press.

Mahoney, M. (1991). *Human Change Processes*. New York: Basic Books.

Nathan, P. (1998). Practice guidelines: not yet ideal. *American Psychologist*, **53**, 290–9.

Nathan, P. and Gorman, J. (1998). *A Guide to Treatments that Work*. New York: Oxford University Press.

Rehm, L. (1995). Psychotherapies for depression. In *Anxiety and Depression in Adults and Children*, ed. K. Craig and K. Dobson, pp. 183–208. Thousand Oaks, CA: Sage.

Robins, C. and Hayes, A. (1993). An appraisal of cognitive therapy. *Journal of Consulting and Clinical Psychology*, **61**, 205–14.

Rutter, M. (1996). Developmental psychopathology: concepts and prospects. In *Frontiers of Developmental Psychopathology*, ed. M. Lenzenweger and J. Haugaard, pp. 209–37. New York: Oxford University Press.

Safran, J. and Greenberg, L. (eds)(1991). *Emotion, Psychotherapy, and Change*. New York: Guilford Press.

Samoilov, A. and Goldfried, M. (2000). Role of emotion in cognitive-behavior therapy. *Clinical Psychology: Science and Practice*, **7**, 373–85.

Searle, J. (2001). *Rationality in Action*. Cambridge, MA: MIT Press.

Segal, Z. (1988). Appraisal of the self-schematic construct in cognitive models of depression. *Psychological Bulletin*, **103**, 147–62.

Segal, Z. and Dobson, K. (1992). Cognitive models of depression: report from a concensus development conference. *Psychological Inquiry*, **3**, 219–24.

Silverman, W. (1996). Cookbooks, manuals, and paint-by-numbers. Psychotherapy in the 90s. *Psychotherapy*, **33**, 207–15.

Strunk, D. and DeRubeis, R. (2001). Cognitive therapy for depression: a review of its efficacy. *Journal of Cognitive Psychotherapy*, **15**(4), 289–97.

Cognitive theory and therapy of depression

Ari Solomon[1] and David A. F. Haaga[2]

[1] Stanford University Medical Center, CA, USA; now at Williams College, Williamstown, MA, USA
[2] American University, Washington, DC, USA

Cognitive theory of depression

Cognitive theory of depression (Beck, 1963) holds a prominent place in the history of clinical psychology as one of the first systematic statements of assumptions that have shaped the cognitive revolution in psychopathology (Clark and Steer, 1996). These tenets have since informed cognitive conceptualizations of many other disorders, as evidenced by the diversity of models described in this volume. Most fundamentally, all cognitive theories of psychopathology assert that people notice, recall, and interpret their experiences idiosyncratically – in accordance with their personal learning histories – and that these cognitive styles play a role in the genesis of specific psychological disorders.

There are numerous cognitive theories of depression (Ellis, 1987; Abramson et al., 1989), and a detailed description and review of each of these models and their implications for treating depression would exceed the scope of this chapter. We have elected to focus specifically on Beck's theory because more than other cognitive models it has both generated substantial empirical research on the psychopathology of depression and led to the development of an empirically supported treatment for depression (Clark et al., 1999).

In cognitive theory of depression, Beck proposed that rigidly negativistic beliefs regarding personal inadequacy or loss (e.g., "I am all alone in the world") in combination with overvaluation of certain outcomes (e.g., "Life is not worth living if I am all alone") are vulnerability factors for the onset and maintenance of depression. Beck (1987) proposed that this vulnerability was relevant only to reactive, nonendogenous depressions, but recent presentations of the model (Clark et al., 1999) do not include this qualifier and imply instead that the model is relevant to understanding major depression in general.

Core dysfunctional beliefs (also sometimes called core assumptions or core schemata) are assumed to be learned primarily through childhood experiences such as neglect or abuse. In one recent taxonomy of core dysfunctional beliefs (Beck, 1995, p. 169), beliefs are divided into two broad categories reflecting assumptions of *helplessness* or *unlovability*. Examples of helplessness core beliefs include "I am trapped" and "I am incompetent;" examples of unlovability beliefs include "I am different" and "I am bound to be abandoned."

Beck proposed that core dysfunctional beliefs become latent during periods of low life stress, but are easily reactivated by negative experiences that resemble the conditions under which the original beliefs were formed. For example, Joanne, who was orphaned at age seven, may have nearly forgotten her childhood belief that she is "all alone in the world" until her husband's request for a divorce brings it suddenly and painfully back into awareness.

Beck proposes that the reactivation of a core dysfunctional belief can have profound effects on both the negative and positive features of cognitive, behavioral, and emotional functioning. First, a reactivated core negative belief can simultaneously inhibit previously available positive cognitions and facilitate awareness of negative cognitions. Immediately after her husband's announcement, for example, Joanne may not endorse the belief that "my friends care about my well-being," even if she previously took that belief for granted. Simultaneously, a range of negative cognitions, emotions, and behaviors may emerge which are uncharacteristic of Joanne except during depressed periods (e.g., she may describe unrealistic expectations of others).

Another consequence of activation of a core negative belief is that appraisals of specific day-to-day experiences (i.e., perception, interpretation, and recollection of experiences) begin to be systematically distorted to conform with the negative belief. In other words, individuals begin to engage in *cognitive distortions* which render their experiences consistent with their underlying negative belief(s). For example, a depressed man who fails to please his wife sexually on one occasion may conclude that he is therefore destined always to displease her sexually. This illustrates the distortion known as *overgeneralization*, i.e., the incorrect assumption that isolated negative experiences are strongly predictive of pervasive and/or persistent negative experiences. Beck et al. (1979) offer a list of other depressotypic cognitive distortions, including *dichotomous thinking* (interpreting experiences as either entirely positive or entirely negative, rather than as "shades of gray"), *magnification* (overestimating and overattending to the negative aspects of one's experiences), and *personalization* (relating negative events to one's self without evidence). The depressive's habitual use of cognitive distortions to reach unrealistically negative conclusions about his or her experience is described by Beck as a "negative filter," whereas the conclusions themselves are called "automatic thoughts" to emphasize their intrusive, repetitive, and seemingly involuntary nature.

Beck proposed that depressotypic automatic thoughts are extremely negative with regard to three domains (a "negative triad") of experience: one's self, one's personal future, and one's personal world (Beck, 1970). He further proposed that these extreme, distorted negative appraisals aggravate other aspects of depressive dysfunction (e.g., they exacerbate lethargy, difficulty concentrating, interpersonal conflict, etc.), which in turn can generate more evidence in favor of the underlying dysfunctional belief, which can result in strengthening of the negative belief and further inhibition of positive beliefs. The strengthening of the negative core belief further amplifies the depressive symptoms. In summary, whenever life circumstances appear to corroborate a latent or underlying dysfunctional belief, a self-amplifying cascade of activated dysfunctional belief(s), resultant negative automatic thoughts, mood symptoms, and behavioral symptoms (and the inhibition of positive beliefs, attitudes, affect, and behaviors) can yield clinical depression.

Beck (1983) described two personality styles – sociotropy and autonomy – which are believed to relate to specific kinds of dysfunctional beliefs about the importance of success in particular domains. Thus, an extreme sociotropic or autonomous personality style is supposed to confer a distinct depressive vulnerability to specific kinds of environmental circumstances. Sociotropy can be defined as extreme investment in positive interpersonal experiences, including human affiliation, approval, and intimacy. Autonomy can be defined as extreme investment in independence, personal rights, mobility, and individual accomplishments. Beck (1983) proposed that predominantly sociotropic or autonomous personality styles render individuals vulnerable to depression in reaction to failings in the domain of primary concern. For example, if an attorney believes that it is essential to excel professionally, he or she will be at particular risk for a depressive reaction to career setbacks. If instead he or she believes that only loving relations are essential, he or she could endure professional setbacks with relative equanimity but be prone to depression in reaction to marital conflict or collegial discord.

Some aspects of cognitive theory of depression are less transparent than others and therefore merit particular attention. First, the theory ascribes a causal role to core dysfunctional beliefs (which are described as always preceding depression onset), but *not* to depressotypic automatic thoughts, which are described only as a concomitant or feature of depression. As discussed later in the chapter, negative automatic thoughts may be a particularly useful feature of depression to target for intervention, but this is not to say that they cause the other depressive symptoms (Haaga et al., 1991a).

Second, as mentioned earlier, the theory incorporates the idea that important cognitive processes can occur outside conscious awareness (Beck, 1967). Indeed, dysfunctional beliefs are expected to recede from consciousness whenever life circumstances fail to arouse the patient's core concerns; the belief(s) are expected to enter awareness again only when primed. (The kind of prime Beck has usually emphasized is negative life events, although other kinds of depression-relevant primes are conceivable: Segal and Ingram, 1994; Beck, 1996).

Third, Beck recently revised the cognitive theory of depression (Beck, 1996), introducing (among other ideas) the construct of a *primal loss mode* in depression (Beck 1996). The concept of a mode refers to a network of congruent cognitive, mood, physiological, and behavioral systems (each composed of multiple elements) which are activated *en masse* whenever a single element in the network is perturbed. Beck employs the mode concept in his restatement of cognitive theory of depression to describe how activation of a depressotypic core belief can inhibit positive beliefs, attitudes, affect, and behaviors while simultaneously facilitating dormant negative beliefs, attitudes, affect, and behaviors:

[T]he schema is activated and, in turn, triggers the rest of the mode to which it is attached. The excitation spreads through the cognitive system of the mode to the affective, motivational, behavioral, and physiological systems (Beck, 1996, p. 12).

It is unclear as yet whether this revision will strongly influence research or further theorizing, generate important new testable hypotheses, or account more adequately for existing findings than did prior statements of the theory.

A final aspect of the theory which merits special consideration is the fact that there is no necessary correspondence between the empirical status of cognitive theory of depression and the effectiveness of cognitive therapy for depression. Certainly, studies of cognitive therapy have provided interesting hypotheses regarding cognitive mechanisms of change (Jacobson et al., 1996). But cognitive therapy could be efficacious for reasons other than those specified by the theory, or it could lack efficacy despite having emerged from a valid causal model of a disorder (Persons, 1991). Thus, in this chapter we will describe separately the empirical status of cognitive therapy for depression and the empirical status of the model from which it emerged. The literature having some bearing on cognitive theory and therapy of depression is vast, and our coverage will be illustrative rather than exhaustive accordingly.

Empirical status

A number of testable hypotheses can be derived from Beck's cognitive theory of depression. Our review begins with descriptive hypotheses (that is, predictions about what should typify currently depressed individuals) and proceeds to causal hypotheses (i.e., predictions about what should predispose people to depressive symptom onset or maintenance).

Descriptive hypotheses

Prominent thoughts of failure or loss

Many studies support the hypothesis that themes of failure, loss, inadequacy, or hopelessness (depressotypic themes) are overrepresented in the thoughts of depressed individuals. Depressed groups score higher on self-report measures of depressotypic thoughts than do a range of psychiatric and nonpsychiatric control groups (Dobson and Breiter, 1983), and higher than themselves when remitted (Eaves and Rush, 1984). Conversely, a number of studies show that depressed people score lower than do nondepressed people on indicators of positive self-referent cognition (Ingram et al., 1990). This finding of a deficiency in positive thinking, while certainly consistent with the excess negativity seen in depression, is not a necessary consequence of negativity but rather an independent empirical result, as positive and negative automatic thoughts appear to be only modestly inversely related (Ingram and Wisnicki, 1988). Depressed groups also score higher than controls in each domain of the negative triad (negative appraisals of self, world, and other). In laboratory cognitive tasks, depressed individuals exhibit more negative interpretation and recall of a range of circumstances, including performance feedback, and rewards and punishments (Gotlib, 1981, 1983). Negative thinking is equally evident in unipolar and bipolar (Hollon et al., 1986), primary and secondary (Norman et al., 1983), endogenous and nonendogenous (Norman et al., 1987), and melancholic and nonmelancholic (Norman et al., 1987) depressions. These studies corroborate Beck's observation that depressive thoughts are elevated across the traditional nosological distinctions among depressions.

Even so, several qualifications are in order. First, while group differences are consistently found, perhaps 50% of clinically depressed individuals (including inpatients) do not report a high frequency of depressotypic thoughts (Hamilton and Abramson, 1983; Miller and Norman, 1986). In other words, there appears to be some overlap in the distributions of depressed versus nondepressed automatic thoughts. What to make of this finding is unclear: uniquely strong depressotypic thoughts are proposed in cognitive theory to be a distinguishing feature of all syndromal depressions, but it may be unrealistic to expect nomothetic self-report measurement techniques to detect such thoughts equally well in all patients; it may also be that prominent negative thoughts should not be defined solely with reference to frequency, but intensity as well. Second, automatic thoughts pertaining to one aspect of the negative triad (self, world, future) do not always predict automatic thoughts pertaining to other aspects. Thus, it is not yet clear which (if any) specific categories of automatic thoughts are necessary features of depression (Haaga et al., 1991b). Finally, depressotypic thoughts do not necessarily reflect distortions of experience. Indeed, under certain very limited circumstances (e.g., certain standardized experimental tasks), depressed individuals are more accurate in self-evaluations than are nondepressed individuals (Alloy and Abramson, 1979). As such, it may be more useful to depict depressive thinking as biased rather than distorted (Haaga and Beck, 1995).

Specificity of thoughts of failure and loss to depression

Cognitive theory of depression also implies that depressed individuals' thinking should have a distinctive profile which distinguishes it from the thinking of individuals with all other disorders (Beck, 1987). This prediction has been called the cognitive specificity hypothesis. In particular, Beck (1967, p. 270) proposes that the themes of failure or loss are uniquely prominent in depressed individuals' thinking across various levels of analysis – across thought content, attention, memory, and interpretive operations – relative to people with other disorders. Because anxiety disorders and depression have particularly high rates of comorbidity (American Psychiatric Association, 1994), a priority has been to determine whether the thinking of depressed individuals can be discriminated from the thinking of anxiety-disordered individuals. According to cognitive theory, whereas depression can be characterized by uniquely high levels of loss or failure cognitions, anxiety disorders should be characterized by uniquely high levels of danger or threat-related thoughts (Beck et al., 1987).

The themes of failure and loss do appear uniquely to characterize the thoughts of clinically depressed individuals, relative to anxiety disorders. However, some studies suggest that themes of danger and threat also appear to be elevated in the depressive disorders – even in noncomorbid depression. For example, self-reported thoughts of failure and hopelessness differentiated pure dysthymic from pure generalized anxiety disorder (GAD) patients, but anxious cognitions were characteristic of both groups (Riskind et al., 1991). Similarly, Clark et al. (1994) found that self-reported thoughts of failure or loss discriminated depressive disorders from GAD, while ostensibly anxiety-related cognitions did not discriminate GAD from depression. Thus, it may be that cognitive themes of loss and failure are typical only of depression, while themes of danger and threat typify depression and GAD alike (Clark et al., 1994).

In addition to distinctive thought *content*, Beck's description of a negative filter implies that depressed individuals' thought *processes* should be distinctive. Specifically, the theory implies that the attention and memory of depressed individuals will be uniquely biased toward excessively noticing and recalling information pertaining to failure or loss. Evidence is fairly strong regarding the existence of such a memory bias in depression. Under a range of encoding conditions and across a range of moods, clinically depressed subjects recall more information regarding failure or loss relative to normals, general psychiatric or anxious controls, while subclinically depressed subjects exhibit balanced recall of positive and negative information (Bellew and Hill, 1990; Matt et al., 1992; Watkins et al., 1992).

Evidence has been largely negative regarding the prediction that the attention of depressed individuals is uniquely focused on stimuli pertaining to themes of loss or failure (relative to anxious individuals). Most studies have failed to detect such a bias (Lang and Craske, 1997; McCabe and Gotlib, 1993; Williams et al., 1996). However, some laboratories have begun to report positive findings for a depression-specific attentional bias using refined experimental strategies such as dichotic attentional tasks under conditions of high cognitive load (Ingram et al., 1994) or pictorial stimuli (Gotlib and Krasnoperova, 1998). Additional studies evaluating the replicability of these recent findings are a high priority for the field.

Causal hypotheses

In addition to implying certain descriptive features of depression, Beck's cognitive theory of depression includes predictions about etiology. Specifically, certain global dysfunctional beliefs should predispose to the onset and recurrence of depression. These cognitive vulnerability factors are viewed as proximal contributory causes of depression (Clark et al., 1999). They are contributory in that, if activated (e.g., by occurrence of relevant negative life events), their presence increases the probability of a depressive episode, but it is acknowledged that they will not inevitably lead to depression and that there are other causes as well. Thus, cognitive vulnerability is seen as neither sufficient nor necessary for the occurrence of depression. Dysfunctional beliefs are "proximal" in the sense that they may interact with stressor occurrence to lead to depression within a relatively short time frame. A further question is what distal causes (genetics, early-childhood experiences, etc.) prompt the development of cognitive vulnerability in the first place, and to date much less research attention has been devoted to this issue than to examining whether cognitive vulnerability indeed serves as a proximal contributory cause of depression.

In general, tests of the causal aspects of Beck's theory of depression attempt to answer one or more of these questions: (1) Do dysfunctional beliefs precede onset of depressive symptoms? (2) Do such beliefs interact with negative life events to yield depression onset? and (3) Are such prospective relations (wherever found) independent of all plausible alternative explanations (such as covarying anxiety symptoms or a prior history of subthreshold depressive symptoms)?

Dysfunctional beliefs and depression onset

Very negative global beliefs about the self such as Beck (1967) describes are clearly more common in depressed than nondepressed individuals (Derry and Kuiper, 1981; Dobson and Shaw, 1986). To merit causal status in the theory, however, such beliefs should also precede depression onset, rather than merely be observed during a depressive episode.

Setting up an adequate test of this temporal sequence is daunting (for a review of the obstacles, see Haaga et al., 1991b). Because of the difficulties of such research, to date there have been no rigorously controlled prospective studies of the cognition–depression temporal sequence using appropriate criteria to define initial onset of clinical symptoms. Instead, much research on cognitive theory has focused on determining whether dysfunctional beliefs persist after remission of an episode of depression. The rationale for such research is that because depression is usually a recurrent and episodic disorder to which many individuals remain prone throughout their lives, individuals with a history of depressive episodes should exhibit uniquely elevated levels of dysfunctional beliefs even when fully remitted.

Early remitted-depressed studies generally did not detect excess dysfunctional beliefs in remitted-depressed individuals (Silverman et al., 1984; Blackburn and Smyth, 1985). Specifically, when traditional self-report measures were administered without priming procedures, dysfunctional beliefs usually appeared to wax and wane with the course of other depressive symptoms, and not persist between episodes. Such findings were usually interpreted as a significant challenge to cognitive accounts of depression, since they suggested that dysfunctional beliefs are a noncausal correlate of depression (Coyne and Gotlib, 1983).

However, cognitive theory specifies that dysfunctional beliefs may be latent during nondepressed periods (Beck, 1964). Thus, between episodes of depression such beliefs may be measurable only after arousing them to consciousness through some kind of priming procedure (Segal and Ingram, 1994). Accordingly, some depression researchers have adapted the remitted-depressed research design to allow for the possibility that depressotypic cognitive processes in remitted individuals are more subtle, latent, or nonconscious than previously assumed. Results of such studies have often (although not universally: Dykman, 1997) been congruent with cognitive theory. For example, following a sad mood induction (Miranda and Persons, 1988) or during naturally occurring sad moods (Miranda et al., 1990; Roberts and Kassel, 1996), remitted-depressed adults report higher levels of dysfunctional beliefs than do never-depressed adults during comparable sad moods. In addition, primed remitted-depressed adults also evidence uniquely strong recall of depressotypic adjectives (Dent and Teasdale, 1988; Hedlund and Rude, 1995), an excess of self-deprecatory solutions to scrambled sentences (Hedlund and Rude, 1995), and may exhibit an attentional bias for depressotypic stimuli on dichotic listening tasks when under a cognitive load (Ingram et al., 1994).

These fairly consistent positive results from second-generation remitted-depressed studies are congruent with the cognitive model, but they by no means confirm the causal aspects of the theory. The remitted-depressed design has a number of shortcomings as a means of testing causal hypotheses (A. Solomon and D. A. F. Haaga, unpublished data). These include the potentially strong demand characteristics of priming procedures; the possibility that cognitive factors in relapse are distinct from cognitive factors in initial depression onset; the difficulty of excluding all plausible alternative explanations for depressotypic ideation (such as comorbid anxiety or chronic interpersonal stressors); and, most basically, the possibility that what has been detected represents cognitive "scars" from prior depressive episodes rather than true vulnerability factors (Rohde et al., 1990). For example, one strategy for priming dysfunctional beliefs in formerly depressed and control subjects involves instructing them to cultivate a sad mood by focusing on sad memories from their past. The demand characteristics of such a procedure are strong, as is the possibility that such an induction is a different imaginal experience for someone who has experienced clinical depression than for someone who has experienced only limited sadness. Coyne (1992) emphasized the risk of confounding cognitive vulnerabilities with cognitive scars in recovered-depressed priming designs, arguing by analogy that "serving in Vietnam may affect responses to a cognitive questionnaire or task, but researchers cannot ipso facto assume that they have isolated the cognitive processes causing someone to serve in Vietnam" (p. 234).

In summary, while priming studies of remitted individuals have provided information that is congruent with cognitive theory, truly prospective studies remain the gold standard for this, as for any, etiological theory. Furthermore, a comprehensive prospective test would involve methodological features such as clinical standards for depression onset; rigorous assessment for past subthreshold symptoms; a long-enough measurement interval (to permit emergence of a relatively low-base-rate disorder); sophisticated controls for environmental influences; and an adequate priming procedure (see Ingram et al., 1998, for more extensive discussion).

In this context, it is not surprising that partial tests of the theory's causal hypotheses are the rule and that the implications of such studies are often clouded by lack of adherence to one or more important methodological criteria. For example, several prospective studies of never-depressed individuals which did not prime participants before measuring cognition (e.g., Lewinsohn et al., 1981; Cole et al., 1998) have essentially failed to find evidence of dysfunctional beliefs prior to depressive symptom onset. Conversely, studies which report evidence of excess premorbid dysfunctional beliefs have not usually controlled rigorously for a history of subthreshold depressive episodes or environmental stressors. Bellew and Hill (1991), for example, report that pregnant women with low self-reported depressive symptoms who exhibited a memory bias for esteem-threatening words experienced higher levels of postpartum depressive symptoms in reaction to stressful life events. These authors did not report data regarding such variables as history of prior depression, anxiety symptoms, possible residual depressive symptoms, or current marital conflict.

Similarly, several studies have reported that residual dysfunctional beliefs in early-remitted individuals predict relapse (Segal et al., 1992; Thase et al., 1992), but none of those studies incorporated measures of both clinical remission and residual self-report symptoms. The one such study which has assessed both recent self-report symptoms and clinical remission (Ilardi et al., 1997) failed to find a relation between pretreatment or follow-up dysfunctional beliefs and relapse risk, but interpretation of that study is complicated by the fact that it did not include a posttreatment (nondepressed) assessment of dysfunctional beliefs. In summary, there is a need for more definitive tests of the temporal sequence implicated by cognitive theory.

The ongoing Temple-Wisconsin Cognitive Vulnerability to Depression (CVD) project (Abramson et al., 1999) comes perhaps closer than any other study to providing a comprehensive test of that temporal sequence. This project has been evaluating risk for onset of clinical depression among college students followed for several years. High and low cognitive risk are defined by freshman year scores in the highest and lowest quartiles respectively on both a measure of dysfunctional beliefs (the Dysfunctional Attitude Scale; A. Weissman and A. T. Beck, unpublished data) and a measure of global negative attributional style (Attributional Style Questionnaire; Peterson et al., 1982). Over the initial 2.5 years of this study, high-risk subjects with no prior history of clinical depression experienced onset of major depression and minor depression at many times the rate of their low-risk counterparts (17% versus 1%, and 39% versus 6% respectively). Importantly, these results essentially replicated across two demographically disparate student populations, and were independent of baseline depressive symptoms.

Similarly, Abramson et al. (1998) report support for a shared tenet of hopelessness theory of depression and cognitive theory of depression – namely, the expectation of a strong predictive relation between hopelessness and suicidality. Such a relation was found and was not explained by several important covariates, including past suicidality, history of depressive disorders, dimensional measures of personality dysfunction, or parental history of depression. This finding is perhaps the strongest description to date of a unique and specific relation between depressotypic cognition and behavioral symptoms, predicted by cognitive theory (Beck et al., 1975).

Again, however, while strongly congruent with cognitive theory of depression, the cognitive high-risk profile for depression and suicide has not yet passed the hurdle of being shown to predict onset of depression independent of other important explanatory constructs, such as a history of subthreshold depression or recent negative life events. A history of clinically significant subthreshold depression, for instance, is a potentially powerful predictor of the onset of clinical depression in its own right (Judd et al., 1997; Lewinsohn et al., 2000). To be sure, controlling for a history of subthreshold depression may represent an unreasonably demanding test of cognitive vulnerability factors, in that these earlier subthreshold depressions may themselves have resulted at least in part from cognitive vulnerability. Nevertheless, ascribing the clinical history to one's preferred causal variable in the absence of direct evidence of this link is conjectural: showing that a hypothesized predisposing factor predicts depression onset apart from its association with clinical history variables is more convincing evidence.

Personality styles, stressful events, and depression onset

In addition to postulating distinctive patterns of premorbid cognition, cognitive theory implies that only particular kinds of stressors will tend to precipitate episodes of depression for individuals with particular kinds of personalities, for example, romantic dissolution or bereavement for sociotropic individuals versus work failure or disabling illness for autonomous individuals. This hypothesis has not been clearly supported. Studies of depression relapse have found the expected personality–stress interactions for sociotropy but not autonomy (Segal et al., 1989), for autonomy but not sociotropy (Hammen et al., 1989), for neither personality style (in a nonclinical, cross-sectional study; Robins and Block, 1988), and for both sociotropy and autonomy with either kind of stressor (Robins et al., 1995).

Several explanations for these inconsistent results have been suggested (Haaga et al., 1991a). For example, sociotropy and autonomy represent very broad constructs, whereas depression may result from failure to achieve much more highly specific ambitions in a particular field of endeavor (such as marriage, job, school). Thus, it is possible that the sociotropy and autonomy constructs are simply too broad to capture the idiographic meaning of any particular single negative outcome (Brown et al., 1995). Studies designed to match specific subtypes of sociotropic or autonomous concerns with highly personally relevant stressors seem most appropriate as tests of the theory. A handful of studies do indeed suggest that the more idiographic a cognitive diathesis-stress design is, the more likely are positive findings. Brown et al. (1995), for example, evaluated undergraduates before and after their first college-level examination. In this sample, the perfectionistic achievement factor of the Dysfunctional Attitude Scale was most strongly associated with depressive symptom increases following poorer-than-expected performance.

Another important consideration is that the scales originally used in studies of sociotropy and autonomy (e.g., Sociotropy–Autonomy Scale; Beck et al., personal communication) may not adequately assess these constructs, especially autonomy, as described in cognitive theory. More theoretically consistent findings may emerge from studies using newer measures such as the Personal Style Inventory (PSI, Robins et al., 1994) or the revised Sociotropy–Autonomy Scale (Clark and Beck, 1991).

The PSI, for example, was designed to improve the validity of measurement of autonomy and to minimize confounding with distress, a problem for some earlier measures of these personality modes (Solomon and Haaga, 1994). Solomon et al. (1998) found large elevations of both PSI sociotropy and autonomy scores in a recovered-depressed population. These results replicated earlier work on sociotropy (Moore and Blackburn, 1996) but were novel with respect to autonomy (Coyne and Whiffen, 1995). That the group differences remained significant after controlling statistically for current depression severity supports the argument by Robins et al. (1997) that associations of sociotropy and autonomy with depression vulnerability are not likely to reflect entirely artifacts of mood-state biases in personality self-ratings. Post-hoc analyses also indicated that group differences in sociotropy and autonomy in this study could not be attributed to the presence of more participants with comorbid anxiety disorders in the remitted-depressed group. Thus, newer measures of personality vulnerability may be more valid, which in turn facilitate stronger tests of the predictions of cognitive theory of depression.

Summary

There is extensive research support for the description of depressive thinking embedded in Beck's cognitive theory. Depressed people, regardless of clinical subtype, exceed nondepressed people, including those with other psychological disorders, in negative thinking about themselves, their personal worlds, and their prospects for the future. It is less clear whether the theory is correct with regard to the etiology of depression. Measurement and research design issues involved in providing adequate tests of the theory are complex, yet there is some promising evidence of latent dysfunctional beliefs among remitted-depressed persons (which could account for their vulnerability to recurrence of depression) and of successful prediction of first onset of depression on the basis of cognitive vulnerability.

Cognitive therapy of depression

We turn now to cognitive therapy for depression, a treatment strategy derived by Beck from his theoretical account of depression. Cognitive therapists target the dysfunctional beliefs hypothesized to contribute to the onset of depression, after first teaching the patient skills for questioning and reevaluating negative automatic thoughts. The intended style of the therapy is collaborative, as therapist and patient work together to examine and evaluate the validity of automatic thoughts associated with depression.

In the early stages of treatment much of this work is carried out via behavioral methods designed both to elevate mood directly and to provide an opportunity to test negative thoughts (e.g., if you think you cannot accomplish anything, test that conceptualization by attempting the following simple tasks, working your way gradually up a graded series of such tasks). Such behavioral experiments are typically debriefed collaboratively to determine whether, for instance, the patient's depressive thinking has led him or her to discount the significance of any accomplishments that may have been made. In standard practice, behavioral activation strategies give way to a focus on teaching skills for evaluating automatic thoughts – questioning the evidence for automatic thoughts, considering whether any equally viable alternative conceptualizations of what has happened are possible, decatastrophizing their implications if true, and looking for whether anything can be done constructively about the sometimes truly dreadful situations the patient confronts. Finally, core beliefs are targeted in an effort to promote maintenance of gains and prevent relapse. Many of the same strategies used in learning to question automatic thoughts are helpful in this phase too. Additionally, patients can learn to question the utility of adhering to dysfunctional beliefs (aside from their accuracy) and can often profit from acting contrary to assumptions as a means of testing beliefs.

In cognitive therapy for other disorders, the use of behavioral strategies and automatic thought-questioning strategies is similar but the content of targeted cognitions differs (e.g., exaggerated expectations of imminent biological catastrophe in panic disorder, of rejection and humiliation in social phobia). Detailed descriptions of cognitive therapy of depression are available (Beck et al., 1979).

Empirical status
Acute efficacy

Cognitive therapy has been evaluated in numerous clinical trials and on the whole appears to be an effective treatment of depression. Numerous reviewers have reached this judgment. For example, published lists of empirically validated treatments identified by the Task Force on Promotion and Dissemination of Psychological Procedures of Division 12 of the American Psychological Association (Chambless et al., 1998) identifies cognitive therapy of depression as meeting the criteria for designation as a "well-established treatment." Cognitive therapy appears to be about equally effective as tricyclic antidepressant medication in achieving acute symptom relief (Hollon et al., 1996).

Maintenance

Several studies have shown an advantage for cognitive therapy relative to (discontinued) antidepressant medication with regard to durability of gains achieved during treatment (Hollon et al., 1996). In the National Institute of Mental Health

(NIMH) Treatment of Depression Collaborative Research Program (TDCRP), cognitive therapy was associated with lower rates of relapse among those achieving remission during treatment than was medication, but the difference was not significant (Shea et al., 1992).

Nevertheless, the evidence that cognitive therapy for depression may have a relapse prevention effect should not be taken to mean that it is a universally enduring cure for depression. Although the number of studies with sizable samples and rigorous recovery/relapse criteria, low attrition rates, and long-term follow-up is small, it appears that only about one-fourth of outpatients with major depression achieve full recovery and then remain remitted continuously through the first 18–24 months posttreatment after receiving cognitive therapy (Gortner et al., 1998).

Such relatively low probabilities of complete success are an old story in areas in which it is common to evaluate treatment success in absolute terms, notably in treating addictive behaviors with a goal of complete abstinence. Absolute success rates have traditionally been obscured, however, in studies of therapies for mood disorders by the custom of evaluating success in terms of mean differences across conditions in average symptom scores (Shaw, 1999). The increasing use of methods for evaluating clinically significant response to treatment (Kendall, 1999), as well as long-term follow-up evaluation, may help promote a more realistic sense of the impact of currently available treatments and of the need for continued improvements in them.

Specificity

There is not convincing evidence that cognitive therapy is more effective than other psychotherapies specifically designed for the treatment of depression. Group cognitive therapy was more effective than psychodynamic group therapy in the study by Covi and Lipman (1987), but several major clinical trials, including the NIMH TDCRP, have found cognitive therapy equivalent to alternative psychotherapies such as interpersonal therapy (for a review, see DeRubeis and Crits-Christoph, 1998). This equivalency of bona fide psychotherapies is by no means unique in the treatment outcome literature (Wampold et al., 1997). Nevertheless, it remains important to keep in mind, especially in evaluating the implications for cognitive theory of the efficacy of cognitive therapy, that cognitive therapy is among the best-documented and most often studied psychotherapies but has not been shown to be superior to plausible alternatives.

For whom is cognitive therapy effective?

In view of the evidence that cognitive therapy is an effective treatment but not universally so, it stands to reason that considerable research attention has been given to the issue of determining for what sorts of patients it is most likely to be helpful. We summarize some of the main findings in this body of research in the following section.

Prognostic factors

Demographics have generally not shown a strong relation with cognitive therapy outcome. Gender (including match of gender with one's therapist; Zlotnick et al., 1998), age, socioeconomic status, and education have usually failed to correlate with treatment outcome in studies of cognitive therapy for depression (Jarrett et al., 1991). However, married patients responded better than did divorced, widowed, or separated patients in cognitive therapy for depression (Sotsky et al., 1991).

It is sometimes thought that high *intelligence* should be associated with favorable response to cognitive therapy because cognitive therapy "requires the understanding of logical arguments and evaluation of beliefs" (Whisman, 1993, p. 256). Nevertheless, Haaga et al. (1991b) found that neither fluid nor crystallized intelligence was significantly predictive of outcome of cognitive therapy for depression.

"Intelligence" may be too general a construct to capture the aptitude useful for deriving benefit from cognitive therapy. Right-ear accuracy for syllables (but not complex tones) in dichotic listening tasks proved to be a strong predictor of favorable response to cognitive therapy for depression (Bruder et al., 1997). Right-ear accuracy for syllables indicates left-hemisphere advantage for verbal processing. The mechanism of this effect is unknown, but the authors proposed that "patients with greater left-hemisphere superiority for verbal processing may have been better able to use the language-dominant hemisphere in learning to reinterpret negative life events" (Bruder et al., 1997, p. 143).

Given that cognitive therapy works, in principle, by challenging dysfunctional thinking, it might seem that patients with high levels of *dysfunctional thinking* would benefit most from this approach. However, it appears that the opposite is true. Patients with *low* levels of dysfunctional attitudes seem to respond best to cognitive therapy (Jarrett et al., 1991; Sotsky et al., 1991). This may be especially the case with respect to perfectionistic, self-critical attitudes, as opposed to dysfunctional beliefs about the need for approval from others (Blatt et al., 1998).

Patients with severely dysfunctional beliefs may be insufficiently flexible in their thinking to make good use of cognitive interventions (Simons et al., 1995). High cognitive dysfunction is associated with severity of depression, poor social support, and a high number of prior depressive episodes, all of which may contribute to poor prognosis in any treatment (Whisman, 1993). Also, the relation between low cognitive dysfunction and favorable response to cognitive therapy for depression may be moderated by variation in the recent occurrence of negative life events. In one study patients with high levels of dysfunctional attitudes who also had experienced a negative life event were likely to respond *well* to cognitive therapy

(Simons et al., 1995). A major negative event combined with biased thinking about it may give the therapist something specific to work with, rather than a general, pervasive dysfunctional belief not tied to specific current setbacks, which may be more intractable (Simons et al., 1995).

Endogenous depression was expected to be less responsive to cognitive therapy on the grounds that it is biologically based and more likely to respond to pharmacotherapy (Whisman, 1993). Some studies corroborate this prediction (McKnight et al., 1992), while others do not (Jarrett et al., 1990). Results may depend on the measure of endogeneity. Abnormal dexamethasone suppression test response has predicted poor outcome (McKnight et al., 1992), and this result appears to be independent of depression severity (Thase et al., 1996).

A *comorbid personality disorder diagnosis* is believed to predict poor response to brief therapy for axis I disorders (Reich and Vasile, 1993). However, whether this is true of cognitive therapy for depression is uncertain. Whereas a diagnosis of borderline personality disorder predicted poor outcome in cognitive therapy for depressed patients (Burns and Nolen-Hoeksema, 1992), the presence of personality disorders in the NIMH TDCRP study did not predict poor response to cognitive therapy (Shea et al., 1990).

Prescriptive factors

For the purpose of treatment selection it is important to know for which types of patients cognitive therapy is the treatment of choice and for which it is inferior to other treatments. In addressing these issues it is necessary to bear in mind the important distinction between the prognostic findings just reviewed, which tell us which patients do best in cognitive therapy, and prescriptive findings, which tell us what treatment (cognitive therapy versus alternatives) is best for a given patient (Hollon and Najavits, 1988), which is not the same issue. If, for example, borderline personality disorder diagnosis predicts poor outcome in cognitive therapy, this does not necessarily mean that cognitive therapy is a poor choice for someone with this diagnosis; such a conclusion would only follow if another treatment were shown to be more effective for patients with this diagnosis.

One potentially useful prescriptive finding is that *marital discord* may contraindicate individual cognitive therapy for depression. Behavioral couples therapy might address the depression just as well, and the relationship problems better, than does individual cognitive therapy (O'Leary and Beach, 1990).

Dispositional resistance might also be an unfavorable prescriptive indicator. Due to the educative and relatively directive style associated with cognitive therapy, it was hypothesized that the resistance of a patient would interfere with therapy, thus leading to poor outcome (Beutler et al., 1991). Studies examining the relationship between a patient's resistance, or a "propensity to resist the influence of authorities"

(p. 20), found that resistance level interacted with treatment condition for group cognitive therapy (Beutler et al., 1993). Cognitive therapy was more effective than self-directed treatments for patients with low resistance potential, while patients with high resistance responded more favorably to self-directed treatments (Beutler et al., 1993). It would be interesting to see this issue pursued in studies of individual cognitive therapy, in which the therapist might be able to be more flexible in adapting to the style of the resistant patient in order to maintain a more collaborative and productive treatment alliance.

The NIMH TDCRP found that *high depression severity* was associated with poorer outcome in cognitive-behavioral therapy relative to antidepressant medication; group differences were not evident among the less severely depressed (Elkin et al., 1995). However, several studies of similar design have failed to replicate this result, and a quantitative review of the NIMH collaborative study along with the other experiements found no significant differences between cognitive-behavioral therapy and antidepressant medication among severely depressed outpatients (DeRubeis et al., 1999). Thus, severity of depression cannot at this time be considered a robust prescriptive indicator.

Learned resourcefulness (Rosenbaum, 1980) refers to people's abilities to use constructive problem-solving strategies, to delay gratification, and to perceive oneself as efficacious in regulating internal events. People scoring high on a measure of learned resourcefulness responded better to cognitive therapy relative to pharmacotherapy for depression, suggesting that it might be a useful prescriptive variable (Simons et al., 1985). Later studies, though, failed to replicate these results (Wetzel et al., 1992). One possible explanation for the mixed results is that learned resourcefulness may be associated with preferential response to cognitive therapy only among the initially more severely depressed patients (Burns et al., 1994).

Learned resourcefulness may be overinclusive as a marker of a favorable prescriptive indicator for cognitive therapy. Several studies suggest that more specific aspects of patients' world views may be relevant. In one study, about one-half of depressed patients responded within 2 weeks, apparently on the basis of finding the cognitive therapy rationale a good fit for making sense of their depressive episodes (Fennell and Teasdale, 1987). These patients did not differ from less responsive ones in symptom severity but did score higher on "depression about depression" (Teasdale, 1985), severely negative reactions to the experience of being depressed itself. Also, patients endorsing abstract, existential reasons for being depressed responded particularly well to cognitive therapy and less so to a component treatment including only behavioral activation strategies (Addis and Jacobson, 1996).

More research is needed before these findings can be employed prescriptively, but a picture seems to be emerging of a subset of depressed patients who are demoralized about the meaningfulness of their lives and discouraged about the implications of their having been depressed, but who react favorably to a cognitive therapy rationale for depression and show a capacity for flexible thinking and constructive, self-directed means of coping with their problems.

How does cognitive therapy work?

Both experimental dismantling studies and correlational process studies have attempted to determine what in particular makes cognitive therapy effective, when indeed it is effective.

Cognitive and behavioral components

A component analysis of cognitive therapy for depression compared the behavioral activation aspect usually emphasized early in treatment, including graded task assignments, mastery and pleasure ratings, pleasant events scheduling, and other efforts to make contact with potential reinforcers, with a second condition in which automatic thoughts evaluation and modification were also included, and a third (full cognitive therapy) condition in which these components were supplemented by efforts to evaluate and challenge core dysfunctional beliefs. All three conditions were equally effective at posttreatment and through 2-year follow-up, suggesting that the behavioral activation component of treatment may be sufficient to serve as the entire therapy (Jacobson et al., 1996; Gortner et al., 1998). These findings, which resemble those of a classic comparative study of cognitive and behavioral (pleasant events scheduling) therapies for depression that obtained nonspecificity of response in terms of both depression and the intermediate targets (cognitive change, behavioral change) of each therapy (Zeiss et al., 1979), may suggest that the specifically cognitive components of cognitive therapy are superfluous; however, such a conclusion would be premature given that treatment time was equated across conditions, and behavioral activation thus may have been superior in the behavioral activation-only condition.

This is an extremely difficult issue for component-analysis studies; if one lets the combination treatments run longer, then "more therapy is better" will be a viable alternative hypothesis able to account for any advantage in efficacy in these conditions, whereas if one holds treatment time constant there is the concern that the common component may be delivered better or more completely when it is the only component. In effect, it is very difficult to compare A + B with A as a means of evaluating the utility of component B, because holding component A truly constant across therapy conditions is not a straightforward task (Haaga and Stiles, 2000).

Technical fidelity

A correlational process-outcome study of cognitive therapy for depression by DeRubeis and Feeley (1990) was more supportive of the idea that the theory-specified treatment components are important determinants of successful cognitive therapy practice. Therapists who implemented the focused, practical techniques of cognitive therapy early in treatment, such as setting and following an agenda, obtained greater reductions in patients' depressive symptoms. This effect was replicated by Feeley et al. (1999).

Therapist empathy

Besides the cognitive and behavioral techniques associated with cognitive therapy, the establishment of a collaborative, productive relationship between therapist and patient is an important factor in outcome. Indeed, a review by Ilardi and Craighead (1994) showed that much of the improvement in depressive symptoms occurred within the first 3 weeks of therapy, before explicitly cognitive techniques become a major focus of cognitive therapy sessions (Beck et al., 1979). Early symptom reduction may therefore depend a great deal on the therapist's credibility in presenting a cognitive therapy rationale and ability to form a positive alliance with patients.

Several studies have examined the role of therapist empathy in particular in promoting positive outcome in cognitive therapy. Persons and Burns (1985) examined mood change during one session of cognitive therapy with depressed and anxious patients. Both negative mood and degree of belief in automatic thoughts significantly decreased during the session. Patients' perceptions of therapist empathy related to mood improvement during the session. However, direction of causality is unclear in this study. Burns and Nolen-Hoeksema (1992) used structural equation modeling in a subsequent study to facilitate clearer inferences about cause and effect. They found that therapist empathy, as rated by patients in a 12-week study of cognitive-behavioral therapy for depression, had a moderate-to-large causal effect on patients' recovery, with patients who rated their therapists as the most warm and empathic showing the greatest improvement. This analysis controlled for the possible reciprocal causality of symptomatic improvement on perceived therapist empathy.

Future directions for cognitive theory and therapy of depression

As we have discussed throughout the chapter, there are many unanswered questions about cognitive theory and therapy of depression requiring further research. We close by highlighting a few issues that seem pressing but that have not to date received sufficient attention.

First, in relation to the etiology of depression, an important question regards the boundaries of the model. Does it apply only to diagnosable depressions, or to all syndromal depressions (diagnosable or otherwise), or to all instances of substantially elevated depressive symptoms? In early statements of the theory, Beck proposed that subclinical affective responses are associated with accurate perceptions of events, whereas psychopathology is associated with a poor correspondence between conceptualization and external reality (Beck, 1971). However, as yet the field lacks a validated means to distinguish subclinical from psychopathological depressive presentations. Indeed, nondiagnosable depressive presentations appear to share many of the clinical correlates of diagnosable presentations (Flett et al., 1997; Lewinsohn et al., 2000), although not necessarily all (Coyne and Downey, 1991). One possible resolution of this issue would be to use criteria other than diagnostic threshold to classify participants. For example, one might investigate whether cognitive distortions are a continuous function of depressive symptom level, or a categorical function of the presence of any clinically significant depressive features (e.g., persistent anhedonia or functional impairment).

Second, the extent to which the model can account for recovery from depression outside the context of cognitive therapy is as yet unknown. Needles and Abramson (1990) extended hopelessness theory to incorporate a recovery model dealing mainly with attributions for positive events that promote the likelihood that such events will restore hopefulness. This model has received empirical support in the context of recovery via antidepressant medication (Johnson et al., 1998). Similar studies would be useful in relation to cognitive theory, as would studies of recovery outside the context of formal intervention altogether, given that the modal person with a psychiatric disorder receives no mental health sector specialty care (Kessler et al., 1994).

Finally, improvements are needed in the measurement of competence in delivering cognitive therapy. The Cognitive Therapy Scale (CTS: J. Young and A. T. Beck, unpublished data) correlates with global quality ratings by experts (Vallis et al., 1986), but as yet there is little evidence of its association with treatment outcome. In the article by Gortner et al. (1998), for instance, CTS ratings by co-author Keith Dobson correlated significantly with outcome, but CTS ratings of the same tapes by two outside experts correlated neither with each other nor with outcome.

Being able to evaluate competence is critically important to interpreting comparative outcome studies, lest any poor findings be explained away as reflecting inadequate implementation of the treatment (Elkin, 1999). Moreover, it would be helpful to know what training procedures are especially effective in enhancing the competence of cognitive therapists. A study of training in manual-guided psychotherapies for cocaine dependence found a training effect for cognitive therapy (unlike comparison therapies) such that therapists did better with subsequent cases in the training phase (Crits-Christoph et al., 1998), but much more needs to be learned about how to maximize such training effects.

REFERENCES

Abramson, L. Y., Metalsky, G. I., and Alloy, L. B. (1989). Hopelessness depression: a theory-based subtype of depression. *Psychological Review*, **96**, 358–72.

Abramson, L. Y., Alloy, L. B., Hogan, M. E., et al. (1998). Suicidality and cognitive vulnerability to depression among college students: a prospective study. *Journal of Adolescence*, **21**, 157–71.

Abramson, L. Y., Alloy, L. B., Hogan, M. E., et al. (1999). Cognitive vulnerability to depression: theory and evidence. *Journal of Cognitive Psychotherapy*, **13**, 5–20.

Addis, M. E. and Jacobson, N. S. (1996). Reasons for depression and the process and outcome of cognitive-behavioral psychotherapies. *Journal of Consulting and Clinical Psychology*, **64**, 1417–24.

Alloy, L. B. and Abramson, L. Y. (1979). Judgment of contingency in depressed and nondepressed students: sadder but wiser? *Journal of Experimental Psychology: General*, **108**, 441–85.

American Psychiatric Association. (1994). *Diagnostic and Statistical Manual of Mental Disorders*, 4th edn. Washington, DC: American Psychiatric Association.

Beck, A. T. (1963). Thinking and depression: I. Idiosyncratic content and cognitive distortions. *Archives of General Psychiatry*, **9**, 324–33.

Beck, A. T. (1964). Thinking and depression: II. Theory and therapy. *Archives of General Psychiatry*, **10**, 561–71.

Beck, A. T. (1967). *Depression: Clinical, Experimental, and Theoretical Aspects*. New York: Harper and Row.

Beck, A. T. (1970). The core problem in depression: the cognitive triad. In *Depression: Theories and Therapies*, ed. J. H. Masserman pp. 47–55. New York: Grune and Stratton.

Beck, A. T. (1971). Cognition, affect, and psychopathology. *Archives of General Psychiatry*, **24**, 495–500.

Beck, A. T. (1983). Cognitive therapy of depression: new perspectives. In *Treatment of Depression: Old Controversies and New Approaches*, ed. P. J. Clayton and J. E. Barrett pp. 265–284. New York: Raven Press.

Beck, A. T. (1987). Cognitive models of depression. *Journal of Cognitive Psychotherapy: An International Quarterly*, **1**, 5–37.

Beck, A. T. (1995). *Cognitive Therapy: Basics and Beyond*. New York: Guilford.

Beck, A. T. (1996). Beyond belief: a theory of modes, personality, and psychopathology. In *Frontiers of Cognitive Therapy*, ed. P. M. Salkovskis, pp. 1–25. New York: Guilford.

Beck, A. T., Kovacs, M., and Weissman, A. (1975). Hopelessness and suicidal behavior: An overview. *Journal of the American Medical Association*, **234**, 1146–9.

Beck, A. T., Rush, A. J., Shaw, B. F., and Emery, G. (1979). *Cognitive Therapy of Depression*. New York: Guilford.

Beck, A. T., Epstein, N., Harrison, R. P., and Emery, G. (1983). *Development of the Sociotropy-Autonomy Scale: A Measure of Personality Factors in Psychopathology.* Unpublished manuscript. Center for Cognitive Therapy, University of Pennsylvania Medical School, Philadelphia.

Beck, A. T., Brown, G., Steer, R. A., Eidelson, J. I., and Riskind, J. H. (1987). Differentiating anxiety and depression: a test of the cognitive content-specificity hypothesis. *Journal of Abnormal Psychology*, **96**, 179–83.

Bellew, M. and Hill, A. B. (1990). Negative recall bias as predictor of susceptibility to induced depressed mood. *Personality and Individual Differences*, **11**, 471–80.

Bellew, M. and Hill, A. B. (1991). Schematic processing and the prediction of depression following childbirth. *Personality and Individual Differences*, **12**, 943–9.

Beutler, L. E., Mohr, D. C., Grawe, K., Engle, D., and MacDonald, R. (1991). Looking for differential treatment effects: cross-cultural predictors of differential psychotherapy efficacy. *Journal of Psychotherapy Integration*, **1**, 121–41.

Beutler, L. E., Machado, P. P., Engle, D., and Mohr, D. (1993). Differential patient x treatment maintenance among cognitive, experiential, and self-directed psychotherapies. *Journal of Psychotherapy Integration*, **3**, 15–31.

Blackburn, I. M. and Smyth, P. (1985). A test of cognitive vulnerability in individuals prone to depression. *British Journal of Clinical Psychology*, **24**, 61–2.

Blatt, S. J., Zuroff, D. C., Bondi, C. M., Sanislow, C. A., and Pilkonis, P. A. (1998). When and how perfectionism impedes the brief treatment of depression: further analyses of the National Institute of Mental Health Treatment of Depression Collaborative Research Program. *Journal of Consulting and Clinical Psychology*, **66**, 423–8.

Brown G. P., Hammen, C. L., Craske, M. G., and Wickens, T. D. (1995). Dimensions of dysfunctional attitudes as vulnerabilities to depressive symptoms. *Journal of Abnormal Psychology*, **104**, 431–5.

Bruder, G. E., Stewart, J. W., Mercier, M. A., et al. (1997). Outcome of cognitive-behavioral therapy for depression: relation to hemispheric dominance for verbal processing. *Journal of Abnormal Psychology*, **106**, 138–44.

Burns, D. D. and Nolen-Hoeksema, S. (1992). Therapeutic empathy and recovery from depression in cognitive-behavioral therapy: a structural equation model. *Journal of Consulting and Clinical Psychology*, **60**, 441–9.

Burns, D. D., Rude, S., Simons, A. D., Bates, M. A., and Thase, M. E. (1994). Does learned resourcefulness predict the response to cognitive behavioral therapy for depression? *Cognitive Therapy and Research*, **18**, 277–90.

Chambless, D. L., Baker, M. J., Baucom, D. H., et al. (1998). Update on empirically validated therapies, II. *Clinical Psychologist*, **51**, 3–16.

Clark, D. A. and Beck, A. T. (1991). Personality factors in dysphoria: a psychometric refinement of Beck's Sociotropy-Autonomy scale. *Journal of Psychopathology and Behavioral Assessment*, **13**, 369–88.

Clark, D. A. and Steer, R. A. (1996). Empirical status of the cognitive model of anxiety and depression. In *Frontiers of Cognitive Therapy*, ed. P. M. Salkovskis, pp. 75–96. New York: Guilford Press.

Clark, D. A., Beck A. T., and Beck, J. (1994). Symptom differences in major depression, dysthymia, panic disorder, and generalized anxiety disorder. *American Journal of Psychiatry*, **151**, 205–9.

Clark, D. A., Beck, A. T., and Alford, B. A. (1999). *Scientific Foundations of Cognitive Theory and Therapy of Depression*. New York: John Wiley.

Cole, D. A., Martin, J. M., Lachlan, G. P., Seroczynski, A. D., and Hoffman, K. (1998). Are cognitive errors of underestimation predictive or reflective of depressive symptoms in children? A longitudinal study. *Journal of Abnormal Psychology*, **107**, 481–96.

Covi, L. and Lipman, R. S. (1987). Cognitive behavioral group psychotherapy combined with imipramine in major depression. *Psychopharmacology Bulletin*, **23**, 173–7.

Coyne, J. C. (1992). Cognition in depression: a paradigm in crisis. *Psychological Inquiry*, **3**, 232–4.

Coyne, J. C. and Downey, G. (1991). Social factors and psychopathology: stress, social support, and coping processes. *Annual Review of Psychology*, **42**, 401–25.

Coyne, J. C. and Gotlib, I. H. (1983). The role of cognition in depression: a critical appraisal. *Psychological Bulletin*, **94**, 472–505.

Coyne, J. C. and Whiffen, V. E. (1995). Issues in personality as diathesis for depression: the case of sociotropy-dependency and autonomy-self-criticism. *Psychological Bulletin*, **118**, 358–78.

Crits-Christoph, P., Siqueland, L., Chittams, J., et al. (1998). Training in cognitive, supportive-expressive, and drug counseling therapies for cocaine dependence. *Journal of Consulting and Clinical Psychology*, **66**, 484–92.

Dent, J. and Teasdale, J. D. (1988). Negative cognition and the persistence of depression. *Journal of Abnormal Psychology*, **97**, 29–34.

Derry, P. A. and Kuiper, N. A. (1981). Schematic processing and self-reference in clinical depression. *Journal of Abnormal Psychology*, **90**, 286–97.

DeRubeis, R. J. and Crits-Christoph, P. (1998). Empirically supported individual and group psychological treatments for adult mental disorders. *Journal of Consulting and Clinical Psychology*, **66**, 37–52.

DeRubeis, R. J. and Feeley, M. (1990). Determinants of change in cognitive therapy for depression. *Cognitive Therapy and Research*, **14**, 469–82.

DeRubeis, R. J., Gelfand, L. A., Tang, T. Z., and Simons, A. D. (1999). Medications versus cognitive behavior therapy for severely depressed outpatients: mega-analysis of four randomized comparisons. *American Journal of Psychiatry*, **156**, 1007–13.

Dobson, K. S. and Breiter, H. J. (1983). Cognitive assessment of depression: reliability and validity of three measures. *Journal of Abnormal Psychology*, **92**, 107–9.

Dobson, K. S. and Shaw, B. F. (1986). Cognitive assessment with major depressive disorders. *Cognitive Therapy and Research*, **10**, 13–29.

Dykman, B. M. (1997). A test of whether negative emotional priming facilitates access to latent dysfunctional attitudes. *Cognition and Emotion*, **11**, 197–222.

Eaves, G. and Rush, A. J. (1984). Cognitive patterns in symptomatic and remitted unipolar major depression. *Journal of Abnormal Psychology*, **93**, 31–40.

Elkin, I. (1999). A major dilemma in psychotherapy outcome research: disentangling therapists from therapies. *Clinical Psychology: Science and Practice*, **6**, 10–32.

Elkin, I., Shea, M. T., Watkins, J. T., et al. (1995). Initial severity and differential treatment outcome in the National Institute of Mental Health Treatment of Depression Collaborative Research Program. *Journal of Consulting and Clinical Psychology,* **63**, 841–7.

Ellis, A. (1987). A sadly neglected cognitive element in depression. *Cognitive Therapy and Research,* **11**, 121–46.

Feeley, M., DeRubeis, R. J., and Gelfand, L. A. (1999). The temporal relation of adherence and alliance to symptom change in cognitive therapy for depression. *Journal of Consulting and Clinical Psychology,* **67**, 578–82.

Fennell, M. J. V. and Teasdale, J. D. (1987). Cognitive therapy for depression: individual differences and the process of change. *Cognitive Therapy and Research,* **11**, 253–71.

Flett, G. L., Vredenburg, K., and Krames, L. (1997). The continuity of depression in clinical and nonclinical samples. *Psychological Bulletin,* **121**, 395–416.

Gortner, E. T., Gollan, J. K., Dobson, K. S., and Jacobson, N. S. (1998). Cognitive-behavioral treatment for depression: relapse prevention. *Journal of Consulting and Clinical Psychology,* **66**, 377–84.

Gotlib, I. H. (1981). Self-reinforcement and recall: differential deficits in depressed and nondepressed psychiatric inpatients. *Journal of Abnormal Psychology,* **90**, 521–30.

Gotlib, I. H. (1983). Perception and recall of interpersonal feedback: negative bias in depression. *Cognitive Therapy and Research,* **7**, 399–412.

Gotlib, I. H. and Krasnoperova, E. (1998). Biased information processing as a vulnerability factor for depression. *Behavior Therapy,* **29**, 603–17.

Haaga, D. A. F. and Beck, A. T. (1995). Perspectives on depressive realism: implications for cognitive theory of depression. *Behaviour Research and Therapy,* **33**, 41–8.

Haaga, D. A. F. and Stiles, W. B. (2000). Randomized clinical trials in psychotherapy research: methodology, design, and evaluation. In *Handbook of Psychological Change: Psychotherapy Processes and Practices for the 21st Century,* ed. C. R. Snyder and R. E. Ingram, pp. 14–39. New York: John Wiley.

Haaga, D. A. F., Dyck, M. J., and Ernst, D. (1991a). Empirical status of cognitive theory of depression. *Psychological Bulletin,* **110**, 215–36.

Haaga, D. A. F., DeRubeis, R. J., Stewart, B. L., and Beck, A. T. (1991b). Relationship of intelligence with cognitive therapy outcome. *Behaviour Research and Therapy,* **29**, 277–81.

Hamilton, E. W. and Abramson, L. Y. (1983). Cognitive patterns and major depressive disorder: a longitudinal study in a hospital setting. *Journal of Abnormal Psychology,* **92**, 173–84.

Hammen, C., Ellicott, A., and Gitlin, M. (1989). Vulnerability to specific life events and prediction of course of disorder in unipolar depressed patients. *Canadian Journal of Behavioural Science,* **21**, 377–88.

Hedlund, S. and Rude, S. S. (1995). Evidence of latent depressive schemas in formerly depressed individuals. *Journal of Abnormal Psychology,* **104**, 517–25.

Hollon, S. D. and Najavits, L. (1988). Review of empirical studies of cognitive therapy. In *American Psychiatric Press Review of Psychiatry,* vol. 7, ed. A. J. Frances and R. E. Hales, pp. 643–66. Washington, DC: American Psychiatric Press.

Hollon, S. D., Kendall, P. C., and Lumry, A. (1986). Specificity of depressotypic cognitions in clinical depression. *Journal of Abnormal Psychology,* **95**, 52–9.

Hollon, S. D., DeRubeis, R. J., and Evans, M. D. (1996). Cognitive therapy in the treatment and prevention of depression. In *Frontiers of Cognitive Therapy*, ed. P. M. Salkovskis, pp. 293–317. New York: Guilford Press.

Ilardi, S. S. and Craighead, W. E. (1994). The role of nonspecific factors in cognitive-behavior therapy for depression. *Clinical Psychology: Research and Practice*, **1**, 138–56.

Ilardi, S. S., Craighead, W. E., and Evans, D. D. (1997). Modeling relapse in unipolar depression: the effects of dysfunctional cognitions and personality disorders. *Journal of Consulting and Clinical Psychology*, **65**, 381–91.

Ingram, R. E. and Wisnicki, K. S. (1988). Assessment of positive automatic cognition. *Journal of Consulting and Clinical Psychology*, **56**, 898–902.

Ingram, R. E., Slater, M. A., Atkinson, J. H., and Scott, W. (1990). Positive automatic cognition in major affective disorder. *Psychological Assessment: A Journal of Consulting and Clinical Psychology*, **2**, 209–11.

Ingram, R. E., Bernet, C. Z., and McLaughlin, S. C. (1994). Attentional allocation processes in individuals at risk for depression. *Cognitive Therapy and Research*, **18**, 317–32.

Ingram, R. E., Miranda, J., and Segal, Z. V. (1998). *Cognitive Vulnerability to Depression*. New York: Guilford Press.

Jacobson, N. S., Dobson, K. S., Truax, P. A., et al. (1996). A component analysis of cognitive-behavioral treatment for depression. *Journal of Consulting and Clinical Psychology*, **64**, 295–304.

Jarrett, R. B., Rush, A. J., Khatami, M., and Roffwarg, H. P. (1990). Does the pretreatment polysomnogram predict response to cognitive therapy in depressed outpatients? A preliminary report. *Psychiatry Research*, **33**, 285–99.

Jarrett, R. B., Eaves, G. G., Grannemann, B. D., and Rush, A. J. (1991). Clinical, cognitive, and demographic predictors of response to cognitive therapy for depression: a preliminary report. *Psychiatry Research*, **37**, 245–60.

Johnson, J. G., Han, Y-S., Douglas, C. J., Johannet, C. M., and Russell, T. (1998). Attributions for positive life events predict recovery from depression among psychiatric inpatients: an investigation of the Needles and Abramson model of recovery from depression. *Journal of Consulting and Clinical Psychology*, **66**, 369–76.

Judd, L. L., Akiskal, H. S., and Paulus, M. P. (1997). The role and clinical significance of subsyndromal depressive symptoms (SSD) in unipolar major depressive disorder. *Journal of Affective Disorders*, **45**, 41–51.

Kendall, P. C. (1999). Clinical significance. *Journal of Consulting and Clinical Psychology*, **67**, 283–4.

Kessler, R. C., McGonagle, K. A., Zhao, S., et al. (1994). Lifetime and 12-month prevalence of DSM-III-R psychiatric disorders in the United States: results from the National Comorbidity Survey. *Archives of General Psychiatry*, **51**, 8–19.

Lang, A. J. and Craske, M. G. (1997). Information processing in anxiety and depression. *Behaviour Research and Therapy*, **35**, 451–5.

Lewinsohn, P. M., Steinmetz, J. L., Larson, D. W., and Franklin, J. (1981). Depression-related cognitions: antecedent or consequence? *Journal of Abnormal Psychology*, **90**, 213–19.

Lewinsohn, P. M., Solomon, A., Seeley, J. R., and Zeiss, A. (2000). The clinical implications of "subthreshold" depressive symptoms. *Journal of Abnormal Psychology*, **109**, 345–51.

Matt, G. E., Vazquez, C., and Campbell, W. K. (1992). Mood-congruent recall of affectively toned stimuli: a meta-analytic review. *Clinical Psychology Review*, **12**, 227–55.

McCabe, S. B. and Gotlib, I. H. (1993). Attentional processing in clinically depressed subjects: a longitudinal investigation. *Cognitive Therapy and Research*, **17**, 359–77.

McKnight, D. L., Nelson-Gray, R. O., and Barnhill, J. (1992). Dexamethasone suppression test and response to cognitive therapy and antidepressant medication. *Behavior Therapy*, **23**, 99–111.

Miller I. W. and Norman, W. H. (1986). Persistence of depressive cognitions within a subgroup of depressed inpatients. *Cognitive Therapy and Research*, **10**, 211–24.

Miranda, J. and Persons, J. B. (1988). Dysfunctional attitudes are mood-state dependent. *Journal of Abnormal Psychology*, **97**, 76–9.

Miranda, J., Persons, J. B., and Byers, C. N. (1990). Endorsement of dysfunctional beliefs depends on current mood state. *Journal of Abnormal Psychology*, **99**, 237–41.

Moore, R. G. and Blackburn, I. (1996). The stability of sociotropy and autonomy in depressed patients undergoing treatment. *Cognitive Therapy and Research*, **20**, 69–80.

Needles, D. J. and Abramson, L. Y. (1990). Positive life events, attributional style, and hopefulness: testing a model of recovery from depression. *Journal of Abnormal Psychology*, **99**, 156–65.

Norman, W. H., Miller I. W., and Klee, S. H. (1983). Assessment of cognitive distortion in a clinically depressed population. *Cognitive Therapy and Research*, **7**, 133–40.

Norman, W. H., Miller, I.W., and Keitner, G. I. (1987). Relationship between dysfunctional cognitions and depressive subtypes. *Canadian Journal of Psychiatry*, **32**, 194–8.

O'Leary, K. D. and Beach, S. R. H. (1990). Marital therapy: a viable treatment for depression and marital discord. *American Journal of Psychiatry*, **147**, 183–6.

Persons, J. B. (1991). Psychotherapy outcome studies do not accurately represent current models of psychotherapy: a proposed remedy. *American Psychologist*, **46**, 99–106.

Persons, J. B. and Burns, D. D. (1985). Mechanisms of action of cognitive therapy: the relative contributions of technical and interpersonal interventions. *Cognitive Therapy and Research*, **10**, 539–51.

Peterson, C., Semmel, A., von Baeyer, C., et al. (1982). The Attributional Style Questionnaire. *Cognitive Therapy and Research*, **6**, 287–301.

Reich, J. H. and Vasile, R. G. (1993). Effect of personality disorders on the treatment outcome of Axis I conditions: an update. *Journal of Nervous and Mental Disease*, **181**, 475–84.

Riskind, J. H., Hohmann, A. A., Beck, A. T., and Stewart, B. (1991). The relation of generalized anxiety disorder to depression in general and dysthymic disorder in particular. In *Chronic Anxiety: Generalized Anxiety Disorder and Mixed Anxiety-Depression*, ed. R. M. Rapee and D. H. Barlow, pp. 153–71. New York: Guilford Press.

Roberts, J. E. and Kassel, J. D. (1996). Mood-state dependence in cognitive vulnerability to depression: the roles of positive and negative affect. *Cognitive Therapy and Research*, **20**, 1–12.

Robins, C. J. and Block, P. (1988). Personal vulnerability, life events, and depressive symptoms: a test of a specific interactional model. *Journal of Personality and Social Psychology*, **54**, 847–52.

Robins, C. J., Ladd, J. S., Welkowitz, J., et al. (1994). The Personal Style Inventory: preliminary validation studies of new measures of sociotropy and autonomy. *Journal of Psychopathology and Behavioral Assessment*, **16**, 277–300.

Robins, C. J., Hayes, A. M., Block, P., Kramer, R. J., and Villena, M. (1995). Interpersonal and achievement concerns and the depressive vulnerability and symptom specificity hypotheses: a prospective study. *Cognitive Therapy and Research*, **19**, 1–20.

Robins, C. J., Bagby, R. M., Rector, N. A., Lynch, T. R., and Kennedy, S. H. (1997). Sociotropy, autonomy, and patterns of symptoms in patients with major depression: a comparison of dimensional and categorical approaches. *Cognitive Therapy and Research*, **21**, 285–300.

Rohde, P., Lewinsohn, P. M., and Seeley, J. R. (1990). Are people changed by the experience of having an episode of major depression? A further test of the scar hypothesis. *Journal of Abnormal Psychology*, **99**, 264–71.

Rosenbaum, M. (1980). A schedule for assessing self-control behaviors: preliminary findings. *Behavior Therapy*, **11**, 109–21.

Segal, Z. V. and Ingram, R. E. (1994). Mood priming and construct activation in tests of cognitive vulnerability to unipolar depression. *Clinical Psychology Review*, **14**, 663–95.

Segal, Z. V., Shaw, B. F., and Vella, D. D. (1989). Life stress and depression: a test of the congruency hypothesis for life event content and depressive subtype. *Canadian Journal of Behavioural Science*, **21**, 389–400.

Segal, Z. V., Shaw, B. F., Vella, D. D., and Katz, R. (1992). Cognitive and life stress predictors of relapse in remitted unipolar depressed patients: test of the congruency hypothesis. *Journal of Abnormal Psychology*, **101**, 26–36.

Shaw, B. F. (1999). How to use the allegiance effect to maximize competence and therapeutic outcomes. *Clinical Psychology: Science and Practice*, **6**, 131–2.

Shea, M. T., Pilkonis, P. A., Beckham, E., et al. (1990). Personality disorders and treatment outcome in the NIMH treatment of depression collaborative research program. *American Journal of Psychiatry*, **147**, 711–18.

Shea, M. T., Elkin, I., Imber, S. D., et al. (1992). Course of depressive symptoms over follow-up: findings from the National Institute of Mental Health treatment of depression collaborative research program. *Archives of General Psychiatry*, **49**, 782–7.

Silverman, J. S., Silverman, J. A., and Eardley, D. A. (1984). Do maladaptive attitudes cause depression? *Archives of General Psychiatry*, **41**, 28–30.

Simons, A. D., Lustman, P. J., Wetzel, R. D., and Murphy, G. E. (1985). Predicting response to cognitive therapy of depression: the role of learned resourcefulness. *Cognitive Therapy and Research*, **9**, 79–89.

Simons, A. D., Gordon, J. S., Monroe, S. M., and Thase, M. E. (1995). Toward an integration of psychologic, social, and biologic factors in depression: effects on outcome and course of cognitive therapy. *Journal of Consulting and Clinical Psychology*, **63**, 369–77.

Solomon, A. and Haaga, D. A. F. (1994). Positive and negative aspects of sociotropy and autonomy. *Journal of Psychopathology and Behavioral Assessment*, **16**, 243–52.

Solomon, A., Haaga, D. A. F., Brody, C., Kirk, L., and Friedman, D. G. (1998). Priming irrational beliefs in formerly depressed individuals. *Journal of Abnormal Psychology*, **107**, 440–9.

Sotsky, S. M., Glass, D. R., Shea, M. T., et al. (1991). Patient predictors of response to psychotherapy and pharmacotherapy: findings of the NIMH treatment of depression collaborative research program. *American Journal of Psychiatry*, **148**, 997–1008.

Teasdale, J. D. (1985). Psychological treatments for depression: how do they work? *Behaviour Research and Therapy*, **23**, 157–65.

Thase, M. E., Simons, A. D., McGeary, J., et al. (1992). Relapse after cognitive behavior therapy of depression: potential implications for longer courses of treatment. *American Journal of Psychiatry*, **149**, 1046–52.

Thase, M. E., Simons, A. D., and Reynolds, C. F. (1996). Abnormal electroencephalographic sleep profiles in major depression: association with response to cognitive-behavioral therapy. *Archives of General Psychiatry*, **53**, 99–108.

Vallis, T. M., Shaw, B. F., and Dobson, K. S. (1986). The Cognitive Therapy Scale: psychometric properties. *Journal of Consulting and Clinical Psychology*, **54**, 381–5.

Wampold, B. E., Mondin, G. W., Moody, M., et al. (1997). A meta-analysis of outcome studies comparing bona fide psychotherapies: empirically, all must have prizes. *Psychological Bulletin*, **122**, 203–15.

Watkins, P. C., Mathew, A., Williamson, D. A., and Fuller, R. D. (1992). Unconscious mood-congruent memory bias in depression. *Journal of Abnormal Psychology*, **105**, 34–41.

Wetzel, R. D., Murphy, G. E., Carney, R. M., Whitworth, P., and Knesevich, M. A. (1992). Prescribing therapy for depression: the role of learned resourcefulness, a failure to replicate. *Psychological Reports*, **70**, 803–7.

Whisman, M. A. (1993). Mediators and moderators of change in cognitive therapy of depression. *Psychological Bulletin*, **114**, 248–65.

Williams, J. M. G., Watts, F. N., MacLeod, C., and Mathews, A. (1996). *Cognitive Psychology and Emotional Disorders*, 2nd edn. Chichester, England: Wiley.

Zeiss, A. M., Lewinsohn, P. M., and Munoz, R. F. (1979). Nonspecific improvement effects in depression using interpersonal skills training, pleasant activity schedules or cognitive training. *Journal of Consulting and Clinical Psychology*, **47**, 427–39.

Zlotnick, C., Elkin, I., and Shea, M. T. (1998). Does the gender of a patient or the gender of a therapist affect the treatment of patients with major depression? *Journal of Consulting and Clinical Psychology*, **66**, 655–9.

3

Cognitive theory and therapy of bipolar disorders

Jan Scott

Gartnavel Royal Hospital, Glasgow, Scotland, UK

This chapter will explore the evolution of cognitive theory and therapy for individuals with bipolar disorders (BP). Unlike most of the other chapters, there is only a small body of research data available on these topics. Until recently, BP were widely regarded as a biological illness best treated with medications (Prien and Potter, 1990; Scott, 1995a). This view is gradually changing for two reasons. First, in the past three decades, there has been a greater emphasis on stress-diathesis models. This has led to the development of new etiological theories of severe mental disorders that emphasize psychological and social aspects of vulnerability and risk. It has also increased the acceptance of brief psychological therapies, such as cognitive therapy (CT), as an adjunct to medication for individuals with treatment-resistant schizophrenia, and severe and chronic depressive disorders (Scott and Wright, 1997). Second, there is a significant efficacy–effectiveness gap for pharmacological treatments for BP (Guscott and Taylor, 1994). Mood stabilizer prophylaxis protects about 60% of individuals against relapse in research settings, but protects only 25–40% of individuals against further episodes in clinical settings (Dickson and Kendall, 1986). The introduction of newer medications has not improved prognosis (Scott, 1995a). This has also increased interest in other treatment approaches in BP.

This chapter explores cognitive models of BP and the empirical support for these models. It comments on the clinical applicability of CT for BP and reviews the outcome studies available. Given the relative lack of data, the final section offers an overview of key areas for further research.

Cognitive models of bipolar disorder

Early descriptions

Beck's original cognitive model (1967) suggests that depressed mood states are accentuated by patterns of thinking that amplify mood shifts. (A detailed review of the model of depression is provided in Chapter 2.) For example, as people become depressed they become more negative in how they see themselves, their world, and their future (called the negative cognitive triad). Hence they tend to jump to negative conclusions, overgeneralize, interpret situations in all-or-nothing terms, and personalize and self-blame to an excessive degree (cognitive distortions). Changes in behavior, such as avoidance of social interaction, may be a cause or a consequence of mood shifts and negative thinking. Cognitive vulnerability to depression centers on prepotent dysfunctional underlying beliefs (e.g., "I'm unlovable") that develop from early learning experiences, and drive thinking and behavior. It is hypothesized that these beliefs may be activated by life events that have specific meaning for that individual. For example, an individual who holds a belief that "I'm unlovable" may experience depression in the face of rejection by a significant other.

Beck's original description suggested that mania was a mirror image of depression and was characterized by a positive cognitive triad of self, world, and future, and positive cognitive distortions. The self was seen as extremely lovable and powerful with unlimited potential and attractiveness. The world was filled with wonderful possibilities, and experiences were viewed as overly positive. The future was one of unlimited opportunity and promise. Hyperpositive thinking (stream of consciousness) was typified by cognitive distortions, as in depression, but in the opposite direction. For example, jumping to positive conclusions, such as "I'm a winner" and "I can do anything;" underestimating risks, such as "there's no danger;" minimizing problems, such as "nothing can go wrong;" and overvaluing immediate gratification, such as "I will do this now." Thus, cognitive distortions provided biased confirmation of the positive cognitive triad of self, world, and future. Positive experiences were selectively attended to, and it was hypothesized that in this way underlying beliefs and self-schemata that guide behaviors, thoughts, and feelings were maintained and strengthened. Examples of such underlying beliefs and self-schemata include: "I'm special" and "Being manic helps me to overcome my shyness."

In contrast to Beck's model of depression, there have been relatively few research attempts to confirm or refute his ideas about mania. Beck's original model of mania was largely derivative, based on the careful observation of individuals in a manic state. It took a traditional stance, viewing mania as the polar opposite of depression. Neither mixed states nor dysphoric mania were considered. Thus gaps are apparent in Beck's original model of the cognitive basis of mania. For example, there is no discussion about the similarities or differences in the specific dysfunctional beliefs held by individuals with BP as compared to unipolar disorders, nor has the role of personality styles (sociotropy and autonomy) been incorporated into his formulation of mania. Also, the nature of life events that may "match" certain beliefs and uniquely precipitate mania as opposed to depression remained unexplored. However, it is important to see the model in context. It was a useful step forward from psychoanalytic models, and has recently provided an important starting point for the research that is now reviewed below.

Empirical evidence

This review of studies of BP is organized into two subgroups: those exploring descriptive components of cognitive models and those exploring the role of "matching" life events in symptom exacerbation in clinical and nonclinical samples.

Descriptive studies

Most studies of cognitive models in BP have used the model of unipolar disorders as a template. As such, the early research comprised cross-sectional studies comparing subjects with BP with other client populations on measures such as dysfunctional beliefs, self-esteem, and cognitive processing.

Apart from one early study, data on dysfunctional attitudes, personality styles, and automatic thoughts in individuals with BP who were not currently manic demonstrate a similar pattern to that seen in individuals in the euthymic (nondepressive) and depressive phases of unipolar disorders. Unfortunately, there are limited data on changes during the manic phase.

Silverman et al. (1984) explored dysfunctional attitudes in a heterogeneous clinical sample and suggested that individuals with BP who were currently euthymic showed lower levels of dysfunctional attitudes than all other diagnostic groups. This finding is not supported by either Bentall et al. (2002) or Scott et al. (2000a). Silverman and colleagues also demonstrated that in a depressive phase, unipolar and BP subjects showed a similar increase in levels of dysfunctional attitudes. This finding was confirmed by Hollon et al. (1986) who reported that, compared to healthy control subjects, individuals with either unipolar or BP depression showed higher levels of dysfunctional attitudes and negative automatic thoughts. However, there were no significant differences between unipolar and BP subjects when depressed or in remission. Alloy et al. (1999) found that attributional style and dysfunctional attitudes were similar in individuals with cyclothymia and dysthymia and were more negative than normal controls. It is not known how these findings relate to major depressive disorders or BP, but individuals with cyclothymia and dysthymia have a greater risk of major affective disorder than individuals in the general population. In a study by Hammen et al. (1992), unipolar and BP subjects who were asymptomatic did not differ on measures of sociotropy or autonomy.

Only two studies have explored mood-congruent or mood-dependent memory in individuals with BP. Weingartner et al. (1977) showed that eight subjects who experienced several cycles of mania and depression were more able to retrieve memories when their mood at retrieval matched their mood at encoding. Recall when mood at testing matched mood at production was twice as high (35% versus 18%) as when there was a mismatch. More recently, Eich et al. (1997) assessed mood-dependent memory in 10 individuals with rapid-cycling BP. They noted, that like healthy controls, their subjects showed mood-dependent changes in autobiographical memory recall. However, their subjects also demonstrated mood-dependent recognition, an effect that healthy controls rarely show. Eich and colleagues propose that this effect may arise because subjects with BP experience stronger, more intense moods.

Scott and colleagues (2000a) explored several aspects of the cognitive model simultaneously, including dysfunctional attitudes, positive and negative self-esteem, autobiographical memory, and problem-solving skills. The sample comprised individuals with BP ($n = 40$) who were rated by an observer as euthymic and a matched control group of healthy subjects ($n = 20$). Interestingly, although reported levels of observer-rated manic and depressive symptoms in BP subjects were minimal, self-rated depression scores suggested significant levels of residual dysphoria and/or ongoing subsyndromal depression.

In comparison to healthy controls, BP clients had more fragile, unstable levels of self-esteem, higher levels of dysfunctional attitudes (particularly related to need for social approval and perfectionism), overgeneral autobiographical memory and poorer problem-solving skills. These statistically significant differences persisted when current depression ratings were taken into account. Within the BP group, those individuals who had multiple previous affective episodes and/or earlier age of onset of BP showed the greatest level of cognitive dysfunction. Scott et al. (2000a) argue that, although it was not possible to determine whether these abnormalities of cognitive style were a cause or a consequence of relapse in BP, it was noteworthy that these differences from healthy controls persisted in clients who were currently adherent with prophylactic medication. This suggests that long-term medication alone may not extinguish cognitive and affective symptoms nor fully protect against relapse. Furthermore, the researchers noted that clients with BP showed a similar cognitive style to individuals with unipolar depression. Preliminary data from a further study comparing subjects with BP and those with severe unipolar disorders appear to support this hypothesis.

Other studies have explored self-esteem, social desirability, and self-representations. Using a repertory grid, Ashworth et al. (1982) demonstrated abnormally high levels of self-esteem during mania, low levels in depression, and a return to normal levels in remission. Winters and Neale (1985) wrote a highly influential article in which they hypothesized that, although subjects with remitted BP do not usually report impaired self-esteem, these subjects possess a cognitive schema of low self-esteem. This idea evolved from data suggesting that, although subjects with BP and healthy controls showed higher levels of self-esteem than individuals prone to unipolar depression, the BP group scored higher than either the unipolar or the healthy control group on measures of social desirability and self-deception. Winters and Neale concluded that subjects with BP might have negative feelings about the self that are not revealed on the typical, explicit self-report measures employed in research settings. Neale (1988) later proposed that unstable self-esteem coupled with unrealistic standards for success may be predisposing factors for BP. Although there is little empirical support for this hypothesis, the study of self-esteem by Pardoen et al. (1993) confirmed the presence of social conformism in BP subjects. A key methodological lesson from these studies is the need to consider the use of implicit as well as explicit measures of cognitive style.

Lyon et al. (1999) used explicit and implicit measures of attributional style and a recall measure of self-schema in BP subjects who were currently manic or currently depressed and compared their results with a group of healthy controls. Manic subjects showed a normal self-serving bias on the explicit attributional style questionnaire, attributing positive events more than negative events to self. As predicted, depressed subjects attributed negative events rather than positive events to self. However, on implicit measures, manic and depressed BP subjects both attributed negative events more than positive events to self. On the self-referent encoding memory task, manic subjects were more likely than depressed subjects to endorse positive words as true of themselves. However, in a surprise recall test, both manic and depressed subjects recalled more negative than positive trait words.

Bentall and colleagues (2000) measured self-discrepancies in BP subjects who were currently manic, currently depressed or currently in remission and compared them with healthy control subjects. Manic subjects showed higher self-actual : self-ideal consistency than healthy controls, whilst depressed BP subjects showed abnormally high self-actual : self-ideal discrepancies. Participants in all four groups showed little evidence of discrepancies between how they viewed themselves and how they thought others viewed them.

As shown from this review, research on cognitive models of BP is at a rudimentary stage. The above studies identify that unipolar and BP disorders are indistinguishable in the depressed phase, sharing a similar cognitive profile that includes abnormalities in information processing, dysfunctional attitudes, and attributional style. Remitted BP subjects show similar cognitive style to remitted unipolar subjects on explicit measures, but this is not always as clear on implicit measures. Data on levels of self-esteem are equivocal as variations may be a function of lability or of differences between implicit and explicit ratings. Scott and colleagues have identified that labile self-esteem as compared with the fixed low level of self-esteem may potentially distinguish BP and subjects with severe unipolar disorders in the depressed or euthymic phases of disorder. However, unstable self-esteem and low level of self-esteem are both known to confer similar levels of risk for depressive relapse (Kernis et al., 1993; Roberts and Munroe, 1994). Alternatively, the discrepancy between explicit and implicit measures of self-esteem or self-representations in remitted unipolar and BP subjects might be explained if we assume that social desirability schemata are activated even in BP subjects in the euthymic state.

Research on subjects experiencing mania is limited, but the evidence available highlights that subjects who are manic do show state-dependent differences from subjects in other phases of BP or unipolar disorders as well as healthy controls. However, differences in attributional style and view of self between unipolar and BP disorders are again less apparent when implicit measures are employed. Finally, the work of Bentall and colleagues demonstrates that transitions between different phases of BP disorder are associated with changes in the cognitive accessibility of discrepancies between self-representations. Bentall and Kinderman (1999) argue that highly labile self-esteem may reflect readily accessible and salient self-representations.

In summary, although there are many similarities in cognitive style between unipolar and BP disorders, there is minimal evidence that the abnormalities in BP individuals are trait vulnerabilities that specifically predispose to onset of BP. It is possible that trait aspects of cognitive style may increase the likelihood of early age of first episode or influence the frequency of recurrence. Without more detailed longitudinal research, little can be said about the stability of cognitive style over time in BP subjects. At this stage many of the identified abnormalities in cognitive processing appear to be state-dependent.

Interaction of life events and cognitive style

According to Beck's model, certain maladaptive core beliefs interact with stressors that carry a specific meaning for the individual, increasing the probability that an affective episode will occur. In their excellent review, Johnson and Miller (1995) confirm the association between adverse life events and either an exacerbation of affective symptoms or relapse into an episode of BP. However, only five studies have explored the interaction between aspects of cognitive style and life events. A small early study (Hammen et al., 1989) failed to find support for a cognitive stress-vulnerability model for individuals with BP. However, a later study by Hammen et al. (1992) reported that individuals with BP who had high levels of sociotropy experienced an exacerbation of affective symptoms in response to negative interpersonal life events. Hammen and colleagues did not identify whether manic or depressive exacerbations were more frequent. In a similar study, Swendsen et al. (1995) explored the relationship between life stress and personality traits known to be associated with negative cognitive style – namely, introversion and obsessionality. They demonstrated that these negative styles interacted with nonspecific stressful life events to predict relapse of BP disorder.

Two other studies have prospectively explored symptom exacerbation in subsyndromal BP or nonclinical populations. Alloy et al. (1999) reported that an internal, stable, global attributional style interacted with life stress to predict increases in affective symptoms in individuals with subsyndromal BP or unipolar disorders. In a further study, Reilly-Harrington et al. (1999) screened a nonclinical sample on the General Behavioral Index (Depue et al., 1989) for BP or the Beck Depression Inventory (Beck et al., 1961) for unipolar disorders. Subjects scoring above the established cut-offs were also administered the Schedule for Affective Disorders and Schizophrenia (Endicott and Spitzer, 1978). Reilly-Harrington and colleagues (1999) initially assessed each individual's attributional style, dysfunctional attitudes, and negative self-referent information processing, then reassessed these factors in subjects 1 month later. In individuals with BP, negative cognitive style at initial assessment interacted significantly with a high number of negative life events to predict an increase in manic or depressive symptoms. The interaction between dysfunctional attitudes and negative life events accounted for a greater proportion of the variance in symptoms (16%) than the interaction between attributional style and negative life events (10%).

In summary, there is a paucity of data on the interaction between specific measures of cognitive vulnerability and specific "matching" life events in BP. The existing studies are either small-scale, or only follow up the sample for a brief time. Measures of cognitive vulnerability, life events, and stress are inconsistent; the assessment tools vary in their reliability and validity, and study samples are heterogeneous. Despite these obvious problems, there is a consistent trend suggesting that negative cognitive style interacts with negative life events or high levels of stress to exacerbate affective symptoms. The evidence is more robust for the prediction of depressive symptoms, but, surprisingly, negative cognitive style, and events may interact to predict increases in manic symptoms. Three key questions remain unanswered from the studies available. First, are the statistically significant changes in reported symptom levels clinically meaningful? Second, is there evidence that specific dysfunctional beliefs are associated with a particular type of life event? Third, why and how might negative cognitive style interact with life events or life stress to predict increases in manic as well as depressive symptoms?

No study undertaken so far has demonstrated unequivocal support for a cognitive stress-vulnerability model of BP. The association between life events, cognitive style, and symptom exacerbation or relapse into manic or depressive phases is most readily explained by assuming that cognitive style and/or life stress interact in a nonspecific or indirect way. Further research is clearly needed to establish the exact mechanisms of any interaction. However, this work will be hampered by the lack of hypotheses about the nature of dysfunctional beliefs held by individuals with BP that, when activated by negative life events, may precipitate a manic as opposed to a depressive episode. This task is further complicated by the fact that some individuals with recurrent depressive episodes will eventually experience a manic episode and be classified as BP as opposed to unipolar cases.

Does cognitive therapy improve outcome?

Despite the lack of a coherent cognitive stress-vulnerability theory of BP, encouraging anecdotal and single case reports on the use of CT in clients with BP have been published over the last 20 years (Chor et al., 1988; Wright and Schrodt, 1992; Scott, 1995b). These have been followed by the publication of treatment and self-help manuals (Basco and Rush, 1995; Lam et al., 1999; Newman et al., 2001; Scott, 2001) and then by eight reports on the use of individual and group CT in small-scale open studies or randomized controlled trials (Cochran, 1984; Palmer et al., 1995; Bauer et al., 1998; Perry et al., 1999; Zaretsky et al., 1999; Lam et al., 2000; Weiss et al., 2000; Scott et al., 2001). This section will give an overview of these studies and then consider the role of CT in individuals with BP.

Studies of group cognitive therapy

The aim of Cochran's study was to add CT to standard clinical care in order to enhance adherence with prophylactic lithium treatment. It compared 28 clients who were randomly assigned to either six sessions of group CT plus standard clinic care or standard clinic care alone (Cochran, 1984). Following treatment, enhanced lithium adherence was reported in the intervention group, with only three patients (21%) discontinuing medication as compared with eight patients (57%) in the standard clinic care group. There were also fewer hospitalizations in the group receiving CT. Unfortunately no information was available on the nature of any affective relapses.

In Palmer and colleagues' (1995) initial exploratory study, six clients with BP were offered CT in a group format. The focus of the program was psychoeducational, recognizing the process of change, enhancing coping strategies, and dealing with interpersonal problems. Overall findings indicated that group therapy combined with mood-stabilizing medications was effective for some but not all of the participants. All participants improved on one or more measures of symptoms or social adjustment, but the pattern of change varied greatly across individuals. A more recent naturalistic study by these investigators (A. Palmer, unpublished data) included a larger number of participants receiving group CT ($n = 25$) and a comparison group ($n = 12$) receiving only treatment as usual. The results showed that, in comparison to the control group, CT reduced nonspecific psychological symptoms and increased social adjustment. There were no significant differences in actual relapse rates in those receiving group CT or those receiving only treatment as usual.

The Life Goals program developed by Bauer and colleagues (1998) is a structured, manual-based intervention that seeks to improve patients' management skills, and their social and occupational functioning. The program utilizes a number of cognitive and behavioral techniques. Although outcome data are not yet available, a recent study of 29 clients suggested the program achieved acceptable retention rates (70% of clients remained in treatment) and resulted in a significant increase in knowledge about BP.

Weiss and colleagues (2000) used a group format to deliver therapy to individuals with comorbid BP and substance dependence. The therapy was described as integrated group therapy, but incorporated a number of cognitive and behavioral elements. Twenty-one individuals receiving group therapy were compared with 24 clients receiving usual treatment and regular assessments. The main outcome measures were severity of addiction and number of months abstinent. The group therapy subjects showed statistically significantly greater improvement on both of these indices at 6-month follow-up.

Studies of individual cognitive therapy

Zaretsky et al. (1999) used a matched case-control design to compare the benefits of 20 sessions of CT plus mood-stabilizer medication for individuals with bipolar depression ($n = 11$) with an equivalent course of CT for individuals with unipolar depression ($n = 11$). Both groups achieved similar reductions in level of depressive symptoms, but Zaretsky and colleagues reported that only subjects with unipolar depression showed a significant posttherapy reduction in levels of dysfunctional attitudes.

Perry and colleagues (1999) undertook the largest study so far ($n = 69$), using cognitive and behavioral techniques to help people identify and manage early warning signs of relapse in a group of clients at high risk of further relapse of BP who were in regular contact with mental health services. The results demonstrated that, in comparison to the control group, the intervention group had significantly fewer manic relapses (27% versus 57%), significantly fewer days in hospital, significantly longer time to first manic relapse, higher levels of social functioning, and better work performance. However, the most fascinating finding was that the intervention did not have a significant impact on depression. The possible reasons for this and the implications of this study are discussed further below.

Lam and colleagues (2000) undertook a small randomized controlled study of 12–20 sessions of outpatient CT for BP. The model particularly utilizes CT techniques to cope with the prodromal symptoms of an affective episode. This has some similarities to Perry et al.'s (1999) model, but Lam and colleagues also targeted longer-term vulnerabilities and difficulties arising as a consequence of the disorder. Twenty-five subjects were randomly allocated to individual CT as an adjunct to mood-stabilizing medication or to usual treatment alone (mood-stabilizers plus outpatient support). Independent assessments demonstrated that, after controlling for gender and illness history, the intervention group had significantly fewer affective relapses than the control group, with a significant reduction in episodes of hypomania, but nonsignificant reductions in the number of episodes of mania and of depression. The intervention group also showed significantly greater improvements in social adjustment and better coping strategies for managing prodromal symptoms.

A pilot study by Scott et al. (2001) examined the effect of 20 sessions of CT in 42 clients with BP. To maximize participation in the study and to increase the data available from a pilot study, Scott and colleagues chose a trial design that offered all subjects the opportunity to receive CT at some point. Individuals initially allocated to the control group ($n = 21$) were therefore offered the opportunity to receive CT after 6 months. Subjects could also enter the study during any phase of BP. Clients were initially randomly allocated to the intervention group or to a "waiting-list" control group. This randomized phase (6 months) allowed assessment of the effects of CT plus usual treatment as compared with usual treatment alone. Individuals from both groups who had received CT and agreed to continue with interview assessments ($n = 29$ of 42) were then monitored for a further 12 months post-CT. Further changes in symptoms, social functioning, relapse, and hospitalization rates were recorded.

Symptoms and functioning were measured using a combination of observer and subjective rating scales. These included self-report questionnaires on medication adherence, views of benefits or drawbacks of CT, work and social adjustment, and simultaneous variations in manic and depressive symptoms. The latter were measured using the Internal State Scale (ISS; Bauer et al., 1991). This comprises 16 items (each rated on a 0–100 Likert scale) that are divided into four subscales: depression, well-being, activation, and perceived conflict. The perceived conflict scale is not easy to interpret, whereas the depression and well-being subscales give indications of mood fluctuations. On the other hand, the activation subscale is of relevance to cognitive therapists since CT of BP must be adapted so that it targets self-regulation. In support of this emphasis, some theories of BP suggest that changes in activation rather than mood may be the key to understanding BP relapse (e.g., Carver and White, 1994).

At initial assessment, 30% of participants met criteria for an affective episode: 11 subjects met diagnostic criteria for depressive disorder, three for rapid cycling disorder, two for hypomania, and one for a mixed state. As is typical of this client population, 12 subjects also met criteria for drug and/or alcohol problems or dependence, two met criteria for other axis I disorders, and about 60% of the sample met criteria for personality disorder. The most prevalent were borderline ($n = 15$) and antisocial personality disorders ($n = 11$), but 14 clients met criteria for more than one personality disorder.

The results of the randomized controlled phase demonstrated that, compared with subjects receiving treatment as usual, those who received additional CT experienced statistically significant improvements in global functioning and work and social adjustment. They also achieved significant improvements in well-being scores and significant reductions in depression and activation levels as measured on the ISS. It is noteworthy that, in the CT plus usual treatment group, reductions in depressive symptoms were more convincing than reductions in manic symptoms.

Data based on the 29 subjects from both groups who received CT and were followed up for 12 months post-CT demonstrated that, although changes in symptoms and functioning immediately after receiving CT were statistically significant, these improvements were not fully maintained after CT had finished. However, changes in relapse and admission rates were encouraging, with a 60% reduction in relapse rates in the 18 months after commencing CT as compared with the 18 months prior to receiving CT. Hospitalization rates showed parallel reductions. Scott et al. concluded that CT plus treatment as usual may offer some benefit and is a highly acceptable treatment intervention to about 70% of clients with BP. The results also suggest that CT plus treatment as usual may help improve self-reported adherence to medication: nonadherence rates in those receiving CT fell from 48% to 21%. Although this difference just failed to reach statistical significance, these improvements in adherence were largely maintained at follow-up. The researchers also sounded a note of caution from their study. It was reported that CT for individuals with BP is often more complex than for unipolar disorders, requiring more flexibility and greater expertise on the part of the therapist.

In summary, no large-scale randomized treatment intervention trials of CT for BP have been published to date. Three are currently underway (two in the UK and one in the USA). From the data above, it appears that the skills-based approach of group CT, although well received, has a greater impact on knowledge about BP and enhancing general coping strategies than reducing relapse rates. However, this is a tentative conclusion based on a limited number of small open pilot studies.

The data on brief CT (Cochran, 1984; Perry et al., 1999) suggests a role for cognitive and behavioral techniques in the self-management of BP. Given the potential benefit of reducing medication nonadherence rates (reported prevalence 50%), it is disappointing that Cochran's study has not been replicated on a larger sample with a longer follow-up. Perry et al.'s study provides useful insight into the potential role and limitations of technique-driven approaches. The study showed that brief CT prevented or delayed the onset only of mania, not of depression. Scott and colleagues (2001) hypothesize that two issues may explain this finding. First, mania has a longer prodrome than depression (median time approximately 3 weeks as compared to 2 weeks), allowing more time, during which an individual can implement a hierarchy of interventions to cope with isolated symptoms. Second, the planned interventions in this brief package usually involve accessing generic psychosocial support and the introduction of additional medications. The pharmacological treatment of the early stages of mania produces a more rapid response and is less hazardous than that of BP depression. Antipsychotic medications act quickly to ameliorate symptoms of mania, whereas antidepressants take about 2 weeks to begin to demonstrate benefit. Thus, in depression, commencing antidepressants during the prodrome may not allow sufficient time for medication to take effect and prevent the escalation into a full episode. Also, the dosage of antidepressants used in BP depression is often subtherapeutic. This is particularly likely in the early stages of an episode of BP depression where dosages have to be increased incrementally in order to avert the risk of precipitating a hypomanic swing.

The other studies reported longer courses of CT and most appeared to begin the therapy with an individualized formulation of the clients' problems. The findings from Lam et al.'s (2000) small but comprehensive study have parallels with those of Perry and colleagues (1999) and also with Zaretsky et al. (2000) and Scott et al. (2001). The course of CT focused on coping with prodromes, but was longer than in Perry et al.'s study. As in the article by Perry et al., the data suggest a more robust effect on hypomanic/manic as compared to other types of BP episode. However, there was also a trend toward fewer depressive relapses. It may be that small sample size reduced the statistical power of Lam et al.'s study, obscuring the beneficial effects on manic and depressive relapses. Alternatively, the data may suggest that, even with more intensive CT approaches, placing a major emphasis on the management of prodromes is less effective in reducing depression than approaches that target cognitive-vulnerability factors in a similar way to CT of unipolar depression. Lam and colleagues are currently conducting a large randomized controlled trial that will hopefully clarify this issue.

Both Zaretsky et al. (2000) and Scott et al. (2001) reported significant reductions in depressive symptoms and the latter study also reported fewer depressive relapses in the 12 months after CT was completed. The difficulty in treating BP depression with antidepressants, plus Scott et al.'s (2000b) findings of high levels of self-rated interepisode depressive symptoms, point to the need to undertake a more comprehensive study of CT for BP depression.

Future developments

The empirical data reviewed in this chapter indicate that research into cognitive theory and therapy for BP is at an embryonic stage. There is no evidence that underlying schemata play a unique causal role in first onset of mania, nor are there differences in the underlying beliefs of those at risk of BP as compared with unipolar disorders. However, there is early evidence that cognitive factors may influence vulnerability to BP relapse. The potential interaction between life events and cognitive style is easier to understand for depressive than for manic relapse. The events associated with the onset of BP depression have many similarities to those linked with unipolar depression. Mania may arise in association with negative life events such as bereavement, but also following events that disrupt an individual's day-to-day social rhythms (Malkoff-Schwartz et al., 1998), for example, following long-haul flights, the sudden cessation of mood-stabilizing medication, or the onset of significant physical disorder. A number of researchers suggest that a common link between these events is that they can all significantly disrupt circadian rhythms (Ehlers et al., 1988; Goodwin and Jamison, 1990). In turn, circadian dysrhythmia may lead to sleep disturbance and affective shifts. This model would suggest that the initial changes in levels of dysfunctional beliefs, attributional style, and thinking processes are epiphenomena of a biologically driven process. In this model, even events with specific personal meaning to an individual would be regarded as a nonspecific factor that can stress or destabilize homeostasis.

Alternatively, Newman and colleagues (2001) have built upon Beck's original linear schematic model (1967) and utilized the concept of modes to explain some of the "beliefs-biology–behavioral" links observed (Beck, 1996). Modes are hypothesized as integrated cognitive-affective-behavioral networks (e.g., powerful combinations of schemata; overlearned behavioural habits; and intensely difficult-to-modulate emotions) that produce synchronous responses to life events and are a mechanism for implementing internally driven goals. When modes are activated predispositional traits are expressed as states. The intensity of the "charge" on a mode determines its threshold for activation. This concept offers an explanation of mood swings and how individuals with BP may endorse extreme views of themselves in different mood states (e.g. "I'm a genius," "I'm a failure"). Negative life events that activate a mode may directly lead to manic swings or activation of modes may lead to further biological dysregulation that can disrupt circadian rhythms, as described in other models. A further consequence of this model is that awareness of modes of different valence may explain the development of the commonly observed moods of irritability, dysphoric mania, or mixed states. These models require further elaboration, and there are still a number of crucial research questions to answer. For example:

- Why do individuals at risk of BP relapse show similar abnormalities in cognitive processing to individuals with unipolar disorders?
- How can differences in ratings by individuals with BP on implicit and explicit measures be explained?
- What other models of self-regulation may help explain the observed phenomena?
- If there is no validity to a cognitive model of BP disorders, why does individual CT appear to be effective?

In trying to elaborate on these issues, it is helpful to consider briefly important findings from general psychiatry research relating to BP. Perhaps the most important idea to challenge is the conventional notion that mania is the polar opposite of depression. There is a considerable body of literature (reviewed by Goodwin and Jamison, 1990) that suggests that the most commonly reported mood during a manic phase is irritability (reported by 80% of subjects), depression/dysphoria (72%), elation/euphoria (71%), or lability (69%). In a factor analytic study of the signs and symptoms of mania, Cassidy et al. (1998) demonstrated five clinically relevant independent factors. The first and strongest factor represented dysphoric mania. The other factors were psychomotor acceleration, psychosis, increased hedonic function, and irritable aggression. These data have led many researchers to conclude that the most important feature of mania may be increased activity rather than elated mood. This model has some resonance with the ideas behind the Behavioral Activation System (Depue and Zald, 1993). This system is thought to control psychomotor activation, incentive motivation, and positive mood. High activity would be synonymous with mania and low activity with depression.

The co-occurrence of manic and depressive symptomatology in mania, along with abnormal implicit style of cognitive processing and self-serving biases in explicit style, has led to other models being proposed. For example, Neale (1988) argues that the abnormalities in implicit and explicit processing are compatible with the notion of a manic defense. He argues that "threats to the vulnerable self-esteem of the patient lead to grandiose ideas that keep distressing thoughts at bay, but lead to mood elevation." Embedded within this concept is the notion that the individual makes a proactive response to the threat of or actual loss of reinforcement.

An alternative or extended version of this model parallels that proposed by Watson et al. (1988). They suggest cognition and emotion are controlled by two independent neural circuits defined as positive activation or affect (PA) and negative activation or affect (NA). According to Watson and colleagues (1988), PA reflects the extent to which an individual feels enthusiastic, active, and alert. High PA is thus a state of high energy and pleasurable engagement, whilst low PA is characterized by lethargy and sadness. In contrast, high NA subsumes a number of aversive mood states (anger, fear, disgust, etc.), whilst low NA represents a state of calm. PA and NA are not necessarily correlated. According to this model, an individual experiencing mania would have high levels of PA and NA. Low PA and high NA would be more typical of depression. Interestingly, Watson et al. suggest that high levels of NA may occur in response to environmental stress, whilst PA may change in response to social stimuli and activities. At this stage, the PA/NA model is unproven in BP, but could account for some of the findings outlined in this chapter. For example, individuals may experience an increase in levels of NA in response to a negative life event. However, if they are also currently experiencing high levels of PA, they may simultaneously experience negative affect with increased motivation and increased goal-directed behaviors. Independently fluctuating levels of PA and NA may also be implicated in the labile mood and variable accessibility of underlying beliefs and self-representations that are characteristic of BP. It is possible to integrate some aspects of this model with Beck's proposal on modes (1996).

Future research could also explore the cognitive aspects of circadian rhythm disruption. As mentioned earlier, circadian rhythm disruption may occur as a consequence of social disruption as circadian rhythms are largely socially entrained. The current data on social rhythm-disrupting life events (Malkoff-Schwartz et al., 1998) do not explore sufficiently the nature of social rhythm-disrupting events or the role of individuals' causal attributions for their initial isolated manic symptoms (e.g., elevated mood or sleep disruption) and how these may in turn influence their actions. For example, up to 43% of social rhythm-disrupting events could also be classified as representing threat of loss or actual loss experiences. To substantiate the "social zeitgebers" model therefore requires further refinement of the concept of social rhythm disruption. Also, as Healy and Williams (1988) stated, if individuals notice that they feel more energetic, happier, and need less sleep, they do not usually attribute such experiences to significant illness but may make dispositional attributions about their own prowess. The acknowledgment that these symptoms were the prodroma of a manic episode may only occur some time later, or through training in self-monitoring and self-management such as undertaken by Perry and colleagues. Healy and Williams hypothesize that an individual who attributes the changes in functioning to dispositional as opposed to illness factors may be at greater risk of entering a vicious cycle leading to manic or depressive relapse. Those who acknowledge the symptom as an early-warning sign of relapse may instigate coping strategies that avert the risk of a further affective episode.

The above models give some clues as to why CT may be useful despite the absence of a definitive cognitive model of BP. Brief CT may facilitate change in an individual's attitudes toward and beliefs about the disorder and its treatment. Alternatively, CT may achieve its effect through other mechanisms. In their study of chronic depression, Scott et al. (2000b) demonstrated that individuals receiving

CT as well as usual treatment experienced fewer depressive relapses despite high levels of residual depressive symptoms. Scott and colleagues argued that this might offer evidence that CT had taught individuals coping strategies to reduce their depression about depression and prevent the cascade of symptoms into an affective episode.

Lam's group and Scott's group have both identified the relevance of teaching self-regulation as a method of reducing instability in circadian rhythms. This is a similar approach to that advocated in interpersonal–social rhythms therapy (IPSRT) for BP (Frank et al., 1997). Facilitating behavior change may also lead to reductions in the use of alcohol and illicit drugs that are known to increase the risk of relapse and worsen prognosis in BP. These problems are not easily overcome by medication and the usual treatments offered by mental health professionals.

The above gives some general reasons why CT may be effective in BP. However, as demonstrated by Scott's group and by Zaretsky and colleagues, there is also a role for CT of BP in the utilization of a cognitive case conceptualization approach. Scott and colleagues particularly target beliefs about social desirability, perfectionism, and autonomy. The evidence so far suggests that this triad may be important in BP subjects. Also, given the extreme thinking styles that characterize depression and mania, it is noteworthy that Teasdale and colleagues (2001) demonstrated that the effect of CT may be mediated by changes in the style rather than content of thinking. The study demonstrated that persistent absolutistic, dichotomous thinking style predicted early relapse in depression. Given that this thinking style is typical of subjects with BP, these data point to important areas of future research into the process of CT in BP.

Given that a more typical course of CT may be particularly beneficial in treating BP depression it is ironic that, despite no unique differences in cognitive style between unipolar and BP depression, individuals with BP have been excluded from treatment studies. Whilst modification of the CT protocol may be needed for BP depression, it is possible that CT will become a crucial alternative to medication for this difficult-to-treat clinical condition. Large-scale trials are warranted. Such research also affords an opportunity to explore further cognitive models of depression and the similarities and differences between individuals with unipolar and BP disorders.

REFERENCES

Alloy, L., Reilly-Harrington, N., Fresco, D., Whitehouse, W., and Zeichmeister, J. (1999). Cognitive styles and life events in subsyndromal unipolar and bipolar mood disorders: stability and prospective prediction of depressive and hypomanic mood swings. *Journal of Cognitive Psychotherapy*, **13**, 21–40.

Ashworth, C. M., Blackburn, I. M., and McPherson, F. M. (1982). The performance of depressed and manic patients on some repertory grid measures. *British Journal of Medical Psychology*, **55**, 247–55.

Basco, M. and Rush, A. J. (1995). *Cognitive Behavior Therapy for Bipolar Disorders*. New York: Guilford Press.

Bauer, M., Crits-Cristoph, P., Ball, W., et al. (1991). Independent assessment of manic and depressive symptoms by self-rating. *Archives of General Psychiatry*, **48**, 807–12.

Bauer, M. S., McBride, L., Chase, C., Sachs, G., and Shea, N. (1998). Manual-based group psychotherapy for bipolar disorder: a feasibility study. *Journal of Clinical Psychiatry*, **59**, 449–54.

Beck, A. T. (1967). *Depression: Clinical, Experimental and Theoretical Aspects*. New York: Harper & Row.

Beck, A. T. (1996). Beyond Belief: A Theory of Modes, Personality and Psychopathology. In *Frontiers of Cognitive Therapy*, ed. P. Salkovskis, pp. 92–108. London: Guilford Press.

Beck, A. T., Ward, C., Mendelson, M., Mock, J., and Erbaugh, J. (1961). An inventory for measuring depression. *Archives of General Psychiatry*, **4**, 561–71.

Bentall, R. P. and Kinderman, P. (1999). Self-regulation, affect and psychosis: the role of social cognition in paranoia and mania. In *Handbook of Cognition and Emotion*, 2nd edn, ed. T. Dalgleish and M. Power, pp. 353–81. Chichester: John Wiley.

Bentall, R. P., Kinderman, P., and Manson, K. (2002). Self-discrepancies in bipolar disorder. *Cognitive Therapy and Research* (in press).

Carver, C. and White, T. (1994). Behavioural inhibition, behavioural activation, and affective responses to impending reward and punishment: the BIS/BAS scales. *Journal of Personality and Social Psychology*, **67**, 319–33.

Cassidy, F., Forest, K., Murry, E., and Carroll, B. J. (1998). A factor analysis of the signs and symptoms of mania. *Archives of General Psychiatry*, **55**, 27–32.

Chor, P. N., Mercier, M. A., and Halper, I. S. (1988). Use of cognitive therapy for the treatment of a patient suffering from a bipolar affective disorder. *Journal of Cognitive Psychotherapy*, **2**, 51–8.

Cochran, S. (1984). Preventing medical non-adherence in the outpatient treatment of bipolar affective disorder. *Journal of Consulting and Clinical Psychology*, **52**, 873–8.

Depue, R. and Zeld, D. (1993). Biological and environmental processes in non-psychotic psychopathology: a neurobehavioural perspective. In *Basic Issues in Psychopatholgy*, ed. C. Costello, pp. 127–237. New York: Guilford Press.

Depue, R., Krauss, S., Spoont, M., and Arbisis, P. (1989). General behavioural inventory identification of unipolar and bipolar affective conditions in a non-clinical university population. *Journal of Abnormal Psychology*, **98**, 117–26.

Dickson, W. and Kendall, R. (1986). Does maintenance lithium therapy prevent recurrence of mania under ordinary clinical conditions? *Psychological Medicine*, **16**, 521–30.

Ehlers, C. L., Frank, E., and Kupfer, D. J. (1988). Social zeitgebers and biological rhythms: a unified approach to understanding the etiology of depression. *Archives of General Psychiatry*, **45**, 948–52.

Eich, E., MacAulay, D., and Lam, R. W. (1997). Mania, depression and mood dependent memory. *Cognition and Emotion*, **11**(5/6), 607–18.

Endicott, J. and Spitzer, R. (1978). A diagnostic interview: the schedule for affective disorders and schizophrenia. *Archives of General Psychiatry*, **35**, 837–44.

Frank, E., Hlastala, S., Ritenour, A., et al. (1997). Inducing lifestyle regularity in recovering bipolar patients: results from the maintenance therapies in bipolar disorder protocol. *Biological Psychiatry*, **41**, 1165–73.

Goodwin, F. and Jamison, K. (1990). *Manic-Depressive Illness*, pp. 101–321. Oxford: Oxford University Press.

Guscott, R. and Taylor, L. (1994). Lithium prophylaxis in recurrent affective illness: efficacy, effectiveness and efficiency. *British Journal of Psychiatry*, **164**, 741–6.

Hammen, C., Ellicott, A., Gitlin, M., and Jamison, K. R. (1989). Sociotropy/autonomy and vulnerability to specific life events in patients with unipolar depression and bipolar disorders. *Journal of Abnormal Psychology*, **98**, 154–60.

Hammen, C., Ellicott, A., and Gitlin, M. (1992). Stressors and sociotropy/autonomy: a longitudinal study of their relationship to the course of bipolar disorder. *Cognitive Therapy and Research*, **16**, 409–18.

Healy, D. and Williams, J. (1988). Moods, misattributions and mania. *Psychiatric Developments*, **1**, 49–70.

Hollon, S., Kendall, P., and Lumry, A. (1986). Specificity of depressive cognitions in clinical depression. *Journal of Abnormal Psychology*, **95**, 52–9.

Johnson, S. and Miller, I. (1995). Negative life events and time to recovery from episodes of bipolar disorder. *Journal of Abnormal Psychology*, **106**, 449–57.

Kernis, M. H., Cornell, D. P., Sun, C. R., Berry, A., and Harlow, T. (1993). There's more to self-esteem than whether it is high or low: the importance of stability of self-esteem. *Journal of Personality and Social Psychology*, **61**, 80–4.

Lam, D. H., Jones, S., Hayward, P., and Bright, J. (1999). *Cognitive Therapy for Bipolar Disorder*. New York: John Wiley.

Lam, D. H., Bright, J., Jones, S., et al. (2000). Cognitive therapy for bipolar illness – a pilot study of relapse prevention. *Cognitive Therapy and Research*, **24**, 503–20.

Leventhal, H., Diefenbach, M., and Leventhal, E. (1992). Illness cognition: using common sense to understand treatment adherence and affect cognition interactions. *Cognitive Therapy and Research*, **16**, 143–63.

Lyon, H. M., Startup, M., and Bentall, R. (1999). Social cognition and the manic defence. *Journal of Abnormal Psychology*, **108** (2), 273–82.

Malkoff-Schwartz, S., Frank, E., Anderson, B., et al. (1998). Stressful life events and social rhythm disruption in the onset of manic and depressive bipolar episodes: a preliminary investigation. *Archives of General Psychiatry*, **55**, 702–7.

Neale, J. M. (1988). Defensive function of manic episodes. In *Delusional Beliefs*, ed. T. F. Oltmanns and B. A. Maher, pp. 48–61. New York: Wiley.

Newman, C., Leahy, R., Beck, A. T., Reilly-Harrington, N., and Gyulia, L. (2001). *Bipolar Disorders: A Cognitive Therapy Approach*. New York: American Psychological Association.

Palmer, A., Williams, H., and Adams, M. (1995). Cognitive behaviour therapy in a group format for bipolar affective disorder. *Behavioural and Cognitive Psychotherapy*, **23**, 153–68.

Pardoen, D., Bauwens, F., Tracy, A., Martin, F., and Mendlewicz, J. (1993). Self-esteem in recovered bipolar and unipolar outpatients. *British Journal of Psychiatry*, **163**, 755–62.

Perry, A., Tarrier, N., Morriss, R., McCarthy, E., and Limb, K. (1999). Randomized controlled trial of efficacy of teaching patients with bipolar disorder to identify early symptoms of relapse and obtain treatment. *British Medical Journal*, **318**, 149–53.

Prien, R. and Potter, W. (1990). NIMH workshop report on the treatment of bipolar disorders. *Psychopharmacology Bulletin*, **26**, 409–27.

Reilly-Harrington, N., Alloy, L., Fresco, D., and Whitehouse, W. (1999). Cognitive style and life events interact to predict unipolar and bipolar symptomatology. *Journal of Abnormal Psychology*, **108**, 567–78.

Roberts, J. and Munroe, S. (1994). A multidimensional model of self-esteem in depression. *Clinical Psychology Review*, **14**, 161–81.

Scott, J. (1995a). Psychotherapy for dipolar disorder: an unmet need? *British Journal of Psychiatry*, **167**, 581–8.

Scott, J. (1995b). Cognitive therapy for clients with bipolar disorder: a case example. *Cognitive and Behavioural Practice*, **3**, 1–23.

Scott, J. (2001). *Overcoming Mood Swings: A Self-help Guide Using Cognitive and Behavioral Techniques.* New York: University Press.

Scott, J. and Wright, J. (1997). Cognitive therapy with severe and chronic mental disorders. In *Review of Psychiatry*, vol. 16, ed. A. Frances and R. Hales, pp. 265–94. Washington: American Psychiatric Association Press.

Scott, J., Stanton, B., Garland, A., and Ferrier, I. (2000a). Cognitive vulnerability in bipolar disorders. *Psychological Medicine*, **30**, 467–72.

Scott, J., Teasdale, J., Paykel, E., et al. (2000b). The effects of cognitive therapy on psychological symptoms and social functioning in residual depression. *British Journal of Psychiatry*, **177**, 440–6.

Scott, J., Garland, A., and Moorhead, S. (2001). A pilot study of cognitive therapy in bipolar disorder. *Psychological Medicine*, **31**, 459–67.

Silverman, J. S., Silverman, J. A., and Eardley, D. A. (1984). Do maladaptive attitudes cause depression? *Archives of General Psychiatry*, **41**, 28–30.

Swendsen, J., Hammen, C., Heller, T., and Giltin, M. (1995). Correlates of stress reactivity in patients with bipolar disorder. *American Journal of Psychiatry*, **152**, 795–7.

Teasdale, J., Scott, J., Moore, R., et al. (2001). How does cognitive therapy prevent relapse in residual depression? Evidence from a controlled trial. *Journal of Consulting and Clinical Psychology*, **69**, 347–57.

Watson, D., Clark, L. A., and Tellegen, A. (1988). Development and validation of brief measures of positive and negative effect: the PANAS scales. *Journal of Personality and Social Psychology*, **76**, 820–38.

Weingartner, H., Miller, H., and Murphy, D. L. (1977). Mood-state-dependent retrieval of verbal associations. *Journal of Abnormal Psychology*, **86**, 276–84.

Weiss, R. D., Griffin, M. L., Greenfield, S. F., et al. (2000). Group therapy for patients with bipolar disorder and substance dependence: results of a pilot study. *Journal of Clinical Psychiatry*, **61**, 361–7.

Winters, K. C. and Neale, J. M. (1985). Mania and low self-esteem. *Journal of Abnormal Psychology*, **94**, 282–90.

Wright, J. and Schrodt, R. (1992). Combined cognitive therapy and pharmacotherapy. In *Handbook of Cognitive Therapy*, ed. A. Freeman, K. Simon, L. Beutler, and H. Arowitz, pp. 234–49. New York: Plenum Press.

Zaretsky, A. E., Segal, Z. V., and Gemar, M. (2000). Cognitive therapy for bipolar disorder: a pilot study. *Canadian Journal of Psychiatry – revue Caanadienne de Psychiatrie*, **44**, 491–4.

Regulation of emotion in generalized anxiety disorder

Douglas S. Mennin,[1] Cynthia L. Turk,[2] Richard G. Heimberg,[3] and Cheryl N. Carmin[4]

[1] Yale University, New Haven, CT, USA
[2] LaSalle University, Philadelphia, PA, USA
[3] Temple University, Philadelphia, PA, USA
[4] University of Illinois-Chicago, Chicago, IL, USA

Introduction

Interest in the study of anxiety disorders has increased dramatically since the publication of the third edition of the *Diagnostic and Statistical Manual of Mental Disorders* (DSM-III; American Psychological Association (APA), 1980). In fact, the 1980s witnessed a 10-fold increase in the number of published articles devoted to the study of anxiety disorders (Norton et al., 1995), and anxiety disorders were the topic of 14% of the articles published in clinical psychology and psychiatry journals between 1990 and 1992 (Cox et al., 1995). The large majority of these studies focused on panic disorder (McNally, 1994) and social phobia (Heimberg et al., 1995). However, investigations of generalized anxiety disorder (GAD) have recently begun to appear with increasing frequency (Borkovec et al., 1991; Brown and Barlow, 1992; Wittchen et al., 1994).

Compared to other anxiety disorders, GAD remains poorly understood. Advances in understanding have been slowed by the evolving definition of the disorder. In DSM-III, GAD was a residual category that could not be diagnosed in the presence of any other anxiety or affective disorder (APA, 1980). Attempts to diagnose GAD according to DSM-III criteria were also characterized by low inter-rater reliability (Barlow, 1987). However, the diagnostic criteria for GAD changed substantially from DSM-III to DSM-IV (APA, 1994). GAD is no longer considered to be a residual category, but a disorder specifically characterized by excessive and uncontrollable worry and somatic symptoms suggestive of central nervous system hyperarousal (e.g., muscle tension).

While the diagnosis of GAD can now be made with adequate reliability (Starcevic and Bogojevic, 1999; Brown et al., 2001), the frequent changes in the diagnostic criteria have made it difficult to maintain a consistent focus in the study of the efficacy of cognitive-behavioral treatments for GAD. As a result, a large percentage of patients continue to experience significant symptoms following treatment (approximately one-third to one-half: Borkovec and Whisman, 1996). Initially, it was difficult to develop a conceptual framework for the treatment of a residual diagnosis. Later, treatments were developed that focused on worry or autonomic hyperarousal. While worry remains central to DSM-IV GAD, autonomic hyperarousal does not. Only now are treatments being developed that target the range of specific deficits and excesses that may underlie GAD. Also, there are few overt behavioral markers for GAD. As a consequence, purely behavioral treatments for GAD have shown only modest efficacy (Gould et al., 1997). Cognitive-behavioral approaches have been more fruitful with respect to understanding and treating GAD, although in many ways GAD defies a traditional cognitive paradigm. The content of automatic thoughts can be a "moving target" since these patients typically alter the focus of their worry as their daily experience changes. This pattern can be contrasted with that of other anxiety disorders such as social phobia and panic disorder, where the content of cognitions is often focused on a recurrent theme such as fear of negative social evaluation or impending physical catastrophe. In addition, these patients often do not always identify clear cognitive antecedents to their anxiety, thereby reflecting the historical description of this syndrome as "free-floating" anxiety.

GAD challenges cognitive-behavioral theorists and practitioners to broaden their conception of psychopathological processes (for an indepth discussion of the need to widen the scope of cognitive therapy, see Safran, 1998). Greenberg and Safran (1987) suggest that the study of emotions as causal entities can provide a unique understanding of the human information-processing system and the ways it can go awry. Conceptualizations of GAD may benefit from attention to recent findings in the field of emotion theory (Ekman and Davidson, 1994), emotion regulation (Gross, 1998), and affective neuroscience (LeDoux, 1996). Likewise, cognitive-behavioral treatment of this disorder may be improved by incorporation of emotion-focused interventions. In fact, a number of cognitive-behavioral therapy variants that directly address emotional experience have begun to gain popularity and acceptance (Safran and Segal, 1990; Linehan, 1993; Mahoney, 1995; Hayes et al., 1999).

In this chapter, we argue for the need to incorporate emotion variables into the study and treatment of GAD. A brief description of the clinical characteristics of the disorder is presented. The avoidance theory of worry developed by Borkovec and colleagues (Borkovec et al., 1998) is then reviewed, along with the supporting empirical findings. Other models have also been proposed but are not presented here because they disregard emotion variables (Rapee, 1991; Tallis and Eysenck, 1994) or because they have only begun to accrue empirical support (Dugas et al., 1998; Wells, 1999). We then describe a model of GAD that attempts to extend the cognitive-behavioral conceptualization of Borkovec and colleagues. This expanded model argues that GAD is best conceptualized as a syndrome that involves deficits in regulation of emotions and overreliance on cognitive resources. After a review of the cognitive-behavioral treatment outcome literature, we discuss the potential advantages of incorporating an emotion-focused perspective into the treatment of GAD.

Clinical characteristics of GAD

According to DSM-IV, the essential feature of GAD is excessive worry occurring more days than not for at least 6 months. The worry may concern a number of different domains or activities (e.g., work, finances, family, health) and must be difficult to control. In addition, the worry or anxiety must be associated with at least three of the following six symptoms: (1) restlessness; (2) fatigue; (3) impaired concentration; (4) irritability; (5) muscle tension; and (6) sleep disturbance. The worry must lead to significant distress or impairment. Furthermore, the anxiety and worry must not be due to another axis I disorder and the anxiety symptoms must not be present solely during the course of a mood disorder, psychotic disorder, or pervasive developmental disorder. In addition, the disorder must not be due to a general medical condition or the direct physiological effects of a substance (APA, 1994).

Lifetime rates of GAD ranged from 4.1% to 6.6% across sites in the Epidemiological Catchment Area Study (Robins et al., 1984) and a similar figure (5.1%) was reported in the National Comorbidity Survey (NCS; Kessler et al., 1994). Additionally, the disorder is prevalent in primary-care medical settings and is one of the most common diagnoses among patients presenting with medically unexplained somatic complaints (Roy-Byrne, 1996). It is also a common condition in psychological and psychiatric practice and is thought by some to be a precursor to other conditions such as depression and panic disorder (Roy-Byrne and Katon, 1997).

Although initially perceived as a relatively mild condition (APA, 1980, 1987), evidence is mounting that GAD is associated with significant disability. Recent studies have demonstrated that it is associated with significantly increased healthcare costs and decreased productivity (Greenberg et al., 1999) and with increased healthcare utilization (Blazer et al., 1991). Wittchen et al. (1994) found that 82% of

NCS respondents with a lifetime diagnosis of GAD experienced significant role impairment (e.g., separated/divorced, unemployed) and interference with daily activities. A majority of these individuals had also sought professional help and received medications for anxiety. Massion et al. (1993), examining subjects from the Harvard/Brown Anxiety Disorders Research Program, found low levels of emotional health, role functioning, social functioning, and overall functioning among patients with GAD. Women with GAD perceive their marriages to be less satisfying than other married women (McLeod, 1994). Lastly, individuals seeking treatment for GAD perceive their quality of life to be extremely low, much lower than that of nonanxious persons (L. L. Turk et al., unpublished data).

The onset of GAD is typically before the age of 20 (Brown and Barlow, 1992). It characteristically follows a chronic course, although the severity of worry and somatic symptoms may fluctuate in response to life stressors (Brown et al., 1994). Between 60% and 80% of patients have reported worrying for their entire life (Barlow, 1988; Rapee, 1991), and the rate of spontaneous remission over a 2-year period is low (Yonkers et al., 1996). Elderly persons also suffer from debilitating generalized anxiety, suggesting that GAD may persist into late adulthood (Beck et al., 1996).

Most individuals with GAD meet criteria for comorbid axis I diagnoses. *Comorbidity* refers to the occurrence of at least two different disorders in the same individual (Brown and Barlow, 1992). Only 20–26% of cases reported by Brown et al. (1994) and Brawman-Mintzer et al. (1993) were not comorbid. Rates of comorbidity above 90% have been reported, both in a clinical sample (Sanderson and Barlow, 1990) and in a community sample (Wittchen et al., 1994). The disorder most commonly comorbid with GAD is social phobia, with rates ranging from 30% to 60% (Sanderson et al., 1990). GAD is also frequently comorbid with mood disorders, with rates ranging from 8% to 39% (Brawman-Mintzer et al., 1993; Brown and Barlow, 1992). In addition, in a study by Sanderson et al. (1994a), 49% of patients with GAD met criteria for at least one personality disorder.

Such high rates of comorbidity in GAD raises the issue of classification. Achenbach (1995) has suggested that high rates of comorbidity may be artifactual if the disorders are different expressions of the same underlying diathesis. Kendler et al. (1992) found that genetic factors were completely shared for major depression and GAD in a twin study. In addition, there were moderate nonfamilial environmental risk factors shared by the two disorders but no evidence for a shared familial environmental factor. Kessler et al. (in press) have argued, however, that this conclusion is based on an assumption that the joint effects of genes and environment are additive. A more interactive model may provide better differentiation between GAD and major depression. None the less, a complete understanding of GAD will most likely include the consideration of these comorbid conditions.

Theoretical models of GAD

Avoidance of worry in GAD

The avoidance theory of worry proposed by Borkovec and colleagues (e.g., Borkovec and Newman, 1998; Borkovec et al., in press) considers cognitive phenomena (e.g., worry, thoughts, images), somatic factors (e.g., autonomic inflexibility, cortical–subcortical activity), emotional factors (e.g., inflexibility/inhibition of subjective emotional experience), and interpersonal dynamics (early attachment history, current relational patterns) in the genesis and maintenance of GAD. This cognitive-behavioral theory is quite comprehensive and, of particular relevance to this chapter, speaks to the importance of emotion variables in worry and GAD.

Worry is a universal experience, but a clear understanding of this phenomenon remains elusive. Borkovec et al. (1983, p. 10) define worry as:

... a chain of thoughts and images, negatively affect-laden and relatively uncontrollable; it represents an attempt to engage in mental problem-solving on an issue whose outcome is uncertain but contains the possibility of one or more negative outcomes; consequently, worry relates closely to the fear process.

Borkovec (1994) also asserts that worry is a mental activity that predominantly involves verbal thought and is less characterized by imagery and autonomic arousal. In support of this assertion, Borkovec and Inz (1990) asked patients with GAD and normal controls to rate whether their mental activity was imagery- or thought-based while in relaxation and worry conditions. The GAD group reported that they engaged in more thought (including negatively valenced thought) than controls during the relaxation period. Furthermore, during the worrying period, both groups displayed large reductions in imagery and substantial increases in thought. Following successful psychological intervention, the ratio of thoughts to images had normalized for the patient group. Borkovec and Lyonfields (1993) found that a majority of participants in both community and college samples reported their worries as predominantly thought-based. Freeston et al. (1996) also noted that excessive worriers reported higher levels of thought compared to ordinary worriers.

Borkovec's theory incorporates the empirical findings that thinking about emotional material leads to very little physiological activity, whereas visualizing images of that same emotional material leads to a significant physiological response (Vrana et al. 1986). As would be expected, worry is not only associated with reduced imagery but also decreased autonomic arousal (Borkovec and Newman, 1998). Borkovec and Hu (1990) found that participants with speech anxiety who worried prior to imagining a phobic scene demonstrated significantly reduced heart rate responses compared with participants instructed to engage in neutral or relaxed thinking. Whereas participants in the relaxation condition habituated to the arousal, those participants in the neutral condition remained consistently aroused. In comparison, participants in the worry condition showed no cardiovascular response at all to the first or subsequent images. These data suggest a complete failure to process the emotional material contained in the image for individuals instructed to worry.

Consistent with these findings, individuals with GAD do not show the same physiological response to threat as do individuals with other anxiety disorders (Borkovec et al., 1998). In studies by Hoehn-Saric and colleagues (Hoehn-Saric and McLeod, 1988; Hoehn-Saric et al., 1989), individuals with GAD demonstrated restricted variability on measures of autonomic arousal such as skin conductance and heart rate. These authors conclude that sympathetic inhibition and autonomic inflexibility often characterize individuals with GAD. More specifically, autonomic inflexibility refers to a reduction in complexity of responding in a range of physiological channels and reflects a system that lacks adaptive responsivity to the environment. In contrast, well-adjusted individuals have been shown to exhibit a strong autonomic response to stress (e.g., large galvanic skin response) but are more flexible in their responding (e.g., quicker return to baseline).

Autonomic inflexibility may reflect a deficiency in vagal tone or parasympathetic activity. Lyonsfield et al. (1995) point out that the vagus nerve is the major determinant of heart rate activity and that low vagal tone is associated with high but stable heart rates. Lyonsfield et al. (1995) compared individuals with a self-reported diagnosis of GAD to normal controls during a rest period, a period of imagery concerning a personally relevant topic of great concern, and a period of worrying about that topic. The individuals with GAD displayed low vagal tone and little cardiac variability during the rest, imagery, and worry periods. In contrast, nonanxious participants demonstrated a significant reduction in variability from rest to imagery and a further reduction from imagery to worry. Similarly, Thayer et al. (1996) compared patients with GAD to nonanxious controls on levels of vagal tone during baseline, relaxation, and worry conditions. As in the Lyonsfield et al. (1995) study, the patients showed lowered vagal tone across all conditions. These authors were also able to show that worry phasically caused this deficiency in both disordered and nonanxious participants. Taken together, these results provide support for the assertion that GAD is characterized by autonomic inflexibility.

While heart rate and heart rate variability data suggest that peripheral nervous system activity is inhibited, other studies suggest that the central nervous system is active during worry. For example, muscle tension has been found to be elevated in individuals with GAD compared to controls (Hoehn-Saric and McLeod, 1988; Hoehn-Saric et al., 1989; Hazlett et al., 1994), and this muscular activation appeared to be mediated by the central nervous system. Indeed, the change in criteria from DSM-III-R to DSM-IV represents a shift from focusing on autonomic symptoms to central nervous system-related symptomatology (Marten et al., 1993).

Borkovec and colleagues synthesize these findings by arguing that worry allows individuals to process emotional topics at an abstract, conceptual level and, consequently, avoid aversive images, autonomic arousal, and intense negative emotions in the short run. In this way, worry is negatively reinforced. Stöber (2000) exemplifies this phenomenon by comparing one's reaction to reading about a horrible accident to looking at a full-color photo of the accident scene. Clearly, the pictorial version is more emotionally evocative. Borkovec et al. (1995) have suggested that worry may have evolved for adaptive purposes, specifically to anticipate future negative events while not being overcome by emotional experience. Although worry allows individuals to deal with emotional material at an abstract, conceptual level, it does not allow the individual completely to quiet emotional distress and "put it aside." Therefore, over the long term, the individual is repeatedly confronted with the emotional material, frequently has a more intense experience of anxiety, and engages in worry in order to dull this experience. In doing so, the person again fails fully to confront the distressing stimuli. The worrier engages in this process again and again in an inadequate attempt to cope with aversive experiences.

Borkovec and colleagues base much of their theory on Lang's (1985) bioinformational account of emotions, as well as examinations of the role of exposure to emotionally arousing stimuli, often termed *emotional processing*, in the treatment of anxiety and mood disorders (Rachman, 1980; Foa and Kozak, 1986). Lang proposes a network model of emotion structures in memory. A fear structure is a memory of a feared situation or event that contains three types of information (stimulus information, response information, and their associated meanings). This structure is activated when present experience matches features of the memory of the feared situation. Foa and Kozak (1986) explain that once the fear structure is accessed, the imagery and physiological arousal associated with that particular emotional meaning must be activated. Absence of physiological arousal and imagery suggests that the entire fear structure stored in memory has not been accessed, and extinction of an aversive response cannot occur. Borkovec et al. (1998, p. 563) state: "We have to confront not only feared situations to overcome our fear of them, but we also have to feel the fear during the confrontations."

Research suggests that worry is likely to prevent full access to fear structures in memory and consequently inhibit the emotional processing necessary for anxiety reduction. Evidence for this assertion comes from a study by Butler et al. (1995), who presented graduate students in health-related fields with distressing films about industrial accidents. Participants who were instructed to worry about the film were found to have reduced anxiety compared to participants who were instructed to form images. However, worrying about the film increased the frequency of intrusive images over the next 3 days. In another study, Wells and Papageorgiou (1995) asked participants to watch a gruesome film of an accident. Thereafter, participants were assigned to different conditions: (1) worry about the film and its implications; (2) focus on images of the film and their implications; (3) distract from the topic; (4) worry about a usual personal topic; or (5) no explicit instructions were given. Worrying about the film (condition 1) led to the most intrusive imagery over the next 3 days. Presumably, in both studies, worry resulted in a failure to process fully emotional material and subsequent failure to extinguish an aversive response.

Although the avoidance theory of worry focuses upon intrapersonal processes, Borkovec and colleagues have recently studied the relationship between interpersonal difficulties and worry (Borkovec and Newman, 1998). Worry topics often center on interpersonal relationships (Borkovec et al., 1991). The cognitions of persons with GAD are more likely to concern interpersonal conflict than are the cognitions of individuals with panic disorder (Breitholtz et al., 1998). Interestingly, recent research suggests that individuals with GAD may interact with others in a manner that imposes stress upon their interpersonal environment. Specifically, they have been shown to be overly nurturing and intrusive and to display rigidity in their interpersonal styles compared to nonanxious individuals (A. L. Pincus and T. D. Borkovec, unpublished data). An example is a former patient who described having many friends and, within her social circle, being viewed as the strong one who could be counted on for sympathy and advice 24 hours a day (e.g., calls from friends in crisis in the middle of the night were welcome). At the same time, she reported having difficulty letting other people know when she was feeling anxious or overwhelmed because she feared being perceived as weak and insecure. Her fear of sharing her feelings with others came at the price of often failing to get her own emotional needs met. For at least some individuals with GAD, problematic interpersonal styles may arise out of a history of role reversal and enmeshment with their primary caregivers, suggesting early attachment difficulties (Cassidy, 1995; A. R. Zuellig et al., unpublished data). These individuals report having unresolved feelings of anger and vulnerability towards their primary caregiver. Furthermore, they may continue to display a pattern of insecure attachment toward others in their adult lives (A. R. Zuellig et al., unpublished data).

An emotion regulation perspective on GAD

Borkovec and colleagues conceptualize worry as avoidance of imagery, physiological arousal, and negative emotion and highlight the need for emotional processing to break the worry cycle and modify negative emotional states over the long run. However, the nature of the emotional experience that prompts individuals with GAD to engage in avoidance strategies such as worry has not been examined. We suggest that understanding how individuals with GAD experience and regulate their emotions will ultimately lead to a better understanding of the disorder and suggest new points for therapeutic intervention.

Our model proposes that emotions are dysregulated among individuals with GAD. That is, individuals with GAD experience marked difficulty understanding their emotional experience and possess few skills to modulate their emotions. These deficits cause persons with GAD to experience emotions as subjectively aversive and to engage in strategies to control, avoid, or blunt emotional experience. In this way, worry can be viewed as a cognitive control strategy employed in attempts to "fix" the regulatory problems associated with subjectively aversive emotional experience. Additionally, individuals with GAD may adopt other maladaptive strategies aimed at controlling emotional experience in addition to worry. We agree with Newman et al. (in press) who suggest that individuals with GAD, in their attempt to avoid painful emotions, engage in behaviors that make negative interpersonal outcomes more likely. From our perspective, individuals with GAD develop an approach to interpersonal relations aimed at obtaining security from others and avoiding feared negative interpersonal outcomes specifically to regulate their own emotional experience. An understanding of emotion regulation deficits in GAD holds the potential for generating a larger framework that integrates what is known about the cognitive, behavioral, interpersonal, and biological aspects of this disorder.

Emotion dysregulation can involve first, difficulties in modulation of emotional experience or expression and/or second, frequent attempts to control or suppress emotional experience or expression (Cole et al., 1994; Cicchetti et al., 1995). Modulation of emotion may be especially difficult for individuals with GAD, because they may have emotional reactions that occur more easily, quickly, and intensely than for most other people. Therefore, experiences that have little effect on other people may trigger an emotional reaction in an individual with GAD. For example, a former patient described being very sensitive to the noise made at night when people in his apartment building would honk their horns to alert the attendant to open the garage door. In contrast, he reported that his wife had no difficulty ignoring this noise. Late one evening when he was feeling particularly tense, he became startled and then intensely angry when someone began honking. The patient ran outside, yelling at his offending neighbor and punching the car window as the neighbor pulled away.

In a recent study examining these hypotheses, individuals who met criteria for GAD by self-report reported higher levels of intensity of emotional experience than control individuals (D. S. Mennin et al., unpublished data). They were also more expressive of negative (but not positive) emotions than control individuals. These findings suggest that individuals with GAD may be particularly motivated to attempt to control their emotional experience.

Difficulties in modulation of emotional experience or expression probably result from a complex combination of heredity and emotionally impoverished environments. In our clinical experience, these emotionally impoverished environments may be ones in which parents spend relatively little time with the children (who are largely expected to fend for themselves and get their own needs met), ones in which a primary caregiver is unreliable, unpredictable, volatile, and/or violent, or ones in which a primary caregiver is intolerant of negative emotions and has difficulty modulating his or her own emotions (and perhaps suffers from GAD). Obviously, such environments are not conducive to teaching the child to understand and modulate emotions. The type of environment in which individuals with GAD learn about emotional experience is well-illustrated by a recent patient who described an experience as a 5-year-old in which he had broken his leg so badly that the bone protruded through his skin. The patient's mother, on seeing the boy's leg, "became hysterical" and was unable to generate an appropriate course of action. The boy, in his wounded state, proceeded to instruct his mother calmly on the best procedure for obtaining treatment for his injury. The patient reported that at an early age he learned that emotions could incapacitate a person and that he needed to be prepared to take care of himself and other people (i.e., worry).

Saarni (1990, 1999) describes the construct of *emotional competence,* which she defines as the ability of individuals to "respond emotionally yet simultaneously and strategically apply their knowledge about emotions and their expression to relationships with others so that they can negotiate interpersonal exchanges and regulate their emotional experiences as well" (1990, p. 116). She identifies eight components (i.e., skills and capabilities) that are crucial to the development of emotional competence during childhood (Saarni, 1999). These components include:

1. awareness of one's emotional state (e.g., presence of multiple emotions);
2. ability to recognize and differentiate others' emotions and their meaning according to situational and expressive cues;
3. use of one's culture's vocabulary for emotion and expression terms;
4. capacity for empathic attunement to others' emotional experiences;
5. ability to distinguish between inner emotional experience and outer emotional expression;
6. the capacity for adaptive coping in response to aversive emotions and distressing circumstances;
7. capacity to communicate emotions within relationships;
8. acceptance and allowance of one's emotional experience such that feelings can occur without suppression, avoidance, or escape.

It may be that individuals with GAD fail to develop many of these skills. If individuals with GAD are highly emotionally sensitive, have difficulty understanding their emotional experience, and possess few skills to modulate their emotions, they may experience emotions as subjectively aversive and feel the need to control their emotional experience. This is most obviously the case for the emotion of anxiety but may also be true for other emotions such as sadness, anger, and even arousal-generating positive emotions such as elation. In essence, individuals with GAD may use worry and other strategies to control or suppress emotional experience ineffectively and inappropriately. In a test of this hypothesis, persons who met criteria for GAD by self-report and control participants underwent either a negative or neutral mood induction (Mennin, 2001). GAD participants displayed greater increases in worry and generalized anxiety symptoms after the negative mood induction than after the neutral mood induction, providing evidence that negative emotions stimulate the cycle of worry among chronic worriers. Interestingly, in response to the negative mood induction, GAD participants were also less likely to accept their emotional experience; reported less clarity about the nature of their emotions, what they were, and why they were having them; and believed that they could do less to repair this mood than did control participants. These results are consistent with other research from our lab which has shown that individuals with self-reported GAD have marked difficulties in their ability to identify, describe, and accept emotional experience (including anxiety, sadness, anger, and positive emotions), and deficits in their ability to soothe themselves when they experienced negative emotions, compared to a control group (D. S. Mennin et al., unpublished data). A study conducted with a clinical sample of persons with DSM-IV GAD and matched community controls produced similar findings (C. L. Turk et al., unpublished data).

These phenomena can be illustrated by a recent patient who described feeling overwhelmed when confronted with the grief displayed by his grandmother as she told him about the death of one of her friends. Although a generally sensitive and caring person, in order to reduce his own distress at her grief, he initially "tuned her out" while she was talking, then attempted to minimize the loss by bringing up her friend's faults, and ultimately ended his visit early. Confronted with difficulty modulating his own emotional experience, the patient quickly attempted to decrease the source of his distress in a maladaptive manner that was most likely distressing to his grandmother and unhealthy for their relationship. He also reported worrying more since the incident. In particular, this interaction fed into his worry about his ability to "handle stress," meet the demands placed upon him by his relationships, and be successful in relationships.

There are a number of adverse consequences that arise as a result of using worry as a means of avoiding emotional experience. As previously discussed, emotional processing is decreased, leaving existing fear structures intact. Furthermore, the worried person continues to focus on apprehension-producing subjects but does not utilize important affective information because of its overwhelming nature. As a result, approaches to problem-solving become inflexible, and perseveration at initial stages of problem generation occurs. Goals for action cannot be accessed because the relevant motivational response tendencies are blocked by avoidance of emotional experience. As such, effective and dynamic functioning cannot occur because all components of experience (i.e., cognition and emotion) are not being utilized.

A number of emotion researchers have argued that an integrated system of cognition and emotion is reflective of adaptive regulatory functioning (Damasio, 1994; Izard, 1993, LeDoux, 1996). LeDoux (1996) explains that there are multiple *bidirectional* connections between limbic cortices that initially process emotional stimuli and cortical centers that regulate this emotional experience. Emotion dysregulation in individuals with GAD may be reflective of a deficit in this normally integrated system. Specifically, cognitive information may be attended at the expense of emotional experience. By decreasing attention to emotional experience, emotion is avoided or blunted. Indeed, worry has been associated with high frontal lobe activity suggestive of increased cognitive activity (Carter et al., 1986). In addition, preliminary results have shown that control individuals have faster access to limbic system processes than do individuals with GAD (as reported in Borkovec et al., 1998). These findings provide initial biological evidence of emotional avoidance in GAD.

Although the cognitive activity of worrying may function to avoid emotional experience, individuals with GAD have not been shown to be "emotionally numb or blunted" as would be more common in disorders such as posttraumatic stress disorder. Rather, as discussed above, these individuals have been shown to report experiencing their emotions in an intense manner (D. S. Mennin et al., unpublished data). This may be reflective of homeostatic mechanisms in the brain that attempt to correct for the maladaptive control strategy of worry. Emotional information initially processed in the amygdala may continue to be transmitted to the cortex, which could further stimulate worry. Put differently, the "volume" of emotional messages may be automatically raised as one attempts to attend only to cognitive information. As a result, the emotional message may intensify and, paradoxically, signal the person of the need to continue to use worry to escape this aversive state.

Future directions for studying the role of emotion regulation in GAD

An emotion regulation perspective may provide a useful direction for understanding emotional phenomena and the worry process in GAD. However, a good deal of research needs to occur before any definitive conclusions can be made about emotion dysregulation in GAD. Additional studies are needed to examine whether individuals with GAD differ from control individuals and individuals with other forms of psychopathology in their perceptions of emotions as aversively stimulating. Furthermore, additional studies that examine emotion regulation strategies in these patients are necessary. More evidence is also necessary to determine if worry is indeed a control strategy for managing emotion and whether this is true for all individuals who worry or only those with GAD. It would also be intriguing to examine the functional brain activity of these patients when they are worrying as opposed to actively engaging emotion to determine if there is differential cortical and subcortical activity. Finally, to what extent can emotion regulation difficulties explain the high rates of comorbidity found in GAD? Gross and Muñoz (1995) have shown that these deficits in emotion regulation are present in many forms of psychopathology. It may be that emotion regulation difficulties are a marker for a common developmental pathway (e.g., poor attachment in relationships with primary caregivers) to many conditions. The authors are currently developing a program of research to address many of these issues among patients with GAD and undergraduate students who are chronic worriers. Preliminary data suggest that these chronic worriers do have more difficulty regulating emotions than control individuals (Mennin, 2001; D. S. Mennin et al., unpublished data; Turk et al., unpublished data).

Treatment of GAD

Review of cognitive-behavioral therapies: components and efficacy

Although progress has been made in understanding GAD and its core feature of worry, the body of research assessing the efficacy of treatment remains relatively small. In this section, we describe the treatment approaches that have been examined in controlled trials. We do not consider studies that grouped patients with GAD together with patients with other primary diagnoses or studies including generally anxious patients who were not formally diagnosed according to either DSM criteria or research diagnostic criteria. Due to early difficulties reliably diagnosing GAD, studies that fail to use stringent diagnostic criteria are likely to include substantial numbers of false-positive cases, reducing the relevance of their findings (Borkovec and Whisman, 1996). Relaxation training, cognitive restructuring, and multicomponent cognitive-behavioral approaches are reviewed and discussed in terms of their relative ability to treat GAD effectively.

The rationale for the application of relaxation training to GAD has been that somatically focused techniques may enhance the patient's ability to cope with internal anxiety cues, an important skill given that clear, stable external triggers for anxiety are lacking for many patients. Most studies have adopted the procedures for progressive muscle relaxation training originally outlined by Bernstein and Borkovec (1973). With this approach, patients learn to relax through exercises involving different muscle groups. Patients learn to notice the difference between the feelings of tension and relaxation, learn to relax by recall, and learn cue-controlled relaxation, in which a word such as "relax" is repeatedly paired with a relaxed state and then used as a cue to begin the process of rapidly relaxing during daily activities. Patients are taught to implement relaxation procedures at the earliest signs of anxiety and when confronting anxiety-provoking internal and external stimuli (i.e., applied relaxation).

The efficacy of relaxation training among individuals with GAD has been evaluated in several studies. Patients receiving training in applied relaxation were more likely to be classified as treatment responders and achieve high end-state functioning than patients assigned to a waiting list (Barlow et al., 1992) or those receiving a nondirective control therapy that generated similar expectations for improvement (Borkovec and Costello, 1993). In both studies, patients receiving applied relaxation maintained their gains at follow-ups ranging from 6 to 24 months. Within-group analysis of change among patients treated with applied relaxation in the Barlow et al. (1992) study indicated that 63% were classified as treatment responders and 56% were classified as having achieved high end-state functioning. Borkovec and Costello (1993) found that 72% of applied relaxation patients were treatment responders at posttreatment and 69% were responders at 12-month follow-up. Additionally, 44% met criteria for high end-state functioning at posttreatment, and 38% met these criteria at 12-month follow-up. Relaxation training (alone or accompanied by a control intervention) has been compared to relaxation training combined with other cognitive-behavioral techniques. In one study (Borkovec et al., 1987), the combined treatment produced more favorable outcomes than relaxation training alone. Two other studies (Barlow et al., 1992; Borkovec and Costello, 1993), however, found equivalent change for relaxation training and relaxation training plus other cognitive-behavioral techniques.

Whether administered alone or combined with other techniques, cognitive therapy has been a frequent component in the treatment of GAD. The approach to cognitive therapy used in almost all the controlled trials has been based on the work of Beck et al. (1985). Beck's approach asserts that negative emotions like anxiety are produced by cognitive processing errors such that patients label, interpret, and evaluate their experiences in a biased, highly personalized, overly arbitrary, or extreme manner (Beck, 1976). Beck's cognitive therapy attempts to correct these errors via logic, Socratic discussion, and empirical testing of negative beliefs through behavioral experiments. The goal of therapy is to remold the patient's rigid, maladaptive ways of thinking into a more accurate, realistic, and flexible style while altering fundamental belief structures (i.e., schemata).

Three studies found that cognitive therapy outperformed a waiting-list condition on most measures after treatment and that patients treated with cognitive therapy maintained their gains at follow-up (Butler et al., 1991; Barlow et al., 1992; White et al., 1992). However, cognitive therapy failed to outperform a placebo treatment in one study (White et al., 1992). In the Barlow et al. (1992) study, 67% of patients receiving cognitive therapy were classified as treatment responders at posttreatment, although only 25% met criteria for high end-state functioning. Butler et al. (1991) found that 32% of patients receiving cognitive therapy reached high end-state functioning at posttreatment and 42% were functioning at this level at 6-month follow-up.

Most commonly, multicomponent cognitive-behavioral treatment packages have been studied. Relaxation and cognitive therapy are usually combined in treatment. In every case, combined cognitive therapy and relaxation have been more efficacious than no treatment (Blowers et al., 1987; Barlow et al., 1992; White et al., 1992). However, combined relaxation and cognitive therapy have failed to show a clear advantage over psychosocial control treatments (Blowers et al., 1987; White et al., 1992; Stanley et al., 1996). Although combined cognitive therapy and relaxation training is the most commonly studied treatment package, additional cognitive and behavioral techniques have been included in some studies. We provide a brief description and efficacy findings of two treatment packages that include procedures in addition to cognitive therapy and relaxation skills (for a more extensive description of these and other cognitive-behavioral techniques as applied to GAD, see Borkovec and Newman, 1998).

Suinn and Richardson's (1971) anxiety management training has been adapted for use in the treatment of GAD. In their version of anxiety management training, Butler and colleagues (1987, 1991) include applied relaxation, reducing subtle avoidance through exposure, identifying and examining anxiety-provoking thoughts, using distraction, and building confidence and combating demoralization by scheduling enjoyable activities. Butler et al. (1987) found that patients receiving anxiety management training made gains superior to patients on the waiting list on all measures at posttreatment. These gains were maintained at 6-month follow-up. Regarding degree of clinically significant change, 51% of patients receiving anxiety management training had achieved high end-state functioning after treatment. In another study that used anxiety management training but without the cognitive elements, Butler et al. (1991) found that patients in this treatment condition had better outcomes than those in the waiting-list condition on a few measures. However, their outcomes were poorer than for patients treated with Beck's cognitive therapy. After treatment, 16% of patients treated with the behavioral version of anxiety management training had achieved high end-state functioning. This figure dropped to 5% at 6-month follow-up.

Borkovec and Costello (1993) tested a cognitive-behavioral package that included applied relaxation, cognitive therapy, and self-control desensitization. During self-control desensitization, the therapist helps the patient to become deeply relaxed. The therapist then presents external and internal cues as the patient vividly imagined the anxiety-provoking situation being described. Patients are instructed to use relaxation skills to cope with the anxiety during the experience being visualized.

After the patient signals that anxiety had been eliminated, the patient continues to imagine coping with the situation for 20 s. Finally, the patient is instructed to stop all imagery and focus on relaxing for 20 s more. This procedure is repeated until the selected situation no longer elicits anxiety or the anxiety is dissipated within 5–7 s. Patients are encouraged to use self-statements and perspective shifts arrived at in cognitive therapy during the coping phase of desensitization. Borkovec and Costello (1993) compared this cognitive-behavioral treatment to applied relaxation and nondirective therapy. Cognitive-behavioral treatment and applied relaxation resulted in more improvement than nondirective therapy on most measures. However, cognitive-behavioral treatment and applied relaxation did not differ on any posttreatment measure. Regarding clinically significant change, 58% of patients receiving cognitive-behavioral treatment were responders after treatment and 84% were responders at 12-month follow-up. Additionally, 26% met criteria for high end-state functioning at posttreatment, and 58% met these criteria at 12-month follow-up.

Recently, Ladouceur and colleagues (2000) examined the efficacy of a multicomponent cognitive-behavioral treatment package for GAD that explicitly excluded relaxation training and specifically targeted worry. In this treatment, patients are introduced to the concept that uncertainty is an important source of worry and anxiety and that accepting and coping with uncertainty will be important for reductions in worry and anxiety to occur. Cognitive therapy is used to target positive beliefs about worry (e.g., "By worrying, I can stop bad things from happening"). Patients are also taught to categorize worries as being of one of two types: those that may be addressed with problem-solving and those that are unlikely to be addressed by problem-solving because they are highly improbable or highly remote in time. For worries amenable to problem-solving, patients practice identifying key elements of the problem without becoming caught up in minor details and then moving ahead with the problem-solving process, even in the face of uncertainty about the strategy that they have chosen. For worries not amenable to problem-solving, cognitive exposure is used. Patients vividly describe the worrisome image, which is recorded on a looped tape for repeated exposure. Patients receiving this treatment package were significantly improved on most posttreatment measures of worry, anxiety, and depression relative to a waitlist control group. Regarding clinically significant change, 65% of patients receiving this package were responders after treatment and 62% were responders at 12-month follow-up. Furthermore, 62% met criteria for high end-state functioning at posttreatment, and 58% met these criteria at 12-month follow-up.

Several metaanalytic studies have examined the efficacy of cognitive-behavioral treatments for GAD. In the first of these efforts, Chambless and Gillis (1993) examined seven studies and found that cognitive-behavioral treatment produced a substantial and enduring impact upon anxiety symptoms, reflected by large uncontrolled within-group pretest–posttest and pretest–follow-up effect sizes. Borkovec and Whisman (1996) examined eight studies and calculated effect sizes based on 17 cognitive and/or behavioral therapy conditions, two psychosocial control conditions, and five waiting-list conditions. All psychosocial treatment conditions, including the psychosocial control conditions, appeared to be superior to waiting list in terms of within-group pretest–posttest effect sizes for measures of anxiety and depression. Improvements were maintained for all conditions at follow-up assessment. More recently, Borkovec and Ruscio (2001) conducted a metaanalysis that included 11 studies and yielded 15 trials of cognitive-behavioral therapy (cognitive therapy plus some form of behavior therapy, most commonly relaxation training), 10 single-component trials (cognitive therapy alone or behavior therapy alone), eight nonspecific/alternative treatment comparison trials (supportive therapy, pill placebo, psychodynamic therapy, diazepam), and four trials of waiting-list conditions. Effect sizes for measures of both anxiety and depression at posttest and follow-up suggested the greatest improvements with combined cognitive-behavioral therapy, followed by nonspecific/alternative treatments, followed by the single-component treatments, followed by the waiting-list conditions. Lastly, Gould et al. (1997) conducted a metaanalysis that included 35 controlled studies examining cognitive-behavioral therapy and/or pharmacotherapy. Cognitive-behavioral treatment and pharmacological treatment both produced effect sizes for symptoms of anxiety and depression that were significantly greater than zero. The effect sizes for cognitive-behavioral therapy and pharmacotherapy were not significantly different from each other for anxiety symptoms. However, cognitive-behavioral therapy did have a significantly greater effect on depression than pharmacotherapy. Cognitive-behavioral therapy also evidenced good maintenance of treatment gains at follow-up, while the limited data available suggested pharmacological treatment was associated with relapse following medication discontinuation. Within the category of cognitive-behavioral therapy, there were no significant differences between interventions, with the exception that combined cognitive-behavioral interventions were superior to relaxation training plus biofeedback. A visual comparison of effect sizes, however, suggested that, in general, combined cognitive-behavioral therapy produced larger effect sizes than relaxation training alone, other behavioral techniques alone, and cognitive therapy alone.

Given that the GAD treatment outcome literature is relatively small, it is not surprising that the literature devoted to addressing the predictors of response to treatment is sparse. In one study, Butler and Anastasiades (1988) found that low levels of initial anxiety and demoralization, coupled with higher levels of initial depression, predicted better outcomes among patients treated with anxiety management training at both posttreatment and 6-month follow-up. However, these results were not replicated in another study that examined patients treated with either cognitive-behavioral therapy or behavior therapy alone (Butler, 1993). For patients treated with behavior therapy, greater anxiety prior to treatment was associated with greater anxiety after treatment. In contrast, for patients treated with cognitive-behavioral therapy, the only significant predictor of treatment outcome was interpretive bias. Specifically, a greater tendency to interpret ambiguous external situations as threatening before treatment was associated with higher anxiety after treatment. Taken together, these results suggest that different factors may be important in predicting treatment outcome and that these factors may be dependent on the nature of treatment administered.

Borkovec and colleagues have examined the relationship of several different process variables to treatment outcome. They have routinely found that first-session patient expectancies predict short- and long-term therapy outcome (Borkovec et al., 1987; Borkovec and Mathews, 1988; Borkovec and Costello, 1993). Although the mechanism by which expectancies are associated with outcome are unknown and not necessarily causal (Chambless et al., 1997), these data raise the possibility that modification of negative expectances may be a worthwhile goal early in treatment. In two studies, they also found that greater anxiety during relaxation training and lower frequency of relaxation practice were associated with poorer outcomes (Borkovec et al., 1987; Borkovec and Mathews, 1988), although these variables bore little relation to outcome in another study (Borkovec and Costello, 1993). Additional research is needed to reveal the extent to which the ability to relax effectively is crucial to good treatment outcome (Borkovec and Mathews, 1988).

Comorbidity is a common feature of GAD, and almost no work has examined the impact of comorbidity on psychosocial treatment outcome. In fact, most treatment outcome studies have excluded patients with a variety of comorbid disorders, including panic disorder (Borkovec and Costello, 1993), obsessive-compulsive disorder (Butler et al., 1987), major depressive disorder (Butler et al., 1987, 1991), and alcohol dependence or abuse (Barlow et al., 1992). Only a few studies are available to shed light upon the impact of comorbidity upon the treatment of GAD. Although their sample excluded patients meeting criteria for major depressive disorder, Butler et al. (1987) found no difference in treatment outcome between GAD patients who met criteria for minor depressive disorder and those who did not. However, Barlow et al. (1992) did find that only pretreatment scores on the Beck Depression Inventory differentiated patients later classified as responders and nonresponders, with responders having significantly lower scores than nonresponders prior to treatment. Thus, the impact of depressive symptomatology on GAD treatment outcome remains unclear. One study has addressed the effect of axis II comorbidity on GAD treatment outcome. Patients with a comorbid personality disorder were found to make treatment gains similar to patients without a comorbid personality disorder but were more likely to drop out of treatment (Sanderson et al., 1994b).

In conclusion, a significant number of patients appear to benefit from existing cognitive-behavioral treatments, and gains generally appear to be maintained over follow-up periods. These findings are consistent across both individual and meta-analytic studies. Unfortunately, it is rare for more than two-thirds of patients with GAD to be functioning within the normal range at the end of treatment. In fact, it is more common for only 50–60% of patients to achieve high end-state functioning. We also have little understanding of the factors that predict a favorable response to the various psychosocial treatments. These findings leave considerable room for new innovations in the treatment of this disorder as well as studies examining variables important to the process of change during treatment.

Incorporation of an emotion regulation perspective to improve cognitive-behavioral therapy for GAD

A focus on emotion regulation may suggest new directions for improving treatment for GAD. A treatment that incorporates this perspective requires that patients learn emotion regulation skills in order to supplant or undermine their need for pathological worry. Patients who increase their identification, acceptance, and understanding of their emotions and their ability to utilize their emotional experiences constructively would be expected to decrease their worrying and associated anxiety. Improved ability to understand and cope with one's own emotions and the emotions of others may also improve interpersonal functioning (e.g., expressing emotion more appropriately to others, greater sensitivity to the emotional reactions of others) and decrease distress and worry in this important domain. Patients would work toward the goal of integrating emotional experience and rational thought. They would learn that feelings can aid in constructive decision-making and action and that energy used to avoid emotions can be utilized in a more functional manner (Greenberg, 1994). Moreover, they should be better equipped to tolerate distress and able to function at a more adaptive level.

Early in treatment, patients need to pay attention to how their emotional responses lead them into a worry cycle and take note of themes that arise as the worry process is engaged (even if the superficial topic of worry is constantly shifting). These themes often include fears of loss of significant others, inability to get one's needs met, failure at their vocation, or health-related concerns. Initially, patients should passively observe and describe their emotional reactions and associated worry, bodily sensations, and automatic thoughts. They are discouraged from attempts to problem-solve their worry concern. Rather, patients are encouraged to develop a sense of "mindfulness," involving stepping back, gaining perspective, and permitting feelings to emerge. Relaxation training skills can be quite useful in helping the patient become more mindful of how emotional reactions can cause tension in their bodies and, as a result, serve to increase anxiety levels. Mindfulness-based meditation techniques (Kabat-Zinn et al., 1992) may also be useful in terms of helping patients to observe, describe, and learn from their emotional experiences.

An important aspect of emotion regulation is learning when introspectively to deepen awareness of one's emotional experience and when this may be counterproductive. Greenberg and Safran (1987) discuss three types of emotional reactions that they label primary, secondary, and instrumental. Primary emotional reactions refer to biologically adaptive emotional responses that provide information about action tendencies, associated meanings, and motivation for behavior. These responses include what have been termed the basic emotions such as fear, joy, anger, and sadness (Plutchik, 1990). Because of their informational value, accessing primary emotions is essential to positive affective change and regulation. As such, patients learn to identify and label different primary emotional experiences. Since patients with GAD are often uncomfortable with affect, they may be quite reluctant to engage their emotional experience. Hence, primary emotions need to be evoked within the session to educate patients about these emotional reactions and the need for acceptance of this experience. Patients may be asked to focus on a salient concern but to remain attentive to their bodily and subjective reactions *in the present moment*. Imaginal exposure or experiential exercises can be utilized to create greater emotional salience and urgency. For example, one GAD patient often had difficulty with experiencing anger. She often began to worry about the ramifications of her anger without letting the anger be experienced or understood. In session, the patient was encouraged to imagine a situation where she felt that her friend had not been supportive of her during a difficult time. Rather than focus on the worry about her friendship, the patient was encouraged to attend to her anger as she envisioned her friend not being supportive. The patient focused on feeling this anger in session, which helped her become more comfortable with this experience and, subsequently, decreased the worry that resulted from her discomfort with anger. Furthermore, by allowing this emotional experience, she developed a greater understanding of her needs concerning her friend and was later able to verbalize them to her.

Although this process may appear similar to "worry exposure" techniques that are presently used in typical cognitive-behavioral packages for GAD (Craske et al., 1995), there are important distinctions between the procedures. Whereas the focus in the traditional cognitive-behavioral approach is to have the patient consistently focus on the consequences of the worried thought (e.g., "If I don't worry about my daughter, she could get hurt"), the focus of the exercise in the present approach is on the associated primary emotional experience. Using worry exposure techniques, patients can remain relatively disconnected from their emotional experience associated with these hypothetical consequences, instead remaining solely cognitively focused. When utilizing an emotion regulation approach, the emotion that the patient experiences when addressing feared consequences is the focus of the exercise. Once this emotion is elicited, the patient learns to be more comfortable and accepting of this experience. However, the patient also gains knowledge about the adaptive value of the emotion and can utilize this information to understand unrecognized motivations and achieve needed goals, thus decreasing the need to instigate a maladaptive worry process. In addition, the traditional cognitive-behavioral approach assumes that patients have the knowledge to recognize and understand their emotions. In an emotion regulation framework, patients directly learn about their emotional experience and develop a new vocabulary for discussing this material.

In contrast to primary emotions, secondary emotions are not direct adaptive responses. Rather, they are problematic expressions of emotion that are typical of most anxiety disorders and are often reactions to primary emotions, that is, "emotions about emotions." For example, a patient may become frustrated with his or her experience of anxiety and, hence, focus on the experience of frustration rather than examining the anxiety. Secondary emotional responses may also occur in response to distorted cognitions. For example, the response of sadness to a belief in one's own essential incompetence would constitute a secondary emotional reaction. As such, the evocation of secondary emotional reactions through experiential exercise is not encouraged (Greenberg and Safran, 1987). Rather, maladaptive beliefs associated with the secondary emotion should be explored through cognitive restructuring. Restructuring can also demonstrate to patients how maladaptive thoughts and beliefs serve to increase negative emotional reactions and instigate the worry process. Patients are then encouraged to confront these beliefs and provide more realistic assessments of the context in question. In addition, patients learn to judge the adaptive value of different thoughts by identifying primary emotions that may be present when these thoughts are evoked. If a primary emotion can be revealed, evocation of this primary response should be encouraged and validated by the therapist.

Instrumental emotional responses refer to emotional patterns that individuals have learned to use to influence, control, or change other people (Greenberg and Safran, 1987). One such response is crying to invoke sympathy. An example is a former patient who experienced frequent, uncontrollable worry about losing her relationship with her boyfriend of 2 years (in addition to other worries). Although they shared similar interests and values and generally got along very well, this patient would intermittently feel overwhelmed by this particular worry and seek reassurance from her boyfriend about his happiness in and commitment to their relationship. When she was not sufficiently soothed by his response to her concern of the moment, she would begin to cry and suggest that they should break up. Not surprisingly, her boyfriend often became frustrated and more distant in response to these emotional displays, which further heightened her worry and anxiety and desire to seek additional reassurance. Patients are encouraged to become more aware of the underlying motivation behind instrumental emotional reactions and are taught alternative methods for meeting their needs, especially in interpersonal situations.

An emotion regulation treatment for GAD is chiefly aimed at amelioration of the suffering associated with pathological worry and anxiety. However, it is our view that recovery from debilitating worry is best achieved when effective emotion regulation skills are attained. Hence, the goal of treatment extends beyond symptom reduction. Newman (2000) has highlighted the need to focus also on improvement in perceived levels of distress, quality of life, and various sources of functionality (e.g., interpersonal relations). To this end, at the close of an emotion regulation treatment of generalized anxiety, patients are expected to have improved in their ability to identify, accept, differentiate, and understand their emotions and associated action tendencies. In addition, it is hoped that patients will have become more attuned to the emotions of others and can use this information to regulate emotional expression effectively to meet the needs of a given environmental context. Finally, in the most general sense, these patients should be able to increase or decrease their attendance to emotional experience effectively as is necessary to adapt properly to life's inevitable challenges.

Future directions for development and validation of emotion-focused treatments

Treatment programs that address emotion regulation difficulties in the treatment of individuals with GAD are currently being developed (D.S. Mennin et al., unpublished data; M. G. Newman et al., unpublished data; Roemer and Orsillo, 2002). The ability of these approaches to demonstrate efficacy in treating GAD will need to be empirically evaluated. It will also be important to examine whether the integration of emotion-focused interventions and cognitive-behavioral interventions results in treatment that is more efficacious than cognitive-behavioral therapy alone.

Another important goal of future research in this area will be to study the process of change in emotion-focused treatments of GAD. Specifically, it will be of interest to determine if therapeutic change occurs as a function of increases in emotion regulation abilities. For example, are decreases in worry commensurate with increases in comfort with emotional experience? Do emotional acceptance and effective emotional regulation mediate the relationship between treatment components and efficacy? These questions can only be answered through a systematic examination of both treatment outcome and process. Toward this goal, assessments that are sensitive to emotional change must be developed and utilized.

Conclusion

GAD has received increased attention in the past decade. However, compared with other anxiety disorders, advances in the understanding and treatment of this syndrome have been limited. We have argued that cognitive-behavioral approaches can be improved through incorporation of an emotion regulation perspective. In particular, GAD is conceptualized as a syndrome that involves deficits in regulation of emotions and attempts to control or avoid affective experience through worrying. In addition, an emotion regulation perspective may inform existing cognitive-behavioral treatments through the incorporation of emotion evocation techniques and emotion regulation skill training. In particular, it is suggested that GAD patients who have improved their ability to modulate their emotional experience and expression and who are able to integrate information from both emotional and cognitive sources will witness decreases in their worrying and associated anxiety.

We have suggested that emotion variables are an important part of a cognitive-behavioral approach to GAD. However, one may question the need to focus on emotion. Skinner (1953, p. 160) directly attacked the importance of emotion when he stated that "'emotions' are excellent examples of the fictional causes to which we commonly attribute behavior." Others have argued that emotion should not be considered separate from cognitive phenomena (Lazarus, 1984). Rather, anxiety and mood disorders should chiefly be considered disorders of cognition (Alloy, 1991). Other theorists describe interpersonal interaction as central to understanding and treating GAD (Safran and Segal, 1990; Crits-Christoph et al., 1995).

By stressing the importance of emotion variables, we are not suggesting that other variables such as cognition, behavior, or interpersonal relations are not vital to the understanding or treatment of GAD. Rather, an emotion regulation perspective may be the "tie that binds" these phenomena together. In fact, the ultimate goal of this approach is an integrated mind that is able to process all levels of information effectively (including both cognitive and emotional characteristics) and act adaptively as a result. Dodge and Garber (1991) have argued that "all information processing is emotional, in that emotion is the energy level that drives, organizes, amplifies, and attenuates cognitive activity and in turn is the experience and expression of that activity" (p. 159). Further research is clearly necessary to determine the relationship between emotional phenomena and other cognitive, behavioral, biological, and interpersonal findings. It will be important to determine how these factors interact in causing and maintaining GAD. In addition, understanding the interaction of these factors may elucidate how GAD is distinguished from other disorders that demonstrate emotion regulation difficulties, such as depression. It is our hope that an emotion regulation perspective can facilitate these integrative goals.

REFERENCES

Achenbach, T. (1995). Diagnosis, assessment, and comorbidity in psychosocial treatment research. *Journal of Abnormal Child Psychology*, **23**, 45–65.

Alloy, L. B. (1991). Depression and anxiety: disorders of emotion or cognition? *Psychological Inquiry*, **2**, 72–74.

American Psychiatric Association. (1980). *Diagnostic and Statistical Manual of Mental Disorders*, 3rd edn. Washington, DC: American Psychiatric Association.

American Psychiatric Association. (1987). *Diagnostic and Statistical Manual of Mental Disorders*, 3rd edn, revised. Washington, DC: American Psychiatric Association.

American Psychiatric Association. (1994). *Diagnostic and Statistical Manual of Mental Disorders*, 4th edn. Washington, DC: American Psychiatric Association.

Barlow, D. H. (1987). The classification of anxiety disorders. In *Diagnosis and Classification in Psychiatry: A Critical Reappraisal of DSM-III*, ed. G. L. Tischler, pp. 223–42. Cambridge, England: Cambridge University Press.

Barlow, D. H. (1988). *Anxiety and its Disorders*. New York: Guilford Press.

Barlow, D. H., Rapee, R. M., and Brown, T. A. (1992). Behavioral treatment of generalized anxiety disorder. *Behavior Therapy*, **23**, 551–70.

Beck, A. T. (1976). *Cognitive Therapy and the Emotional Disorders*. New York: New American Library.

Beck, A. T., Emery, G., and Greenberg, R. L. (1985). *Anxiety Disorders and Phobias: A Cognitive Perspective*. New York: Basic Books.

Beck, J. G., Stanley, M. A., and Zebb, B. J. (1996). Characteristics of generalized anxiety disorder in older adults: a descriptive study. *Behaviour Research and Therapy*, **34**, 225–34.

Bernstein, D. A. and Borkovec, T. D. (1973). *Progressive Relaxation Training*. Champaign, IL: Research Press.

Blazer, D. G., Hughes, D., and George, L. K. (1991). Generalized anxiety disorder. In *Psychiatric Disorders in America: The Epidemiological Catchment Area Study*, ed. L. N. Robins and D. A. Regier, pp. 180–203. New York: Free Press.

Blowers, C., Cobb, J., and Mathews, A. (1987). Generalised anxiety: a controlled treatment study. *Behaviour Research and Therapy*, **25**, 493–502.

Borkovec, T. D. (1994). The nature, functions, and origins of worry. In *Worrying: Perspectives on Theory, Assessment and Treatment*, ed. G. C. L. Davey and F. Tallis, pp. 5–33. Chichester, England: John Wiley.

Borkovec, T. D. and Costello, E. (1993). Efficacy of applied relaxation and cognitive-behavioral therapy in the treatment of generalized anxiety disorder. *Journal of Consulting and Clinical Psychology*, **61**, 611–19.

Borkovec, T. D. and Hu, S. (1990). The effect of worry on cardiovascular response to phobic imagery. *Behaviour Research and Therapy*, **28**, 69–73.

Borkovec, T. D. and Inz, J. (1990). The nature of worry in generalized anxiety disorder: a predominance of thought activity. *Behaviour Research and Therapy*, **28**, 153–8.

Borkovec, T. D. and Lyonfields, J. D. (1993). Worry: thought suppression of emotional processing. In *Attention and Avoidance: Strategies in Coping with Aversiveness*, ed. H. W. Krohne, pp. 101–18). Goettingen, Germany: Hogrefe & Huber.

Borkovec, T. D. and Mathews, A. M. (1988). Treatment of nonphobic anxiety disorders: a comparison of nondirective, cognitive, and coping desensitization therapy. *Journal of Consulting and Clinical Psychology*, **56**, 877–84.

Borkovec, T. D. and Newman, M. G. (1998). Worry and generalized anxiety disorder. In *Comprehensive Clinical Psychology*, vol. 6, ed. A. S. Bellack and M. Hersen, pp. 439–59. New York: Pergamon Press.

Borkovec, T. D. and Ruscio, A. M. (2001). Psychotherapy for generalized anxiety disorder. *Journal of Clinical Psychiatry*, **62** (suppl. 11), 37–45.

Borkovec, T. D. and Whisman, M. A. (1996). Psychosocial treatment for generalized anxiety disorder. In *Long-term Treatments of Anxiety Disorders*, ed. M. R. Mavissakalian and R. F. Prien, pp. 171–99. Washington, DC: American Psychiatric Press.

Borkovec, T. D., Robinson, E., Pruzinsky, T., and DePree, J. A. (1983). Preliminary exploration of worry: some characteristics and processes. *Behaviour Research and Therapy*, **21**, 9–16.

Borkovec, T. D., Mathews, A. M., Chambers, A., et al. (1987). The effects of relaxation training with cognitive or nondirective therapy and the role of relaxation-induced anxiety in the treatment of generalized anxiety. *Journal of Consulting and Clinical Psychology*, **55**, 883–8.

Borkovec, T. D., Shadick, R. N., and Hopkins, M. (1991). The nature of normal and pathological worry. In *Chronic Anxiety: Generalized Anxiety Disorder and Mixed Anxiety–Depression*, ed. R. M. Rapee and D. H. Barlow, pp. 29–51. New York: Guilford Press.

Borkovec, T. D., Roemer, L., and Kinyon, J. (1995). Disclosure and worry: opposite sides of the emotional processing coin. In *Emotion, Disclosure, and Health*, ed. J. W. Pennebaker, pp. 47–70. Washington, DC: American Psychiatric Association.

Borkovec, T. D., Ray, W. J., and Stöber, J. (1998). Worry: a cognitive phenomenon intimately linked to affective, physiological, and interpersonal behavioral processes. *Cognitive Therapy and Research*, **22**, 561–76.

Borkovec, T. D., Alcaine, O., and Behar, E. (in press). Avoidance theory of worry and generalized anxiety disorder. In *Generalized Anxiety Disorder: Advances in Research and Practice*, ed. In R. G. Heimberg, C. L. Turk, and D. S. Mennin. New York: Guilford Press.

Brawman-Mintzer, O., Lydiard, R. B., Emmanuel, N., et al. (1993). Psychiatric comorbidity in patients with generalized anxiety disorder. *American Journal of Psychiatry*, **150**, 1216–18.

Breitholtz, E., Westling, B. E., and Öst, L.-G. (1998). Cognitions in generalized anxiety disorder and panic disorder patients. *Journal of Anxiety Disorders*, **12**, 567–77.

Brown, T. A. and Barlow, D. H. (1992). Comorbidity among anxiety disorders: implications for treatment and DSM-IV. *Journal of Consulting and Clinical Psychology*, **60**, 835–44.

Brown, T. A., Barlow, D. H., and Liebowitz, M. R. (1994). The empirical basis of generalized anxiety disorder. *American Journal of Psychiatry*, **151**, 1272–80.

Brown, T. A., DiNardo, P. A., Lehman, C. L., and Campbell, L. A. (2001). Reliability of DSM-IV anxiety and mood disorders: implications for the classification of emotional disorders. *Journal of Abnormal Psychology*, **110**, 49–58.

Butler, G. (1993). Predicting outcome after treatment for generalised anxiety disorder. *Behaviour Research and Therapy*, **31**, 211–13.

Butler, G. and Anastasiades, P. (1988). Predicting response to anxiety management in patients with generalised anxiety disorder. *Behaviour Research and Therapy*, **26**, 531–4.

Butler, G., Cullington, A., Hibbert, G., Klimes, I., and Gelder, M. (1987). Anxiety management for persistent generalised anxiety. *British Journal of Psychiatry*, **151**, 535–42.

Butler, G., Fennell, M., Robson, P., and Gelder, M. (1991). Comparison of behavior therapy and cognitive behavior therapy in the treatment of generalized anxiety disorder. *Journal of Consulting and Clinical Psychology*, **59**, 167–75.

Butler, G., Wells, A., and Dewick, H. (1995). Differential effects of worry and imagery after exposure to a stressful stimulus: a pilot study. *Behavioural and Cognitive Psychotherapy*, **23**, 45–56.

Carter, W. R., Johnson, M. C., and Borkovec, T. D. (1986). Worry: an electrocortical analysis. *Advances in Behaviour Research and Therapy*, **8**, 193–204.

Cassidy, J. (1995). Attachment and generalized anxiety disorder. In *Emotion, Cognition, and Representation. Rochester Symposium on Developmental Psychopathology*, vol. 6, ed. D. Cicchetti and S. L. Toth, pp. 343–370. Rochester, NY: University of Rochester Press.

Chambless, D. L. and Gillis, M. M. (1993). Cognitive therapy of anxiety disorders. *Journal of Consulting and Clinical Psychology*, **61**, 248–60.

Chambless, D. L., Tran, G. Q., and Glass, C. R. (1997). Predictors of response to cognitive-behavioral group therapy for social phobia. *Journal of Anxiety Disorders*, **11**, 221–40.

Cicchetti, D., Ackerman, B. P., and Izard, C. E. (1995). Emotions and emotion regulation in developmental psychopathology. *Development and Psychopathology*, **7**, 1–10.

Cole, P. M., Michel, M. K., and O'Donnell-Teti, L. (1994). The development of emotion regulation and dysregulation: a clinical perspective. *Monographs of the Society for Research in Child Development*, **59**, 73–100.

Cox, B. J., Wessel, I., Norton, G. R., Swinson, R. P., and Direnfeld, D. M. (1995). Publication trends in anxiety disorders research: 1990–1992. *Journal of Anxiety Disorders*, **9**, 531–8.

Craske, M. G., Barlow, D. H., and Zinbarg, R. E. (1995). *Mastery of your Anxiety and Worry*. Albany, NY: Graywind.

Crits-Christoph, P., Crits-Christoph, K., Wolf-Palacio, D., Fichter, M., and Rudick, D. (1995). Brief supportive-expressive psychodynamic therapy for generalized anxiety disorder. In *Dynamic Therapies for Psychiatric Disorders (Axis I)*, ed. J. P. Barber and P. Crits-Christoph, pp. 43–83. New York, NY: Basic Books.

Damasio, A. R. (1994). *Descartes' Error: Emotion, Reason, and the Human Brain*. New York: Avon.

Dodge, K. A. and Garber, J. (1991). Domains of emotion regulation. In *The Development of Emotion Regulation and Dysregulation*, ed. J. Garber and K. A. Dodge, pp. 3–14. Cambridge, England: Cambridge University Press.

Dugas, M. J., Gagnon, F., Ladouceur, R., and Freeston, M. H. (1998). Generalized anxiety disorder: a preliminary test of a conceptual model. *Behaviour Research and Therapy*, **36**, 215–26.

Ekman, P. and Davidson, R. J. (eds) (1994). *The Nature of Emotion: Fundamental Questions*. New York: Oxford University Press.

Foa, E. B. and Kozak, M. J. (1986). Emotional processing of fear: exposure to corrective information. *Psychological Bulletin*, **99**, 20–35.

Freeston, M. H., Dugas, M. J., and Ladouceur, R. (1996). Thoughts, images, worry, and anxiety. *Cognitive Therapy and Research*, **20**, 265–73.

Gould, R. A., Otto, M. W., Pollack, M. H., and Yap, L. (1997). Cognitive behavioral and pharmacological treatment of generalized anxiety disorder: a preliminary meta-analyis. *Behavior Therapy*, **28**, 285–305.

Greenberg, L. S. (1994). Acceptance in experiental therapy. In *Acceptance and Change: Content and Context in Psychotherapy*, ed. S. C. Hayes, N. S. Jacobson, V. M. Follette, and M. J. Dougher, pp. 53–67. Reno, NV: Context Press.

Greenberg, L. S. and Safran, J. D. (1987). *Emotion in Psychotherapy: Affect, Cognition, and the Process of Change*. New York: Guilford Press.

Greenberg, P. E., Sisitsky, T., Kessler, R. C., et al. (1999). The economic burden of anxiety disorders in the 1990s. *Journal of Clinical Psychiatry*, **60**, 427–35.

Gross, J. J. (1998). The emerging field of emotion regulation: an integrative review. *Review of General Psychology*, **2**, 271–99.

Gross, J. J. and Muñoz, R. F. (1995). Emotion regulation and mental health. *Clinical Psychology: Science and Practice*, **2**, 151–64.

Hayes, S. C., Strosahl, K. D., and Wilson, K. G. (1999). *Acceptance and Commitment Therapy: An Experiental Approach to Behavior Change*. New York: Guilford Press.

Hazlett, R. L., McLeod, D. R., and Hoehn-Saric, R. (1994). Muscle tension in generalized anxiety disorder: elevated muscle tonus or agitated movement? *Psychophysiology*, **31**, 189–95.

Heimberg, R. G., Liebowitz, M. R., Hope, D. A., and Schneier, F. R. (eds) (1995). *Social Phobia: Diagnosis, Assessment, and Treatment*. New York: Guilford Press.

Hoehn-Saric, R. and McLeod, D. R. (1988). The peripheral sympathetic nervous system: its role in normal and pathologic anxiety. *Psychiatric Clinics of North America*, **11**, 375–86.

Hoehn-Saric, R., McLeod, D. R., and Zimmerli, W. D. (1989). Somatic manifestations in women with generalized anxiety disorder: psychophysiological responses to psychological stress. *Archives of General Psychiatry*, **46**, 1113–19.

Izard, C. E. (1993). Four systems for emotion activation: cognitive and noncognitive processes. *Psychological Review*, **100**, 68–90.

Kabat-Zinn, J., Massion, A. O., Kristeller, J., et al. (1992). Effectiveness of a meditation-based stress reduction program in the treatment of anxiety disorders. *American Journal of Psychiatry*, **149**, 936–43.

Kendler, K. S., Neale, M. C., Kessler, R. C., and Heath, A. C. (1992). Major depression and generalized anxiety disorder: same genes, (partly) different environments? *Archives of General Psychiatry*, **49**, 716–22.

Kessler, R. C., McGonagle, K. A., Zhao, S., et al. (1994). Lifetime and 12-month prevalence of DSM-III-R psychiatric disorders in the United States: results from the National Comorbidity Survey. *Archives of General Psychiatry*, **51**, 8–19.

Kessler, R., Walters, E. E., and Wittchen, H. U. (in press). The epidemiology of generalized anxiety disorder. In *Generalized Anxiety Disorder: Advances in Research and Practice*, ed. R. G. Heimberg, C. L. Turk, and D. S. Mennin. New York: Guilford Press.

Ladouceur, R., Dugas, M. J., Freeston, M. H., et al. (2000). Efficacy of a new cognitive-behavioral treatment for generalized anxiety disorder: evaluation in a controlled clinical trial. *Journal of Consulting and Clinical Psychology*, **68**, 957–64.

Lang, P. J. (1985). The cognitive psychophysiology of emotion: fear and anxiety. In *Anxiety and the Anxiety Disorders*, ed. A. H. Tuma and J. D. Maser, pp. 131–70. Hillsdale, NJ: Erlbaum.

Lazarus, R. S. (1984). On the primacy of cognition. *American Psychologist*, **39**, 124–9.

LeDoux, J. E. (1996). *The Emotional Brain: The Mysterious Underpinnings of Emotional Life.* New York: Simon & Schuster.

Linehan, M. M. (1993). *Cognitive-Behavioral Treatment of Borderline Personality Disorder.* New York: Guilford Press.

Lyonfields, J. D., Borkovec, T. D., and Thayer, J. F. (1995). Vagal tone in generalized anxiety disorder and the effects of aversive imagery and worrisome thinking. *Behavior Therapy*, **26**, 457–66.

Mahoney, M. J. (1995). *Cognitive and Constructivist Psychotherapies: Theory, Research, and Practice.* New York: Springer.

Marten, P. A., Brown, T. A., Barlow, D. H., et al. (1993). Evaluation of the ratings comprising the associated symptom criterion of DSM-III-R generalized anxiety disorder. *Journal of Nervous and Mental Disease*, **181**, 676–82.

Massion, A. O., Warshaw, M. G., and Keller, M. B. (1993). Quality of life and psychiatric morbidity in panic disorder and generalized anxiety disorder. *American Journal of Psychiatry*, **150**, 600–7.

McLeod, J. D. (1994). Anxiety disorders and marital quality. *Journal of Abnormal Psychology*, **103**, 767–76.

McNally, R. J. (1994). *Panic Disorder: A Critical Analysis.* New York: Guilford Press.

Mennin, D. S. (2001). *Examining the Relationship between Emotion and Worry: A Test of the Avoidance Theory of Generalized Anxiety Disorder.* Doctoral dissertation. Temple University, Philadelphia, PA.

Newman, M. G. (2000). Recommendations for a cost-offset model of psychotherapy allocation using generalized anxiety disorder as an example. *Journal of Consulting and Clinical Psychology*, **68**, 549–55.

Newman, M. G., Castonguay, L. G., Borkovec, T. D., and Molnar, C. (in press). Integrative therapy for generalized anxiety disorder. In *Generalized Anxiety Disorder: Advances in Research and Practice*, ed. R. G. Heimberg, C. L. Turk, and D. S. Mennin, New York: Guilford Press.

Norton, G. R., Cox, B. J., Asmundson, G. J. G., and Maser, J. D. (1995). The growth of research on anxiety disorders in the 1980s. *Journal of Anxiety Disorders*, **9**, 75–85.

Plutchik, R. (1990). Emotions and psychotherapy: a psychoevolutionary perspective. In *Emotion: Theory, Research, and Experience*, vol. 5, ed. R. Plutchik and H. Kellerman, pp. 3–41. San Diego, CA: Academic Press.

Rachman, S. (1980). Emotional processing. *Behaviour Research and Therapy*, **18**, 51–60.

Rapee, R. M. (1991). Generalized anxiety disorder: a review of clinical features and theoretical concepts. *Clinical Psychology Review*, **11**, 419–40.

Robins, L. N., Helzer, J. E., Weissman, M. M., et al. (1984). Lifetime prevalence of specific psychiatric disorders in three sites. *Archives of General Psychiatry*, **41**, 949–58.

Roemer, L. and Orsillo, S. M. (2002). Expanding our conceptualization of and treatment for generalized anxiety disorder: integrating mindfulness/acceptance-based approaches with existing cognitive-behavioral models. *Clinical Psychology: Science and Practice*, **9**, 54–68.

Roy-Byrne, P. P. (1996). Generalized anxiety and mixed anxiety–depression: association with disability and health care utilization. *Journal of Clinical Psychiatry*, **57**, 86–91.

Roy-Byrne, P. P. and Katon, W. (1997). Generalized anxiety disorder in primary care: the precursor/modifier pathway to increased health care utilization. *Journal of Clinical Psychiatry*, **58**, 34–40.

Saarni, C. (1990). Emotional competence: how emotions and relationships become integrated. In *Socioemotional Development. Nebraska Symposium on Motivation, 1988*, ed. R. A. Thompson, pp. 115–82. Lincoln, NE: University of Nebraska Press.

Saarni, C. (1999). *The Development of Emotional Competence*. New York: Guilford Press.

Safran, J. D. (1998). *Widening the Scope of Cognitive Therapy: The Therapeutic Relationship, Emotion, and the Process of Change*. Northvale, NY: Jason Aronson.

Safran, J. D. and Segal, Z. V. (1990). *Interpersonal Process in Cognitive Therapy*. New York: Jason Aronson.

Sanderson, W. C. and Barlow, D. H. (1990). A description of patients diagnosed with DSM-III-R generalized anxiety disorder. *Journal of Nervous and Mental Disease*, **178**, 588–91.

Sanderson, W. C., DiNardo, P. A., Rapee, R. M., and Barlow, D. H. (1990). Syndrome comorbidity in patients diagnosed with a DSM-III–R anxiety disorder. *Journal of Abnormal Psychology*, **99**, 308–12.

Sanderson, W. C., Wetzler, S., Beck, A. T., and Betz, F. (1994a). Prevalence of personality disorders among patients with anxiety disorders. *Psychiatry Research*, **51**, 167–74.

Sanderson, W. C., Beck, A. T., and McGinn, L. K. (1994b). Cognitive therapy for generalized anxiety disorder: significance of comorbid personality disorders. *Journal of Cognitive Psychotherapy: An International Quarterly*, **8**, 13–18.

Skinner, B. F. (1953). *Science and Human Behavior*. New York: Free Press.

Stanley, M. A., Beck, J. G., and Glassco, J. D. (1996). Treatment of generalized anxiety disorder in older adults: a preliminary comparison of cognitive-behavioral and supportive approaches. *Behavior Therapy*, **27**, 565–81.

Starcevic, V. and Bogojevic, G. (1999). The concept of generalized anxiety disorder: between the too narrow and too wide diagnostic criteria. *Psychopathology*, **32**, 5–11.

Stöber, J. (2000). Worry, thoughts, and images: a new conceptualization. In *Generative Mental Processes and Cognitive Resources: Integrative Research on Adaptation and Control*, ed. U. von Hecker, S. Dutke, and G. Sedek, pp. 223–44. Dordrecht, Netherlands: Kluwer.

Suinn, R. M. and Richardson, F. (1971). Anxiety management training: a nonspecific behavior therapy program for anxiety control. *Behavior Therapy*, **2**, 498–510.

Tallis, F. and Eysenck, M. W. (1994). Worry: mechanisms and modulating influences. *Behavioural and Cognitive Psychotherapy*, **22**, 37–56.

Thayer, J. F., Friedman, B. H., and Borkovec, T. D. (1996). Autonomic characteristics of generalized anxiety disorder and worry. *Biological Psychiatry*, **39**, 255–66.

Vrana, S. R., Cuthbert, B. N., and Lang, P. J. (1986). Fear imagery and text processing. *Psychophysiology*, **23**, 247–53.

Wells, A. (1999). A cognitive model of generalized anxiety disorder. *Behavior Modification*, **23**, 526–55.

Wells, A. and Papageorgiou, C. (1995). Worry and the incubation of intrusive images following stress. *Behaviour Research and Therapy*, **33**, 579–83.

White, J., Keenan, M., and Brooks, N. (1992). Stress control: a controlled comparative investigation of large group therapy for generalized anxiety disorder. *Behavioural Psychotherapy*, **20**, 97–113.

Wittchen, H.-U., Zhao, S., Kessler, R. C., and Eaton, W. W. (1994). DSM-III-R generalized anxiety disorder in the National Comorbidity Survey. *Archives of General Psychiatry*, **51**, 355–64.

Yonkers, K. A., Warshaw, M. G., Massion, A. O., and Keller, M. B. (1996). Phenomenology and course of generalised anxiety disorder. *British Journal of Psychiatry*, **168**, 308–13.

5

Cognitive theory and therapy of obsessions and compulsions

David A. Clark[1] and Christine Purdon[2]

[1] University of New Brunswick, Fredericton, Canada
[2] University of Waterloo, Waterloo, Ontario, Canada

Introduction

Obsessive-compulsive disorder (OCD) is one of the major anxiety disorders in the fourth edition of *Diagnostic and Statistical Manual of Mental Disorders* (DSM-IV: American Psychiatric Association, 1994). The disorder is characterized by persistent obsessions and compulsions that are time-consuming or cause marked distress or impairment and are perceived by the patient to be excessive or unreasonable. Obsessions are intrusive, recurrent, and persistent thoughts, images, or impulses that are unacceptable, unwanted, and usually associated with subjective resistance (Rachman and Hodgson, 1980). The content of the obsession is egodystonic in that it deals with themes that are inconsistent or even alien to one's sense of self, values, or usual ways of behaving (Purdon and Clark, 1999). Because of this the occurrence of the obsession is highly distressing for individuals with OCD, even though they may acknowledge that the intrusion is senseless and irrational (Rachman and Hodgson, 1980). The most common obsessions involve concerns about dirt/disease contamination, accidents, unintended aggression or violence towards others, inappropriate sexual acts, mistakes, doubt, blasphemous thoughts, orderliness and symmetry, and hoarding.

Compulsions are repetitive, stereotypic, and intentional behavioral or mental responses that are subjectively experienced as an urge or pressure to act. The OCD patient may view the compulsion as excessive or exaggerated but the urge to act is not necessarily resisted in all cases. Compulsions are usually triggered by the occurrence of a distressing obsession. Although there is a sense of reduced volition over the compulsion, it is strengthened by relatively quick but temporary reduction in anxiety associated with the obsession once the compulsive act is executed to completion (Rachman and Hodgson, 1980; American Psychiatric Association, 1994;

Rachman and Shafran, 1998). The main types of compulsions are washing, checking, ordering, reassurance-seeking, and hoarding (Rachman and Shafran, 1998). Checking, cleaning/washing, and covert or mental rituals are the most common types of compulsions, followed by repeating, ordering, hoarding, and counting (Foa and Kozak, 1995). A typical obsessive-compulsive cycle is exemplified by the compulsive washer who has the obsession "Maybe I am contaminated with cancer germs from touching this doorknob" and then proceeds to wash his or her hands repeatedly (compulsion) until he or she feels relieved that he or she is no longer in danger of contamination. In the DSM-IV field trial, Foa and Kozak (1995) found that 96% of individuals with OCD had both obsessions and compulsions, 2% had mainly obsessions, and 2% had predominantly compulsions.

OCD generally follows a chronic, fluctuating clinical course with little evidence of spontaneous remission of symptoms (Rasmussen and Eisen, 1992). Onset is usually gradual and most often occurs in early adolescence to young adulthood (Rasmussen and Tsuang, 1986). Chronic waxing and waning of symptoms is typical, with first treatment sought many years (average is 7 years) after the initial onset of significant symptoms. Gender distribution is approximately equal, with the disorder associated with significant impairment in psychosocial and occupational functioning. There is a high rate of comorbidity for major depression, panic disorder, social phobia, and generalized anxiety disorder (Crino and Andrews, 1996; Antony et al., 1998). Based on the Epidemiological Catchment Area (ECA) study (Karno and Golding, 1991), the lifetime prevalence of OCD has been estimated at 2–3%, although Antony et al. (1998) have questioned whether this is an overestimate because the interview schedule used in the ECA, the Diagnostic Interview Schedule, may overdiagnosis anxiety disorders and be unreliable and invalid for detecting OCD.

Until the mid-1960s there were no effective psychological or pharmacological treatments for OCD. Psychoanalysis and early behavioral interventions such as systematic desensitization, modeling, operant conditioning, aversion relief, and re-laxation therapy produced at best modest and rather mixed benefits (Emmelkamp, 1982; Foa et al., 1998). Given the chronic nature of the disorder, this meant that individuals with OCD could suffer for decades without relief from their debilitating symptoms. In the last 20 years this situation has changed dramatically. There is now considerable evidence that certain medications, in particular, clomipramine, fluox-etine, fluvoxamine, sertraline, and paroxetine, are effective in producing a 25–35% reduction in OC symptoms and so are considered efficacious in the treatment of the acute phase of the disorder (for reviews see March et al., 1997; Pigott and Seay, 1998, 2000). As well, a number of well-controlled clinical trials have shown that a behavioral treatment consisting of exposure and response prevention (ERP) can produce even greater symptom reduction and longer-lasting results than medication alone in

60–85% of OCD patients who complete a trial of ERP (for reviews and metaanalyses see Rachman and Hodgson, 1980; Emmelkamp, 1982; Foa et al., 1985; van Balkom et al., 1994; Stanley and Turner, 1995; Foa and Kozak, 1996; Abramowitz, 1998; Kozak et al., 2000). Although there is considerable optimism given the advances made in the treatment of OCD, a number of thorny treatment issues persist, leading researchers to search for ways to enhance conventional treatments of OCD.

This chapter is divided into two main sections. In the first part we examine cognitive theory and research on OCD. We begin by considering problems with the prevailing behavioral theory of OCD advanced by Rachman and colleagues in the mid-1970s. We then consider the empirical evidence for the more contemporary cognitive-behavioral models of OCD proposed by Salkovskis, Rachman, and others, and whether these proposals do in fact provide a better account of OCD. We will also briefly review information-processing studies that have searched for general processing deficits in OCD. In the second section of the chapter we examine reasons for the dissatisfaction with ERP and the empirical evidence for cognitive interventions as augmentation for standard ERP. The chapter concludes with a summary and consideration for future directions.

Cognitive theory and research on OCD

Behavioral theory of OCD

Early behavioral accounts of OCD were rooted in Mowrer's (1939, 1953, 1960) two-stage learning theory of fear and avoidance. Obsessions, like other phobic stimuli, were considered noxious conditioned stimuli that cause personal pain or distress and persist because of the patient's increased responsiveness (i.e., sensitization) and failure to habituate to the obsession (Rachman, 1971, 1976a, 1978). Compulsive responses or neutralizing activities are strengthened because of avoidance learning. The compulsive act temporarily reduces the anxiety associated with the obsession (Rachman and Hodgson, 1980; Emmelkamp, 1982). Because fear reduction is reinforcing, the compulsive activity becomes powerfully linked to the obsession as a strategy for reducing distress.

The behavioral theory of obsessions and compulsions was an intuitively appealing explanation for the persistence, if not etiology, of obsessional phenomena. There was considerable empirical evidence that obsessions had phobic-like qualities and that most compulsions served to bring temporary relief from the distressing obsessions (see Rachman and Hodgson, 1980; Clark, 2004 for reviews). Moreover, adaptations of Victor Meyer's (1966) ERP therapy, with its behavioral orientation, proved to be a very effective intervention for OCD. By the end of the 1970s, a credible explanation and highly efficacious treatment were available for OCD that were both based on a learning paradigm.

By 1980 and the publication of Rachman and Hodgson's seminal work on OCD entitled *Obsessions and Compulsions*, inconsistencies were beginning to emerge in the behavioral account of OCD. There was evidence: (1) that most obsessions are not the result of traumatic learning; (2) that several obsessions can occur simultaneously; (3) that the content and focus of obsessions can regularly change; (4) that in some cases compulsions result in no change to or an increase in subjective discomfort; (5) that factors like presence of therapist can change an individual's experience of the obsession; (6) of the nonrandom distribution of obsessional content; and (7) that, contrary to predictions, obsessions without overt compulsions are more severe than obsessions with compulsions. All of these features of the disorder were difficult to accommodate with the standard behavioral explanation for OCD. In addition, criticisms raised with the two-factor theory of fears and phobias (Rachman, 1976b, 1977), more generally, were applicable to the behavioral account of OCD. These shortcomings, along with the obvious prominence of dysfunctional cognition in OCD, led to the conclusion that obsessional phenomena were not adequately explained by the behavioral theory. This resulted in a switch in focus to a more cognitive perspective in theory and research on OCD.

General cognitive deficit theory

Some of the earliest research on cognitive dysfunction in OCD proposed that the uncontrolled, repeated occurrence of rather bizarre thoughts and behaviors is the result of deficits or biases in certain cognitive processes. Research focused on whether recurrent obsessions and repetitive compulsions are the result of: (1) heightened attentional bias for threatening material leading to more elaborated encoding of this material; (2) poor general memory for actions or a reality-monitoring deficit; or (3) lowered confidence or bias in memory functioning, resulting in reduced decision-making ability (McNally, 2000). Neuropsychological investigations have been conducted on OCD to determine whether the disorder is associated with declines in general intellectual functioning, memory, frontal lobe functioning, or underinclusive bias on category formation tasks (for review, see Tallis, 1995).

Rachman and Shafran (1998) noted two main questions that have spurred research on general cognitive deficits in OCD. Why are people with OCD so sensitive to certain "threat" stimuli, and why do they appear to have such poor memory for their compulsive actions (i.e., "did I really lock the door?")? The heightened attentional bias for threat in OCD is similar to the attentional bias noted more generally for anxiety disorders (Williams et al., 1997). This attentional bias is considered a preconscious, automatic scanning of the environment for threat-related stimuli. Once detected, threatening stimuli are given attentional priority that results in the activation and hypervalence of danger and threat memory structures or schemas (Beck and Emery, 1985). Activation of these schemas causes further deliberate and effortful elaboration of the threatening material that is evident in the form of worry and various escape and avoidance strategies designed to eliminate exposure to the threat or danger and reinstate a sense of safety (Beck and Clark, 1997).

Experimental studies involving dichotic listening, modified dot probe detection, Stroop color naming, and lexical decision-making tasks have found that OCD patients do show a heightened attentional bias for threat cues but only if they are related to their primary OC-related concerns (Foa and McNally, 1986; Foa et al., 1993; Sauteraud et al., 1995; Tata et al., 1996). That is, compulsive washers, for example, will show heightened sensitivity to contamination words but not to more general threat stimuli like death, illness, or injury (McNally, 2000). Tata et al. (1996) employed a modified dot probe detection task to show that OCD patients had automatic vigilance for threat but only for contamination threat words, whereas the high-trait anxious group exhibited vigilance for social anxiety words but not contamination words. The authors concluded that individuals with OCD do have an automatic preconscious vigilance for threat but, unlike clinically anxious or high-trait anxious individuals, this threat bias is confined to content-specific threat cues directly related to the individual's primary obsessional concern. However, other studies have failed to find a content-specific threat bias in OCD (J. E. Calamari et al., unpublished data; Kyrios and Andrews, 1998). Given these mixed findings, Summerfeldt and Endler (1998) concluded in their review that evidence of attentional threat bias in OCD was not as robust as seen in other anxiety disorders, whereas McNally (2000) concluded that "patients with OCD exhibit both context-dependent and context-independent abnormalities in attentional processing" (pp. 113–114).

McNally (2000) also concluded that OCD patients may have a general inability to inhibit the processing of irrelevant information. Clinically this would be evident in the obsessional person's overinclusiveness or tendency to give excessive focus on unimportant environmental details (Enright and Beech, 1990, 1993). Clayton et al. (1999) found that, compared to individuals with panic disorder and nonclinical controls, OCD patients showed a reduced ability to ignore unimportant external (sensory) and internal (cognitive) stimuli.

Given that individuals with OCD, especially those with checking compulsions, often complain that they cannot clearly remember whether they performed certain actions (i.e., did I check the light switch?), there has been considerable research interest in the possibility of memory impairment in OCD. One possibility is that compulsive checkers have a poor memory for their actions. Sher et al. (1983), for example, found that students with high scores on the Maudsley Obsessive-Compulsive Inventory Checking subscale had poorer recall of their actions on seven separate tasks than noncheckers. Since then a number of studies have replicated this memory-for-action deficit in nonclinical checkers and individuals with diagnosable checking compulsions. Ecker and Engelkamp (1995) found poorer free recall of motorically encoded actions for clinical OCD checkers but not for the high-checking nonclinical group. Tallis (1995) concluded from his review of the literature that there is evidence of memory-for-action and nonverbal memory deficits in OC checking. On the other hand, McNally (2000) concluded that there are no demonstrated memory deficits in OCD.

A number of studies have investigated whether obsessional checkers have impaired reality monitoring, that is, difficulty in determining whether a memory is from a perception or one's imagination (McNally, 2000). Ecker and Engelkamp (1995) found a trend for OC checkers to have a higher frequency of confusion between motor ("doing something") and motor-imaginal ("imagine that you did something") encoding than the low-checking control group. McNally (2000), however, reviewed a number of studies that failed to find reality-monitoring deficits in OC checkers.

Two further considerations are possible concerning memory functioning in OCD. First, it may be that real memory deficits are not present but rather obsessional individuals may have less confidence in their memory ability. Reduced confidence in memory function could trigger the doubting, checking, and repetitions that are characteristic of OCD. MacDonald et al. (1997) found that OCD patients with excessive checking performed similar to nonchecking OCD and nonclinical controls on a recognition and recall memory task. However, the OC checkers had significantly lower confidence ratings in their recognition memory judgments than the other two groups. McNally (2000) and Rachman and Shafran (1998) both concluded that there is mounting evidence that OC patients may suffer from a lack of confidence in their memory performance. Finally, in a recent study, Radomsky and Rachman (1999) found that individuals with diagnosable OCD and a fear of contamination actually showed an enhanced memory bias for contaminated objects rather than for clean ones. This memory bias was not evident in the general anxiety and nonclinical control groups.

Over the years a number of cognitive deficits have been proposed to explain obsessive-compulsive phenomena. Despite concerted efforts to find general memory deficits, or impairments in the encoding, organization, and integration of information (Reed, 1985) there appears to be little consistent evidence of cognitive deficits at the general or nonspecific level. There does appear to be attentional and possibly memory biases for threatening material that is specifically linked to the OC patients' primary symptomatic concerns. Individuals with OCD may also have greater difficulty inhibiting irrelevant stimuli (could this result in poorer thought suppression? McNally, 2000), and they probably have lower confidence in their memory ability. Moreover, Salkovskis (1996) noted that general deficit theories cannot account for key aspects of OC phenomenology. Individuals with OCD do not show information processing or memory impairments outside the primary concerns related to their OCD. For this reason cognitive-clinical researchers have turned to more specific, content-based constructs derived from the clinical theories of Beck (1967) and Rachman and Hodgson (1980) to explain the psychological basis of OCD.

Specific cognitive content theories
Salkovskis' responsibility theory of OCD

Salkovskis is credited with proposing one of the first comprehensive and detailed cognitive-behavioral models of OCD that attempted to address key aspects of obsessional phenomenology. The initial theory and associated therapy was first published in *Behaviour Research and Therapy* in 1985 and advocated an amalgamation of behavioral theory and therapy of OCD with elements from Beck's cognitive therapy of depression. The primary focus was on the development of a theory and treatment for obsessional ruminations that would address shortcomings with the current behavioral approach. The model has since been elaborated in a number of publications (Salkovskis, 1985, 1989, 1996, 1998; Salkovskis et al., 1995), including the current chapter by Salkovskis and Wahl (Chapter 7). Based on research by Rachman and de Silva (1978), Salkovskis' model begins with the assertion that all individuals experience unwanted, somewhat distressing, ego-alien intrusive thoughts, images, or impulses that are similar in content to clinical obsessions. However the key process that transforms a normal mental intrusion into a recurrent, persistent obsession is the meaning attached to the intrusion by individuals predisposed to OCD. Individuals with a predisposition to misinterpret the occurrence and content of their unwanted intrusive thoughts as indicating personal *responsibility* will in turn experience greater discomfort and an urge to neutralize or eliminate this inflated sense of responsibility. These appraisals of personal responsibility for preventing subjectively crucial negative outcomes erroneously ascribed to certain unwanted mental intrusions are derived from the activation of enduring, more general beliefs concerning responsibility for harm. According to Salkovskis' model, psychological vulnerability for OCD is found in these underlying responsibility beliefs that have been instilled in predisposed individuals because of childhood upbringing and experiences that erroneously reinforced the view that one's thoughts, actions, or inactions contributed to a serious misfortune (Salkovskis et al., 1999). Once personal responsibility beliefs and interpretations for the occurrence or prevention of harm or threat to self or others are activated in response to an unwanted intrusive thought, image, or impulse, a whole cascade of obsessional phenomenology occurs. The intrusive thought is felt to be more discomforting, attention is directed toward the intrusion and its triggers, the intrusion itself becomes more salient or accessible, and covert or overt neutralization responses are instigated designed to reduce this inflated sense of responsibility. The end result is that obsessional individuals try too hard to control their unwanted thoughts, which turns out to be futile and counterproductive, resulting in a further escalation in the recurrence, intensity, and duration of the obsession (Salkovskis and Wahl, 2001).

Responsibility beliefs and appraisals have probably received more empirical investigation than any other cognitive-clinical construct proposed by contemporary cognitive-behavioral therapy theories of OCD. A number of studies have found that responsibility beliefs and appraisals are elevated in individuals with OCD compared to nonobsessional anxious and nonclinical controls, and that measures of responsibility are specifically associated with OC symptom measures independent of anxiety and depression level (Rhéaume et al., 1994, 1995; Steketee et al., 1998; Salkovskis et al., 2000; Obsessive Compulsive Cognitions Working Group, 2001, 2002). However, other studies have not found elevated scores on responsibility measures to differentiate OCD, or to show a particularly strong or specific relation with OC symptom measures (Wells and Papageorgiou, 1998; Wilson and Chambless, 1999). In fact, other cognitive constructs, like thought–action fusion (TAF), may be more characteristic of obsessional thinking than general responsibility beliefs and appraisals (Rachman et al., 1995; Emmelkamp and Aardema, 1999). Experiments in which level of perceived personal responsibility was manipulated have shown that high perceived responsibility over negative outcomes can lead to an increase in obsessional behaviors, estimates of perceived threat and unwanted intrusive thinking (Ladouceur et al., 1995; Bouchard et al., 1999; Menzies et al., 2000). Based on an experimental manipulation involving a sample of 30 OCD patients, Lopatka and Rachman (1995) found that a decrease in perceived responsibility resulted in a significant decline in the urge to check, whereas an increase in perceived responsibility led to a nonsignificant increase in checking urges.

Generally the research is somewhat supportive of Salkovskis' proposition that perceived responsibility for the occurrence or prevention of negative outcomes thought to be associated with obsessions may be critical in OCD. However, its role and function in the pathogenesis of obsessions may be more limited than proposed by Salkovskis. The importance of inflated responsibility may be confined to certain subtypes of OCD such as compulsive checkers (Rhéaume et al., 1995; Rachman and Shafran, 1998). Although–TAF and inflated responsibility are theoretically linked (Rachman, 1993; Rachman and Shafran, 1999), none the less TAF may be a more precise cognitive construct with a stronger relation to obsessionality than the broader concept of inflated responsibility (Rassin et al., 1999). In other words, there is no evidence that appraisals of responsibility have a more prominent role in the pathogenesis of obsessions than other dysfunctional beliefs and appraisals such as TAF, overimportance and control of thoughts, perfectionism, intolerance of uncertainty, or overestimation of threat (Freeston et al., 1996). Furthermore, we do not know whether beliefs and appraisals of responsibility are a cause or consequence of OCD, whether the function of compulsive rituals and other forms of neutralization is to reduce perceived responsibility, whether maladaptive responsibility beliefs are an enduring vulnerability factor for obsessional rumination, and whether the active ingredient in cognitive-behavioral therapy for OCD is the modification of responsibility beliefs and appraisals. Until research is conducted on these issues, the empirical evidence for Salkovskis' responsibility theory of OCD remains largely untested.

Rachman's significance model

Rachman (1997, 1998) proposed a cognitive-behavioral model of OCD that emphasizes four key elements in the development and persistence of obsessional problems. First, he notes that the important themes of all moral systems (e.g., aggression, sex, and blasphemy) are reflected in the main themes of obsessions/intrusive thoughts. As such, obsessions are particularly vulnerable to being experienced as sinful, disgusting, alarming, or threatening. This "catastrophic misinterpretation" of obsessional thoughts will lead to the escalation and persistence of obsessions by many of the same processes involved in the development of panic disorder, which involves a "catastrophic misinterpretation" of bodily sensations (Rachman, 1997). Rachman (1998) proposed that a cognitive bias he labels "thought–action fusion" is especially apt to promote misinterpretations of significance. TAF includes beliefs that having an unacceptable thought increases the likelihood of the negative event represented in the thought coming true (TAF–likelihood) and that having a morally repugnant thought is the moral equivalent to committing a morally repugnant deed (TAF–moral). Closely linked to the TAF bias is the belief that when one is responsible for an outcome, things are more likely to go wrong. This particular bias contributes to anxious feelings and increases threat-sensitivity. Finally, negative mood states like dysphoria can also lead to an escalation and maintenance of obsessions by increasing the accessibility of negative interpretations of the thought as well as the thought itself. In sum, Rachman identifies four vulnerability factors in the development of OCD: elevated moral standards, particular cognitive biases such as TAF, depression, and anxiety.

A key element in Rachman's model is his proposal that vulnerable persons have a tendency to engage in TAF when interpreting the content of their unwanted mental intrusions, and this biased interpretation will be a primary contributor to the catastrophic misinterpretation of personal significance which is pathognomonic to the etiology and persistence of obsessions. Shafran et al. (1996) developed a questionnaire on TAF with three subscales that assessed fusion of thoughts and actions as morally equivalent (TAF–moral), that thoughts could increase the likelihood of negative events happening to friends/relatives (TAF–likelihood other) and that thoughts could raise the probability of negative events happening to one's self (TAF–likelihood self). OCD patients scored significantly higher on all three TAF subscales than nonclinical community adults, but they did not score higher than nonclinical students on TAF–moral or TAF–likelihood self. In the OCD sample, TAF–likelihood others was the only subscale to show a significant correlation with obsessional symptoms after controlling for depression level. Other studies have also found that TAF has a significant relationship with obsessional symptoms (Rachman et al., 1995; Emmelkamp and Aardema, 1999).

TAF has also been investigated by a Dutch research group led by Rassin and colleagues. In their first study nonclinical participants were assigned to either a TAF–likelihood other manipulation condition or a control condition (Rassin et al., 1999). Individuals in the high TAF condition (i.e., a thought of "apple" will cause an unpleasant shock for a "yoked" confederate) experienced significantly more intrusive thoughts, discomfort, anger, and effort to avoid thinking the target thought than those in the control condition. In a second study, Rassin et al. (2000) subjected the TAF scale, White Bear Suppression Inventory and Maudsley Obsessional-Compulsive Inventory to structural equation analysis based on 173 undergraduates. They found that the best-fitting model represented TAF associated with an increase in thought suppression efforts which, in turn, led to more obsessive-compulsive symptoms. Finally, Rassin et al. (2001) examined pre- and posttreatment TAF beliefs and suppression effort in a sample of individuals with OCD and a clinical sample of individuals with other anxiety disorders. They found that TAF beliefs were endorsed equally by both groups pre- and posttreatment, and that TAF scores correlated with general anxiety and mood symptoms in both groups.

The Obsessive Compulsive Cognitions Working Group (OCCWG) is an international group of researchers whose purpose is to investigate the dysfunctional beliefs and appraisals that are characteristic of OCD (OCCWG, 1997). They developed two questionnaires, the Obsessive Beliefs Questionnaire (OBQ) and the Interpretation of Intrusions Inventory (III), whose Importance of Thoughts subscales primarily contain items that reflect TAF. In two separate studies involving large samples of OCD patients, nonobsessional anxious controls, and nonclinical community adults and students, the obsessional group scored significantly higher than all other groups on the OBQ Control of Thoughts, Importance of Thoughts and Responsibility subscales (OCCWG, 2001). As well, Importance of Thoughts beliefs and appraisals were significantly correlated with measures of OC symptoms, although they also showed a strong correlation with depression, anxiety, and worry symptoms, and were very highly correlated with other cognitive domains of OCD such as tolerance of uncertainty, control of thoughts, and overestimation of threat. Finally, in our own research on the appraisal and control of unwanted obsessive-like intrusive thoughts in nonclinical samples, we found that ratings involving

TAF–likelihood were the strongest predictors of the frequency and perceived controllability of unwanted mental intrusions (Purdon and Clark, 1994a, 1994b; Clark et al., 2000).

The above findings, then, indicate that TAF–likelihood, in particular, may be a critical variable that is differentially related to OC symptomatology and so may be an important contributor to overinterpreting the significance and threatening nature of one's unwanted intrusive thoughts. Rachman and Shafran (1999), however, indicated that TAF may not be specific to OCD, and Thordarson and Shafran (2002) concluded that beliefs about the overimportance of thoughts may be a more robust and predictive factor in OCD than TAF. Certainly Rachman's formulation is too recent and relatively untested to draw any firm conclusions about the role and function of TAF in relation to the other variables implicated by the model in the pathogenesis of obsessions.

Failed thought control model

Clark and Purdon (Clark and Purdon, 1993; Purdon and Clark, 1999) are in general agreement with the models proposed by Salkovskis and Rachman, but they argue that beliefs about thought control and its consequences, and the egodystonic nature of the thought, may have a greater role in the pathogenesis of obsessions than previously acknowledged. First, they suggest that individuals may be vulnerable to developing obsessions if they possess rigid, unrealistic, and dysfunctional beliefs about thought control. For example, metacognitive beliefs (i.e., beliefs about one's thought processes) that perfect control over thoughts is possible and desirable, that failing to control thoughts is a sign of mental weakness and instability, and that failures in thought control potentiate loss of control over any or all other domains of functioning, may be particularly relevant to OCD. Second, Purdon and Clark (1999) observe that one distinguishing cardinal feature of obsessions is that they are typically experienced as being egodystonic, or inconsistent with: (1) specific and important schemata about the self; (2) one's past behavior; (3) expectations about one's thoughts; or (4) one's norms and values. For example, an obsession of stabbing or harming a loved one is egodystonic in that it is inconsistent with the person's explicit feelings about the loved one, as well as with his or her values and sense of morality. An obsession that one has left an appliance on and caused a fatal accident is egodystonic in that it violates the individual's sense of him- or herself as a conscientious, reliable, caring, and cautious person. Finally, an obsession that one has become contaminated is egodystonic because it violates that individual's sense of him- or herself as a clean person. Insight into the irrationality of the obsessional doubt can also violate a person's sense of him- or herself as a rational, sane person.

An obsessional thought, then, represents a threat to the self-view and the individual must reconcile the thought's occurrence with the self-view. Drawing from information-processing theory, Purdon and Clark (1999) suggest that one strategy for resolving the inconsistency would be to accommodate the self-schema to incorporate the experience of the thought (e.g., "I suppose even a person like me can have a thought like this, but of course a person like me would never act on this thought"). This may characterize the response of the majority of individuals to their obsessional thoughts. The alternative strategy would be to assimilate the thought (e.g., "Maybe I am the kind of person who would stab a loved one;" "Maybe I actually am a careless person;" "Maybe I am not a rational, sane person"). Given that the thought itself is initially the only evidence that the undesirable personality qualities exist, the individual is likely to assume that absence of the thought would signify that the trait is not present. This, in combination with preexisting beliefs about control, TAF, and responsibility, will result in the individual developing an enormous stake in controlling the thought. By the same token, failures in thought control will be perceived as catastrophic and the individual is likely to increase attempts to control thoughts. The individual's conviction that such undesirable personality characteristics may exist will be strengthened in the face of failures in thought control. Failures in thought control in turn will be experienced as catastrophic, and will result in escalating attempts at thought control and a subsequent decline in mood state. In sum, Purdon and Clark argue that it is not the thought itself that is appraised catastrophically, but rather the meaning of failures in thought control.

Is there any empirical evidence that clinical obsessions are the result of maladaptive beliefs and appraisals about the importance of controlling unwanted egodystonic intrusive thoughts because of the perceived dire consequences of failed thought control? Clark and Purdon (1995) investigated thought control beliefs in a large nonclinical sample and a small sample of individuals with OCD. They found that beliefs about the necessity and importance of thought control predicted obsessional symptomatology in nonclinical individuals, and that individuals with OCD had significantly higher scores on this scale than did the nonclinical sample. Emmelkamp and Aardema (1999) administered a large series of items that assessed OC appraisals and beliefs to a nonclinical community sample and conducted a factor analysis of this item pool. Fourteen separate domains were identified, including beliefs about control (a four-item factor). Beliefs about control, in addition to concern over mistakes, magical thinking, rigidity/morality, and decision-making, were not found to predict OCD symptoms over and above the other belief domains. However, the Control scale consisted of only four items which together do not adequately represent the range of themes contained in our understanding of

OCD-relevant thought control beliefs (Clark and Purdon, 1993; D. A. Clark and C. L. Purdon, unpublished data; Purdon and Clark, 1999).

Based on their own self-report OC belief measure, Steketee et al. (1998) found that all belief scales, except the Coping scale, but including the Control scale, were strongly correlated with each other, affirming that there is significant overlap between the belief/appraisal domains in OCD. The OCD sample showed higher scores than the anxious and nonclinical control groups on all six scales. The anxious controls did not score higher than the nonclinical controls on the Control, Responsibility, and Threat Estimation scales, suggesting that these domains of belief are unique to OCD as opposed to general beliefs characteristic of anxiety. Finally, data from the OCCWG also suggest that control beliefs and appraisals are important predictors of OCD. Once again, the Control of Thoughts subscale of the OBQ and the III, to a lesser extent, was significantly elevated in the OCD sample and correlated with OC symptom measures, although moderate correlations were also evident with depression and anxiety, and the Control subscales were highly intercorrelated with other OC cognition domains (OCCWG, 2001, 2002).

Purdon (2001) developed a questionnaire entitled the Concern over Failures in Thought Control Questionnaire which assesses participants' in vivo appraisal of the meaning of thought *recurrences* whilst control efforts are in operation. This measure includes appraisals reflecting concerns about the need to control thoughts (e.g., "The more I had the thought, the more important it seemed that I try to control it;" "I had the thought more often than I expected;" "The more I had the thought the more strategies I used to control it") as well as appraisals relevant to the domains of TAF and egodystonicity (e.g., "The more I had the thought, the more concerned I became that I secretly wanted it to come true," ". . . the more concerned I became that I was going to cause it to come true"). She found that the perceived need to control thoughts was a significant unique predictor of immediate and subsequent suppression effort, even after controlling for other domains of general thought appraisal. At the same time, appraisals of TAF/egodystonicity emerged as significant unique predictors of anxiety over thought occurrences, thought frequency, and negative mood state.

At this time, there is some preliminary empirical evidence to support at least an association between the main appraisals and beliefs emphasized by leading models of OCD as factors in the development and persistence of obsessions. Moreover, certain cognitive domains like TAF–likelihood may be a particularly robust predictor of obsessional symptoms. As well, there is some emerging evidence that beliefs and interpretations related to the importance of controlling one's thoughts and avoiding perceived negative consequences of failed thought control may be related to obsessionality. However, for the most part these relationships are correlational in nature, they have shown a moderate association with general anxiety and depression symptoms, and the distinctiveness of each domain is questionable given their high subscale intercorrelations. Future work is required to establish the specificity of appraisal in OCD as well as its causal role in the development and maintenance of the disorder.

Cognitive-behavioral treatment of OCD

Exposure and response prevention

In 1966 Victor Meyer published the first case report on the use of ERP for the treatment of OCD. Based on the behavioral learning theory of fears and phobias, the aim of ERP is to extinguish the distress associated with an obsession by systematic, repeated exposure to anxiety-provoking situations that trigger the obsession followed by prevention or blocking of the anxiety-reducing compulsive ritual (Rachman et al., 1970). For example, ERP for compulsive washing would involve repeated, approximately 90-min daily exposure sessions to a hierarchy of situations that would trigger the patient's fear of contamination (e.g., touch floor, dirty clothes, doorknobs, public telephones, toilet seats, etc.). These situations are normally arranged in a hierarchical fashion beginning with moderately distressing situations and proceeding to extremely troubling situations. Kozak and Foa (1997) describe tasks where the compulsive washer carries around toilet paper with a smudge of feces on it or shakes hands with street people. Of course the success of the exposure sessions depends on the person not carrying out any compulsive or neutralizing activities. Patients are verbally encouraged by the therapist to refrain from performing compulsive rituals, avoidance, or reassurance-seeking. Modeling may be used to demonstrate the ERP sequence which is the hallmark of the treatment (Rachman and Hodgson, 1980; Kozak and Foa, 1997). Because most ERP is now done on an outpatient basis with the voluntary participation of the patient, considerable attention is devoted to explaining the behavioral rationale (i.e., extinction of anxiety with prolonged exposure and blocking of neutralizing responses) in order to promote compliance with the treatment program.

ERP has been one of the great success stories for the treatment of an anxiety disorder, thanks in large part to the long and distinguished clinical research of Jack Rachman, Edna Foa, and their colleagues. A number of well-designed treatment outcome studies have shown that ERP produces significant and lasting reductions in obsessive and compulsive symptoms (see reviews by van Balkom et al., 1994; Stanley and Turner, 1995; Steketee and Shapiro, 1995; Foa and Kozak, 1996; Abramowitz, 1998; Foa et al., 1998). In 12 outcome studies an average of 83% were responders at posttreatment and 76% maintained their gains over mean follow-up intervals of 29 months (Foa and Kozak, 1996; Kozak et al., 2000). Foa et al. (1985) reported that 51% of OCD patients treated with ERP were symptom-free or much improved at posttreatment. Hiss et al. (1994) concluded that 15–25% of patients will relapse after completing a course of ERP, which is lower than the relapse rate after discontinuation of pharmacotherapy. Moreover, ERP is at least as effective as, and in most cases superior to pharmacotherapy at posttreatment. When follow-up is considered, patients treated with behavior therapy maintain their gains much better than patients discontinued from their medication, although less advantage is evident if patients are maintained on their medication regimen (Rachman and Hodgson, 1980; van Balkom et al., 1994; Stanley and Turner, 1995; Foa and Kozak, 1996). In a recent National Institute of Mental Health (NIMH)-sponsored collaborative study comparing ERP and clomipramine, Kozak et al. (2000) reported preliminary findings that ERP was superior to clomipramine alone immediately following treatment, but the combination of medication plus ERP was not more successful than ERP alone. Furthermore, at 3-month follow-up ERP was still superior to clomipramine alone after treatment discontinuation. Franklin et al. (2000) reported that the treatment effectiveness of ERP generalized to a more diagnostically heterogeneous OCD fee-for-service outpatient sample who may be more representative of the broader population of OCD patients.

Given the clinical effectiveness of ERP for the treatment of obsessions and compulsions, why have OCD researchers and clinicians explored the inclusion of cognitive interventions in order to augment the effects of traditional behavior therapy? Although ERPs are still considered the essential ingredients for the effective treatment of OCD, a broader cognitive-behavioral treatment perspective has been advocated for a number of reasons. First, approximately 20–30% of individuals with OCD refuse to begin ERP or terminate treatment prematurely, while another 20–30% who complete treatment are nonresponders to either ERP or pharmacotherapy (Stanley and Turner, 1995). Possibly cognitive strategies could be used to deal with dysfunctional attitudes that might interfere with the acceptance or response to ERP. Second, ERP is much less effective for obsessional ruminations than it is for patients with clear-cut compulsive rituals (Beech and Vaughan, 1978; Rachman, 1983; Salkovskis and Kirk, 1997; Freeston and Ladouceur, 1999). Freeston and his colleagues have had some success in using a cognitive-behavioral treatment package for obsessional ruminations that combines cognitive restructuring with exposure and covert response prevention (Freeston and Ladouceur, 1999; Freeston et al., 1997). Third, the inclusion of cognitive intervention may be more important with certain OCD subtypes where ERP may be less successful, such as compulsive hoarders (Frost and Steketee, 1999), primary obsessional slowness (Rachman, 1985), or those with symmetry and ordering compulsions where the compulsion does not fulfill a strict anxiety-reduction function. Fourth, the presence of comorbid severe depression or personality disorders or high levels of stress may reduce the efficacy of ERP (Rachman, 1983; Abramowitz et al., 2000; Steketee et al., 2000). Cognitive therapy, especially for depression, may be helpful in these comorbid conditions. Fifth, certain therapy issues such as low motivation, negative treatment expectancies, noncompliance and failure to complete homework assignments, or presence of overvalued ideation (i.e., strong belief that one's fears are realistic and that compulsive rituals prevent actual disasters; Foa, 1979), may be more effectively addressed by a cognitive therapy intervention (Salkovskis and Warwick, 1985). And finally, as noted by current cognitive theories of OCD, cognitive biases, dysfunctional beliefs, and erroneous thinking play a key role in the pathogenesis of the disorder. Thus cognitive strategies should be included to target directly the cognitive component of OCD.

Cognitive-behavioral treatment

The inclusion of cognitive interventions in the treatment of OCD is a rather late development that can be traced to Salkovskis' (1985) seminal paper in which he proposed that the cognitive therapy approach developed by Beck for the treatment of depression (Beck et al., 1979) might be combined with exposure and response prevention to treat obsessional problems more effectively. Since then, CBT for obsessions and compulsions has developed in three stages. In the late 1980s a few studies investigated the effectiveness of standard cognitive therapy approaches such as rational-emotive therapy (RET) or Beck's cognitive therapy in the treatment of OCD. Then, with the development of more refined and elaborated cognitive models of OCD (i.e., Salkovskis, 1985; Rachman, 1997, 1998), newer cognitive-behavioral treatment packages were proposed that were tailored to the cognitive biases and dysfunctional beliefs and appraisals that were thought to characterize the disorder. Finally we are beginning to see clinical trials on the efficacy of this new generation of cognitive-behavioral therapy for obsessions and compulsions.

Emmelkamp and colleagues (Emmelkamp et al., 1988; Emmelkamp and Beens, 1991) found that RET was equivalent to ERP in reducing obsessive-compulsive symptoms. In addition, various single and multiple case studies have reported that the combination of ERP plus cognitive restructuring resulted in clinically significant improvement in OC symptoms (Salkovskis and Warwick, 1985; Kearney and Silverman, 1990; Ladouceur et al., 1993, 1995b; O'Kearney, 1993). Although some have found less positive results with cognitive and behavioral treatment (Enright, 1991), nevertheless most of these earlier studies suggested that a combination of cognitive and behavioral strategies might be the more optimal treatment for OCD (for reviews see Foa et al., 1998; van Oppen and Emmelkamp, 2000).

Based on more recent cognitive theories of OCD, slightly different variations of a cognitive-behavioral therapy treatment have been proposed by Salkovskis (Salkovskis and Warwick, 1988; see also Chapter 7), van Oppen and Arntz (1994),

Freeston (Freeston and Ladouceur, 1999), Rachman (1998) and Whittal and McLean (1999). Because Salkovskis and Wahl (2001) have provided a detailed and authoritative description of cognitive-behavioral therapy for obsessions and compulsions in their chapter, we shall keep our own comments on cognitive-behavioral therapy brief. There are, however, several elements of cognitive-behavioral therapy that are common across the various treatment protocols. These include: (1) educating the patient about the cognitive model of OCD; (2) identifying the patient's faulty appraisals, neutralization, and avoidance strategies; (3) teaching individuals to challenge cognitively their erroneous appraisals and maladaptive beliefs of obsessions; (4) developing behavioral experiments that include ERP in order to challenge the exaggerated importance and catastrophic interpretations associated with the obsession; (5) offering alternative explanations for the persistence of the obsession; (6) correcting dysfunctional core beliefs; and (7) providing relapse prevention strategies (see also Clark, 1999).

Too few empirical studies have been conducted utilizing these new cognitive-behavioral therapy interventions to conclude whether or not they improve on the effectiveness of standard ERP treatment. In the first published empirical study of cognitive-behavioral therapy based on the writings of Beck and Emery (1985) and Salkovskis (1985), van Oppen et al. (1995) found a slight to moderate superiority of cognitive-behavioral therapy over ERP. Freeston et al. (1997) found that 77% of a sample of obsessional ruminators obtained significant symptomatic improvement after treatment with cognitive-behavioral therapy compared to a waitlist control condition. Moreover improvement was maintained at 6-month follow-up. In a small sample of OCD patients, O'Connor et al. (1999) found that cognitive-behavioral therapy alone and cognitive-behavioral therapy after a period of medication were effective in reducing OC symptoms and strength of belief in the primary obsession.

Despite these encouraging findings, a number of reviewers have concluded that the inclusion of cognitive therapy may not significantly increase the effectiveness of treatment for OCD beyond that achieved by ERP alone. Kozak (1999) concluded there is no differential efficacy in studies that directly compared exposure and cognitive therapy. He argued that many of these studies used suboptimal exposure procedures, and when effect sizes are calculated, there may be no advantage for adding cognitive interventions to ERP. Foa et al. (1998) suggested that the issue of whether cognitive therapy improves the efficacy of ERP may be a moot point because clinicians will routinely discuss dysfunctional thinking as part of the rationale for exposure therapy. Notwithstanding, it must be concluded that the incremental effectiveness of the cognitive components of cognitive-behavioral therapy has not been empirically verified, while at the same time ERPs have been shown to be essential in the psychological treatment of OCD.

Conclusions and future directions

In the last decade there has been a renewed interest in theory, research, and treatment of the cognitive biases and dysfunctions of OCD. Although behavioral theory, and especially behavior therapy consisting of ERP, proved remarkably successful in treating obsessional states with an overt compulsive feature, theoretical and therapeutic limitations of the behavioral perspective led to the recent focus on the cognitive concomitants of OCD. Behavioral learning theory proved unable to account for important aspects of the phenomenology and pathogenesis of obsessions in particular. Gaps became apparent in the ability of ERP to deal with obsessional ruminations, poorly motivated or treatment-resistant patients, or obsessional states complicated by major depression, high stress, or personality disorders. Cognitive interventions were introduced into standard ERP treatment in order to broaden the efficacy of behavior therapy for OCD and to deal with aspects of the disorder that weaken the effectiveness of behavioral techniques.

Behavioral theory did not provide a full account of critical psychological processes involved in the etiology and persistence of OCD. The refocus on the cognitive concomitants of OCD led some researchers to search for general cognitive deficits in memory or attentional bias as the source of obsessional phenomenology, whereas other researchers took a more content-based approach, searching for specific thinking patterns, biases, and beliefs that might account for the pathogenesis of obsessions. As noted previously, empirical evidence suggests that individuals with OCD may have lower confidence in their memory ability but their actual memory functioning appears quite normal. There is evidence that OC individuals have an automatic preconscious attentional bias for threatening stimuli that is directly related to their primary symptomatic concerns, and that they may have trouble inhibiting irrelevant information. Moreover, Radomsky and Rachman (1999) found that compulsive washers may have enhanced memory for contaminated objects. Together these findings suggest that the cognitive biases evident in OCD probably involve both preconscious automatic and voluntary effortful processes that are highly specific to the primary symptom concerns of the patient.

Another stream of cognitive-clinical research has taken a somewhat different direction by investigating specific thematic cognitions, beliefs, and interpretations that are thought to be defining features of the cognitive dysfunction of OCD. A number of key cognitive constructs have been proposed, such as inflated responsibility, TAF, overimportance and control of thoughts, intolerance of uncertainty, thought–event fusion, overestimation of threat and egodystonicity (Salkovskis, 1985; Clark and Purdon, 1993; Freeston et al., 1996; OCCWG, 1997; Rachman, 1997, 1998; Wells, 1997; Salkovskis and Wahl, 2001). Each of these cognitive viewpoints assumes that unwanted intrusive thoughts, images, and impulses, which are normal byproducts of an active, creative mind, escalate into persistent, recurrent obsessions when the individual interprets or appraises the unwanted mental intrusion in a pathological fashion. For example, an unwanted intrusion may gain obsessive-like qualities if it is misinterpreted as indicating the possibility that one is responsible for the occurrence or the prevention of some highly threatening or unwanted event that might befall one's self or others (Rachman, 1997, 1998; Salkovskis and Wahl, 2001). Preexisting dysfunctional beliefs in personal responsibility, overimportance and control of thoughts, intolerance of uncertainty, perfectionism, and threat estimation are considered an underlying vulnerability that may predispose individuals to misinterpret their unwanted intrusive thoughts in a pathogenic fashion.

As noted above, there is empirical evidence that inflated responsibility, threat estimation, and TAF are cognitive distortions, beliefs, and appraisals that are evident in OCD. Fewer studies have investigated beliefs and appraisals of overimportance of thoughts, control of thoughts, and egodystonicity so the role of these constructs in OCD remains to be determined. It is less certain whether any of these cognitive constructs are specific to OCD, or whether they may also be found in other types of anxiety disorders, or even in psychopathology more generally. As well, it may be that some constructs, like inflated responsibility, may be more applicable to specific subtypes of OCD, such as compulsive checkers (and harming obsessions), and less applicable to others, like those with washing compulsions (Rachman and Shafran, 1998). Ultimately, longitudinal studies are needed to determine whether these OC-related thoughts, beliefs, and appraisals are causal agents of the disorder or whether they are mere consequences of the acute phase of OCD.

It is also assumed in cognitive theories of OCD that nonclinical individuals appraise their unwanted intrusive thoughts very differently from obsession-prone individuals. Even though the content of nonclinical intrusions and obsessions is quite similar, it is assumed that the nonclinical person interprets the intrusion as insignificant or mere "mental flotsam" (Rachman, 1993) and promptly ignores the thought. However it is not at all clear that nonclinical individuals completely avoid the faulty responsibility, threat, importance, and control beliefs and appraisals that are seen in OCD. Certainly there is considerable evidence that nonclinical individuals appraise their unwanted intrusive thoughts negatively and that they do engage in deliberate thought control efforts in response to these intrusions (Parkinson and Rachman, 1981; Clark and de Silva, 1985; Freeston et al., 1991; Purdon and Clark, 1994a, 1994b). Although the faulty appraisals of OC patients are more extreme than the appraisals generated by nonclinical individuals (J. E. Calamari and A. S. Janeck, unpublished data) it is unknown whether this difference in degree rather than kind is due to the increased frequency and salience of clinical obsessions. Clearly much more research is needed to clarify the nature of the "normal" appraisal and response pattern to obsessive-like intrusive thoughts, images, and impulses of nonclinical individuals. Only when the normative response to unwanted egodystonic intrusions is understood will we be in a position to explore the distinctive pathological dimension of the obsessional response to intrusions.

There can be little doubt that cognitive therapy has finally had a profound impact on current behavioral treatment of OCD. Standard ERP has been redefined as cognitive-behavior therapy (Kozak et al., 2000), and behavioral-oriented practitioners are now advocating the inclusion of direct cognitive interventions in the treatment of OCD. Cognitively oriented treatment packages have been introduced by Rachman (1998), Salkovskis (Salkovskis and Warwick, 1988) and Freeston (Freeston and Ladouceur, 1999). Moreover, there is evidence that cognitive interventions can be effective in the treatment of obsessions and compulsions. However, many critical questions remain unanswered. It is unclear whether the inclusion of cognitive intervention strategies significantly increases treatment effectiveness beyond that achieved by exposure and response prevention. Kozak (1999) argues that ERP is still the core treatment ingredient for OCD. Also there is no evidence that cognitive interventions are effective in addressing the shortcomings noted with standard ERP. For example, we don't know whether CBT is more effective than standard ERP in reducing treatment resistance or noncompliance, or in dealing with comorbid depression. There is also no evidence on which particular cognitive intervention strategies are most effective, or whether the effectiveness of CBT is attributable to change in the key cognitive constructs postulated by cognitive theorists (i.e., reductions in responsibility appraisals). Moreover, there is disagreement over the sequencing of the treatment components, with Salkovskis and Wahl (2001) emphasizing the use of cognitive techniques to modify responsibility beliefs and appraisals prior to ERP, and Freeston and Ladouceur (1999) focusing on ERP prior to more formal cognitive restructuring interventions. Although the cognitive perspective on OCD is a recent development, with many outstanding issues that remain to be resolved, nevertheless the flurry of cognitive-behavioral research has resulted in remarkable progress in clarifying the cognitive basis of this complex, heterogeneous, but debilitating disorder. Moreover, the cognitive-behavioral perspective on OCD provides an excellent example of how theory and research can inform the development and implementation of promising treatment innovations for a challenging emotional disorder.

REFERENCES

Abramowitz, J. S. (1998). Does cognitive-behavioral therapy cure obsessive-compulsive disorder? A meta-analytic evaluation of clinical significance. *Behavior Therapy*, **29**, 339–55.

Abramowitz, J. S., Franklin, M. E., Street, G. P., Kozak, M. J., and Foa, E. B. (2000). Effects of comorbid depression on response to treatment for obsessive-compulsive disorder. *Behavior Therapy*, **31**, 517–28.

American Psychiatric Association. (1994). *Diagnostic and Statistical Manual of Mental Disorders*, 4th edn. DSM-IV. Washington, DC: American Psychiatric Association.

Antony, M. M., Downie, F., and Swinson, R. P. (1998). Diagnostic issues and epidemiology in obsessive-compulsive disorder. In *Obsessive-Compulsive Disorder: Theory, Research and Treatment*, ed. R. P. Swinson, M. M. Antony, S. Rachman, and M. A. Richter, pp. 3–32. New York: Guilford Press.

Beck, A. T. (1967). *Depression: Causes and Treatment*. Philadelphia: University of Pennsylvania Press.

Beck, A. T. and Clark, D. A. (1997). An information processing model of anxiety: automatic and strategic processes. *Behaviour Research and Therapy*, **35**, 49–58.

Beck, A. T., Rush, A. J., Shaw, B. F., and Emery, G. (1979). *Cognitive Therapy of Depression*. New York: Guilford Press.

Beck, A. T., Emery, G., and Greenberg, R. (1985). *Anxiety Disorders and Phobias: A Cognitive Perspective*. New York: Basic Books.

Beech, H. R. and Vaughan, M. (1978). *Behavioural Treatment of Obsessional States*. Chichester: Wiley.

Bouchard, C., Rhéaume, J., and Ladouceur, R. (1999). Responsibility and perfectionism in OCD: an experimental study. *Behaviour Research and Therapy*, **37**, 239–48.

Clark, D. A. (1999). Cognitive behavioral treatment of obsessive-compulsive disorders: a commentary. *Cognitive and Behavioral Practice*, **6**, 408–15.

Clark, D. A. (2004). Cognitive behavioral therapy of OCD. New York: Guilford Press.

Clark, D. A. and de Silva, P. (1985). The nature of depressive and anxious thoughts. Distinct or uniform phenomena? *Behaviour Research and Therapy*, **23**, 383–93.

Clark, D. A. and Purdon, C. L. (1993). New perspectives for a cognitive theory of obsessions. *Australian Psychologist*, **28**, 161–7.

Clark, D. A., Purdon, C., and Byers, E. S. (2000). Appraisal and control of sexual and non-sexual intrusive thoughts in university students. *Behaviour Research and Therapy*, **38**, 439–55.

Clayton, I. C., Richards, J. C., and Edwards, C. J. (1999). Selective attention in obsessive-compulsive disorder. *Journal of Abnormal Psychology*, **108**, 171–5.

Crino, R. D. and Andrews, G. (1996). Obsessive-compulsive disorder and axis I comorbidity. *Journal of Anxiety Disorders*, **10**, 37–46.

Ecker, W. and Engelkamp, J. (1995). Memory for actions in obsessive-compulsive disorder. *Behavioural and Cognitive Psychotherapy*, **23**, 349–71.

Emmelkamp, P. M. G. (1982). *Phobic and Obsessive-Compulsive Disorders: Theory, Research and Practice*. New York: Plenum Press.

Emmelkamp, P. M. G. and Aardema, A. (1999). Metacognition, specific obsessive-compulsive beliefs and obsessive-compulsive behaviour. *Clinical Psychology and Psychotherapy*, **6**, 139–45.

Emmelkamp, P. M. G. and Beens, H. (1991). Cognitive therapy with obsessive-compulsive disorder: a comparative evaluation. *Behaviour Research and Therapy*, **29**, 293–300.

Emmelkamp, P. M. G., Visser, S., and Hoekstra, R. J. (1988). Cognitive therapy vs exposure in vivo in the treatment of obsessive-compulsives. *Cognitive Therapy and Research*, **12**, 103–14.

Enright, S. J. (1991). Group treatment of obsessive-compulsive disorder: an evaluation. *Behavioural Psychotherapy*, **19**, 183–92.

Enright, S. J. and Beech, A. R. (1990). Obsessional states: anxiety disorders or schizotypes? An information processing and personality assessment. *Psychological Medicine*, **20**, 621–7.

Enright, S. J. and Beech, A. R. (1993). Reduced cognitive inhibition in obsessive compulsive disorder. *British Journal of Clinical Psychology*, **32**, 67–74.

Foa, E. B. (1979). Failure in treating obsessive compulsives. *Behaviour Research and Therapy*, **17**, 169–76.

Foa, E. B. and Kozak, M. J. (1995). DSM-IV field trial: Obsessive-compulsive disorder. *American Journal of Psychiatry*, **152**, 90–6.

Foa, E. B. and Kozak, M. J. (1996). Psychological treatment for obsessive-compulsive disorder. In *Long-Term Treatments of Anxiety Disorders*, M. R. Mavissakalian and R. F. Prien, pp. 285–309. Washington, DC: American Psychiatric Press.

Foa, E. B. and McNally, R. J. (1986). Sensitivity to feared stimuli in obsessive-compulsives: a dichotic listening analysis. *Cognitive Therapy and Research*, **10**, 477–85.

Foa, E. B., Steketee, G. S., and Ozarow, B. J. (1985). Behavior therapy with obsessive-compulsives: from theory to treatment. In *Obsessive-Compulsive Disorder: Psychological and Pharmacological Treatment*, ed. M. Mavissakalian, S. M. Turner, and L. Michelson, pp. 49–129. New York: Plenum Press.

Foa, E. B., Ilai, D., McCarthy, P. R., Shoyer, B., and Murdock, T. (1993). Information processing in obsessive-compulsive disorder. *Cognitive Therapy and Research*, **17**, 173–89.

Foa, E. B., Franklin, M. E., and Kozak, M. J. (1998). Psychosocial treatments for obsessive-compulsive disorder: literature review. In *Obsessive-Compulsive Disorder: Theory, Research and Treatment*, ed. R. P. Swinson, M. M. Antony, S. Rachman, and M. A. Richter, pp. 258–76. New York: Guilford Press.

Franklin, M. E., Abramowitz, J. S., Kozak, M. J., Levitt, J. T., and Foa, E. B. (2000). Effectiveness of exposure and ritual prevention for obsessive-compulsive disorder: randomized compared with nonrandomized samples. *Journal of Consulting and Clinical Psychology*, **68**, 594–602.

Freeston, M. H. and Ladouceur, R. (1999). Exposure and response prevention for obsessional thoughts. *Cognitive and Behavioral Practice*, **6**, 362–83.

Freeston, M. H., Ladouceur, R., Thibodeau, N., and Gagnon, F. (1991). Cognitive intrusions in a non-clinical population. I. Response style, subjective experience, and appraisal. *Behaviour Research and Therapy*, **29**, 585–97.

Freeston, M. H., Rhéaume, J., and Ladouceur, R. (1996). Correcting faulty appraisals of obsessional thoughts. *Behaviour Research and Therapy*, **34**, 433–46.

Freeston, M. H., Ladouceur, R., Gagnon, F., et al. (1997). Cognitive-behavioral treatment of obsessive thoughts: a controlled study. *Journal of Consulting and Clinical Psychology*, **65**, 405–13.

Frost, R. O. and Steketee, G. (1999). Issues in the treatment of compulsive hoarding. *Cognitive and Behavioral Practice*, **6**, 397–407.

Hiss, H., Foa, E. B., and Kozak, M. J. (1994). Relapse prevention program for treatment of obsessive-compulsive disorder. *Journal of Consulting and Clinical Psychology*, **62**, 801–8.

Karno, M. and Golding, J. M. (1991). Obsessive compulsive disorder. In *Psychiatric Disorders in America: The Epidemiologic Catchment Area Study*, ed. L. N. Robins and D. A. Regier, pp. 204–19. New York: Free Press.

Kearney, C. A. and Silverman, W. K. (1990). Treatment of an adolescent with obsessive-compulsive disorder by alternating response prevention and cognitive therapy: an empirical analysis. *Journal of Behavior Therapy and Experimental Psychiatry*, **21**, 39–47.

Kozak, M. J. (1999). Evaluating treatment efficacy for obsessive-compulsive disorder: caveat practitioner. *Cognitive and Behavioral Practice*, **6**, 422–6.

Kozak, M. J. and Foa, E. B. (1997). *Mastery of Obsessive-Compulsive Disorder: A Cognitive-Behavioral Approach. Therapist Guide.* San Antonio: TX: Graywind Publications.

Kozak, M. J., Liebowitz, M. R., and Foa, E. B. (2000). Cognitive behavior therapy and pharmacotherapy for obsessive-compulsive disorder: the NIMH-sponsored collaborative study. In *Obsessive-Compulsive Disorder: Contemporary Issues in Treatment*, ed. W. K. Goodman, M. V. Rudorfor, and J. D. Maser, pp. 501–30. Mahweh, NJ: Lawrence Erlbaum.

Kyrios, M. and Andrew, M. (1998). Automatic and strategic processing in obsessive-compulsive disorder: attentional bias, cognitive avoidance or more complex phenomena? *Journal of Anxiety Disorders*, **12**, 271–92.

Ladouceur, R., Freeston, M. H., Gagnon, F., Thibodeau, N., and Dumont, J. (1993). Idiographic considerations in the behavioral treatment of obsessional thoughts. *Journal of Behavior Therapy and Experimental Psychiatry*, **24**, 301–10.

Ladouceur, R., Rhéaume, J., Freeston, M. H., et al. (1995a). Experimental manipulations of responsibility: an analogue test for models of obsessive-compulsive disorder. *Behaviour Research and Therapy*, **33**, 937–46.

Ladouceur, R., Freeston, M. H., Gagnon, F., Thibodeau, N., and Dumont, J. (1995b). Cognitive-behavioral treatment of obsessions. *Behavior Modification*, **19**, 247–57.

Lopatka, C. and Rachman, S. (1995). Perceived responsibility and compulsive checking: an experimental analysis. *Behaviour Research and Therapy*, **33**, 673–84.

MacDonald, P. A., Antony, M. M., MacLeod, C. M., and Richter, M. A. (1997). Memory and confidence in memory judgments among individuals with obsessive compulsive disorder and non-clinical controls. *Behaviour Research and Therapy*, **35**, 497–505.

March, J. S., Frances, A., Carpenter, D., and Kahn, D. A. (1997). Expert consensus guideline for treatment of obsessive-compulsive disorder. *Journal of Clinical Psychiatry*, **4** (suppl. 4), 5–72.

McNally, R. J. (2000). Information-processing abnormalities in obsessive-compulsive disorder. In *Obsessive-Compulsive Disorder: Contemporary Issues in Treatment*, ed. W. K. Goodman, M. V. Rudorfor, and J. D. Maser, pp. 105–16. Mahweh, NJ: Lawrence Erlbaum.

Menzies, R. G., Harris, L. M., Cumming, S. R., and Einstein, D. A. (2000). The relationship between inflated personal responsibility and exaggerated danger expectancies in obsessive-compulsive concerns. *Behaviour Research and Therapy*, **38**, 1029–37.

Meyer, V. (1966). Modifications of expectations in cases with obsessional rituals. *Behaviour Research and Therapy*, **4**, 273–80.

Mowrer, O. H. (1939). A stimulus-response analysis of anxiety and its role as a reinforcing agent. *Psychological Review*, **46**, 553–65.

Mowrer, O. H. (1953). Neurosis, psychotherapy, and two-factor learning theory. In *Psychotherapy Theory and Research*, ed. O. H. Mowrer, pp. 140–9. New York: Ronald Press.

Mowrer, O. H. (1960). *Learning Theory and Behavior*. New York: Wiley.

Obsessive Compulsive Cognitions Working Group. (1997). Cognitive assessment of obsessive-compulsive disorder. *Behaviour Research and Therapy*, **35**, 667–81.

Obsessive Compulsive Cognitions Working Group. (2001). Development and initial validation of the Obsessive Beliefs Questionnaire and the Interpretation of Intrusions Inventory. *Behaviour Research and Therapy*, **39**, 987–1006.

Obsessive Compulsive Cognitions Working Group. (2002). Psychometric validation of the Obsessive Beliefs Questionnaire and the Interpretation of Intrusions Inventory: Part I. Manuscript submitted for publication.

O'Connor, K., Todorov, C., Robillard, S., Borgeat, F., and Brault, M. (1999). Cognitive-behaviour therapy and medication in the treatment of obsessive-compulsive disorder: a controlled study. *Canadian Journal of Psychiatry*, **44**, 64–71.

O'Kearney, R. (1993). Additional considerations in the cognitive-behavioral treatment of obsessive-compulsive ruminations – a case study. *Journal of Behavior Therapy and Experimental Psychiatry*, **24**, 357–65.

Parkinson, L. and Rachman, S. (1981). Part II: The nature of intrusive thoughts. *Advances in Behaviour Research and Therapy*, **3**, 101–10.

Pigott, T. A. and Seay, S. (1998). Biological treatments for obsessive-compulsive disorder: literature review. In *Obsessive-Compulsive Disorder: Theory, Research and Treatment*, ed. R. P. Swinson, M. M. Antony, S. Rachman, and M. A. Richter, pp. 298–326. New York: Guilford Press.

Pigott, T. A. and Seay, S. (2000). Pharmacotherapy of obsessive-compulsive disorder: overview and treatment-refractory strategies. In *Obsessive-Compulsive Disorder: Contemporary Issues in Treatment*, ed. W. K. Goodman, M. V. Rudorfor, and J. D. Maser, pp. 277–302. Mahweh, NJ: Lawrence Erlbaum.

Purdon, C. (2001). Appraisal of obsessional thought recurrences: impact on anxiety, active resistance and mood state. *Behavior Therapy*, **32**, 47–64.

Purdon, C. L. and Clark, D. A. (1994a). Obsessive intrusive thoughts in nonclinical subjects. Part II. Cognitive appraisal, emotional response and thought control strategies. *Behaviour Research and Therapy*, **32**, 403–10.

Purdon, C. L. and Clark, D. A. (1994b). Perceived control and appraisal of obsessional intrusive thoughts: a replication and extension. *Behavioural and Cognitive Psychotherapy*, **22**, 269–85.

Purdon, C. L. and Clark, D. A. (1999). Metacognition and obsessions. *Clinical Psychology and Psychotherapy*, **6**, 102–10.

Rachman, S. J. (1971). Obsessional ruminations. *Behaviour Research and Therapy*, **9**, 229–35.

Rachman, S. J. (1976a). The modification of obsessions: a new formulation. *Behaviour Research and Therapy*, **14**, 437–43.

Rachman, S. J. (1976b). The passing of the two-stage theory of fear and avoidance: fresh possibilities. *Behaviour Research and Therapy*, **14**, 125–31.

Rachman, S. (1977). The conditioning theory of fear-acquisition: a critical examination. *Behaviour Research and Therapy*, **15**, 375–87.

Rachman, S. J. (1978). An anatomy of obsessions. *Behaviour Analysis and Modification*, **2**, 253–78.

Rachman, S. J. (1983). Obstacles to the successful treatment of obsessions. In *Failures in Behavior Therapy*, ed. E. B. Foa and P. M. G. Emmelkamp, pp. 35–57. New York: Wiley.

Rachman, S. J. (1985). An overview of clinical and research issues in obsessional-compulsive disorders. In *Obsessive-Compulsive Disorder: Psychological and Pharmacological Treatment*, ed. M. Mavissakalian, S. M. Turner, and L. Michelson, pp. 1–47. New York: Plenum.

Rachman, S. J. (1993). Obsessions, responsibility and guilt. *Behaviour Research and Therapy*, **31**, 149–54.

Rachman, S. J. (1997). A cognitive theory of obsessions. *Behaviour Research and Therapy*, **35**, 793–802.

Rachman, S. J. (1998). A cognitive theory of obsessions: elaborations. *Behaviour Research and Therapy*, **36**, 385–401.

Rachman, S. J. and de Silva, P. (1978). Abnormal and normal obsessions. *Behaviour Research and Therapy*, **16**, 233–48.

Rachman, S. J. and Hodgson, R. J. (1980). *Obsessions and Compulsions*. Englewood Cliffs, NJ: Prentice-Hall.

Rachman, S. J. and Shafran, R. (1998). Cognitive and behavioral features of obsessive-compulsive disorder. In *Obsessive-Compulsive Disorder: Theory, Research and Treatment*, ed. R. P. Swinson, M. M. Antony, S. Rachman, and M. A. Richter, pp. 51–78. New York: Guilford Press.

Rachman, S. and Shafran, R. (1999). Cognitive distortions: thought–action fusion. *Clinical Psychology and Psychotherapy*, **6**, 80–5.

Rachman, S. J., Hodgson, R., and Marzillier, J. (1970). Treatment of an obsessional-compulsive disorder by modeling. *Behaviour Research and Therapy*, **8**, 385–92.

Rachman, S., Thordarson, D. S., Shafran, R., and Woody, S. R. (1995). Perceived responsibility: structure and significance. *Behaviour Research and Therapy*, **33**, 779–84.

Radomsky, A. S. and Rachman, S. (1999). Memory bias in obsessive-compulsive disorder (OCD). *Behaviour Research and Therapy*, **37**, 605–18.

Rasmussen, S. A. and Eisen, J. L. (1992). The epidemiology and clinical features of obsessive compulsive disorder. *Psychiatric Clinics of North America*, **15**, 743–58.

Rasmussen, S. A. and Tsuang, M. T. (1986). Clinical characteristics and family history in DSM-III obsessive-compulsive disorder. *American Journal of Psychiatry*, **143**, 317–22.

Rassin, E., Merckelbach, H., Muris, P., and Saan, V. (1999). Thought–action fusion as a causal factor in the development of intrusions. *Behaviour Research and Therapy*, **37**, 231–7.

Rassin, E., Muris, P., Schmidt, H., and Merckelbach, H. (2000). Relationships between thought–action fusion, thought suppression and obsessive-compulsive symptoms: a structural equation modeling approach. *Behaviour Research and Therapy*, **38**, 889–97.

Rassin, E., Diepstraten, P., Merckelbach, H., and Muris, P. (2001). Thought–action fusion and thought suppression in obsessive-compulsive disorder. *Behaviour Research and Therapy*, **39**, 757–64.

Reed, G. F. (1985). *Obsessional Experience and Compulsive Behavior: a Cognitive-Structural Approach*. Orlando, FL: Academic Press.

Rhéaume, J., Ladouceur, R., Freeston, M. H., and Letarte, H. (1994). Inflated responsibility in obsessive-compulsive disorder: psychometric studies of a semiidiographic measure. *Journal of Psychopathology and Behavioral Assessment*, **16**, 265–76.

Rhéaume, J., Freeston, M. H., Dugas, M. J., Letarte, H., and Ladouceur, R. (1995). Perfectionism, responsibility and obsessive-compulsive symptoms. *Behaviour Research and Therapy*, **33**, 785–94.

Salkovskis, P. M. (1985). Obsessional-compulsive problems: a cognitive-behavioural analysis. *Behaviour Research and Therapy*, **23**, 571–83.

Salkovskis, P. M. (1989). Cognitive-behavioural factors and the persistence of intrusive thoughts in obsessional problems. *Behaviour Research and Therapy*, **27**, 677–82.

Salkovskis, P. M. (1996). Cognitive-behavioral approaches to the understanding of obsessional problems. In *Current Controversies in the Anxiety Disorders*, ed. R. M. Rapee, pp. 103–33. New York: Guilford Press.

Salkovskis, P. M. (1998). Psychological approaches to the understanding of obsessional problems. In *Obsessive-compulsive Disorder: Theory, Research and Treatment*, ed. R. P. Swinson, M. M. Antony, S. Rachman, and M. A. Richter, pp. 33–50. New York: Guilford Press.

Salkovskis, P. M. and Kirk, J. (1997). Obsessive-compulsive disorder. In *Science and Practice of Cognitive Behaviour Therapy*, ed. D. M. Clark and C. G. Fairburn, pp. 179–208. Oxford: Oxford University Press.

Salkovskis, P. M. and Warwick, H. M. C. (1985). Cognitive therapy of obsessive-compulsive disorder: treating treatment failures. *Behavioural Psychotherapy*, **13**, 243–55.

Salkovskis, P. M. and Warwick, H. M. C. (1988). Cognitive therapy of obsessive-compulsive disorder. In *Cognitive Psychotherapy: Theory and Practice*, ed. C. Perris, I. M. Blackburn, and H. Perris, pp. 376–395. Berlin: Springer-Verlag.

Salkovskis, P. M., Richards, H. C., and Forrester, E. (1995). The relationship between obsessional problems and intrusive thoughts. *Behavioural and Cognitive Psychotherapy*, **23**, 281–99.

Salkovskis, P. M., Shafran, R., Rachman, S., and Freeston, M. H. (1999). Multiple pathways to inflated responsibility beliefs in obsessional problems: possible origins and implications for therapy and research. *Behaviour Research and Therapy*, **37**, 1055–72.

Salkovskis, P. M., Wroe, A. L., Gledhill, A., et al. (2000). Responsibility attitudes and interpretations are characteristic of obsessive compulsive disorder. *Behaviour Research and Therapy*, **38**, 347–72.

Sauteraud, A., Cottraux, J., Michel, F., Henaff, M. A., and Bouvard, M. (1995). Processing of obsessive, responsibility, neutral words and pseudo-words in obsessive-compulsive disorder: a study with lexical decision test. *Behavioural and Cognitive Psychotherapy*, **23**, 129–43.

Shafran, R., Thordarson, D. S., and Rachman, S. (1996). Thought–action fusion in obsessive-compulsive disorder. *Journal of Anxiety Disorders*, **10**, 379–91.

Sher, K. J., Frost, R. O., and Otto, R. (1983). Cognitive deficits in compulsive checkers: an exploratory study. *Behaviour Research and Therapy*, **21**, 357–63.

Stanley, M. A. and Turner, S. M. (1995). Current status of pharmacological and behavioral treatment of obsessive-compulsive disorder. *Behavior Therapy*, **26**, 163–86.

Steketee, G. and Shapiro, L. J. (1995). Predicting behavioral treatment outcome for agoraphobia and obsessive compulsive disorder. *Clinical Psychology*, **15**, 317–46.

Steketee, G. S., Frost, R. O., and Cohen, I. (1998). Beliefs in obsessive-compulsive disorder. *Journal of Anxiety Disorders*, **12**, 525–37.

Steketee, G., Henninger, N. J., and Pollard, C. A. (2000). Predicting treatment outcome for obsessive-compulsive disorder: effects of comorbidity. In *Obsessive-Compulsive Disorder: Contemporary Issues in Treatment*, ed. W. K. Goodman, M. V. Rudorfor, and J. D. Maser, pp. 257–74. Mahweh, NJ: Lawrence Erlbaum.

Summerfeldt, L. J. and Endler, N. S. (1998). Examining the evidence for anxiety-related cognitive biases in obsessive-compulsive disorder. *Journal of Anxiety Disorders*, **12**, 579–98.

Tallis, F. (1995). *Obsessive Compulsive Disorder: A Cognitive and Neuropsychological Perspective.* Chichester, UK: John Wiley.

Tata, P. R., Leibowitz, J. A., Prunty, M., Cameron, M., and Pickering, A. D. (1996). Attentional bias in obsessional compulsive disorder. *Behaviour Research and Therapy*, **34**, 53–60.

Thordarson, D. S. and Shafran, R. (2002). Importance of thoughts. In *Cognitive Approaches to Obsessions and Compulsions: Theory, Assessment and Treatment*, ed. R. O. Frost and G. Sketee, pp. 15–28. Oxford: Elsevier.

van Balkom, A. J. L. M., van Oppen, P., Vermeulen, A. W. A., Nauta, M. C. E., and Vorst, H. C. M. (1994). A meta-analysis on the treatment of obsessive compulsive disorder: a comparison of antidepressants, behavior, and cognitive therapy. *Clinical Psychology Review*, **14**, 359–81.

van Oppen, P. and Arntz, A. (1994). Cognitive therapy for obsessive-compulsive disorder. *Behaviour Research and Therapy*, **32**, 79–87.

van Oppen, P. and Emmelkamp, P. M. G. (2000). Issues in cognitive treatment of obsessive-compulsive disorder. In *Obsessive-Compulsive Disorder: Contemporary Issues in Treatment*, ed. W. K. Goodman, M. V. Rudorfor, and J. D. Maser, pp. 117–32. Mahweh, NJ: Lawrence Erlbaum.

van Oppen, P., de Haan, E., van Balkom, A. J. L. M., et al. (1995). Cognitive therapy and exposure in vivo in the treatment of obsessive compulsive disorder. *Behaviour Research and Therapy*, **33**, 379–90.

Wells, A. (1997). *Cognitive Therapy of Anxiety Disorders: A Practice Manual and Conceptual Guide.* Chichester: John Wiley.

Wells, A. and Papageorgiou, C. (1998). Relationships between worry, obsessive-compulsive symptoms and meta-cognitive beliefs. *Behaviour Research and Therapy*, **36**, 899–913.

Whittal, M. L. and McLean, P. D. (1999). CBT for OCD: the rationale, protocol, and challenges. *Cognitive and Behavioral Practice*, **6**, 383–96.

Williams, J. M. G., Watts, F. N., MacLeod, C., and Mathews, A. (1997). *Cognitive Psychology and Emotional Disorders*, 2nd edn. Chichester, UK: John Wiley.

Wilson, K. A. and Chambless, D. L. (1999). Inflated perceptions of responsibility and obsessive-compulsive symptoms. *Behaviour Research and Therapy*, **37**, 325–35.

6

The cognitive model of panic

Stefan G. Hofmann

Boston, University, Boston, MA, USA

Introduction

Findings from the National Comorbity Survey indicate that the 12-month preva-lence rate for panic disorder is 2.3% (Kessler et al., 1994). To meet *Diagnostic and Statistical Manual of Mental Disorders,* fourth edition (DSM-IV: American Psychi-atric Association, 1994) criteria for panic disorder (with or without agoraphobia) a person must experience an unexpected panic attack and develop substantial anx-iety over the possibility of having another attack or its implications. The DSM-IV defines a panic attack as a discrete period of intense fear that is accompanied by at least four of 13 somatic or cognitive symptoms (e.g., palpitations, chest pain, fear of dying). The typical attack has a sudden onset, which builds to a peak rapidly and is accompanied by a sense of imminent danger or impending doom and an urge to escape. The worry about future attacks or its implications is the primary reason why panic-disorder patients use medical treatment facilities seven times more frequently than the general population (Siegal et al., 1990). Even those with panic attacks not meeting full diagnostic criteria for panic disorder (subclinical panic) have been found to manifest substantial disability in perceived physical and emotional health, occupational functioning, and incapacity for financial independence (Klerman et al., 1991). Compared to the general population, individuals with subclinical panic are also at higher risk for other comorbid mental disorders, particularly for major depressive disorder, alcohol, and other drug abuse. Further-more, panic disorder is associated with significantly elevated risks of poor marital functioning, impaired social functioning, and suicide attempts (see Hofmann and Barlow, 1999, for review).

Cost-effectiveness studies show significant reductions in indirect costs if panic disorder is successfully treated (Salvador-Carulla et al., 1995). One of the most efficacious treatments, cognitive-behavioral therapy (CBT), is based on the cogni-tive model of panic disorder. This model of panic has sparked nothing less than a cognitive revolution within the field of anxiety disorders. David M. Clark's article A cognitive approach to panic (Clark, 1986), a brief theoretical paper published in *Behaviour Research and Therapy*, was the second most frequently cited article in the entire field of psychology among more than 50 000 articles published between 1986 and 1990 (Garfield, 1992). Other prominent proponents of the model include Beck and Emery (1985), Barlow (1988), and Margraf et al. (1993).

Based on this approach, a number of similar CBT protocols have been developed and tested in clinical trials (Clark et al., 1985, 1994, 1999; Barlow et al., 1989; Klosko et al., 1990, 1995; Craske et al., 1991; Beck et al., 1992; Telch et al., 1993; Clark et al., 1994).

These treatment protocols are based on the same basic treatment rationale but vary in the number of treatment sessions, length of treatment, and emphasis on the particular treatment components (such as the amount and type of exposure). One of the most frequently cited CBT protocols is the panic control treatment (PCT). It combines, similar to other CBT protocols, a number of treatment components, including cognitive restructuring, psychoeducation, relaxation, controlled breathing procedures, and exposure techniques (Barlow and Craske, 1994; Craske and Barlow, 1994; Hofmann and Spiegel, 1999). PCT first teaches patients about the nature and function of fear and its nervous system substrates. In addition to normalizing and demystifying panic attacks, PCT then teaches patients a breathing technique designed to slow respiration rate and promote diaphragmatic breathing. This approach aims to reduce the frequency of panic attacks by helping patients to attribute their symptoms to overbreathing and by teaching patients correct breathing habits that attenuate the intensity of such symptoms. To reduce anxiety-exacerbating thoughts and images, patients are taught as part of the PCT protocol to examine critically, based upon past experience and logical reasoning, their estimations of the likelihood that a feared event will occur, the probable consequences if it should occur, and their ability to cope with it. In addition, they are assisted in designing and conducting behavioral experiments to test their predictions. Finally, to change maladaptive anxiety and fear behaviors, patients are taught to engage in graded therapeutic exposure to cues they associate with panic attacks. The exposure component focuses primarily on internal cues, specifically, frightening bodily sensations (interoceptive exposure). During exposure, patients deliberately provoke physical sensations like smothering, dizziness, or tachycardia by means of exercises such as breathing through a straw, spinning, or vigorous exercise. These exercises are done initially during treatment sessions with therapist modeling, and subsequently by patients at home. As patients become less afraid of the sensations, more naturalistic activities are assigned, such as drinking caffeinated beverages, or watching scary movies.

PCT was found to be superior to a waitlist condition and relaxation training (Barlow et al., 1989). In an intent-to-treat analysis, approximately 80% of patients assigned to CBT were panic-free at posttreatment, compared to 40% of patients assigned to applied relaxation, and 30% of waitlist patients. Similar results were reported by Klosko and colleagues, who demonstrated that PCT was superior to either the waitlist condition or drug placebo as well as alprazolam in the treatment for panic disorder (Klosko et al., 1990, 1995). The authors found that 87% of patients in the CBT group were panic-free by the end of treatment, compared to 50% in the alprazolam condition, 36% in the placebo group, and 33% in the waitlist group. A 2-year follow-up of PCT completers found that gains were maintained (Barlow, 1990; Craske et al., 1991). Subsequently, Telch and colleagues (1993) found a similar treatment to be effective when administered in an 8-week group therapy format. At posttreatment, 85% of the treated patients were panic-free, versus 30% in a waitlist condition. When more stringent outcome criteria were used, including measures of panic frequency, general anxiety, and agoraphobic avoidance, 63% of treated patients and only 9% of waitlist subjects were classified as improved. In an attempt to increase the cost-effectiveness of CBT for panic disorder even further, Clark and colleagues (1999) created an abbreviated version of CBT which reduced the therapist contact time to 6.5 h. This intervention was as effective as a standard CBT protocol administered in 12–15 1-h sessions.

Similar results were reported in a large multicenter clinical trial comparing the efficacy of PCT to imipramine, a pill placebo, and combinations of PCT with imipramine or a pill placebo (Barlow et al., 2000). The results showed that imipramine was clearly superior to placebo after acute treatment, 3 months after the beginning of the study, with drug–placebo differences even larger at the end of maintenance treatment 9 months after the beginning of the study. The efficacy of PCT was comparable to imipramine on nearly all measures during treatment, with better maintenance of gains after treatment discontinuation. Furthermore, more than a third of all eligible patients refused participation in the study because they were unwilling to take imipramine. In contrast, only one out of 308 potential participants refused the study because of the possibility of receiving psychotherapy (Hofmann et al., 1998).

The efficacy of CBT for panic disorder has been officially recognized by both the American Psychiatric Association and the American Psychological Association. For example, the practice guidelines for the treatment of panic disorder by the American Psychiatric Association (1998) concluded that panic-focused CBT and medications are both effective treatments for panic disorder. Moreover, PCT was classified as a "well-established" intervention for panic disorder by the Task Force on Promotion and Dissemination of Psychological Procedures of the American

Psychological Association, Division of Clinical Psychology (American Psychological Association, 1993; Chambless et al., 1996). For a treatment to be classified as "well-established," four stringent criteria had to be met: (1) the efficacy of the intervention had to be demonstrated in at least two clinical trials conducted by different investigators or in a large series of well-designed single case studies; (2) treatment had to be delivered in accordance with a manual; (3) the characteristics of the subject sample had to be clearly delineated; and (4) the treatment had to be either as efficacious as an already established treatment or superior to a placebo or other treatment.

Given these data, why revisit the cognitive model of panic again? The treatment obviously works. What is there to criticize? As I will outline in the following sections, there are at least three problems with the cognitive approach to panic in its current formulation: (1) the cognitive approach implies a scientific theory that is difficult to test; (2) the cognitive model does not explain differences in the prevalence rates and phenomenology of panic between subgroups of people; and (3) the success of CBT does not necessarily validate the cognitive model of panic because we still know very little about the active ingredients of the treatment approach.

The goal of this chapter is not to discount the obvious success of the cognitive model of panic but to identify weaknesses with the goal to improve further the scientific and practical value of this approach. In my critique, I will focus primarily on David M. Clark's theoretical view of panic, which has been the most influential and prominent formulation of this model. After briefly summarizing Clark's model, I will present a critique of the underlying theoretical views and discuss alternative models and specific directions for future research.

The cognitive model

The original conceptualization of panic disorder is based on a medical illness model which assumes the existence of distinct and mutually exclusive syndromes with an inherently organic etiology and specific treatment indications (Klein, 1964; Klein and Klein, 1989). Clark (1986) even introduced his cognitive model by referring to pharmacological studies: "Paradoxically, the cognitive model of panic attacks is perhaps most easily introduced by discussing work which has focused on neurochemical and pharmacological approaches to the understanding of panic" (p. 462).

According to Clark's (1986) model, panic attacks are viewed as resulting from the catastrophic misinterpretation of certain bodily sensations, such as palpitations, breathlessness, dizziness, etc. An example of such a catastrophic misinterpretation would be a healthy individual perceiving palpitations as evidence of an impending heart attack. The vicious cycle of the cognitive model suggests that various external (i.e., the feeling of being trapped in a supermarket) or internal stimuli (i.e., body sensations, thoughts, or images) trigger a state of apprehension if these stimuli are perceived as a threat. It is assumed that this state is accompanied by fearful bodily sensations which, if interpreted in a catastrophic fashion, further increases the apprehension and the intensity of bodily sensations. This model further states that the attacks appear to come from "out of the blue" because patients fail to distinguish between the triggering body sensations and the subsequent panic attack and the general beliefs about the meaning of an attack.

For example, if an individual believes that there is something wrong with his heart, he is unlikely to view the palpitation which triggers an attack as different from the attack itself. Instead he is likely to view both as aspects of the same thing – a heart attack or near miss (Clark, 1986, p. 463).

The model does not rule out biological factors in panic. Rather, it is assumed that biological variables may contribute to an attack by triggering benign bodily fluctuations or intensifying fearful bodily sensations. For example, the model assumes that pharmacological treatments can be effective in reducing the frequency of panic attacks if they reduce the frequency of bodily fluctuations, which can trigger panic, or if they block the bodily sensations, which accompany anxiety. However, if the patient's tendency to interpret bodily sensations in a catastrophic fashion is not changed, discontinuation of drug treatment should be associated with a high rate of relapse.

Although this claim has not been directly tested, there is strong evidence in the literature that cognitive variables do in fact influence the results of biological challenge procedures. For example, it has been shown that panic patients who were informed about the effects of CO_2 inhalation reported less anxiety and fewer catastrophic thoughts than uninformed individuals (Rapee et al., 1986). Furthermore, nonanxious individuals who were told that lactate infusion would produce unpleasant bodily sensations experienced more anxiety than nonanxious subjects who were told that lactate would induce pleasant feelings (van der Molen et al., 1987). Moreover, panic patients who believed they had control over the amount of CO_2 they inhaled by turning an inoperative dial were less likely to panic than individuals who knew that they had no control over it (Sanderson et al., 1989). Similarly, panic patients who underwent a CO_2 challenge were less anxious in the presence of their "safe person" than patients without their "safe person" present (Carter et al., 1995). Finally, a study by Schmidt et al. (1997a) suggested that cognitive-behavioral treatment of panic disorder significantly reduces CO_2-induced panic attacks. These data suggest that cognitive variables can in fact moderate the effects of panic provocation procedures and therefore provide evidence for some important aspects of Clark's cognitive model of panic.

The scientific value of the cognitive model of panic

Terminology

Before examining the scientific value of the cognitive approach to panic, it will be necessary first to define two terms that are often used interchangeably in the literature, namely the terms *model* and *theory*. A model can be defined as a simplified representation of the world (that is, of the part of the world that is of interest to us). In contrast, a theory contains, in addition, the causal structure of the world, and the entities and processes underlying phenomena (Hesse, 1966). Developing a theory implies constructing a model to help us "visualize" the complex of explanations contained in a theory and it also implies developing concepts which help us reduce the infinitude of observed events to a small number of variables tied together by rules or laws. A good scientific theory consists of a simple set of propositions that explain past phenomena and predict future events that are compatible with this theory but incompatible with alternative theories. Given this definition, is Clark's cognitive approach to panic a good "cognitive theory" of panic?

Epistemological considerations

Theories can vary in their scientific value. Scientific value can be determined by examining the characteristics of the hypotheses that are deduced from a theory (Popper, 1992). Hypotheses are predictive statements about an outcome that we would expect to be true if our theory (and other assumptions) were correct. The value of a theory is therefore high if its hypotheses possess high informative content, high predictive power, and if they withstand critical testing. In contrast, the value of a theory is low if no clear hypotheses can be derived from it, or if the theory is untestable because different experimental outcomes can be predicted by the same theory, or because the same outcome can be predicted by many different theories (Popper, 1992). Therefore, a good theory should lead to implausible (i.e., counter-intuitive) rather than plausible predictions (Hofmann, 1999a) because plausibility of a hypothesis and informative content of its theory vary inversely (Popper, 1992). Many (Popperian) philosophers would further agree that the goal of science is not only to find satisfactory explanations of phenomena but also to improve the degree of satisfactoriness of the explanations by improving their degree of testability, which then leads science to the creation of theories of ever richer content, of higher degree of universality, and higher degree of precision.

Although this view is not shared by all members of the philosophical community (e.g., Lakatos, 1974; Feyerabend, 1978), Popper has been one of the most influential philosophers for contemporary science, and falsification has been the guiding principle since the beginning of psychology. For example, Hull (1930) noted:

If a hypothesis be so vague and indefinite, or so lacking in relevance to the phenomena which it seems to explain that the results neither of previous experiments nor those of experiments subsequently to be performed may be deduced from it, it will be difficult indeed to prove it false.... Unfortunately, because of its very sterility and barrenness in the above deductive sense, such an hypothesis should have no status whatever in science. It savors more of metaphysics, religion, or theology (p. 252).

Critique 1: The cognitive approach implies a theory that is difficult to test

Since its formulation in the 1980s, a number of objections have been raised against the cognitive model of panic (see also McNally, 1990, 1994). For example, Klein and Klein (1989) argued that, if the "theory" was correct, imipramine should actually worsen panic disorder because its side-effects include bodily sensations that are likely to be catastrophically misinterpreted (e.g., increased heart rate). Proponents of the cognitive model replied that the antipanic effects of imipramine are probably indirect by modulating noradrenergic dysregulation which reduces the frequency of symptoms that patients are prone to misinterpret. Furthermore, only a small percentage of panic patients who take imipramine complain of intolerable side-effects, and these individuals do not respond to treatment (Pohl et al., 1988).

Klein and Klein (1989) further stated that nocturnal panic attacks are inconsistent with the cognitive model. Proponents of the cognitive model, on the other hand, argued that catastrophic misinterpretations may well occur during sleep when sleepers monitor their body for significant stimuli (e.g., heart rate increase), just as sleepers monitor the external environment for important stimuli.

Seligman (1988) also raised the question as to why panic patients persistently misinterpret symptoms of panic attacks as catastrophic events after having repeatedly survived such episodes. Salkovskis (1988) responded that panic patients continue to misinterpret their symptoms catastrophically because they typically take protective actions to avoid the feared (and catastrophic) event.

Finally, it has been argued that the catastrophic misinterpretation of bodily sensations is neither a sufficient nor a necessary criterion for experiencing panic attacks (Rachman et al., 1988; Teasdale, 1988; Rachman, 1997). For example, Aronson et al. (1989) reported cases of panic patients who panicked in response to lactate but who did not experience fears of dying, going crazy, or losing control despite intense levels of fear. Similarly, Rachman and colleagues (1988) found that 27% of the attacks experienced by panic patients were not accompanied by catastrophic misinterpretations.

Clark's response to this critique was that catastrophic misinterpretations need not be conscious (Clark, 1986) because "in patients who experience recurrent attacks, catastrophic misinterpretations may be so fast and automatic that patients may not always be aware of the interpretive process" (Clark, 1986, p. 76). This argument, however, was criticized by McNally (1994) who pointed out that it is implausible that thoughts of such imminent disaster do not at some point become conscious. Furthermore, McNally (1994) argued:

> Although catastrophic misinterpretation may indeed occur outside of awareness, postulation of unconscious catastrophizing seems to threaten the falsifiability of Clark's theory. It is unclear what could possibly count for evidence against the hypothesis that catastrophic misinterpretations necessarily precede panic attacks. For any given attack, one can maintain that the patient ipso facto catastrophized, either consciously or unconsciously (p. 114).

These examples illustrate an important weakness of the cognitive model: The underlying theory is difficult to test, and it remains uncertain what empirical evidence could possibly falsify the underlying "theory." The experimental literature provides only limited information. Information-processing studies indicate that panic disorder is characterized by interpretive, attentional, memory, and interoceptive biases for processing threat (see McNally, 1994, for review). However, the results of these studies are often difficult to replicate. One of the most robust (or the least unreliable) findings is the attentional bias using the modified Stroop color-naming test. In the original Stroop test (Stroop, 1935), subjects are asked to name the color of color words printed in antagonistic colors (e.g., the word "blue" printed in red). Subjects typically perform more slowly on tasks involving such incongruent stimuli than on naming solid-color squares. During the modified Stroop test for panic patients, subjects typically have to name the color of neutral and panic-related (threat) words (e.g., "stroke").

Studies utilizing this modified Stroop test suggest that panic patients in fact show an attentional bias for processing threat cues because they take longer to name the colors of threat words than to name the colors of nonthreat words (Ehlers et al., 1988; McNally et al., 1990, 1992, 1994). However, this interference effect does not seem to be restricted to panic patients or to the processing of threat cues alone. In fact, panic patients also exhibit interference for material related to their personal content regardless of whether the concern is positive or negative (e.g., McNally, 1994). This suggests that panic patients selectively process threat cues primarily because their attention is captured by information related to material with either positive or negative valence as long as this information has direct personal relevance.

Although information-processing studies highlight the importance of automatic processing biases, the results are of little theoretical or practical relevance for the cognitive model. McNally (1994) attributes this problem partly to the growing divide between experimentalists and practitioners which diminishes cross-fertilization between basic and applied research.

Critique 2: The cognitive model does not explain differences in the prevalence rates and phenomenology of panic between subgroups of people

Individuals with panic disorder vary greatly in age, demographic characteristics, and comorbid diagnoses. Are the panic attacks that are experienced by children caused by the same cognitive misinterpretation of bodily sensations as the attacks that are reported by a severely disturbed schizophrenic patient? And why are panic attacks particularly common in certain age groups, females, and people with certain additional diagnoses?

For example, while panic disorder is uncommon prior to the peripubertal period, retrospective reports of adults suggest that panic disorder often begins during adolescence or young adulthood (von Korff et al., 1985; Moreau and Follett, 1993). Bernstein et al. (1996) even concluded that adolescence is the peak period for onset of panic disorder. After reviewing the literature, Ollendick et al. (1994) stated:

> We conclude that panic attacks are common among adolescents, while both panic attacks and Panic Disorder appear to be present, but less frequent, in children. Furthermore, it is evident that both adolescents and children who report panic attacks describe the occurrence of cognitive symptoms, although with less frequency than physiological ones. Consistent with the cognitive model of panic, it seems that at least some youngsters are capable of experiencing the physiological symptoms of panic accompanied by the requisite catastrophic cognitions. However, a more complete understanding of the cognitive manifestation of panic attacks/disorder among children awaits further investigation (p. 131).

The cognitive model predicts that panic attacks can only develop after a certain developmental age is reached when an individual possesses the required knowledge base to misinterpret certain bodily symptoms (only people who know that a pain in the left arm can be due to a cardiovascular disease can misinterpret a pain in their arm as a signal for a heart attack). However, panic attacks commonly occur in developmentally delayed people who seem to lack the cognitive capacities to generate catastrophic misinterpretations as suggested by the cognitive model. Similarly, the cognitive model does not explain the gender differences. The incidence rate of panic is approximately twice as common in women than in men in community and clinical studies around the world (Wittchen et al., 1992). Finally, the cognitive model does not explain why panic attacks commonly co-occur with other mental disorders, most notably schizophrenia. Data from the Epidemiological Catchment Area survey indicate that, depending on the site, the 6-month prevalence of panic attacks in patients with schizophrenia is between 28% and 63% (Boyd, 1986). Other studies report that between 16% (P. C. Bermanzohn et al., unpublished data) and 42% (Moorey and Soni, 1994) of patients with schizophrenia report panic attacks as defined by DSM-III-R (American Psychiatric Association, 1987) or DSM-IV (American Psychological Association, 1994). Furthermore, between 11%

(Bermanzohn et al., 1996) and 20% of patients with schizophrenia meet current criteria for panic disorder (Argyle, 1990). In contrast, the lifetime prevalence rate of panic disorder in a community sample is only between 2% (Eaton et al., 1991) and 3.8% (Katerndahl and Realini, 1993).

It might be possible that the schizophrenic thought disorder is directly associated with the misinterpretation of bodily sensations. It might also be possible that panic and schizophrenia are connected via certain biochemical substances that are important factors in both domains of psychopathology (Hofmann, 1999b). For example, it has been suggested that noradrenergic hyperactivity, dopaminergic hypoactivity, or both are the common underlying mechanisms (Iruela et al., 1991). It has also been hypothesized that cholecystokinin (CCK), a gut-brain peptide that exists in high concentrations in the mammalian brain, may be a possible biological link between panic attacks and certain schizophrenic symptoms (Bourin et al., 1996). A review of the literature (Bourin et al., 1996), which included animal experiments and studies on humans, suggests that CCK is implicated in the pathophysiology of schizophrenic symptoms via its neuroanatomical association with dopamine. In addition, CCK probably induces panic anxiety through the CCK-B receptors. Further studies are needed to examine the validity of the cognitive model for various subgroups of panic patients, and to clarify the contribution of biological factors in order to integrate the cognitive perspective with findings from developmental, genetic, and neuropsychological research.

Critique 3: Success of cognitive-behavior therapy does not necessarily validate the cognitive model of panic

As outlined at the beginning of this chapter, treatment approaches that are based on the cognitive model are clearly effective. However, there is still room for improvement. The reported efficacy data from nearly all treatment studies to date have been based on cross-sectional assessments. Although such assessments show good maintenance of gains *on average* following CBT, longitudinal data reveal that many patients have a fluctuating posttreatment course, with periods of symptom recrudescence. For example, Brown and Barlow (1995) found that 40% of subjects met criteria for high end-state functioning at 3 months posttreatment and 57% at 24 months posttreatment, but only 27% met the criteria at both 3 and 24 months.

More importantly, even in cases that showed clear and stable improvement, we know very little about the active ingredient of treatment and the mechanism of action (i.e., mediators of change). Mediators of change are those characteristics of the individual that are changed by the treatment and that, in turn, produce the observable treatment effects (Baron and Kenny, 1986). For a variable to be a mediator, it must therefore covary with variables indicating therapeutic change.

Although there is evidence to suggest that cognitive variables can influence the subjective experience of panic attacks, it remains unclear whether CBT (and other therapies) are actually mediated by cognitive variables. For example, Rachman (1997) noted:

> There are prickly questions of causality, and the results of cognitive behaviour therapy are open to alternative interpretations: cause, consequences, or correlate? . . . The decline in cognitions, and/or in bodily sensations, may produce the reduction of the panics. But it is possible that the decline in cognitions, and in bodily sensations, are consequences of the reduced episodes of panic, and not the cause. It is also possible that the decline of cognitions is a correlate of the reduction in the episodes of panic (p. 19).

Furthermore, little is known about the relative efficacy of the various CBT components in isolation. Studies suggest that cognitive intervention is an important aspect in the treatment of panic disorder. For example, the effectiveness of breathing retraining is diminished without cognitive restructuring (Hibbert and Chan, 1989). Furthermore, the fearful responding during interoceptive exposure exercises seems to be a function of perceived stimulus intensity and other cognitive variables, such as perceived controllability of the stimulus (Hofmann et al., 1999). However, it is difficult to estimate the efficacy of cognitive techniques for reducing panic attacks because cognitive restructuring is typically combined with other treatment components, such as education about panic, breathing retraining, and exposure to feared bodily sensations.

In an attempt to study the relative efficacy of cognitive therapy that specifically focuses on "catastrophic misinterpretation," Brown et al. (1997) randomly assigned 40 patients to either 12–18 sessions of standard cognitive therapy which primarily addressed cognitions and beliefs relevant to interpersonal concerns, or focused cognitive therapy which was designed specifically to target catastrophic misinterpretation and included some interoceptive exposure exercises. The results showed that the majority of patients (more than 80%) improved as a result of treatment, but no difference was found between the two treatment groups in the degree of improvement at the posttreatment assessment or the 6- and 12-month follow-ups. The authors concluded that interoceptive exposure exercises are not necessary for improvement. However, the results of a metaanalysis (Gould et al., 1995) suggest that both the cognitive component and the interoceptive exposure component are necessary to produce the best results in treatment of panic disorder because the combination reached the highest overall mean effect size (effect size $= 0.88$, $n = 7$ studies). More well-designed and systematic dismantling studies are sorely needed to isolate and study changes of cognitions, panic symptoms, and other relevant (mediating) variables at various intervals during the course of treatment.

Alternative panic models

At least three other prominent approaches have been previously discussed in the literature, namely the expectancy theory (Reiss and McNally, 1985; Reiss, 1991), the interoceptive conditioning model (Goldstein and Chambless, 1978) and, more recently, the modern learning perspective (Bouton et al., 2001).

Anxiety sensitivity and expectancy theory

The expectancy model (Reiss and McNally, 1985; Reiss, 1991) states that anxiety and avoidance are a function of the expectations (what one thinks might happen in a situation), and sensitivities (why one is afraid of the anticipated event). In the case of panic disorder, it has been suggested that panic patients tend to fear anxiety symptoms because of greater anxiety sensitivity. Anxiety sensitivity is conceptualized as a dispositional construct that determines the tendency to respond fearfully to anxiety symptoms (Reiss and McNally, 1985; Reiss, 1991; Taylor et al., 1991, 1992; McNally, 1994; Taylor, 1999). Specifically, Reiss (1991) stated:

Anxiety sensitivity is indicated by beliefs about the personal consequences of experiencing anxiety. People with high anxiety sensitivity believe that anxiety leads to heart attacks, causes mental illness, or causes additional anxiety. People with low anxiety believe that anxiety is a harmless emotion (p. 145).

Reiss (1991) acknowledges that, because anxiety sensitivity is defined in terms of irrational beliefs, the concept has similarities to the cognitive model of panic (Clark, 1986), and some individuals with high anxiety sensitivity may misinterpret bodily sensations catastrophically. Furthermore, McNally (1994) stated that "anxiety sensitivity resembles the 'enduring tendency' to misinterpret bodily sensations catastrophically postulated by Clark (1986)" (p. 116). However, in contrast to the cognitive model, the expectancy model predicts that individuals with high anxiety sensitivity also believe that high arousal itself can lead to harmful consequences without necessarily misinterpreting any physical sensations.

Reiss' expectancy model led to the development of the 16-item Anxiety Sensitivity Index (ASI; Peterson and Reiss, 1992). Considerable research supports the utility and validity of the ASI (see McNally, 1994 for a review). Furthermore, recent data suggest that ASI scores predict the development of spontaneous panic attacks after controlling for the history of panic attacks and trait anxiety (Schmidt et al., 1997b). However, it is uncertain whether the ASI is a valid instrument to measure the patients' beliefs about their anxiety symptoms as proposed by the expectancy model. Specifically, the ASI instructs subjects to indicate how *scared* they are when they feel shaky (item 3), faint (item 4), nauseous (item 8), short of breath (item 10), nervous (item 16), when their heart beats rapidly (item 6), or when they feel unusual body sensations (item 14). Four items determine the subject's *beliefs about the consequence of bodily sensations* (e.g., item 9: "when I notice my heart beating rapidly, I worry that I might be having a heart attack"). These items are classic catastrophic misinterpretations and are therefore also consistent with Clark's cognitive model of panic. Surprisingly, the ASI does not provide any items specific to the expectancy model by measuring the beliefs that symptoms which are associated with anxiety may lead to physical or mental catastrophes (e.g., "I believe that the pounding heart that I feel when I am anxious may eventually lead to a heart attack"). Furthermore, the items of the ASI are highly overlapping with the 18-item Body Sensations Questionnaire (Chambless et al., 1984) which was developed to measure "fear of fear," a construct that will be described in more detail in the next paragraph. Consequently, findings from studies that validate the ASI not only provide corroborating evidence for Reiss's expectancy model, but also for Clark's cognitive model and Chambless and Goldstein's interoceptive conditioning model.

Interoceptive conditioning model

Goldstein and Chambless (1978) suggested that certain internal bodily sensations become the conditioned stimuli for the conditioned response of a panic attack which then results in the development of fear of fear, a process that has also been labeled as interoceptive conditioning. Specifically, Goldstein and Chambless stated:

> Having suffered one or more panic attacks, these people become hyperalert to their sensations and interpret feelings of mild to moderate anxiety as signs of upcoming panic attacks and react with such anxiety that the dreaded episode is almost invariably induced. This is analogous to the phenomenon described by Razran (1961) as interoceptive conditioning in which the conditioned stimuli are internal bodily sensations. In the case of fear of anxiety, a client's own physiological arousal becomes the conditioned stimuli for the powerful conditioned response of a panic attack (Goldstein and Chambless, 1978, p. 55).

Reiss (1988) and McNally (1994) argued that the fear of fear concept in panic disorder is difficult to describe in terms of interoceptive conditioning because it is unclear how to identify and separate the conditioned stimulus from the conditioned response and the unconditioned stimulus from the unconditioned response. Furthermore, unlike in classical conditioning, the unconditioned stimulus does not reflexively lead to panic. This model therefore leads to an overprediction of panic, because a fear of panic response should theoretically occur every time the conditioned stimulus (e.g., increased heart rate) is perceived (Clark, 1988). Finally, this model does not explain why the panic response does not seem to be subject to extinction after repeated trials to the conditioned stimulus (Rachman, 1991). McNally (1994) concluded that the interoceptive-conditioning hypothesis in its original formulation "constitutes little more than a misleading metaphor for the mechanism underlying panic" (p. 108).

Modern learn-theory perspective

Recently, Bouton et al. (2001) discussed a revised learning model of panic disorder. The authors distinguish between *anxiety*, an anticipatory emotional state that functions to prepare the individual for a threatening event, and *panic*, an emotional state designed to deal with a threatening event that is already in progress. This model assumes that panic disorder develops because exposure to panic attacks causes the conditioning of anxiety to exteroceptive and interoceptive cues. The presence of conditioned anxiety then potentiates the next panic attack. Anxiety therefore becomes a precursor of panic. The model considers a number of general and specific vulnerability factors that might influence the person's susceptibility to conditioning, such as early experiences with uncontrollable and unpredictable events, and vicarious learning events that focused on certain bodily sensations, which can be measured by the physical harm factor of ASI.

The model of Bouton et al. incorporates supporting data of other theoretical accounts and attempts to correct some of the weaknesses of previous models. However, it is still unable to explain differences between subgroups of individuals in the prevalence of the disorder. Furthermore, it tends to be at times unspecific and overinclusive, which limits its testability. For example, with respect to the role of cognitions, the authors stated:

> Although a causal role for catastrophic cognition is ... not outside the scope of a learning theory analysis, we are less convinced than other theorists that catastrophic thoughts are necessary to generate panic attacks. Whether they are sufficient remains to be determined (p. 22).

Discussion and future research directions

CBT for panic disorder is one of the great success stories in clinical psychology. However, our knowledge about the underlying cognitive model has improved very little since Clark's article was published in 1986. A similar critique applies to Goldstein and Chambless's interoceptive conditioning model (1978) and Reiss's expectancy theory (1988). These alternative views of panic share many of the same characteristics of the cognitive model and also many of the same problems. The following weaknesses of the cognitive model of panic were identified:

1. The cognitive approach to panic is difficult to test. In order to advance the scientific progress in this domain, it will be necessary to transform the cognitive *model* of panic into a cognitive *theory* of panic by improving the degree of testability (i.e., by formulating specific falsifiable predictions). Modifying a

particular model post hoc in order to make it applicable to all panic patients has little empirical value because it immunizes the underlying theory from experimental falsification. Programmatic experiments are needed to test the cognitive model systematically. Information-processing paradigms could be used to study changes in cognitive biases during the course of the illness (e.g., as part of a longitudinal study in a high-risk population) and during therapy.

2. It is assumed that the cognitive model is applicable to all subgroups of patients. However, the cognitive model does not offer an explanation for the differences in the prevalence of panic disorder among certain subgroups of patients. For example, why is panic disorder more common in women than in men? Why does it often begin during adolescence or young adulthood? Why is it particularly common among patients with other mental disorders, such as schizophrenia? Are there differences in prevalence or phenomenology of panic between different ethnic groups? The sparse literature on this topic suggests that cultural issues are indeed important variables (Freedman, 1997). After reviewing the evidence, Kirmayer (1997) concluded:

> Anxiety disorders should not be conceived of as entirely within the skin of the individual. Like all psychological phenomena, they take part in the networks of interpersonal interaction that are embedded in larger social structures. The whole is sustained by cultural knowledge and practice. Culturally, responsive treatment is based on assessment of this wider social network, which can then be mobilized through family and other social interactions (p. 245).

Moreover, even within the same culture, different factors seem to be important for different people. Not every patient with panic disorder develops agoraphobia, not every panic patient avoids caffeine, not every patient hyperventilates during an attack, and not every patient can identify catastrophic thoughts during an attack. The cognitive model (or any other model) does not account for such differences between individuals and diagnostic subgroups. Future research is required to identify the specific vulnerability factors leading to panic disorder.

3. The success of CBT does not validate the cognitive model of panic because we still know very little about the active ingredients of the treatment approach. It is unclear whether cognitive variables are in fact responsible for the treatment gains. Alternatively, changes in cognitions may simply be a consequence of changes in the (yet undiscovered) mediating variables. Well-designed and systematic dismantling studies in combination with appropriate assessment instruments and statistical techniques would provide valuable information to clarify some of these issues. Mediators (the mechanism of action) and moderators (predictors of treatment outcome) are typically studied by using analyses of variance, regression models, and structural equation models (Judd and Kenny, 1981; Baron and Kenny, 1986; Holmbeck, 1997).

In conclusion, the cognitive model of panic is one of the most important developments in contemporary clinical psychology. This model led to the development of highly efficacious psychosocial treatments, and it offered an alternative approach to the original medical illness model of panic disorder. However, despite the obvious success of the cognitive treatment approach to panic, relatively little progress has been made in the further development of the underlying theory of panic. To advance the psychological model of panic, it will be necessary to convert the psychological model of panic into a scientifically valuable theory of panic. This could be achieved by improving the testability of the model, by identifying and specifying the subgroups of panic patients for which the model is applicable, and by studying the mechanism of treatment change.

Acknowledgment

This research was supported in part by NIMH grant MH-57326 and a grant from NARSAD.

REFERENCES

American Psychiatric Association. (1987). *Diagnostic and Statistical Manual of Mental Disorders*, 3rd edn, revised. Washington, DC: American Psychiatric Association.

American Psychological Association. (1993). *Task Force on Promotion and Dissemination of Psychological Procedures. A Report to the Division 12 Board of the American Psychological Association.* Washington, DC: American Psychological Association.

American Psychiatric Association. (1994). *Diagnostic and Statistical Manual of Mental Disorders*, 4th edn. DSM-IV. Washington, DC: American Psychiatric Association.

American Psychiatric Association. (1998). Practice guideline for the treatment of patients with panic disorder. *American Journal of Psychiatry*, **155**, 1–34.

Argyle, N. (1990). Panic attacks in chronic schizophrenia. *British Journal of Psychiatry*, **157**, 430–3.

Aronson, T. A., Whitaker-Azmitia, P., and Caraseti, I. (1989). Differential reactivity to lactate infusions: the relative role of biological, psychological, and conditioning variables. *Biological Psychiatry*, **25**, 469–81.

Barlow, D. H. (1988). *Anxiety and its Disorders.* New York: Guilford Press.

Barlow, D. H. (1990). Long-term outcome for patients with panic disorder treated with cognitive-behavioral therapy. *Journal of Clinical Psychology*, **51**, 17–23.

Barlow, D. H. and Craske, M. G. (1994). *Mastery of your Anxiety and Panic II.* Albany, New York: Graywind.

Barlow, D. H., Craske, M. G., Cerny, J. A., and Klosko, J. S. (1989). Behavioral treatment of panic disorder. *Behavior Therapy*, **20**, 261–82.

Barlow, D. H., Gorman, J. M., Shear, M. K., and Woods, S. W. (2000). Cognitive-behavioral therapy, imipramine, or their combination for panic disorder: a randomized control trial. *Journal of the American Medical Association*, **283**, 2529–36.

Baron, R. M. and Kenny, D. A. (1986). The moderator-mediator variable distinction in social psychological research: conceptual, strategic, and statistical considerations. *Journal of Personality and Social Psychology*, **51**, 1173–82.

Beck, A. T. and Emery, G. (1985). *Anxiety Disorders and Phobias: A Cognitive Perspective*. New York: Basic Books.

Beck, A. T., Sokol, L., Clark, D. A., Berchick, R., and Wright, F. (1992). A crossover study of focused cognitive therapy for panic disorder. *American Journal of Psychiatry*, **149**, 778–83.

Bernstein, C. A., Borchardt, C. M., and Perwien, A. R. (1996). Anxiety disorders in children and adolescents: a review of the past 10 years. *Journal of the American Academy of Child and Adolescent Psychiatry*, **35**, 1110–19.

Bourin, M., Malinge, M., Vasar, E., and Bradwejn, J. (1996). Two faces of cholecystokinin: anxiety and schizophrenia. *Fundamentals of Clinical Pharmacology*, **10**, 116–26.

Bouton, M. E., Mineka, S., and Barlow, D. H. (2001). A modern learning theory perspective on the etiology of panic disorder. *Psychological Review*, **108**, 4–32.

Boyd, J. H. (1986). Use of mental health services for the treatment of panic disorder. *American Journal of Psychiatry*, **143**, 1569–74.

Brown, T. A. and Barlow, D. H. (1995). Long-term outcome of cognitive-behavioral treatment of panic disorder: clinical predictors and alternative strategies for assessment. *Journal of Consulting and Clinical Psychology*, **63**, 754–65.

Brown, G. K., Beck, A. T., Newman, C. F., Beck, J. S., and Tran, G. Q. (1997). A comparison of focused and standard cognitive therapy for panic disorder. *Journal of Anxiety Disorders*, **11**, 329–45.

Carter, M. M., Hollon, S. D., Carson, R., and Shelton, R. C. (1995). Effects of a safe person on induced stress following a biological challenge in panic disorder with agoraphobia. *Journal of Abnormal Psychology*, **104**, 156–63.

Chambless, D. L., Caputo, G. C., Bright, P., and Gallaher, R. (1984). Assessment of fear of fear in agoraphobics: the Body Sensations Questionnaire and the Agoraphobic Cognitions Questionnaire. *Journal of Consulting and Clinical Psychology*, **52**, 1090–7.

Chambless, D. L., Sanderson, W. C., Shoham, V., et al. (1996). An update on empirically validated therapies. *Clinical Psychologist*, **49**(2), 5–18.

Clark, D. M. (1986). A cognitive approach to panic. *Behaviour Research and Therapy*, **24**, 461–70.

Clark, D. M. (1988). A cognitive model of panic attacks. In *Panic: Psychological Perspectives*, ed. S. Rachman and J. D. Maser, pp. 71–89. Hillside, NY: Erlbaum.

Clark, D. M., Salkovskis, P. M., and Chalkley, A. J. (1985). Respiratory control as a treatment for panic attacks. *Journal of Behavior Therapy and Experimental Psychiatry*, **16**, 23–30.

Clark, D. M., Salkovskis, P.M., Hackman, A., et al. (1994). A comparison of cognitive therapy, applied relaxation, and imipramine in the treatment of panic disorder. *British Journal of Psychiatry*, **164**, 759–69.

Clark, D. M., Salkovskis, P. M., Hackman, A., et al. (1999). Brief cognitive therapy for panic disorder: a randomized controlled trial. *Journal of Consulting and Clinical Psychology*, **67**, 583–9.

Craske, M. G. and Barlow, D. H. (1994). *Agoraphobia Supplement to the MAP II Program*. Albany, New York: Graywind.

Craske, M. G., Brown, T. A., and Barlow, D. H. (1991). Behavioral treatment of panic disorder: a two-year follow-up. *Behavior Therapy*, **22**, 289–304.

Eaton, W. W., Dryman, A., and Weissman, M. M. (1991) Panic and phobia. In *Psychiatric Disorders in America*, ed. L. N. Robins and D. A. Regier, pp. 155–79. New York: Free Press.

Ehlers, A. (1993). Somatic symptom and panic attacks: a retrospective study of learning experiences. *Behaviour Research and Therapy*, **31**, 269–78.

Ehlers, A., Margraf, J., Davies, S., and Roth, W. T. (1988). Selective processing of threat cues in subjects with panic attacks. *Cognition and Emotion*, **2**, 201–19.

Feyerabend, P. (1978). *Science in a Free Society*. London: New Left Books.

Freedman, S. (1997). *Cultural Issues in the Treatment of Anxiety*. New York, NY: Guilford Press.

Garfield, E. (1992). A citationist perspective of psychology. Part 1: Most cited papers, 1986–1990. *APS Observe*, **5**(6), 8–9.

Goldstein, A. J. and Chambless, D. L. (1978). A reanalysis of agoraphobia. *Behaviour Research and Therapy*, **9**, 47–59.

Gould, R. A., Otto, M. W., and Pollack, M. H. (1995). A meta-analysis of treatment outcome for panic disorder. *Clinical Psychological Review*, **15**, 810–44.

Hesse, M. B. (1966). *Models and Analogies in Science*. Notre Dame: University Press.

Hibbert, G. A. and Chan, M. (1989). Respiratory control: its contribution to the treatment of panic attacks: a controlled study. *British Journal of Psychiatry*, **154**, 232–6.

Hofmann, S. G. (1999a). Introducing the grandmother test into psychological science. *Journal of Theoretical and Philosophical Psychology*, **19**, 167–76.

Hofmann, S. G. (1999b). Relationship between panic and schizophrenia. *Depression and Anxiety*, **9**, 101–6.

Hofmann, S. G. and Barlow, D. H. (1999). The costs of anxiety disorders: implications for psychosocial interventions. In *Cost-Effectiveness of Psychotherapy*, ed. N. E. Miller and K. M. Magruder, pp. 224–34. Oxford, UK: Oxford University Press.

Hofmann, S. G. and Spiegel, D. A. (1999). Panic control treatment and its applications. *Journal of Psychotherapy Practice and Research*, **8**, 3–11.

Hofmann, S. G., Barlow, D. H., Papp, L. A., et al. (1998). Pretreatment attrition in a comparative treatment outcome study on panic disorder. *American Journal of Psychiatry*, **155**, 43–7.

Hofmann, S. G., Bufka, L., and Barlow, D. H. (1999). Panic provocation procedures in the treatment of panic disorder: early perspectives and case studies. *Behavior Therapy*, **30**, 307–19.

Holmbeck, G. N. (1997). Toward terminological, conceptual, and statistical clarity in the study of mediators and moderators: examples from the child-clinical and pediatric psychology literatures. *Journal of Consulting and Clinical Psychology*, **4**, 599–610.

Hull, C. L. (1930). Simple trial-and-error learning: a study in psychological theory. *Psychological Review*, **37**, 241–56.

Iruela, L. M., Ibanez-Rojo, V., Oliveros, S. C., and Caballero, L. (1991). Panic attacks in schizophrenia. *British Journal of Psychiatry*, **158**, 436–7.

Judd, C. M. and Kenny, D. A. (1981). Process analysis: estimating mediation in evaluation research. *Evaluation Research*, **5**, 602–19.

Katerndahl, D. A. and Realini, J. P. (1993). Lifetime prevalence of panic states. *American Journal of Psychiatry*, **150**, 246–9.

Kessler, R. C., McGonagle, K. A., Zhao, S., et al. (1994). Lifetime and 12-month prevalence of DSM-III-R psychiatric disorders in the United States: results from the National Comorbidity Survey. *Archives of General Psychiatry*, **51**, 8–19.

Kirmayer, L. J. (1997). Culture and anxiety: a clinical and research agenda. In *Cultural Issues in the Treatment of Anxiety*, ed. S. Friedman, pp. 225–51. New York, NY: Guilford Press.

Klein, D. F. (1964). Delineation of two drug-responsive anxiety syndromes. *Psychopharmacologia*, **5**, 397–408.

Klein, D. F. and Klein, H. M. (1989). The definition and psychopharmacology of spontaneous panic and phobia. In *Psychopharmacology of Anxiety*, ed. P. Tyrer, pp. 135–62. New York, NY: Oxford University Press.

Klerman, G. L., Weissman, M. M., Ouellette, R., Johnson, J., and Greenwald, S. (1991). Panic attacks in the community. Social morbidity and health care utilization. *Journal of the American Medical Association*, **265**, 742–6.

Klosko, J. S., Barlow, D. H., Tassinari, R., and Cerny, J. A. (1990). A comparison of alprazolam and cognitive-behavior therapy in treatment of panic disorder. *Journal of Clinical and Consulting Psychology*, **58**, 77–84.

Klosko, J. S., Barlow, D. H., Tassinari, R., and Cerny, J. A. (1995). "A comparison of alprazolam and cognitive-behavior therapy in treatment of panic disorder": correction. *Journal of Clinical and Consulting Psychology*, **63**, 830.

Lakatos, I. (1974). The role of crucial experiments in science. *Studies in History and Philosophy of Science*, **4**, 309–25.

Margraf, J., Barlow, D. H., Clark, D. M., and Telch, M. J. (1993). Psychological treatment of panic: work in progress on outcome, active ingredients, and follow-up. *Behaviour Research and Therapy*, **31**, 1–8.

McNally, R. J. (1990). Psychological approaches to panic disorder: a review. *Psychological Bulletin*, **108**, 403–19.

McNally, R. J. (1994). *Panic Disorder. A Critical Analysis.* New York: Guilford Press.

McNally, R. J., Riemann, B. C., and Kim, E. (1990). Selective processing of threat cues in panic disorder. *Behaviour Research and Therapy*, **28**, 407–12.

McNally, R. J., Riemann, B. C., Louro, C. E., Lukach, B. M., and Kim, E. (1992). Cognitive processing of emotional information in panic disorder. *Behaviour Research and Therapy*, **30**, 143–9.

McNally, R. J., Amir, N., Louro, C. E., et al. (1994). Cognitive processing of idiographic emotional information in panic disorder. *Behaviour Research and Therapy*, **32**, 119–22.

Moorey, H. and Soni, S. D. (1994). Anxiety symptoms in stable chronic schizophrenics. *Journal of Mental Health*, **3**, 257–62.

Moreau, D. and Follett, C. (1993). Panic disorder in children and adolescents. *Child and Adolescent Psychiatric Clinics of North America*, **2**, 581–602.

Ollendick, T. H., Mattis, S. G., and King, N. J. (1994). Panic in children and adolescents: a review. *Journal of Child Psychology and Psychiatry*, **35**, 113–34.

Peterson, R. A. and Reiss, S. (1992). *Test Manual for the Anxiety Sensitivity Index*, 2nd edn. Orlando Park., IL: International Diagnostic Systems.

Pohl, R., Yeregani, V. K., Balon, R., and Lycaki, H. (1988). The jitteriness syndrome in panic disorder patients treated with antidepressants. *Journal of Clinical Psychiatry*, **49**, 100–4.

Popper, K. R. (1992). *Realism and the Aim of Science. Postscript to the Logic of Scientific Discovery.* London: Routledge.

Rachman, S. (1991). Neo-conditioning and the classical theory of fear acquisition. *Clinical Psychology Review*, **11**, 155–73.

Rachman, S. (1997). The evolution of cognitive behaviour therapy. In *Science and Practice of Cognitive Behaviour Therapy*, ed. D. F. Clark and C. G. Fairburn, pp. 3–26. Oxford, England: Oxford University Press.

Rachman, S., Lopatka, C., and Levitt, K. (1988). Experimental analyses of panic: II. Panic patients. *Behaviour Research and Therapy*, **26**, 33–40.

Rapee, R. M., Mattick, R., and Murrell, E. (1986). Cognitive mediation in the affective components of spontaneous panic attacks. *Journal of Behavior Therapy and Experimental Psychiatry*, **17**, 245–54.

Razran, G. (1961). The observable unconscious and the inferable conscious in current Soviet psychophysiology: interoceptive conditioning, semantic conditioning, and the orienting reflex. *Psychological Review*, **68**, 81–147.

Reiss, S. (1988). Interoceptive theory and fear of anxiety (letter to the editor). *Behavior Therapy*, **19**, 84–5.

Reiss, S. (1991). Expectancy model of fear, anxiety and panic. *Clinical Psychology Review*, **11**, 141–53.

Reiss, S. and McNally, R. J. (1985). Expectancy model of fear. In *Theoretical Issues in Behavior Therapy*, ed. S. Reiss and R. R. Bootzin, pp. 107–21. San Diego, CA: Academic Press.

Salkovskis, P. M. (1988). Phenomenology, assessment, and the cognitive model of panic. In *Panic: Psychological Perspectives*, ed. S. Rachman and J. D. Maser, pp. 111–36. Hillsdale, NJ: Erlbaum.

Salvador-Carulla, L., Segui, J., Fernandez-Cano, P., and Canet, J. (1995). Costs and offset effect in panic disorder. *British Journal of Psychiatry*, **116** (suppl. 27), 23-8.

Sanderson, W. C., Rapee, R. M., and Barlow, D. H. (1989). The influence of an illusion of control on panic attacks induced via inhalation of 5.5% carbon dioxide-enriched air. *Archives of General Psychiatry*, **46**, 157–62.

Schmidt, N. B., Trakowski, J. H., and Staab, J. P. (1997a). Extinction of panicogenic effects of a 35% CO_2 challenge in patients with panic disorder. *Journal of Abnormal Psychology*, **106**, 630–8.

Schmidt, N. B., Lerew, D. R., and Jackson, R. J. (1997b). The role of anxiety sensitivity in the pathogenesis of panic: prospective evaluation of spontaneous panic attacks during acute stress. *Journal of Abnormal Psychology*, **106**, 355–64.

Seligman, M. E. P. (1988). Competing theories of panic. In *Panic: Psychological Perspectives*, ed. S. Rachman and J. D. Maser, pp. 321–9. Hillsdale, NJ: Erlbaum.

Siegal, L., Jones, W. C., and Wilson, J. O. (1990). Economic and life consequences experienced by a group of individuals with panic disorder. *Journal of Anxiety Disorders*, **4**, 201–11.

Stroop, J. R. (1935). Studies of interference in serial verbal reactions. *Journal of Experimental Psychology*, **18**, 643–61.

Taylor, S. (1999). *Anxiety Sensitivity: Theory, Research, and Treatment of the Fear of Anxiety*. Mahwah, NJ: Lawrence Erlbaum.

Taylor, S., Koch, W. J., and Crockett, D. J. (1991). Anxiety sensitivity, trait anxiety, and the anxiety disorders. *Journal of Anxiety Disorders*, **5**, 293–311.

Taylor, S., Koch, W. J., and McNally, R. J. (1992). Conceptualizations of anxiety sensitivity. *Psychological Assessment*, **4**, 245–50.

Teasdale, J. (1988). Cognitive models and treatments of panic: a critical evaluation. In *Panic: Psychological Perspectives*, ed. S. Rachman and J. D. Maser, pp. 189–203. Hillsdale, NJ: Erlbaum.

Telch, M. J., Lucas, J. A., Schmidt, N. B., et al. (1993). Group cognitive-behavioral treatment of panic disorder. *Behaviour Research and Therapy*, **31**, 279–87.

van der Molen, P. J., van den Hout, M. A., Vromen, J., Lousberg, H., and Griez, E. (1987). Cognitive determinants of lactate induced anxiety. *Behaviour Research and Therapy*, **24**, 677–80.

von Korff, M. R., Eaton, W. W., and Keyl, P. M. (1985). The epidemiology of panic attacks and panic disorder: results of three community surveys. *American Journal of Epidemiology*, **122**, 970–81.

Wittchen, H. –U., Essau, C. A., Von Zerssen, D., Krieg, J. –C., and Zaudig, M. (1992). Lifetime and six-month prevalence of mental disorders in the Munich follow-up study. *European Archives of Psychiatry and Clinical Neuroscience*, **241**, 247–58.

7

Treating obsessional problems using cognitive-behavioral therapy

Paul M. Salkovskis[1] and Karina Wahl[2]

[1] Institute of Psychiatry, London, UK
[2] University of Oxford, Oxford, UK

The earliest description of behavioral treatment of obsessive-compulsive disorder (OCD) was by Vic Meyer (1966), in a paper titled Modification of expectations in cases with obsessional rituals. This work formed the nucleus of what came to be known as exposure and response prevention (ERP) (Rachman and Hodgson, 1980). This cognitive emphasis in the earliest description of behavioral treatment reflects a recurring theme throughout the theoretical, experimental, and clinical development of this line of psychological treatment. However, the importance of cognitive factors was reflected in a more diffuse understanding of their likely significance rather than a specific recognition of their nature. For example, Marks in 1981 pointed out that:

Obsessives develop a more elaborate set of beliefs around their rituals than phobics develop around their fears. Cognitions seem to play a larger role in obsessives than in phobics. Minor changes in obsessives' perception of a situation can therefore produce a marked change in their behaviour (Marks, 1981, p. 40).

In 1976, Rachman and colleagues had more systematically identified a similar phenomenon as an intriguing observation during experiments on the "spontaneous decay" of compulsive urges. In this ground-breaking series of experiments, the researchers both predicted and demonstrated that behavioral rituals were associated with an immediate reduction in discomfort and urge to ritualize further rather than an increase (as predicted by other theories current at that time). A subsequent reduction of discomfort and the urge to wash in people who did not engage in their ritual over the longer term was also noted. Roper and Rachman (1976) extended this work in a field setting (that is, in the patients' own homes rather than the laboratory) and demonstrated that the elicitation of discomfort was substantially blocked by the presence of the experimenter during the provocation phase. They also suggested that this effect may have been the result of the patient transferring responsibility to the experimenter. This observation has been of particular importance in the development of an integrated cognitive-behavioral approach to OCD. Salkovskis (1985) proposed a cognitive-behavioral approach to obsessional problems which represented an integration of cognitive theories of anxiety and existing behavioral conceptualizations of OCD, particularly that of Rachman (1978). This cognitive-behavioral approach seeks to build on and enhance existing behavioral theories and treatment (Clark and Purdon, 1993; Freeston et al., 1993; Rachman, 1993, 1997, 1998).

Cognitive-behavioral theory as applied to OCD

Cognitive-behavioral theory is predicated on the idea that obsessional thinking has its origins in normal intrusive thoughts rather than being qualitatively different. Intrusive thoughts (indistinguishable in terms of content from clinical obsessions) occur in almost 90% of the general population (Rachman and de Silva, 1978; Salkovskis and Harrison, 1984). According to cognitive-behavioral theory, the crucial difference between normal intrusive thoughts and obsessions lies in the meaning attached by obsessional patients to their intrusions as an indication first, that harm to themselves or to others is a serious risk and second, that they may be responsible for such harm (or its prevention). There are close parallels to other cognitive conceptualizations of anxiety problems, such as the cognitive hypothesis of panic (Clark, 1988; Salkovskis, 1988), in which panic attacks are said to occur as a result of the misinterpretation of normal bodily sensations, particularly the sensations of normal anxiety. Most normal people experience such sensations, but only people who have an enduring tendency to interpret them in a catastrophic fashion will experience repeated panic attacks. By the same token, intrusive thoughts, impulses, images, and doubts are normal, but only people who have an enduring tendency to misinterpret their own mental activity as indicating personal responsibility will experience the pattern of discomfort and neutralizing characteristic of OCD.

The *interpretation* of the occurrence and content of intrusions as indicating increased responsibility has a number of important effects in people suffering from OCD: (1) increased discomfort, including, but not confined to, anxiety and depression; (2) the focusing of attention to both the intrusions themselves and to triggers in the environment which may increase their occurrence; (3) increased accessibility to and preoccupation with the original thought and other related ideas; (4) behavioral responses, including neutralizing reactions in which individuals seek to reduce or escape responsibility (such behaviors can be overt or covert, and include compulsive behavior, avoidance of situations related to the obsessional thought, seeking reassurance, thus diluting or sharing responsibility, and attempts to get rid of or exclude the thought from their mind).

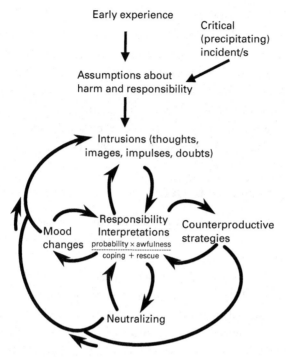

Figure 7.1   Current cognitive-behavioral model of the development and maintenance of obsessional problems.

Distress is therefore seen as a relatively automatic result of the person's interpretation of the content and occurrence of intrusive thoughts, whilst behavioral reactions are motivated reactions. Both types of reactions can have the effect of increasing the subsequent occurrence of intrusions and further enhancing the negative interpretations made. The inflated sense of responsibility which sufferers attach to their activities (including intrusive thoughts and memories as well as overt behavior) leads them to attempt to engage in a pattern of mental and behavioral effort characterized both by *overcontrol* and preoccupation. (Salkovskis et al., 2000; Wroe and Salkovskis, 2000; Salkovskis and Freeston, 2001; Salkovskis and Forrester, 2002). The current cognitive-behavioral model of the development and maintenance of obsessional problems incorporates each of these variables and processes (Salkovskis, 1999), and is presented in Figure 7.1.

The immediate basis of obsessional problems is the occurrence of intrusive cognitions. Such intrusive cognitions mostly occur as an *automatic process*, but these are often linked to an individual's current concerns and probably play an important part in normal psychological mechanisms related to creativity and problem-solving. Intrusive cognitions acquire emotional significance as a result of the way in which they are appraised and the specific meanings that are attached to them. It therefore follows that intrusions are initially emotionally neutral, but can take on positive, negative, or no emotional significance, depending on the person's prior experience and the context in which intrusions occur (Edwards and Dickerson, 1987; England and Dickerson, 1988).

If the intrusion is appraised as having no adaptive implications, further processing is unlikely. At least two aspects of the intrusion are subject to appraisal: the *occurrence* and *content*. If appraisal suggests a specific reaction (including attempts to suppress or avoid the thought), *controlled processing* will follow. Behavioral reactions (overt or covert) to intrusive cognitions result in such cognitions becoming salient and therefore acquiring priority of processing. Thus, when an intrusive cognition or its content has some direct implications for the reactions of the individual experiencing it, processing priority will increase and further appraisal and elaboration become more likely. In addition, such appraisals lead to the deployment of strategic attention towards the control of mental activity. Effort will be directed towards a range of responses, including attempts to be sure of the accuracy of one's memory, to take account of all factors in one's decisions, to prevent the occurrence of unacceptable material, to ensure that an outcome has been achieved when the difference between achieving it and not achieving it is imperceptible (for example, getting rid of perceived contamination which cannot be seen or felt). Personally relevant ideas will therefore tend to persist and be the subject of further thought and action; irrelevant ideas can be considered but no further thought or action will ensue.

Appraisal of responsibility and consequent neutralizing can arise from a sensitivity to responsibility arising from a failure to control thoughts, and from an increase in the level of perceived personal responsibility (Salkovskis and Forrester, 2002). The majority of nonclinical subjects do not regard the occurrence of intrusive thoughts as being of special significance. Once neutralizing responses to intrusive thoughts are established they are maintained by the association with the perception of reduced responsibility and discomfort, whilst the recurrence of the intrusive cognitions becomes more likely as a result of the other processes described above. Obsessional experiences may, as such, arise from normal cognitive processes. It appears, for example, that the occurrence of recurrent, intrusive thoughts about harm can affect an individual's emotional reactions to neutral events. Recent research indicates that, when provided with details about ambiguous situations and a negative intrusive thought about that situation, both obsessional patients and controls demonstrate a higher intensity of behavioral and emotional response than when the intrusive thought is neutral. Obsessional patients demonstrated a stronger emotional reaction overall than did the controls, with obsessional patients showing higher levels of perceived responsibility (Forrester et al., 2002). Thus, obsessional problems will occur in individuals who are distressed by the occurrence of intrusions and also believe the occurrence of such cognitions indicates personal responsibility for distressing harm unless corrective action is taken.

The appraisal of intrusive thoughts as having implications for responsibility for harm to self or others is therefore seen as important because appraisal links the intrusive thought with both distress and the occurrence of neutralizing behavior and other deliberate responses to the intrusion. An obsessional pattern would be particularly likely in vulnerable individuals when intrusions are regarded as self-initiated (e.g., resulting in appraisals such as "these thoughts might mean I want to harm the children; I must guard against losing control"). As described above, the importance of responsibility was clearly demonstrated by the experiments originally conducted by Rachman's research group (Roper et al., 1973; Roper and Rachman, 1976) and continued more recently (Shafran, 1997). In these important experiments, situations which usually provoked checking rituals in obsessional patients (such as locking the door) produced little or no discomfort or checking when the therapist was present, in sharp contrast to the effects of having to deal with such situations when alone.

The central point of the model, and the element which marks the transition from "normal" to "abnormal" obsessions, is therefore to be found in responsibility appraisals which are in turn linked to more general beliefs concerning responsibility for harm. A group of researchers working on obsessions recently defined the "responsibility" appraisals of obsessionals as:

The belief that one has power which is pivotal to bring about or prevent subjectively crucial negative outcomes. (P. M. Salkovskis et al., unpublished data).

"Responsibility" as used in cognitive conceptualizations means that the person believes that he or she may be, or come to be, the cause of harm (to self or others); implicit in this definition is the need to take some preventive or restorative action. It is this appraisal of the occurrence and content of intrusions as indicating personal responsibility which results in repeated neutralizing behavior.

Neutralizing includes both overt compulsions (such as washing and checking) (Rachman, 1976; Salkovskis, 1985, 1989b) or mental checking and restitution activity (such as "putting right" by saying prayers, thinking "good thoughts" in response to "bad thoughts," repeatedly running over details of events in memory) (Rachman, 1971; Salkovskis and Westbrook, 1989). The problem behaviors in obsessions therefore include not only obvious compulsive activities such as repeated checking and washing and their mental equivalents, but also attempts at thought suppression (which paradoxically may increase intrusions and preoccupation; see below). Neutralizing is defined as voluntarily initiated activity *which is intended to have the effect of reducing the perceived responsibility* and can be overt or covert (compulsive behavior or thought rituals). These responsibility-motivated neutralizing efforts reduce discomfort in the short term but have the longer-term effect of increasing preoccupation and triggering further intrusions. Attempts both to suppress and to *neutralize* the thought, image, or impulse can be counterproductive, in that they can both sustain and/or increase responsibility beliefs and increase the occurrence of intrusive thoughts. As a consequence of neutralizing activity, intrusive cognitions become more salient and frequent, they evoke more discomfort, and the probability of further neutralizing increases. By the same token, attempts to suppress the thought increase the likelihood of recurrence.

OCD is a problem caused by inflated responsibility and maintained by trying too hard. OCD is therefore conceptualized as a problem which arises because the patient tries too hard (to remember, to be clean, to be certain, to stop intrusive thoughts from occurring, to ensure that avoidable harm does not occur). People suffering from OCD try too hard to exert control over mental processes and activity in a variety of counterproductive and therefore anxiety-provoking ways. Efforts at overcontrol increase distress because: (1) direct and deliberate attention to mental activity can modify the contents of consciousness; (2) efforts deliberately to control a range of mental activities apparently and actually meet with failure and even opposite effects; (3) attempts to prevent harm and responsibility for harm increase the salience and accessibility of patients' concerns with harm; (4) neutralizing directed at preventing harm also prevents disconfirmation, (i.e., prevents patients from discovering that the things they are afraid of will not occur); this means that exaggerated beliefs about responsibility and harm do not decline.

Why do obsessional patients try too hard?

Cognitive theories specify that both anxiety and avoidant/escape behaviors (including attempts to (over)control mental activity) arise from threat beliefs (Beck et al., 1985): emotional reactions as an involuntary response, behaviors as a motivated response. The perception of threat leads both to anxiety and to active attempts to achieve safety. In anxiety, appraisal is not confined to the perceived probability of danger, but can be represented as:

$$\text{Anxiety} = \frac{\begin{array}{c}\text{Perceived likelihood} \\ \text{of anticipated danger}\end{array} \times \begin{array}{c}\text{Perceived awfulness/cost} \\ \text{of anticipated danger}\end{array}}{\begin{array}{c}\text{Perceived ability} \\ \text{to cope with danger}\end{array} + \begin{array}{c}\text{Perceived external} \\ \text{factors which would} \\ \text{assist ("rescue")}\end{array}}$$

The top line summarizes what is often referred to as primary appraisal, the bottom line secondary appraisal. In fact, the view presented here (derived from Beck et al., 1985) differs somewhat from that of Lazarus in that the appraisal of coping and rescue is regarded as being part of the initial appraisal of threat. Despite being virtually instantaneous, the appraisal of threat in a particular situation is clearly a complex process, based on a combination of past experience, present context, mood state, and so on. Although not truly mathematical, this equation neatly summarizes the idea that very low probabilities of danger may become very anxiety-provoking if associated with very high cost, and that efforts to control and cope with danger are part of the overall perception of threat.

The cognitive theory proposes that people are predisposed to making particular appraisals because of assumptions which are learned over longer periods from childhood onwards or which may be formed as a result of unusual or extreme events and circumstances. These assumptions result in negative appraisals when intrusive thoughts occur. Some assumptions which apparently characterize OCD patients are:

- "Having a thought about an action is like performing the action."
- "Failing to prevent (or failing to try to prevent) harm to self or others is the same as having caused the harm in the first place."
- "Responsibility is not reduced by other factors such as something being improbable."
- "Not neutralizing when an intrusion has occurred is similar or equivalent to seeking or wanting the harm involved in the intrusion to happen."
- "One should (and can) exercise control over one's thoughts."

Thus, the person who believes that thinking something is the same a doing it (a thought–action fusion assumption) has no problems as long as any intrusive thoughts remain relatively benign. However, if the person were to experience a thought such as "I would like to kill my baby," it would be expected that he or she would become much more distressed than someone who does not have the thought–action fusion assumption.

The effects of these type of assumptions is often described in terms of "thinking errors" (Beck, 1976); thinking errors are characteristic distortions which influence whole classes of reactions. Thinking errors are not of themselves pathological; in fact, most people make judgments by employing a range of heuristics, that can be adaptive under some circumstances. Many, however, can be maladaptive and some can be fallacious (Nisbett and Ross, 1980). The cognitive hypothesis suggests that OCD patients show a number of characteristic thinking errors which link to their obsessional difficulties; probably the most typical and important is the idea that:

any influence over outcome = responsibility for outcome

The belief that "*any* influence over outcome = responsibility for outcome" could be expected to increase concern with *omissions*. Consideration of the phenomenology of obsessional problems suggests several ways in which omissions may become relatively more important. An important factor in judgments concerning responsibility is the perception of agency, meaning that one has chosen to bring something about. Particular importance is usually given to *premeditation* in the sense of being able to foresee possible harmful outcomes. Thus, if a person can anticipate a real possibility of causing harm, and does not act to prevent it, the act or the omission would be regarded as blameworthy. In addition, responsibility tends to be linked to the idea that one *should* be aware of the possibility of harm. Clearly, this everyday notion leads to the conclusion that one has a duty to anticipate harmful outcomes (Salkovskis, 1996b; Salkovskis and Forrester, 2002). Unfortunately, it is in the nature of obsessional problems that patients are troubled by intrusions which appear to represent foresight of a range of possible negative outcomes. That is, the intrusive thoughts often concern things that could go wrong unless dealt with (such as passing on contamination, having hurt someone accidentally, having left the door unlocked, or the gas turned on). As described above, some people consider it their duty to try to foresee negative outcomes. However, if in any case a negative outcome *is* foreseen, even as an intrusive thought, responsibility is established, because to do nothing the person would have to decide not to act to prevent the harmful outcome. That is, deciding *not* to act despite being aware of possible disastrous consequences becomes an active decision, making the person a causal agent in relation to those disastrous consequences. Thus, the occurrence of intrusive/obsessional thoughts transforms a situation where harm can only occur by omission into a situation where the person has "actively" chosen to allow the harm to take place. This might mean that the apparent absence of omission bias in obsessionals is mediated by the occurrence of obsessional thoughts. There is now some evidence supporting such a view (Wroe and Salkovskis, 2000; Wroe et al., 2000).

Deciding not to do something results in a sense of agency; thus, patients will not be concerned about sharp objects they have not seen, and will not be concerned if they did not consider the possibility of harm. However, if something is seen and it occurs to them that they could or should take preventive action, the situation changes because not acting becomes an active decision. In this way, the actual occurrence of intrusive thoughts of harm and/or responsibility for it come to play a key role in the perception of responsibility for their contents. Recent research from our group has found evidence consistent with this, in that it was noted that the inclusion of an intrusive thought in a situation increased individuals' distress and involvement in it whether or not they suffered from OCD, and that obsessional patients show a heightened sensitivity to omission bias in those areas most directly related to their problems relative to both nonclinical and anxious controls (Wroe and Salkovskis, 2000).

Treatment implications of the cognitive-behavioral theory

Marks (1981) has highlighted both the unstructured application of cognitive techniques and the limitations of the exposure-based approach when he argued that "calm, gentle, yet firm persuasion is helpful, but if the patient resists strongly, little can be done" (p. 97). Cognitive therapy can bring a systematic approach to the solution of this problem for the substantial proportion of patients in whom behavioral treatment can do little (Salkovskis and Westbrook, 1987). Usually, where it is concluded that "little can be done," this in fact means that something *completely different* needs to be done. If, as seems likely, exposure is effective through bringing about belief change, cognitive strategies which *combine and interact* with behavioral techniques would seem an optimal strategy. Such an approach would therefore not only involve identifying and modifying the thoughts and beliefs which prevent the patient from engaging in or benefiting from exposure treatment but also take a general form indicated by the cognitive conceptualization (Salkovskis and Warwick, 1985, 1988; Salkovskis, 1989a). Modification of anxious or depressed mood concurrent with the obsessions can also be helpful (Salkovskis and Warwick, 1988). There is also evidence that self-esteem may impact on obsessional symptoms, both in general terms and more specifically (Ehntholt et al., 1999). These findings suggest that some obsessional patients may benefit from work directed at changing self-esteem.

The cognitive theory therefore predicts that successful treatment requires modification both of beliefs involved in and leading to the misinterpretation of intrusive thoughts as indicating heightened responsibility and of the associated behaviors involved in the maintenance of these beliefs. Prior to treatment, obsessional patients are distressed because they have a particularly threatening perception of their obsessional experience; for example, that their thoughts mean that they are a child molester, or that they are in constant danger of passing disease on to other people, and so on. (This is similar to the treatment of panic patients who believe that their palpitations mean that they are dying. Therapy is intended to help them to form and test a psychological model of their problem as arising from their misinterpretation.) The essence of treatment is helping sufferers to construct and test a new, less threatening model of their experience. Obsessional washers are helped to shift their view of their problem away from the idea that they might be contaminated and therefore must ensure that they do not pass this on to someone else or come to harm themself on to the idea that they have a specific problem which concerns their *fears* of contamination. That is, patients are helped to understand their problem as one of *thinking* and deciding rather than the "real-world" risks which they fear. The therapist and patient work to construct, agree, and actively test a coherent alternative and less threatening explanation of their problem. This shared understanding of the mechanism of obsessional problems is directly and explicitly contrasted with the beliefs they had previously held and which had motivated their obsessional and avoidance behavior. Thus, the mother who has intrusive ideas about harming her children is helped to consider that this may be because she loves her children so much that she dwells on and worries about the worst thing imaginable. This explanation is clearly quite different from the idea that she has these intrusions because she is a wicked person and bad mother who is in imminent danger of harming her children.

The main elements of treatment are as follows:

1. working with patients to develop a comprehensive cognitive-behavioral model of the maintenance of their obsessional problems as an alternative to the fears that they have. This process involves the identification of key distorted beliefs and the collaborative construction of a nonthreatening alternative account of their obsessional experience to allow patients to evaluate the validity of this alternative;

2. detailed identification and self-monitoring of obsessional thoughts and patients' appraisal of these thoughts combined with strategies designed to help patients to modify their responsibility beliefs;

3. discussion of techniques and behavioral experiments intended to challenge negative appraisals and basic assumptions upon which these are based. The aim is modification of patients' negative beliefs about the extent of their own personal responsibility (for example, by having patients describe all contributing factors for a feared outcome and then dividing the contributions in a piechart);

4. behavioral experiments to test directly appraisals, assumptions, and processes hypothesized to be involved in patients' obsessional problems (e.g., demonstrating that attempts to suppress a thought lead to an increase in the frequency with which it occurs, or showing that beliefs such as "If I think it, I therefore want it to happen" are incorrect). Each behavioral experiment is idiosyncratically devised in order to help patients test their previous (threatening) explanation of their experience against the new (nonthreatening) explanation worked out with their therapist;

5. helping patients to identify and modify underlying general assumptions (such as "not trying to prevent harm is as bad as making it happen deliberately") which give rise to their misinterpretation of their own mental activity.

It is necessary not only to tailor treatment to the specific shared understanding reached between therapist and patient concerning the particular idiosyncratic pattern of maintaining factors, but also to follow well-defined general principles concerning the way therapy is conducted. These general principles and several of the more important specific techniques are described below. Several other sources provide further details of these and other techniques in the treatment of obsessional problems (Salkovskis, 1989a, 1998; Salkovskis and Kirk, 1997; Salkovskis and Warwick, 1985, 1988; Salkovskis and Westbrook, 1987, 1989).

The style and format of cognitive-behavioral therapy

The style, format, and organization of cognitive-behavioral therapy for OCD (Salkovskis, 1999) is essentially similar to that used in treating other disorders (Beck, 1995). A sound and trusting therapeutic relationship in which the therapist seeks to maximize the extent to which the patient feels understood and wishes to engage actively in changing how he or she reacts to the problem serves as a foundation for effective treatment. The use of normalizing is particularly important in assisting patients with OCD, in that patients are helped to see that their reactions are not as unusual, strange, or crazy, as they had previously thought, but can be readily understood in terms of their own experience. This normalizing and empathic approach is particularly helpful in terms of restoring or boosting sufferers' self-esteem, and in helping to engage them in the active exploration and modification of their problem.

Therapy sessions are routinely audiotaped, and patients are given the tape to listen to as homework. Audiotapes are used for two main reasons. First, therapy sessions are relatively long, and patients are likely to have problems recalling all that was discussed. Second, if therapy is well-conducted, patients will frequently become upset, because therapy focuses on eliciting and modifying negative beliefs and behaviors which are central to patients' concerns. The emotion experienced can make it difficult for patients to process fully what went on during the therapy session. Listening to the tape allows individuals to assimilate fully what occurred in therapy, and to benefit more fully from the new ideas discussed and discovered in the session.

Cognitive therapy is conducted as part of a process of guided discovery, in which questioning and discussion are used to help patients to understand the nature of their problem and the factors involved in its persistence. Guided discovery almost inevitably leads patients to reach an understanding of the changes which they need to make in order to overcome their problems. This socratic style often incorporates the use of metaphors, stories, and analogies as a way of normalizing patients' experiences. Treatment techniques can be broadly split into discussion techniques and behavioral experiments. These two types of strategy are very closely linked, and are complementary. In discussion, the patient and therapist work on achieving a better understanding of the problem, considering evidence, past and present, for the patient's key beliefs and interpretations. As such discussion proceeds as a process of guided discovery, it will become clear that information important to answering crucial questions is simply not available. At such points, the aim is to devise behavioral experiments which have the effect of providing information relevant to these questions. Sometimes such experiments can fully answer key questions, as in experiments which provide patients with disconfirmation of their feared consequences (Salkovskis, 1991, 1996a, 1999). On completion of the behavioral experiment, the focus returns to discussion. In this way, good cognitive therapy involves the interweaving of discussion and behavioral experiments.

As described above, assessment and treatment have the aim of helping patients to consider and evaluate an alternative view of their situation, such as: "Maybe you are not dangerous, but are very worried about being dangerous." Much of the early part of therapy involves the explicit identification of the two contrasting views of the patient's problem, together with a detailed exploration of the implications of each, sometimes referred to as theory A/theory B. The patient and therapist work together to construct and test a new, less threatening explanation of the patient's experience, and then to examine explicitly the validity of the contrasting accounts. The early part of therapy therefore seeks to pose a general question of the form: "Which explains things best: that you are a child molester, or that you fear being a child molester?" From early in therapy, therapists make it clear that they do not expect patients simply to change their views as a result of discussions and the construction of an alternative explanation. "Don't trust me, test it out for yourself" is the explicit theme of therapy sessions subsequent to the therapist and patient agreeing on a possible, anxiety-based alternative account of the problem.

Reaching a shared understanding therefore involves the identification of key distorted beliefs and the collaborative construction of a nonthreatening *alternative account* of their obsessional experience and preoccupations. This alternative explanation is important because it allows patients to consider and explicitly test beliefs about the nature of their problem. Such beliefs emphasize the role of an inflated sense of responsibility for harm (to themselves and/or others) in generating and motivating compulsive and avoidant behaviors, and the way in which such neutralizing and avoidant behavior can in turn sustain or increase distorted beliefs concerning responsibility. One of the implications of such an approach is that it leads not only to verbal change strategies but also to a variant of ERP in which belief change is the guiding principle: the two types of strategy, verbal and behavioral, are closely interwoven. That is, ERP strategies are used as a way of helping patients discover the way in which neutralizing behavior acts to maintain their beliefs and the associated discomfort, and that stopping such behaviors is beneficial. Discussion helps patients understand how their problem works and directs them both to particular behavioral experiments and to ways of conducting these so as to maximize their understanding, which is consolidated in further discussion.

Assessment

Assessment, case formulation, and the presentation of a parsimonious cognitive-behavioral rationale to the patient are essential steps in treating obsessional disorders (Salkovskis, 1999). The first step in any program of cognitive-behavioral therapy is to establish a good rapport with the sufferer. This is usually done as part of a general assessment, which typically involves reviewing the history of the problem. During the more focused assessment, therapist and patient begin by identifying a recent episode during which the person's obsessional problem occurred or intensified. The context is primed (When was this? What were you doing at that time? What else was happening? How did you feel just before it began to be problematic?). Careful questioning and discussion about this episode are used to identify the *particular intrusion* (thought, image, impulse, or doubt) and the *significance* that the person attached to it (i.e., the way the intrusion was interpreted/appraised). The therapist then helps the patient focus on the way his or her particular interpretation, at the time in question, resulted in both distress and the desire (compulsion) to prevent or put right any possible harm which the patient has foreseen. Thus, discussion helps the patient and therapist identify the specific sequence of:

Intrusion → Interpretation → Reactions to the → Effects of these reactions both
                                  interpretation   on the interpretation and on
                                                            the occurrence of intrusions

The importance of negative evaluation is explored by asking patients if they can recall an occasion when the intrusion occurred, but they were *not* bothered by it. Discussion focuses on what was different on that occasion. Almost invariably, the difference lies in the fact that the person attached little or no significance to the occurrence of the intrusion. This discussion is critical in that it helps the patient to realize that an intrusion which is not negatively interpreted does not result in either distress or attempts to neutralize. Patients come to see that it is the meaning they attach to the intrusive thought that leads to their distress, not the thought itself. Patients are asked what they think they can learn from this comparison in terms of understanding the problems they experience when an intrusion occurs.

Having identified the fact that negative beliefs (particularly concerning responsibility for harm to oneself or others) account for the experience of distress, the therapeutic focus shifts to understanding the other implications of the way in which the person interprets intrusions. It is particularly useful to help the person put these factors together in a formulation of the type depicted in Figure 7.1. As in cognitive-behavioral therapy for other disorders socratic questioning and discussion are the main techniques used. When patients believed that they may have harmed a passerby, how did that make them feel? When they became depressed and afraid, what effect did those emotions have on their thinking? What did they try to *do*? What was the effect of trying to push the intrusions out of their mind? Did seeking reassurance make them feel more or less sure? What about in the longer term? And so on. It is important to check whether this was a typical episode. If not, or if the patient believes that there are different types of episode, repeat the assessment with another specific episode, seeking to identify both commonalities and differences.

Assessment is seldom entirely straightforward or easy. Probably the commonest difficulty experienced in assessment is when it is not clear what the intrusions are. In such instances, patients may often refer to "my thoughts" repeatedly in session, but will not specify what they are. Patients often are reluctant to describe intrusions due to beliefs about what might happen if they did describe their thoughts (e.g., the therapist will think they are mad or bad, will laugh, or simply saying things out loud will make the thoughts worse, the feared outcomes more likely to happen, and so on). It is relatively easy to identify such factors. The therapist indicates a degree of understanding ("Many people with this type of problem find it difficult to mention what their thoughts are about, often because they think that it is risky to do so. Does that type of idea ever cross your mind? What do you think is the worst thing which would happen if you mentioned them to me?"). It can often be helpful to second-guess the type of thoughts by giving clinical examples which the therapist judges are likely to be similar to the present patient's experience. The therapist might, for example, note: "I saw a patient last week who was bothered by thoughts of being violent to his family; he was worried that I might think that he wanted to do these things, which of course I did not."

In some patients with prominent, frequent, or long-standing compulsive behavior or neutralizing, no obvious negative interpretations or evaluations may be apparent. This typically happens because the avoidance and neutralizing behaviors have become relatively automatic responses which preempt the perception of threat. As such responses are used, awareness of threat recedes. To help patients consider what is being sought, a simple metaphor can be useful. Patients are asked why they stop at red traffic lights. What *actually* runs through their mind each time they stop? In fact, few people call to mind the danger involved. How could they identify their beliefs? What would run through their mind if they found that their brakes were not working as they approached lights? Is it possible that something similar is happening when they check or wash at the moment? How could they find out? Such a discussion almost inevitably leads to a simple behavioral experiment in which patients refrain from their ritual or other neutralizing in order to identify the implicit negative evaluations motivating their obsessional behavior.

Finally, home visits can be a particularly useful adjunct to assessment, often helping the therapist to observe and work with patients to explore the full scope of their problem.

Goal setting

As the therapist gains a better understanding of patients' problems, it is important to agree with patients their principal goals. This can be divided into: (1) short-term goals: goals which can reasonably be achieved in two to four sessions; (2) medium-term goals: what can reasonably be achieved by the end of therapy; and (3) long-term goals: what the patient would like to do over the next few years. It is important to note that getting rid of all intrusive thoughts is not a helpful or achievable goal (because such thoughts are known to be both common and normal: Rachman and de Silva, 1978; Salkovskis and Harrison, 1984).

Beginning treatment

A range of cognitive and behavioral interventions can be used in treating obsessional disorders (Salkovskis and Westbrook, 1987; Salkovskis and Kirk, 1997; Salkovskis, 1999). These approaches will only be successful, however, if patients are actively engaged in a collaborative relationship which has the explicit aim of changing their reactions to obsessional intrusions and the situations which provoke them. Such an aim can conflict with patients' initial goals, which are often to be reassured, to find more effective ways of washing, checking, or overcoming doubts. This conflict of goals is usually not an issue once a shared understanding has been reached. Much of the more specific engagement work involves helping patients shift perspective. A good way of doing this is to help patients to identify the full balance of costs and benefits involved in their obsessional behavior, not just the immediate ones. Many patients will be reluctant to change the way they react to obsessional fears unless they are provided with a guarantee from the therapist that the catastrophes they fear being responsible for will not happen. Bad things happen, though, and guarantees that catastrophes will not strike cannot be made. Living without undue anxiety requires the acceptance of risk. Early in therapy, there is no point in seeking to work with the probabilities of disaster (which in any case often tend to seem very low but very awful to them), but rather to have them refocus. For example, a woman who seeks assurance that her house will not be burgled if she reduces her checking is told: "I can't guarantee that your house will be safe if you don't check. I *can* guarantee that you will continue to suffer from obsessional problems, probably for the rest of your life, if you continue to check." "How much would you pay to get rid of your obsessional problem?" "How much *are* you paying to make sure that you are clean/sure."

A major aim of therapy is to help patients to identify why they are distressed by their obsessional problem (because they believe that they are in danger of being responsible for harm). Treatment helps them to consider an alternative, altogether more benign explanation (that they are so sensitive to ideas of being responsible for harm that they take unnecessary precautions, which then have counterproductive effects). This comparison can be used in a theory A/theory B contrast. For example: "There are two ways of thinking about your problem. The first possibility is that your problem is that *you are contaminated*, and that you have to wash repeatedly because you believe that your failure to wash to your complete satisfaction could result in you being responsible for your family falling ill and possibly dying. The alternative way of looking at it is that you are someone who, for understandable reasons, is sensitive to *worries* about being contaminated and who reacts to those worries in ways which tend actually to increase your concerns and which disrupt your life (for example, by washing excessively)."

Some patients will agree that the alternative makes sense of what is happening to them, and agree that this is the sensible way to work with their problems. Some patients will find this more difficult, initially suggesting that it is too difficult or dangerous for them to change their obsessional patterns of thinking and behaving. In such instances, it is helpful to contrast their previous counterproductive ways of coping with the possibility of change. The patient can be asked: "How much effort have you put into dealing with the problem *as if* you were a danger to those around you?" Most patients are aware that this is the *only* way they have sought to deal with their obsessional concerns, so this is followed up with "How helpful has that been?" This discussion reaches the conclusion that any relief they have obtained from being obsessional has been short-lived at best, and that trying to obsess one's way out of an obsession almost always results in a worsening of the problem.

This discussion is followed by further questioning which aims to have the patient consider the possibility for change and its likely consequences: "Have you ever tried to deal with the problem *as if* it were a problem of excessive concern and worry?" Few, if any, patients have done this at all. The therapist suggests that, as the assessment indicates that this is now an obvious alternative way of dealing with their current problems: "Would you give it a wholehearted try for 3 months, then review it with me?" Assuming the answer is yes, it is then helpful to ask: "How do you think it would be most helpful to begin to change things?" This last question is a very helpful way of beginning things, as it usually results in patients making active suggestions for changes in the way they respond to their intrusions.

Given that most obsessional problems reflect patients' sensitivity to fears that they will cause or fail to prevent harm, it is not surprising that some patients express the concern that changing their behavior as part of therapy might result in an overreaction, so that they become excessively careless, dirty, irreligious, and so on (Salkovskis, 1999). If such fears are expressed, the therapist will want to address them directly. This can be accomplished through socratic questioning. The therapist might, for example, ask: "In your experience, how easy is it to get less obsessional? How easy to get more obsessional?" Without exception, obsessional patients will indicate that it is all too easy to become more obsessional, and thus far has been extremely difficult to reduce their OCD. On the basis of this discussion, the therapist promises to help the person to become more obsessional in the unlikely event that, as treatment draws to an end, there have been unacceptable negative effects. That is, if some aspect of the changes they have made has resulted in a significant and, to the patient, undesirable reversal of obsessional behavior (that a cleaner has become dirty, that a checker has become careless). This has not so far been requested in the author's practice.

Changing the way intrusions are interpreted by normalizing them

Given that the focus of treatment is on helping patients to adopt and test an alternative, less threatening explanation of their problems, most therapy techniques focus on reappraisal. A key component of this is *normalizing* the experience of intrusions, helping patients to change their understanding of the significance of the occurrence and content of intrusions (Salkovskis, 1999). These approaches are important in so far as studies indicate that provision of a rational normalization of intrusive thoughts and reappraisal of notions of responsibility over the course of cognitive-behavioral therapy are associated with reductions in the severity of OCD symptoms (Williams et al., 2002). Some normalizing will have taken place in the course of the assessment, through the fact that the therapist is clearly aware of the type of intrusive thoughts which occur and the use of simple empathic statements (e.g., "So it's not surprising that you felt uncomfortable in that situation, because the thought 'I'll kill my baby' came to your mind just as you were cuddling him, and you thought that this might mean that you wanted to kill him"). As treatment begins, the therapist uses more explicit normalizing strategies, often beginning this phase by saying something like "people suffering from obsessions often wrongly believe that their thoughts are abnormal, insane, or unusual. I'd like to examine whether that really is so." Guided discovery is used to help patients consider several important questions, as follows.

Who has obsessional thoughts?

It is helpful to ask patients who is likely to be troubled by intrusions concerning a range of obsessional themes, starting with some which they are *not* currently experiencing. Who is likely to be bothered by blasphemous obsessions? Obsessions of harming children? Violent obsessions? When might a positive thought be upsetting? The patient is asked to consider the effect on someone of a thought about having a pleasant holiday if it occurs in the context of a close friend being lowered into the grave. This discussion is used to emphasize the idea that it is not the intrusion itself which causes discomfort, but the way in which it is interpreted. By definition, negative interpretations are most likely in those who hold personal beliefs which are the opposite of the content of intrusions. Religious people are bothered and worried by blasphemous thoughts, gentle people by violent thoughts, careful people by thoughts of carelessness and so on. The discussion can also turn to consideration of the similarity between obsessional thoughts and worry. When people worry, what do they worry about? Do people worry more about good things not happening or terrible things happening? What does the patient think the therapist might worry about? What intrusive thoughts might the therapist have? Once the patient concludes that obsessions usually concern areas in which one is particularly sensitive, the discussion refocuses on their own obsessional intrusions.

How common are intrusive thoughts? Do they only occur in people suffering from OCD?

Patients are invited to consider how common negative intrusive thoughts might be. Research findings indicating that almost everyone experiences unwanted and unacceptable intrusions are discussed (Rachman and de Silva, 1978; Salkovskis and Harrison, 1984). Intrusions as a general phenomenon are discussed (including the fact that intrusions can be positive, negative, and neutral intrusions). The patient is asked to consider what it would be like never to have intrusions: "Imagine that you had to plan every thought you were going to have; what would that be like?"

Why are intrusions so common? Are they any use?

Following on from the previous question, the patient is asked whether intrusive thoughts might be useful. The discussion leads to the ideas that intrusions play an important role in problem-solving and creativity. If one is seeking to problem-solve, what's the best way to generate solutions? Should you only try to consider solutions which you think are good? The creative function of brainstorming is highlighted. When might violent thoughts be helpful? How about when one's family were being threatened? If a boy were on the point of accidentally drinking something poisonous, might it be helpful to knock the cup from his hand as the quickest way of stopping him? This discussion might turn to consideration of how helpful or otherwise it might be only to have positive thoughts when someone directly threatens the patient or his or her family. The aim of this discussion is to conclude that intrusive thoughts are not only normal, but are also an important part of daily life.

Linking the individual's history to the formulation

People with a history of OCD are likely to maintain a heightened sense of responsibility for events which may not be completely within their control. Sometimes there are very obvious links between the patient's early experience and their heightened sensitivity to responsibility. A more detailed assessment of the origins of such beliefs can be helpful as a way of challenging these ideas in the present, especially in cases where dysfunctional assumptions about responsibility are extremely difficult to change. For example, patients can respond to a strongly held unconditional belief by reminding themselves that this is a product of "brainwashing." That is, beliefs which they learned from important authority figures as a child are returning and that they are responding to these as if they were still a child. An alternative is to challenge the idea from an adult perspective and consider whether these beliefs first, were true then and second, are still true now.

It has been suggested that there are several characteristic patterns of experience involved in the development of an inflated sense of responsibility (Salkovskis et al., 1999). These are: (1) patients who have, from an early age, believed themselves to be crucially responsible, usually as a result of excessive responsibility being placed upon them due to absence, actions, or incompetence of others, e.g., the eldest child of a depressed mother and alcoholic father who assumes responsibility for siblings; (2) patients who have been overprotected to the point of seldom having felt responsible for even minor actions; (3) people who have had an experience which they erroneously believe indicates that they have caused harm, e.g., wishing someone dead followed by their actual death a short time later; (4) people who have had an experience which has indeed contributed to harm (e.g., the person who left the television on by mistake and whose house subsequently burned down).

Understanding and testing counterproductive strategies

Having worked on decatastrophizing the occurrence and content of intrusions, the therapist then turns attention to helping the patient understand and deal with responses which are involved in the maintenance of his or her negative beliefs. These factors fall into several broad categories, including selective attention and vigilance, the effects of mood (anxiety and depression), physiological arousal, neutralizing behaviors and other counterproductive safety-seeking strategies (including overt avoidance, thought suppression and cognitive avoidance, reassurance-seeking, the use of inappropriate criteria for stopping a behavior, and so on: Salkovskis, 1999). Much of this part of therapy focuses on those responses to intrusive thoughts, impulses, images, and doubts in which patients actively engage as part of their safety-seeking efforts. Such efforts are, of course, usually directed at attempts to ensure that harm does not come to themselves or others, and that they can be sure that they are not responsible (or risking being responsible) for such harm.

It is particularly important that patients be helped to understand the impact of counterproductive strategies. Several metaphors are clinically helpful here, including the idea that these activities (such as thought suppression and ritualizing) are rather like digging to get out of a hole, trying to put out a fire with gasoline. That is, the action that one believes is making things better is actually making them worse. The patient is helped to question whether obsessional behavior is a good way of dealing with an obsessional problem, or whether the things the person is doing as part of the "solution" to obsessional worries have in fact become a major part of the problem and its maintenance. For some patients, the discussion of the history of the development of their problem helps them to understand that, in the past, the harder they have tried to check, wash, or otherwise neutralize, the worse their problem has become. It is suggested that it may not be appropriate to try to get out of a hole by digging faster or finding a bigger shovel. Another helpful strategy is briefly to describe the spontaneous decay experiments of Rachman and colleagues (Rachman et al., 1976). The short-term benefits of ritualizing such as anxiety relief are contrasted with the longer-term effects of obsessional fears, avoidance, and behavior. This discussion will inevitably lead to consideration of behavioral experiments involving elements of exposure and response prevention.

Consideration of the formulation leads to closely interwoven discussion and behavioral experiments designed to help patients gather further evidence for the way in which the mechanisms identified affect them. For example, patients are asked to consider what usually happens to someone who tries to avoid thinking about something which is important to him or her. Have they themselves ever had the experience of trying not to think of something? Could they try now, in the office, not to think of giraffes? What happens? Why would trying not to think of something make this thing come to mind more both now and later? The discussion focuses on the fact that, if you wish to avoid something, you have to keep in mind what is being avoided! Follow-up homework experiments involving an alternating treatments single case experimental design can be helpful in gathering further evidence for the importance of the paradoxical effects of thought suppression (Salkovskis, 1999). Patients keep a daily diary of intrusive thoughts, also recording the amount of effort they put into suppression in the course of the day. They are then asked to try very hard to get rid of their intrusions by suppressing them on some days (for example, on Monday, Wednesday, Friday, and Sunday), and simply to record the occurrence of thoughts without making any special attempts at suppression on the other days. The frequency of intrusions is set out in a graph with the two types of days interspersed. Figure 7.2 shows an example from an actual patient. The patient recorded her intrusion during intervals of the day on a diary for a week, then alternated suppression/recording for a further week (Salkovskis, 1999). Ratings of suppression were also recorded, and indicated that the patient had indeed suppressed more on the days when she had been instructed to do this. The thought frequency information was then set out in a graph, as shown in Figure 7.2. Patients are shown their graph, and asked what they make of the results. This patient concluded that attempts to push the thoughts out of her mind were worse than useless, and agreed to stop any efforts to resist, suppress, or neutralize her intrusions.

The Oxford OCD group have highlighted the importance of the use of unusual criteria in the decision to stop an activity (i.e., to stop checking, washing, and so on).

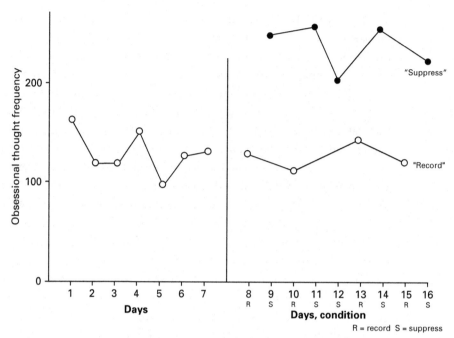

Figure 7.2   Example of an actual patient of frequency of intrusions. Reproduced from Salkovskis. P. M. (1999). Understanding and treating obsessive-compulsive disorder. *Behaviour Research and Therapy*, 37, S29–S52, with permission.

Preliminary evidence has been obtained which suggests that obsessional patients make simple decisions (such as whether or not the light switch is off, or whether or not one's hands are clean) using the type of criteria which would be typical of nonobsessionals *when they are making a particularly important decision*. If this is confirmed, it is entirely consistent with the cognitive-behavioral theory, in that obsessional patients are evaluating simple decisions as being more serious than they really are. Important decisions are usually made on the basis of as wide a range of evidence as is available; given that the evidence may be relatively complicated (and possibly even somewhat contradictory), obsessional patients are more likely to use difficult-to-achieve internal states (being sure of something, feeling certain, and so on) as the criteria for ceasing repetition (see also Salkovskis et al., 1998, p. 50).

The leading explanation for these phenomena involves the assumption that patients with OCD have "elevated evidence requirements" to make a stopping decision. The elevated evidence requirement means that multiple criteria have to be fulfilled in order to stop the compulsion. We expect that initially multiple *external* criteria have to be fulfilled and that, towards the end of the compulsion, *additional internally referenced* criteria become more and more important. In other words, the pattern we expect to find in patients with OCD could be a hierarchical pattern with external criteria being important all the time and internal criteria becoming more and more important when the compulsion progresses. For each of these criteria it is assumed that they have to meet an increased threshold compared to thresholds involved in decision-making for noncompulsive behavior.

The decision-making process involved in compulsive behavior is therefore not qualitatively different from decision-making processes in noncompulsive behavior. Under certain conditions every decision-making process can be based on elevated evidence requirements. These conditions are believed to be characterized by a perception of harm threatening yourself or others and the belief that by acting in a certain way you can prevent or reduce this harm. Individuals with OCD thus make use of *strategic* decision-making processes in order to stop a compulsion. These processes are assumed to require mental capacity, conscious awareness, and they can be voluntarily started and finished. By contrast, in order to initialize or terminate short noncompulsive behavior, less mental effort is spent on it, and it can occur without awareness (but we assume it is subject to voluntary control).

These counterproductive decision-making strategies are modified in therapy in similar ways to thought suppression, including the use of behavioral experiments using an alternating treatments design. For example, a client who agreed to use only his "feeling-sure" strategy for determining whether his alarm was set on some days of the week, and only his "intellectual recognition that the switch was up" on the remainder, for instance, swiftly discovered that *trying* to feel sure actually made him more uncomfortable and decreased his perceived certainty. Such behavioral experiments require careful setting-up and the client has to record the outcomes in ways which are then used to illustrate how these apparently helpful strategies are actually maintaining the problem.

A similar sequence of discussion and behavioral experiments is used for each factor identified, including other safety-seeking behaviors and mood. Behavioral experiments are used wherever possible to discover or demonstrate the effects of the patients' anxiety-based reactions to intrusions, with the basis for such experiments being drawn from discussion with the patient. Other examples include the use of mood induction procedures (Clark, 1983) if patients do not understand the effects of negative mood on their thinking and beliefs. The negative impact of reassurance-seeking and obsessional ritualizing can be illustrated in similar ways. Discussion, in which the patient is reminded of the formulation previously identified, provides a detailed alternative account which highlights the way in which ritualistic behavior is counterproductive in the long term, even though it often feels beneficial in the short term (e.g., in helping the patient reduce immediate discomfort). A helpful metaphor is to compare the obsessional problem to a playground bully. Again, questioning and guided discovery are the preferred mode of discussion. The bully may begin by making relatively small demands for money, and the victim feels relieved once he or she has bought the bully off. Does that mean that the victim is now free from any further threat? Why not? What happens next? How is that similar to the demands imposed by OCD? How can one break free of the demands of the bully? Will that feel comfortable at first? How will matters progress? The discussion aims to have patients conclude that they need to take the offensive against their obsessional problems, challenging their beliefs rather than seeking to be safe from them. Again, the use of behavioral experiments to demonstrate the effects of reassurance-seeking or ritualizing is a helpful development from that discussion. Once patients are, in their heart, convinced that obsessional ritualizing is maintaining and/or increasing their problems, systematic and self-initiated response prevention follows naturally. Often such a course of action is suggested by patients themselves.

Challenging responsibility appraisals

The assessment, formulation, discussion, and behavioral experiments described above all serve to reveal beliefs focused on an inflated sense of responsibility for harm. Such beliefs are crucial as they motivate patients' efforts to neutralize, check that they have not caused harm, or to undo any harm which they may have triggered. Assisting patients to understand the role of such beliefs in their OCD can be helpful. This knowledge will not, however, necessarily result in them being able to resist the urge to neutralize. Modifying these maladaptive beliefs about responsibility is a central focus of treatment in so far as changes in beliefs about responsibility appear to be associated with clinical improvement among patients with OCD (Williams et al., 2002).

Typically, more direct and assertive responsibility modification strategies are needed. One of the most helpful of these is the piechart, in which therapist and patient work together to learn a strategy to deal with one of the commonest assumptions found in obsessional problems. Cognitive distortions, such as all-or-nothing thinking (Beck, 1995), lead the patient with OCD to believe that "if in any way you can influence a harmful outcome, then you are responsible for it." Such distortions are particularly difficult to deal with if they concern past events where, with hindsight, it is remotely possible that the patient could have prevented the negative event from happening. The fact that such prevention would have required foresight and unusual reactions to mundane situations is not usually regarded by the patient as in any way helpful. The piechart is used as a way of tackling all-or-nothing thinking whilst at the same time allowing the therapist to avoid debating the intrusion and thereby buying into the patient's attempt to neutralize and seek reassurance.

The therapist draws a piechart which represents responsibility for the negative event in question. Patients are then asked to draw up a list of all possible influences contributing to such responsibility, *starting with their own actions or failure to act*. All other influences are then listed, with as much time as necessary being taken in order to ensure a thorough list. Once this is completed, patients are asked to assign proportions of the responsibility to each factor in turn, *starting at the bottom of the list*. This means, of course, that the patient's own contribution is the last one dealt with. Note that the therapist does not seek to reassure the patient; the elements in the list come from the patient, with occasional prompting from the therapist, whose main job is to provide the structure in this discussion. Note also that the aim is not to convince patients that they are *not* responsible, but rather to draw their attention to the fact that responsibility is multifaceted and characterized by shades of gray rather than black and white. Note also that such a strategy helps counteract obsessional patients' tendency towards overlooking the role of those alternative explanations for which they do not have any responsibility. This exercise can also be helpful in making the point that it is seldom possible to prove that one had no influence whatsoever over a past event, and that reviewing such events in great detail will lead to an increase in doubt rather than to certainty that you were not responsible. A helpful way of providing a counterpoint to such a discussion is to ask patients to consider whether they could, by a reversal of their obsessional behavior, bring about the feared consequences. Could a washer assassinate someone by deliberately not washing his or her hands after going to the bathroom? Would not washing be a good way of committing murder?

Exposure and behavioral experiments

The techniques described above are all designed to help patients reach the conclusion that they should cease their counterproductive strategies. As cognitive-behavioral therapy progresses, the notion of ERP becomes self-evident, and a more planned and detailed program is initiated (Salkovskis and Kirk, 1989). Such a program is discussed with patients as the logical extension of the previous belief change strategies, with an appropriate combination of explicit aims: (1) to deal with compulsive/neutralizing behaviors as a factor which maintain their negative beliefs; (2) as a way of demonstrating to themselves that the formulation is indeed correct, as it predicts that reducing neutralizing will result in decreases in both anxiety and in negative beliefs; (3) as a confrontation and disconfirmation of their negative expectancies where appropriate (i.e., to help them to discover that their feared consequences do not occur when they stop their safety-seeking behaviors when such disconfirmation is possible); (4) to begin the process of regaining control over those aspects of their life which have come to be dominated by compulsive and neutralizing behavior, that is, to deal with compulsive behavior as a problem rather than as a way of preventing harm. Exposure tasks are planned and set up with the explicit aim of bringing about such belief changes. Early on, therapist-aided tasks are used to begin the process of challenging the negative appraisals activated by the person not neutralizing. Discussion after the task is completed is used to consolidate and extend such belief change, particularly with respect to patients' perceptions of the alternative account of their problems.

The importance of patients assuming responsibility for their own actions (rather than simply complying with the suggestions made by the therapist) is emphasized. This is best achieved by the therapist modeling exposure exercises in the early stages, but rapidly moving to having the patient do things without modeling, then having patients assume the role of identifying and planning exposure exercises themselves. Subsequently, patients are asked to plan and execute exposure tasks and to describe their responses without describing the task itself. Doing this removes the reassurance involved in having the therapist know about the details of the task undertaken by the patient. If the task is described, this serves as reassurance, as patients believe that, had they undertaken something truly dangerous, then the therapist will react, making the absence of a reaction reassuring in itself. Note also that the rationale for the shift of responsibility to the patient is explained and reviewed in detail.

Direct or subtle reassurance-seeking tends to occur in the course of therapy, most commonly without patients being aware that "just mentioning" something they did as part of therapy to the therapist is problematic. To deal with this, the therapist first discusses the way that this works: "When you mention things like that, are you interested in my reaction? Why is that?" In patients who find it hard to understand why such reassurance is not being offered, a simple discussion strategy can be helpful: "You can have as much reassurance as you need. I'll cancel my remaining appointments for today, and we'll just work on reassurance. In turn, you have to promise me that the reassurance will last for the rest of the year." In this situation, the patient almost invariably points out that it is not possible, and on questioning will say that the effects of reassurance are only very temporary, often lasting only minutes. The therapist can then ask whether the patient believes that seeking reassurance is actually a helpful strategy. In this way, *the patient tells the therapist* that reassurance-seeking is at best ineffective and at worst counterproductive and anxiety-provoking. Again, this discussion is related back to the formulation.

More reappraisal and belief change strategies

Other cognitive therapy techniques are used to help the patient to become more aware of the presence and role of threat and responsibility beliefs. These include modifications (Salkovskis et al., 1998) of the Dysfunctional Thought Record (Beck, 1979). The downward arrow and two-column technique are used as appropriate in the context of particular issues arising in therapy (Salkovskis, 1989a; Salkovskis and Warwick, 1988; Salvoskis et al., 1998). The use of the downward arrow is tailored to the specific appraisals the person makes, which can be of the occurrence or the content of the intrusion, or both (Salkovskis et al., 1995). Figure 7.3 shows a previously

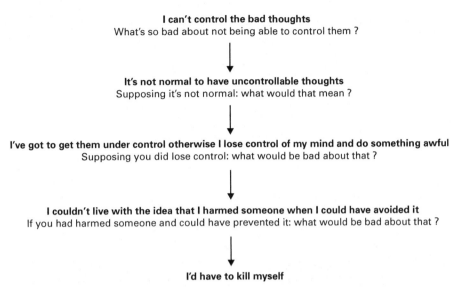

I can't control the bad thoughts
What's so bad about not being able to control them ?

It's not normal to have uncontrollable thoughts
Supposing it's not normal: what would that mean ?

I've got to get them under control otherwise I lose control of my mind and do something awful
Supposing you did lose control: what would be bad about that ?

I couldn't live with the idea that I harmed someone when I could have avoided it
If you had harmed someone and could have prevented it: what would be bad about that ?

I'd have to kill myself

Figure 7.3   Using the vertical arrow to access assumptions. Reproduced from Salkovskis. P. M. (1999). Understanding and treating obsessive-compulsive disorder. *Behaviour Research and Therapy*, 37, S29–S52, with permission.

published version of such a downward arrow, in which both the occurrence and content of the intrusions form the focus (Salkovskis and Westbrook, 1987). Both responsibility and metacognitive beliefs were identified here.

Therapy would aim: (1) to help the patient to understand the way in which an apparently innocuous thought can evoke so much discomfort ("so when you think 'I can't control the bad thoughts,' this means you might have to kill yourself because you believe you might have harmed someone"); (2) to challenge the assumptions at each level (see Salkovskis and Warwick, 1988, for examples of this) using conventional cognitive therapy challenges towards the end of the sequence; and (3) having identified key assumptions on the basis of downward arrows and specific questionnaires such as the Responsibility Attitudes scale (Salkovskis et al., 2000), seeking to modify these more directly. Wells (1996, p. 91) identifies a further novel use of the downward arrow. Rather than probing for threat cognitions in the usual way when the person identifies the wish to engage in a safety-seeking behavior (i.e., by responding to "I've got to check" with "What do you think is the worst thing that would happen if you failed to check at that time?"), the therapist probes the consequences of the safety-seeking behavior itself by responding to "I've got to check" with "What's bad about that?" (Wells, 1996). Such a procedure has the effect of highlighting the negative consequences of being obsessional, and can serve as a useful engagement strategy supplementing the procedures described above. Interestingly, rather than examining patients' beliefs about their thoughts as described here, this procedure examines their thoughts about the consequences of their behaviors, for example, by using the downward arrow (see Salkovskis, 1989a/b, 1999).

Although the type of cognitive challenge strategies described here are specific to each patient, the outcomes of the challenge are always referred back to the formulation. In OCD the therapist pays particular attention to the possibility that such techniques and their discussion with the therapist may become a form of subtle neutralizing behavior or may begin to take on characteristics of obsessional reassurance-seeking.

Evaluation of cognitive theory of OCD and cognitive-behavioral therapy for OCD

Most aspects of the cognitive-behavioral theory of OCD have now been subjected to experimental evaluation. Such research has, for example, established that beliefs directly and indirectly related to responsibility are elevated in obsessional patients relative to both nonclinical and anxious controls (Freeston and Ladouceur, 1993; Rheaume et al., 1994; Wilson and Chambless, 1999). In a large study conducted by our group, responsibility assumptions and interpretations in obsessional patients, anxious controls, and community volunteers found not only that responsibility beliefs were higher in obsessional patients than in controls, but these were also strong predictors of obsessional symptoms (Salkovskis et al., 2000). The impact of responsibility appraisals has also been shown in the effect of responsibility manipulations on systematically increasing and decreasing obsessional behaviors (Lopatka and Rachman, 1995; Ladouceur et al., 1995, 1997; Bouchard et al., 1999; Shafran, 1997) and on intrusive thinking (Rassin et al., 1999). The parallel between covert neutralizing and overt rituals has been established (Rachman et al., 1996), as has the effect of neutralizing on increasing discomfort and decreasing resistance to further neutralizing (Salkovskis et al., 1997). Numerous studies have demonstrated the paradoxical effect of thought suppression on the occurrence of intrusions in both the short term (Wegner et al., 1987; Clark et al., 1991; Salkovskis and Campbell, 1994) and the long term (Trinder and Salkovskis, 1994). Our group has found that a major component of the effects seen in suppression studies may be related to the effects of self-monitoring; this is an important observation, as it is clear that obsessional patients tend to become highly focused on their own thought processes, particularly to the occurrence of intrusions.

Although the effectiveness of therapeutic interventions based on a particular theory does not provide evidence in support of that theory, the failure of such interventions, assuming that they were properly conducted, would call the theory into serious question. Thus far, the results of treatment studies have consistently demonstrated the effectiveness of cognitive interventions.

Effectiveness of cognitive-behavioral strategies

Cognitive treatment without the incorporation of exposure has, surprisingly, been shown to be at least as effective as behavioral treatment (Van Oppen et al., 1995). It has also been shown to be as effective as a combination of cognitive treatment with fluvoxamine or behavioral treatment with fluvoxamine. (van Balkom et al., 1994). A number of studies are now under way in which cognitive-behavioral therapy is compared with behavior therapy; the results of these should illuminate the relative contribution of explicit cognitive elements.

Whilst some indication of the contribution of cognitive as opposed to purely behavioral treatments is of academic and theoretical interest, clinical interest has tended to focus on the issue of drug versus cognitive-behavioral treatment, and whether it is likely to be helpful to combine these. Over the last few years, it has often been suggested that pharmacotherapy and psychotherapy operate through different mechanisms. It would therefore follow that their effects would be additive in combination. On the basis of this, combination therapy has been proposed as the treatment of choice. Kozak et al. (2000) have recently reported preliminary results of a particularly well-conducted two-center study investigating this issue. Cognitive-behavioral therapy, pharmacotherapy, placebo, and their combination are evaluated. In the short term, cognitive-behavioral therapy adds to the effectiveness of pharmacotherapy but not vice versa. In the longer term, pharmacotherapy is associated with a high relapse rate, with very similar relapse in both cognitive-behavioral therapy and combination treatments. If the results of this interim analysis prove to hold on completion of the study, they suggest that the mechanisms of action may be more similar than had previously been thought. This raises the interesting prospect of investigations involving a microanalysis of the cognitive and behavioral changes which occur in pharmacotherapy and which are reversed by medication cessation. Such an analysis could lead to more efficient combinations, in which pharmacotherapy is used for brief periods in order to enhance psychological changes, which would be expected to be more enduring once established and medication has been withdrawn.

Future directions

The next 5 years are likely to see the completion of a substantial number of individual difference and experimental studies designed to investigate the contribution of cognitive factors in OCD, particularly studies emanating from the international Obsessive-Compulsive Cognitions Working Group (1997), and randomized controlled trials systematically investigating the contribution of cognitive components in the treatment of OCD, as opposed to the sterile comparison of purely cognitive versus purely behavioral treatments. Particularly exciting is the prospect of the completion of the National Institute of Mental Health (NIMH) two-center cognitive-behavioral therapy/pharmacotherapy study, for which the preliminary results are outlined above. Assuming that the preliminary results hold for the full sample, this study will dispel the long-standing clinical myths that psychological and pharmacological treatments should be combined and that pharmacological treatments are sufficient when cognitive-behavioral therapy is not available. Those responsible for the provision of treatment for patients suffering from OCD are likely to be confronted by the necessity of providing good-quality cognitive-behavioral therapy, despite the very limited availability of competent therapists. This problem is also likely to highlight a further problem, which is the extent to which cognitive-behavioral therapy in OCD simply represents the addition of cognitive restructuring elements to behavior therapy (Foa and Franklin, 2000), or whether the use of cognitive elements constitutes a set of guiding principles resulting in a substantially different and more cognitively elaborated treatment as described here (see also Salkovskis, 2000).

The tension between biological and psychological understanding and treatment of OCD is not confined to the treatment arena. Although a variety of biological mechanisms have been proposed to account for obsessional problems, none has received consistent experimental validation. It has been suggested (Salkovskis, 1996b) that this problem at least in part arises from the type of theories of OCD currently used in biological psychiatry, which tend to rely on overly simplistic "lesion" or "biochemical imbalance"-type models. Most commonly, there is a failure of such theories to account for the *phenomenology* of OCD; that is, there is little correspondence between the pattern of symptoms which patients report and the biological mechanisms which are supposed to account for them. By contrast, the main psychological theories adopt a continuum/normal processes-type approach to OCD, explicitly specifying that there is no distinctive pathophysiology involved. However, even from such a normalizing perspective it could be argued that identifying brain mechanisms involved in the key psychological processes, particularly in the way OCD-relevant stimuli are processed, would have at least epistemological value. From such a perspective, it could be argued that a sensible (nonlesion-based) neuroscience approach should take as its starting point an understanding of the psychological processes involved in OCD. The limited success of pharmacotherapy and the extraordinarily high relapse rates suggest an important direction of such an approach. This type of approach would involve a microanalysis, in which OCD is not seen as a "lump," but rather as a complex (but readily definable) interaction between cognitive processes and products. For example, it is possible to define separately the occurrence of intrusions, their vividness, the associated meaning, the strength of any urge to neutralize, the degree of resistance experienced, the intensity of any neutralizing, and so on. The components of the model shown in Figure 7.1 can be characterized in terms of an assessment of at least 30 items. Based on such an approach, a microanalysis of the psychological changes associated with effective treatment with medication could be used to identify which components change in the course of successful treatment, and which revert to their original levels when medication is withdrawn and patients relapse. Such analyses should allow identification of a relatively smaller number of specific components of OCD which could usefully be dealt with following effective pharmacotherapy and should reduce relapse rates. By the same token, a comparable microanalysis should allow the idenfication of patients in whom the response to cognitive-behavioral therapy has been less than complete, and who are likely to benefit from the addition of medication. Although complex to implement, the results of such a program of research would inform both theoretical and clinical issues. Clearly, for such a program to become a reality, there is a need for some further elaboration of cognitive factors in OCD, although considerable progress has been made in this respect already. More problematic is the way in which biological theories have become both fragmented and have been built on the assumption that OCD must involve some fundamental disturbance of brain functioning. Paradoxically, then, helping biological researchers to achieve a more sophisticated view of OCD is probably the greatest challenge facing those working from a cognitive-behavioral therapy perspective.

REFERENCES

Beck, A. T. (1976). *Cognitive Therapy and the Emotional Disorders*. New York: International Universities Press.

Beck, A. T. (1979). *Cognitive Therapy of Depression*. New York: Guilford Press.

Beck, J. (1995). *Cognitive Therapy: Basics and Beyond*. New York: Guilford Press.

Beck, A. T., Emery, G., and Greenberg, R. L. (1985). *Anxiety Disorders and Phobias: A Cognitive Perspective*. New York: Basic Books.

Bouchard, C., Rheaume, J., and Ladouceur, R. (1999). Responsibility and perfectionism in OCD: an experimental study. *Behaviour Research and Therapy*, **37**(3), 239–48.

Clark, D. M. (1983). On the induction of depressed mood in the laboratory: evaluation and comparison of the Velten and musical procedures. *Advances in Behaviour Research and Therapy*, **5**, 27–49.

Clark, D. M. (1988). A cognitive model of panic. In *Panic: Psychological Perspectives*, ed. S. J. Rachman and J. Maser, pp. 71–90. Hillsdale: Erlbaum.

Clark, D. A. and Purdon, C. (1993). New perspectives for a cognitive theory of obsessions. *Australian Psychologist*, **28**(3), 161–7.

Clark, D. M., Ball, S., and Pape, D. (1991). An experimental investigation of thought suppression. *Behaviour Research and Therapy*, **29**(3), 253–7.

Edwards, S. and Dickerson, M. (1987). On the similarity of positive and negative intrusions. *Behaviour Research and Therapy*, **25**, 207–11.

Ehntholt, K. A., Salkovskis, P. M., and Rimes, K. A. (1999). Obsessive-compulsive disorder, anxiety disorders, and self-esteem: an exploratory study. *Behaviour Research and Therapy*, **37**(8), 771–81.

England, S. L. and Dickerson, M. (1988). Intrusive thoughts; unpleasantness not the major cause of uncontrollability. *Behaviour Research and Therapy*, **26**(3), 279–82.

Foa, E. B. and Franklin, M. E. (2000). Psychotherapies for obsessive-compulsive disorder. In *Obsessive Compusive Disorder*, ed. M. Maj, N. Sartorius, A. Okash, and J. Zohar, pp. 93–115. Chichester: Wiley.

Forrester, E., Wilson, C., and Salkovskis, P. M. (2002). The occurrence of intrusive thoughts transforms meaning in ambiguous situations: an experimental study. *Behavioural and Cognitive Psychotherapy*, **30**(2), 143–52.

Freeston, M. H. and Ladouceur, R. (1993). Appraisal of cognitive intrusions and response style: replication and extension. *Behaviour Research and Therapy*, **31**(2), 185–91.

Freeston, M. H., Ladouceur, R., Gagnon, F., and Thibodeau, N. (1993). Beliefs about obsessional thoughts. *Journal of Psychopathology and Behavioural Assessment*, **15**(1), 1–21.

Kozak, M., Liebowitz, M. R., and Foa, E. B. (2000). Cognitive behavior therapy and pharmacotherapy for obsessive-compulsive disorder: the NIMH-sponsored collaborative study. In *Obsessive-Compulsive Disorder: Contemporary Issues in Treatment*, ed. W. K. Goodman, M. V. Rudorfer, and J. D. Maser, pp. 501–30. Mahwah, NJ: Lawrence Erlbaum.

Ladouceur, R., Rheaume, J., Freeston, M. H., et al. (1995). Experimental manipulations of responsibility: an analogue test for models of obsessive-compulsive disorder. *Behaviour Research and Therapy*, **33**(8), 937–46.

Ladouceur, R., Rheaume, J., and Aublet, F. (1997). Excessive responsibility in obsessional concerns: a fine-grained experimental analysis. *Behaviour Research and Therapy*, **35**(5), 423–7.

Lopatka, C. and Rachman, S. (1995). Perceived responsibility and compulsive checking: an experimental analysis. *Behaviour Research and Therapy*, **33**(6), 673–84.

Marks, I. M. (1981). *Cure and Care of Neurosis*. Chichester: Wiley.

Meyer, V. (1966). Modification of expectations in cases with obsessional rituals. *Behaviour Research and Therapy*, **4**(4), 273–80.

Nisbett, R. and Ross, L. (1980). *Human Inference; Strategies and Shortcomings of Social Judgement*. Englewood Cliffs, NJ: Prentice-Hall.

Obsessive-Compulsive Cognitions Working group (1997). Cognitive assessment of obsessive-compulsive disorder. *Behaviour Research and Therapy*, **35**(7), 667–81.

Rachman, S. (1971). Obsessional ruminations. *Behaviour Research and Therapy*, **9**(3), 229–35.

Rachman, S. (1976). The modification of obsessions: a new formulation. *Behaviour Research and Therapy*, **14**(6), 437–43.

Rachman, S. (1978). An anatomy of obsessions. *Behavioural Analysis and Modification*, **2**, 253–78.

Rachman, S. (1993). Obsessions, responsibility and guilt. *Behaviour Research and Therapy*, **31**(2), 149–54.

Rachman, S. (1997). A cognitive theory of obsessions. *Behaviour Research and Therapy*, **35**(9), 793–802.

Rachman, S. (1998). A cognitive theory of obsessions: elaborations. *Behaviour Research and Therapy*, **36**(4), 385–401.

Rachman, S. and de Silva, P. (1978). Abnormal and normal obsessions. *Behaviour Research and Therapy*, **16**(4), 233–48.

Rachman, S. J. and Hodgson, R. J. (1980). *Obsessions and Compulsions*. Englewood Cliffs, NJ: Prentice Hall.

Rachman, S., De Silva, P., and Roper, G. (1976). The spontaneous decay of compulsive urges. *Behaviour Research and Therapy*, **14**(6), 445–53.

Rachman, S., Shafran, R., Mitchell, D., Trant, J., and Teachman, B. (1996). How to remain neutral: an experimental analysis of neutralization. *Behaviour Research and Therapy*, **34**(11–12), 889–98.

Rassin, E., Merckelbach, H., Muris, P., and Spaan, V. (1999). Thought–action fusion as a causal factor in the development of intrusions. *Behaviour Research and Therapy*, **37**(3), 231–7.

Rheaume, J., Ladouceur, R., Freeston, M. H., and Letarte, H. (1994). Inflated responsibility in obsessive-compulsive disorder: psychometric studies of a semiidiographic measure. *Journal of Psychopathology and Behavioural Assessment*, **16**(4), 265–76.

Roper, G. and Rachman, S. (1976). Obsessional-compulsive checking: experimental replication and development. *Behaviour Research and Therapy*, **14**(1), 25–32.

Roper, G., Rachman, S., and Hodgson, R. (1973). An experiment on obsessional checking. *Behaviour Research and Therapy*, **11**(3), 271–7.

Salkovskis, P. M. (1985). Obsessional-compulsive problems: a cognitive-behavioural analysis. *Behaviour Research and Therapy*, **23**, 571–83.

Salkovskis, P. M. (1988). Phenomenology, assessment and the cognitive model of panic. In *Panic: Psychological Perspectives*, ed. S. J. Rachman and J. Maser, pp. 111–36. Hillsdale, NJ: Erlbaum.

Salkovskis, P. M. (1989a). Obsessions and compulsions. In *Cognitive Therapy: A Clinical Casebook*, ed. J. Scott, J. M. G. Williams, and A. T. Beck, pp. 50–77. London: Croom Helm.

Salkovskis, P. M. (1989b). Obsessive and intrusive thoughts: clinical and non-clinical aspects. In *Fresh Perspectives on Anxiety Disorders*, ed. P. M. G. Emmelkamp, W. T. A. M. Everaerd, and M. J. M. van Son. Amsterdam: Swets and Zeitlinger.

Salkovskis, P. M. (1991). The importance of Behaviour in the maintenance of anxiety and panic: a cognitive account. *Behavioural Psychotherapy*, **19**(1), 6–19.

Salkovskis, P. M. (1996a). The cognitive approach to anxiety: threat beliefs, safety seeking Behaviour, and the special case of health anxiety and obsessions. In *Frontiers of Cognitive Therapy*, ed. P. M. Salkovskis, pp. 48–74. New York: Guilford.

Salkovskis, P. M. (1996b). Cognitive-Behavioural approaches to the understanding of obsessional problems. In *Current Controversies in the Anxiety Disorders*, ed. R. Rapee, pp. 103–33. New York: Guilford.

Salkovskis, P. M. (1999). Understanding and treating obsessive-compulsive disorder. *Behaviour Research and Therapy*, **37**, S29–S52.

Salkovskis, P. M. (2000). Obsessional problems: newer cognitive behavioural approaches are a work in progress. In *Obsessive Compulsive Disorder*, ed. M. Maj, N. Sartorius, A. Okasha, and J. Zohar, pp. 131–4. Chichester: Wiley.

Salkovskis, P. M. and Campbell, P. (1994). Thought suppression in naturally occurring negative intrusive thoughts. *Behaviour Research and Therapy*, **32**, 1–8.

Salkovskis, P. M. and Forrester, E. (2002). Responsibility. In *Cognitive Approaches to Obsessions and Compulsions: Theory, Assessment and Treatment*, ed. R. Frost and G. Steketee, pp. 45–61. Amsterdam, Netherlands: Pergamon/Elsevier Science.

Salkovskis, P. M. and Freeston, M. H. (2001). Obsessions, compulsions, motivation, and responsibility for harm. *Australian Journal of Psychology*, **53**(1), 1–6.

Salkovskis, P. M. and Harrison, J. (1984). Abnormal and normal obsessions – a replication. *Behaviour Research and Therapy*, **22**, 549–52.

Salkovskis, P. M. and Kirk, J. (1989). Obsessional disorders. In *Cognitive Behaviour Therapy for Psychiatric Problems: A Practical Guide*, ed. K. Hawton, P. M. Salkovskis, J. Kirk, and D. M. Clark, pp. 129–68. Oxford: Oxford University Press.

Salkovskis, P. M. and Kirk, J. (1997). Obsessive-compulsive disorder. In *The Science and Practice of Cognitive-Behaviour Therapy*, ed. D. M. Clark and C. G. Fairburn, pp. 200–13. Oxford: Oxford University Press.

Salkovskis, P. M. and Warwick, H. M. (1985). Cognitive therapy of obsessive-compulsive disorder: treating treatment failures. *Behavioural Psychotherapy*, **13**(3), 243–55.

Salkovskis, P. M. and Warwick, H. M. C. (1988). Obsessional problems. In *The Theory and Practice of Cognitive Therapy*, ed. C. Perris, I. M. Blackburn, and H. Perris. Berlin: Springer Verlag.

Salkovskis, P. M. and Westbrook, D. (1987). Obsessive-compulsive disorder: clinical strategies for improving Behavioural treatments. In *Clinical Psychology: Research and Developments*, ed. H. R. Dent, pp. 200–13. London: Croom Helm.

Salkovskis, P. M. and Westbrook, D. (1989). Behaviour therapy and obsessional ruminations: can failure be turned into success? *Behaviour Research and Therapy*, **27**(2), 149–60.

Salkovskis, P. M., Richards, H. C., and Forrester, E. (1995). The relationship between obsessional problems and intrusive thoughts. *Behavioural and Cognitive Psychotherapy*, **23**, 281–99.

Salkovskis, P. M., Westbrook, D., Davis, J., Jeavons, A., and Gledhill, A. (1997). Effects of neutralizing on intrusive thoughts: an experiment investigating the etiology of obsessive-compulsive disorder. *Behaviour Research and Therapy*, **35**(3), 211–19.

Salkovskis, P. M., Forrester, E., Richards, H.C., and Morrison, N. (1998). The devil is in the detail: conceptualising and treating obsessional problems. In *Cognitive Therapy with Complex Cases*, ed. N. Tarrier, pp. 46–80. Chichester: Wiley.

Salkovskis, P., Shafran, R., Rachman, S., and Freeston, M. H. (1999). Multiple pathways to inflated responsibility beliefs in obsessional problems: possible origins and implications for therapy and research. *Behaviour Research and Therapy*, **37**(11), 1055–72.

Salkovskis, P. M., Wroe, A., Gledhill, A., et al. (2000). Responsibility attitudes and interpretations are characteristic of obsessive-compulsive disorder. *Behaviour Research and Therapy*, **38**, 347–72.

Shafran, R. (1997). The manipulation of responsibility in obsessive-compulsive disorder. *British Journal Clinical Psychology*, **36**, 397–407.

Trinder, H. and Salkovskis, P. M. (1994). Personally relevant intrusions outside the laboratory: long-term suppression increases intrusion. *Behaviour Research and Therapy*, **32**(8), 833–42.

van Balkom, A. J. L. M., van Oppen, P., Vermeulen, A. W. A., et al. (1994). A meta-analysis on the treatment of obsessive compulsive disorder: a comparison of antidepressants, behavior, and cognitive therapy. *Clinical Psychology Review*, **14**(5), 359–81.

Van Oppen, P., de Haan, E., Van Balkom, A. J. L. M., et al. (1995). Cognitive therapy and exposure in vivo in the treatment of obsessive compulsive disorder. *Behaviour Research and Therapy*, **33**(4), 379–90.

Wegner, D. M., Schneider, D. J., Carter, S. R., and White, T. L. (1987). Paradoxical effects of thought suppression. *Journal of Personality and Social Psychology*, **53**, 5–13.

Wells, A. (1996). *Cognitive Therapy of Anxiety: A Practical Guide*. Chichester, UK: Wiley.

Williams, T. I., Salkovskis, P. M., Forrester, E. A., and Allsopp, M. A. (2002). Changes in symptoms of OCD and appraisal of responsibility during cognitive behavioural treatment: a pilot study. *Behavioural and Cognitive Psychotherapy*, **30**(1), 69–78.

Wilson, K. A. and Chambless, D. L. (1999). Inflated perceptions of responsibility and obsessive-compulsive symptoms. *Behaviour Research and Therapy*, **37**(4), 325–35.

Wroe, A. and Salkovskis, P. M. (2000). Causing harm and allowing harm: a study of beliefs in obsessional problems. *Behaviour Research and Therapy*, **38**, 1141–62.

Wroe, A. L., Salkovskis, P. M., and Richards, H. C. (2000). "Now I know it could happen, I have to prevent it": a clinical study of the specificity of intrusive thoughts and the decision to prevent harm. *Behavioural and Cognitive Psychotherapy*, **28**, 63–70.

8

Narcissistic personality disorder

Cory F. Newman[1] and Christine L. Ratto[2]

[1]University of Pennsylvania, Philadelphia, PA, USA
[2]Albert Einstein College of Medicine, New York, NY, USA

Self-interest, in moderation, is necessary for healthy functioning. From an evolutionary perspective, the desire to thrive and succeed has survival value, and is likely to be genetically selected (Stone, 1998). Indeed, it is widely held (most notably in modern western cultures) that self-esteem is a desirable trait, and that the pursuit of "the good life" is a worthy path in order to make the most out of one's time on earth. There is some evidence that those who like and respect themselves are less vulnerable to the kinds of life stressors that might otherwise cause others to lapse into despair (Seligman, 1991; Ryff and Singer, 1996, 1998). In addition, it has been proposed that a prerequisite to giving true love to another is the ability to give acceptance and compassion to oneself (Erikson, 1964). From this standpoint, it would seem that clinicians do their clients – and society at large – a service by helping clients develop higher regard for themselves, along with improved moods and motivations.

However, like almost everything else in our delicately balanced existence, the *overabundance* of a seemingly good thing can become a problem. For example, too much individual freedom without regulations and laws can threaten to become destructive anarchy. Likewise, a medication that can alleviate an illness, when taken to excess can lead to premature death. Similarly, a child who receives too many material benefits without a commensurate sense of efficacy or mastery may learn to have little gratitude, and may spend his or her life in a state of perceived deprivation and longing for more. Indeed, extremity – in and of itself – is often a sign of potential dysfunction in a world where it is generally healthier to be "within normal limits."

Hence, we discuss the phenomenon designated in the fourth edition of the *Diagnostic and Statistical Manual of Mental Disorders* (DSM-IV) (American Psychiatric Association, 1994) known as narcissistic personality disorder (NPD). The term derives from Narcissus of Greek mythology, who fell in love with his own reflection, and was doomed to waste away while transfixed with his own image. In modern diagnostic nomenclature, NPD refers to pervasive, long-standing patterns of functioning, deemed (by implication) to be dysfunctional, immature, and difficult to modify. Specifically, NPD persons have an inflated sense of self-importance, along with a concomitant lack of appreciation and empathy for others. In spite of their overt grandiosity, many NPD sufferers actually demonstrate a very fragile self-esteem. Thus, they are quick to become enraged and humiliated if reproached even in mild ways, and prone to envy and to begrudge the accomplishments of others (it is not enough that they succeed; other people must fail).

Individuals with NPD believe that they stand apart from others, thus the rules that are meant for the masses should not pertain to them. Accordingly, a sense of entitlement is prominent. Interpersonal relationships are often problematic, owing in part to NPD persons' (1) lack of empathy, (2) excessive demands for attention and deference, (3) propensity for jealousy, (4) failure to reciprocate acts of care and kindness, (5) emotional shallowness, (6) overemphasis on physical attractiveness and social standing rather than the capacity for loyalty, bonding, and other components of good character, and (7) a ready willingness to discard people who do not serve their needs. They are very easily dissatisfied, as they want the absolute best out of life, and little else will do. Their fantasies of wealth, fame, and love with the perfect person are not so much a diversion from the realities of everyday life as an imperative for how things *should* be.

Consider the following summary descriptions of clients of ours who were diagnosed with NPD, with sufficient disguises in place so as to protect their anonymity:

1. "Spence" was a 19-year-old student at a small local college who was brought into therapy by his frightened parents. Spence had punched a hole in the wall of his home, and threatened his father with doing the same to him. He also promised he would commit suicide if his complaint – specifically, that he was unjustly denied a new car – was not heeded. This followed Spence's having crashed his third car in less than a year, and the father stating that he would not buy a fourth car for Spence.

   When he presented for his first session, Spence looked quite dashing in his "cool" clothes, and acted in a charming manner. He insisted that he was not suicidal, completed all of his mood inventories with nary an endorsed symptom, and assured the therapist that his parents were "hysterical overreactors." Later, however, when he ascertained that the therapist had supported the father's decision to hold off on buying a fourth car, Spence turned nasty. He accused the therapist of pandering to the parents, and promised that he would immediately *become* depressed if the therapist did not change his stance, thus "proving" to all that the therapist was guilty of malpractice. In spite of his C average in college, Spence bragged that he would some day become world-famous as the preeminent lawyer specializing in the rights of adolescents against their parents.

2. "Rayna" was a 40-year-old widow, whose 72-year-old husband had died 3 months earlier. She did not present for therapy with grief issues. Instead, she was distressed over her relationship with her 58-year-old boyfriend, who would not buy her everything she desired. Still, she felt quite dependent on him, explaining that her access to influential people and celebrities hinged on her accompanying him to his various gala functions. Thus, she was very frustrated, and suffered from anxiety. In addition, Rayna was preoccupied with and angry about the ongoing litigation war she was waging with her deceased husband's adult children from a previous marriage, over his will.

   Rayna often disregarded the ground rules of therapy. She consistently arrived late to session, and assumed that the hour would be extended to accommodate her pressing need for a full session. She phoned the therapist on a frequent basis, often to complain (at great length, and in excruciating detail) about her stepdaughter's latest act of "cruelty" and her boyfriend's most recent demonstration of "stinginess." Rayna did not desist when told that such calls did not constitute clinical emergencies, and therefore she should refrain from calling. Rayna also was inconsistent in paying for sessions. Her behavior in session was pretentious, and she treated the therapist as one might a personal valet (for example, asking him to make various phone calls on her behalf during the session).

3. "Ellison" was a 53-year-old businessman who presented with an acute depression following a professional setback. He admitted that he routinely took out his anger on his wife and four children, but justified this behavior by saying that his problems were by far the most severe of anyone he knew. He demanded that his family give him audience for his daily diatribes, and professed that this was the only way that he would get sufficient sympathy for his plight. Ellison expressed the belief that the only way he could recover from his depression would be to receive his just due in his professional life, to earn substantially more money, and to get revenge on all those who had laughed at him.

4. "Tabitha" was a 35-year-old female who presented with a severe mood disorder. Although she acknowledged being highly suicidal, she was dressed and made up for every session as if she were attending a photo shoot, and her outward demeanor was unfailingly upbeat. Although she implored her therapist to see her five times a week for treatment, she claimed that she already knew all there was to know about cognitive therapy as a result of her personal readings. Tabitha often bragged that she had a gift for relating to others, but complained that she was lonely and ignored, and therefore wanted to die. She emphatically claimed that her depression was unique, and therefore could not be understood through any textbook (except perhaps those read through her eyes!). Likewise, she maintained that therapy homework did not pertain to her, and she rejected all attempts to encourage her to engage in self-help exercises between sessions.

As the above cases illustrate, clients who are diagnosed with NPD demonstrate some degree of heterogeneity, reflecting their demographic, cultural, and developmental differences. Although NPD clients share the basic characteristics that comprise the official criteria of the diagnosis, they may present with somewhat different dysfunctional beliefs, emotions, and behaviors, reminding us of the importance of an individualized case conceptualization for understanding and treating clients (Beck, 1995).

The construct of the narcissistic personality

The concept of the narcissistic personality has been difficult to explicate in a consistent manner, thus making its measurement a challenge to researchers. Narcissism was originally described by psychoanalytic writers, who viewed the disorder as stemming from a developmental arrest or disturbed object relations (Millon, 1969; Kohut, 1971; Kernberg, 1975). The result was a person who later would demonstrate characteristics such as shame-based rage, entitlement, and an absence of healthy bonding with others. Later successive versions of the DSM attempted to categorize the disorder in atheoretical terms, choosing a cluster of observable symptoms as the benchmark (Clark et al., 1997). Further problems have arisen owing to the confusion between measuring personality disorders in terms of *dimensions* (such as the Minnesota Multiphasic Personality Inventory (MMPI)), versus discrete *categories* (as the DSM-IV attempts to do). Clark et al. (1997) believe that this is a false dichotomy, explaining that these apparently conflicting models can exist in hierarchical relation to one another, "with dimensions being the blocks from which categories may be built" (p. 206).

Questions have also been raised as to whether NPD can be viewed as a reliably diagnosable condition having distinguishable features from other personality disorders (Vaillant and Perry, 1985). Concern with these issues resulted in substantial changes in the NPD criteria in DSM-IV (Gunderson et al., 1995). However, these revisions were incorporated into the DSM-IV without first being subjected to empirical evaluation (Blais et al., 1997). Not surprisingly, it is very difficult to find a person who exhibits only symptoms of NPD. Overlap with other diagnosable disorders – especially other axis II disorders – is substantial. For example, Widiger and Rogers' (1989) review of the personality disorder literature found that the average percent of multiple axis II diagnoses was 85%. Similarly, the review by Gunderson et al. (1991) of 11 studies that used structured assessments concluded that the diagnosis of NPD without at least one accompanying personality disorder was the rarest of exceptions to the rule.

Since then, the validity and specificity of some of the overt features of NPD have been supported by a number of empirical studies (Blais et al., 1997; Holdwick et al.,

1998; Morey and Jones, 1998). These characteristics include grandiosity, desire for uniqueness, a need for admiration and attention, and arrogance. Other empirical studies have examined the validity and utility of other NPD characteristics besides those included in the DSM. Ronningstam and Gunderson (1990) found the following features to discriminate NPD clients from other psychiatric clients: (1) boastful and pretentious behavior; (2) self-centered and self-referential behavior; and (3) marked envy of others.

Efforts have been made to systematize and describe clinical features of NPD by devising assessment measures that may aid in differentiating NPD from both nonclinical samples and other personality disorders. These measures have included interviews, including the Diagnostic Interview for Narcissism (DIN: Ronningstam and Gunderson, 1991), and, more commonly, self-report measures, such as the Minnesota Multiphasic Personality Inventory – 2nd edition (MMPI-2) and Millon Clinical Multiaxial Inventory (MCMI) (Chatham et al., 1993; Hilsenroth, 1997). Although these measures have been successful in differentiating narcissists from nonnarcissists, they have had a poor track record in distinguishing *between* personality disorders. The Narcissistic Personality Inventory (NPI: Raskin and Hall, 1979), derived from DSM-III criteria (American Psychiatric Association, 1980), has become the most frequently used measure of narcissism in empirical studies. Factor analyses conducted on this measure have identified both maladaptive and adaptive psychological indices (Emmons, 1987; Raskin and Terry, 1988). Although positive factors, such as leadership and self-sufficiency, have been identified, the majority of factors – including exploitiveness/entitlement, superiority/arrogance, vanity, and exhibitionism – tap maladaptive aspects of narcissism. Below, we will look at the manner in which cognitive theorists have attempted to construct taxonomies of cognitive characteristics that identify and distinguish clients with NPD.

Given the high degree of comorbidity between NPD and other personality disorders (Morey and Jones, 1998), it may also be useful to study differential *secondary* diagnosis on axis II, especially in relation to demographic differences. Our clinical examples above are cases in point. Spence had a secondary diagnosis of antisocial personality disorder (AsPD), whereas Ellison's was obsessive-compulsive personality disorder (OCPD). Likewise, Rayna was also diagnosed with dependent personality disorder (DPD), and Tabitha met almost every criterion for histrionic personality disorder (HPD). These cases raise interesting issues about the impact of demographics – such as gender – on the NPD phenomena, and their accompanying diagnostic conditions.

There have been inconsistent findings in research studies examining the gender distribution of NPD. Some studies indicate that NPD is more common in males than in females (Millon, 1990; Ronningstam and Gunderson, 1990), with the DSM-IV indicating that as many as 75% of those diagnosed with NPD are male. Other studies, however, have reported no gender differences in the prevalence of NPD (Plakun, 1990). Reichman and Flaherty (1990) posit that the present conceptualization of NPD, as depicted in DSM-IV, is somewhat biased toward male symptoms. Men, for example, may manifest a greater sense of uniqueness, entitlement, explosiveness, and lack of empathy, whereas women may react more intensely to slights from others. Similarly, Tschanz et al. (1998) found that exploitative tendencies and feelings of entitlement were less central to the construct of narcissism in females than in males. The authors suggest that for females such displays may carry a greater possibility of negative social sanction, as they would violate stereotypical gender role expectancies for women.

In the general population, the prevalence of NPD is estimated to be less than 1% (Reich et al., 1989; Zimmerman and Coryell, 1990). However, in western culture, individuals exhibiting a narcissistic personality style or narcissistic traits may be more common (Stone, 1993; Sperry, 1995). Lasch (1979) postulated that the emphasis on individual achievement, productivity, and autonomy in western society may contribute to the development of narcissism. However, there is no empirical evidence that these factors have a direct causal relationship with the prevalence of NPD.

Developmental factors in NPD

The literature on narcissistic personality has been overwhelmingly represented by writers working from psychoanalytic, object-relations, and attachment theory perspectives (Rosenfeld, 1964; Kohut, 1971; Bowlby, 1973; Kernberg, 1975, 1980, 1984; Masterson, 1981). Although each of these authors has emphasized a different aspect of the problem, a common theoretical thread is that they view narcissism as stemming from maladaptive early relationships that impair the developing child's sense of self and comfort in bonding with others. For example, at least one parent tries to get his or her emotional needs met through the child rather than through the spouse, who is aloof and distant. The doting parent sets insufficient limits, overindulges the child, and communicates to the child that he or she is "special" and "unique," and therefore is expected to accomplish great things. Unfortunately, the child accurately perceives that he or she must please this parent in a way that gratifies the ego of the parent, rather than in a way that supports the development of the child. Failure to do so results in rejection.

Although cognitive theory does not assume the same etiology for NPD (in terms of specific family relationships and internal dynamics) as traditional psychodynamic theories, it does assert that harmful, faulty lessons are lived and learned in the households where NPD children grow up. Still, it has only been fairly recently that the field of cognitive therapy has turned its attention to this clinical problem

(Beck et al., 1990; Bux, 1992; Young, 1994, 1999; Young and Flanagan, 1998). There are a number of possible reasons for this delay in focusing on NPD. First, it was not until personality disorders were operationalized in the latter versions of the DSM that they came to be seen as amenable to empirical evaluation. Second, cognitive therapy was developed as a model for brief psychotherapy, whereas the treatment of personality disorders was seen as requiring significantly longer periods of time to effect therapeutic progress. Third, the tradition of cognitive therapy (Beck et al., 1979) maintained that a stance of collaborative empiricism was necessary and sufficient for the formation of a therapeutic relationship conducive to change. However true this may be of the nonpersonality-disordered client, it is far less an accurate descriptor of the working alliance with NPD clients. Given that interpersonal relationship problems are very much at the core of axis II disorders, such as NPD, a greater focus must be placed on the therapeutic relationship than is commonly afforded in standard cognitive therapy (Layden et al., 1993; Peyton and Safran, 1998). In fact, it may be argued that the study of NPD and its treatment would necessitate an integrative approach between cognitive therapy and models that emphasize the therapeutic relationship as a key vehicle of change. We will address this point later.

In spite of much theorizing, very little empirical work has examined the developmental aspects of NPD. A recent attempt to investigate the role of parenting in the development of NPD comes from Lyons (1998), who used the NPI (Raskin and Hall, 1979) in studying a group of preadolescents from intact families. She found that, for both mothers and fathers, there was an important interaction between the independent variables of permissiveness and nurturance. Specifically, nurturing parents were less likely to have children who possessed narcissistic characteristics than those who were significantly less nurturing, but only if the parents were not excessively permissive. These findings suggest that parental permissiveness weakens the protective effect of nurturance in preventing narcissism in preadolescents. Lyons also found that highly narcissistic children were lacking in empathy and social responsibility, and were more likely to be verbally and physically aggressive, even toward their closest friends. These findings dovetail with a study by Bushman and Baumeister (1998), who reported that narcissistic college students were characterized not only by an inflated view of themselves and a vulnerability to criticism, but also by a penchant to be aggressive even toward people who ostensibly gave them positive feedback. This fits conceptually with the view that narcissists have unstable self-esteem that they fight to preserve, and a tendency to fail to reciprocate positive behaviors in relationships.

In a study examining the role of empathy deficiency in NPD (Leventhal, 1995), college students were classified via the Structured Clinical Interview for the DSM-IV (SCID-II) into four groups: (1) narcissistic; (2) avoidant/dependent; (3) personality-disordered control; and (4) normal control. All were exposed to videotapes depicting three different degrees of empathy between a mother and her daughter. Narcissists evidenced greater levels of grandiosity, power-seeking, and anger after viewing the low-empathy tape. Although there are limitations in this study (e.g., sample consisting of college students), the results suggest that individuals with NPD demonstrate a hypersensitivity to perceived lapses in empathy to which they respond by exhibiting symptomatic behavior.

The cognitive characteristics of NPD

The DSM-III, III-R, and IV tend to emphasize affective and behavioral symptoms that comprise each personality disorder. Cognitive theorists have contributed to our understanding of personality disorders, such as NPD, by hypothesizing *cognitive* characteristics and processing deficits associated with each disorder. The assessment and treatment of NPD can be greatly aided by developing a cognitive case conceptualization (Beck, 1995; Greenberger and Padesky, 1995). In the case of NPD, Beck et al. (1990) have posited a number of characteristic maladaptive beliefs. These include (p. 361):

- "Since I am so superior, I am entitled to special treatment and privileges."
- "Other people should satisfy my needs."
- "Other people should recognize how special I am."
- "People have no right to criticize me."
- "I have every reason to expect grand things."

An interesting question (that has yet to be addressed satisfactorily) is *how* these beliefs – once formed – are *maintained* over the course of development. Narcissistic clients have a child-like egocentrism whereby they see the world predominantly through their own eyes, and have a difficult time taking the perspective of another person. Hence, they lack empathy, and are deficient in taking stock of themselves as others might. Over the course of normative development, children come to learn that the world does not revolve around them, that they can give as well as receive nurturance, and that their opinions are subjective, and not necessarily synonymous with fact. NPD clients seem not to have made sufficient strides in maturing toward these viewpoints.

This poses an interesting – and, arguably, apropos – challenge to the field of cognitive therapy. Clients who meet criteria for NPD often present with a seemingly unshakable confidence in the validity of their points of view. They fail to distinguish subjective from objective perspectives. Thus, the notion of engaging in changing their thought processes – which is at the core of cognitive therapy – may seem anathema to NPD clients. Yet this may be one of the most important skills that they need to develop, and what better approach to facilitate this process than cognitive therapy? (It goes without saying that therapists cannot expect to teach their NPD clients a skill against their will. A strong therapeutic alliance must be in place, thus allowing therapists to take the risk of focusing on areas the NPD clients would just as soon ignore. Indeed, the future directions of cognitive therapy for NPD – and perhaps for most axis II clients – will need to address methods for enhancing the therapeutic alliance as a vehicle of change, including cognitive change.)

One hypothesis as to why NPD clients have difficulty reflecting upon their own cognitive processing of information may be that they lack objective self-evaluation skills that enable them to tell how poorly they are performing and, as a result, they come to hold inflated views of their performance and ability. Kruger and Dunning (1999) found a link between what they term "incompetence" and deficits in accurate self-evaluation in a set of four empirical studies. They propose that those who are deficient in a skill are prone to overestimate their performance relative to those who are competent at a given task. Incompetent individuals appear to be less able to gain insight into their true level of performance by means of social comparison information than their more competent peers. Although these studies were conducted with college students, it may have implications for NPD clients as well, who are notorious for overestimating their abilities and performance relative to objective criteria.

The Personality Beliefs Questionnaire

The examples of NPD beliefs presented above represent a number of assumptions that these clients typically maintain about themselves and their relationships with others. A more comprehensive, clinically generated overview of the most common beliefs endorsed by clients with axis II disorders can be found in the Personality Beliefs Questionnaire (PBQ). The PBQ is a measure of dysfunctional beliefs associated with personality disorders, and is similar in form to the Dysfunctional Attitudes Scale (DAS: Beck et al., 2001) a measure of tacit beliefs associated with depression. The PBQ represents an attempt to construct a taxonomy of beliefs that will indicate and distinguish personality disorders. It also serves as a means by which to formulate a cognitive case conceptualization in clinical practice (Beck, 1995).

The PBQ consists of clinically derived sets of beliefs that are hypothesized to correspond to specific personality disorders, allowing for the likelihood that clients will endorse items that cross traditional diagnostic lines. A methodological strength of the PBQ is its scrupulous avoidance of items that directly map on to DSM-IV symptoms, or that reflect general distress. Thus, correlations between the self-report PBQ and interviewer-based DSM-IV diagnoses would be more robust indicators of the criterion validity of the PBQ, rather than an artifact of item overlap.

Beck et al. (2001) found that five of the PBQ scales (including the NPD scale) demonstrated reliabilities near 0.90. Across all comparisons, clients with specific axis II diagnoses scored higher on the corresponding belief scale than did the collection of clients with other axis II disorders. It is worth noting that the NPD subjects also received elevated scores on PBQ scales for paranoid personality disorder and OCPD. The authors propose that this may reflect the NPD subjects' intolerance of imperfection, their investment in the unassailable "rightness" of their views, and their perceived vulnerability to slights against their self-image.

The Schema Questionnaire

A similar cognitive model of personality disorders has been proffered by Young and his associates (Young, 1990; Schmidt et al., 1995). Young's (1990) approach is termed the "schema-focused" model of cognitive therapy for personality disorders. Schemata are hypothesized to be the basic building blocks of cognitive-affective perception, formed during childhood as a result of repeated, problematic interactions (or lack of interactions) with primary caregivers. As the person develops, incoming information is processed on the basis of preexisting schemata. Information is assimilated to fit with preexisting beliefs, making it difficult for clients with maladaptive schemata to learn from mistakes, or to reconstrue a situation more adaptively. Young's (1990) schema theory is largely consistent with the aforementioned model of Beck et al. (1990).

Young and Flanagan (1998) review and explicate some of the "early maladaptive schemas" that are present in NPD clients. These include: (1) entitlement; (2) emotional deprivation; (3) defectiveness; (4) mistrust; and (5) unrelenting standards, among others. These are not the only schemata that can be found among NPD clients, nor are they found only in NPD. As with the higher-order beliefs mentioned above, schemata tend to overlap the various axis II categories. What identifies the schemata as being part and parcel of the NPD thinking style is the level of severity of the schemata, the particular configuration of schemata, and (arguably) the primacy or availability of specific schemata.

Analogous to the PBQ (Beck et al., 2001), Young (1990, 1994) has developed the Schema Questionnaire (SQ), a 205-item self-report inventory designed to measure early maladaptive schemata. Each item is rated on a continuum from a low score of 1 ("completely untrue of me") to a high score of 6 ("describes me perfectly"). Sample items include "I am inherently flawed and defective" and "I must be the best at what I do; I can't accept second best." Schmidt et al. (1995) factor-analyzed the SQ and found strong support for 15 main categories of early maladaptive schemata. These schemata, including "entitlement," "emotional deprivation," and "mistrust," are strikingly similar to those posited by the Beck model. Interestingly, even after Schmidt et al. (1995) deleted SQ items hypothesized to be associated with specific symptoms and stress, they still found a significant effect on the Stroop task. Specifically, the Stroop task was modified to include color-naming of schema-specific words. As the authors note, "subjects scoring high on the SQ, compared to those scoring low on the SQ, showed significantly greater Stroop interference for schema-specific words. These data provide preliminary evidence that the SQ factors may also be assessed by information processing paradigms" (p. 318).

Let us examine more closely each of the schemata that Young and Flanagan (1998) posit are most salient in the NPD client. The *entitlement* schema manifests itself in the adult belief, "Since I am so superior, I am entitled to special treatment and privileges" (Beck et al., 1990, p. 361). It is hypothesized to develop as a result of chronic, pervasive, poor limit-setting by parents. The NPD child comes to believe that privileges, material advantages, and praise are birthrights. The NPD adult expects to get what he or she wants, without having to reciprocate. In a related vein, NPD adults may believe they have been so mistreated and deprived in their lives that the world now owes them major compensation, hence the entitled stance.

NPD children may receive very little by way of mature, altruistic parental affection, thus leading to the development of the *emotional deprivation* schema. Consequently, no matter what freedoms and material possessions the adult NPD person may accumulate, there is always a sense of emptiness. "Love" may be sought through frequent sex with the most attractive partners one can find, but a true sense of connection is missing. This continually frustrates the NPD sufferer, leading him or her to continue to seek the "perfect" mate, rather than to change him- or herself. Accordingly, NPD clients do not develop a capacity for mature empathy, as they remain preoccupied with *getting* their needs for love met. The idea of selflessly *giving* love as a part of the equation is lacking.

The *defectiveness* schema is often compensated for by the NPD clients' arrogance and grandiosity. However, they are extremely sensitive to criticism, which highlights their fragile sense of self. In order to cope with their fears of being "no good," they require constant attention and accolades. However much they want to be praised and admired, it is rarely enough to satisfy them, because the basic sense of defectiveness overrides the fleeting interpersonal interaction that otherwise gives them a "quick fix" of worthiness. Thus, NPD individuals seem quite demanding, but others cannot give them enough. In response, NPD individuals may escalate their demands, rather than try to find ways to work earnestly and nonjudgmentally on self-improvement. Consistent with the Bushman and Baumeister (1998) data, we may posit that, although NPD clients try to prop up their self-image, they are vulnerable to "schema activation," in which their defectiveness schema is triggered by a given situation. Thus, the NPD clients' self-esteem appears unstable and fragile.

Clients with NPD also manifest excessive *mistrust*. This fits conceptually with findings on the PBQ (Beck et al., 2001), suggesting that NPD sufferers show signs of paranoid thinking style. They tend, for example, to view their romantic partners as possessions who must be kept within view, lest they stray or be stolen away.

Thus, NPD clients tend to be excessively jealous in relationships. Another example of their mistrust is seen in their frequent lack of faith that others will meet their needs. For example, they may grill their therapists about the latter's credentials, doubting that anybody but "the best" could possibly help them. Unfortunately, the NPD person's definition of "best" is not simply about the other person possessing competency – it is also about whether or not the other person will repeatedly "prove" his or her worth and loyalty. Narcissistic clients will insist that others jump through hoops for them, and will express strong disapproval if the other person does not comply.

Yet another schema observed in NPD clients is that of *unrelenting standards*, consistent with the Beck et al. (2001) data indicating the high loading of NPD clients on obsessive-compulsive beliefs. As NPD clients are prone to primitive, all-or-nothing thinking, "good enough" is not good enough; it is instead "terrible." They have low tolerance for human frailties or mistakes, both in themselves and in others. To be "at the top" is a necessity. To be anything else is to be "average" at best, and a failure at worst. Some NPD clients will threaten suicide as a result of their lives not meeting the lofty standards they demand, reasoning that a life of mediocrity is not worth living. This puts therapists in quite a bind, as they must walk the fine line between coaxing the NPD clients off their high horse, without having them break their necks in a fall. We will discuss some of the problems and opportunities that arise in the therapeutic relationship with NPD clients below.

Treatment issues

As cognitive therapists, we place strong emphasis on identifying and modifying maladaptive beliefs and attitudes. We do not, however, overlook the importance of affect, interpersonal factors, environmental contingencies, genetic and biological contributions, and other variables. It is worth acknowledging that if we help personality-disordered clients to reduce the frequency of their engaging in self-defeating behaviors, this will be a benefit to their lives. The techniques and strategies described here are geared to achieve just that sort of change, and to teach useful psychological skills in the process.

The presenting problems of NPD clients

Why do NPD clients enter treatment? A glance at their typical comorbid, axis I diagnoses offers a clue. For example, 42–50% of clients with NPD also suffer from dysthymia or major depression (Ronningstam and Gunderson, 1988, 1990), perhaps after experiencing failures, losses, along with boredom, emptiness, and aloneness (Ronningstam, 1999). In fact, narcissistic clients may be particularly vulnerable to suicide (Perry, 1990; Maltsberger, 1998). Comorbid NPD in borderline personality disorder (BPD) is associated with an increased risk of suicide as compared to pure BPD clients (McGlashan and Heinssen, 1989; Stone, 1989). In addition, substance abuse has been implicated in 24–50% of NPD clients (Ronningstam, 1998a). The relationship between NPD and mood disorders may suggest a vulnerability in NPD clients for developing these syndromes due to the constant discrepancies between their grandiose expectations for themselves and reality (Ronninsgstam, 1996).

The brittle, pathologic self-image of the NPD client is highly vulnerable to collapse. Affective disorders can easily be the result. The following frameworks may be used in conceptualizing the NPD clients' depressive states:

- They feel betrayed by life. They had expectations that they would be much more successful, wealthy, loved, famous, and happy than they are, and they view this as a function of the world having been unfair and unjust toward them. They become angry, bitter, and envious of others.
- They are quick to feel humiliated and ashamed. Unable to accept gracefully the hurdles, setbacks, and criticisms that are intrinsic to the trial-and-error struggle for a better life, NPD clients instead quickly feel thwarted and harshly judged. They may abandon their pursuits, and spend inordinate amounts of time ruminating about their tragic misfortunes on the one hand, and their wished-for triumphs on the other.
- As NPD clients seek pleasure in abundance, they are vulnerable to overindulging in hedonistic behaviors such as sex, drugs, spending, gambling, and the like. Thus, they are quite vulnerable to developing addictions that come to warrant treatment. An example is the man who gambles because he magically believes that the odds (which always favor the house) do not apply to him because he is special and gifted. Along the same lines, NPD clients do not tolerate frustration well, and thus may enter treatment out of anger, and with the expectation that therapists will do their bidding to get their richly deserved needs met at once. For example, an NPD client who aspired to become a psychiatrist wanted his therapist to "pull strings" to get him into medical school at the university where they were meeting for therapy.
- They recognize that they are at risk for failure, which they fear enormously. Therefore, they avoid engaging in the necessary pursuits to achieve success in an enduring fashion, believing instead that good things will gravitate toward them naturally, free of risk. As time goes on, they watch their contemporaries – whom they consider to be inferior to them – achieve relatively more and get more out of life. This angers and frustrates the NPD clients, as their sense of failure becomes more and more difficult to avoid. Their relationships with successful friends become strained, which can lead to further isolation and despair. All the while, the NPD clients continue to fear failure, so they do not extend themselves in ways that might bring about a sense of accomplishment. Thus, the disparity

between their ideal self and real self widens as they get older, leading to profound bitterness and hopelessness.

- Of course, as with many clients suffering from personality disorders, NPD clients sometimes enter treatment at the mandate of someone else, such as a disgruntled spouse, an exasperated employer, or the courts. When this occurs, the NPD clients may or may not experience distress independent of their forced treatment. If they do not believe the treatment is warranted, the therapist and client will have a most difficult time forging a mutually acceptable agenda.

The therapeutic relationship

From a cognitive therapy perspective, a constructive, meaningful therapeutic relationship is essential for successful therapy (Newman, 1998). In and of itself, however, a healthy therapeutic alliance is *not sufficient* for change with clients whose problems are as serious and pervasive as those who suffer from NPD. The therapeutic relationship must be managed very carefully as even minor ruptures can result in a premature end to the enterprise of treatment if the clients experience schema activation. (For example, a therapist may change the time of the client's appointment owing to an academic meeting. The client may feel disrespected and rejected, based on the activation of schemata of entitlement, mistrust, and emotional deprivation. Such clients may choose never to return to therapy, rather than be rescheduled against their wishes.) It is not uncommon for therapists to become frustrated with NPD clients who make repeated unreasonable demands, demean them on a routine basis, make threats, fail to pay for sessions, and require tremendous professional attention with little apparent benefit (Curtis, 1999). In short, a positive, productive therapeutic relationship with NPD clients is difficult to create, and easy to lose.

Lest we paint an entirely negative picture, let us reiterate that the interpersonal lessons that can be learned from the ebb and flow of the therapeutic relationship can be extremely valuable to NPD clients. Significant shifts in cognitive style – along with affect – can occur as a result of standing back and evaluating the vicissitudes of how the client and therapist interact, and how they experience and understand each other (Safran and Muran, 2000). This learning experience comes to full fruition when the clients apply their new beliefs about themselves and their relationships in everyday life, outside the therapist's office.

However, therapists of NPD clients must possess the knowledge, motivation, self-awareness, technical skill, and emotional wherewithal to survive the discomfort and tumult that usually accompany this process. In this way, therapists distinguish themselves from most others with whom the NPD clients have interacted in their lives, because the therapists remain composed, accepting, goal-focused, and collaborative (Safran and Segal, 1990; Safran and Muran, 2000). If therapists meet these goals, they can serve the much-needed function of creating a stable, secure environment for the NPD client to do the arduous and sometimes painful work of therapy.

Narcissistic clients often interact with their therapists in ways that test the mettle and professionalism of the clinician (Newman, 1997; Curtis, 1999). Therapists of NPD clients need to be self-confident enough to deal with devaluation, and astute enough to conceptualize the process. Spence, our 19-year-old adolescent of car-crashing fame, lamented in a vulnerable moment that he felt "all alone." The therapist noted that Spence unwittingly prevented himself from having true friends because he was so preoccupied with thoughts such as, "Who is better than me?" and "Who am I better than?" To Spence, all relationships involved a hierarchy of personal importance. With thoughts such as these, Spence could not be on the *same* level as another individual, hence the experience of loneliness. The therapist suggested that Spence ponder the question, "Who are my peers – who are the people I could bond with more, on my own level?" Spence's response was that the therapist's suggestion was one of the "stupidest things" he had ever heard. The therapist had to work hard to compose himself, and to be nondefensive while continuing to probe for Spence's more substantive reactions to what he had just heard.

Therapists of NPD clients also have to be on guard to set limits and maintain appropriate boundaries. Sometimes the situation can be handled with humor, such as when Spence put his feet up on the therapist's desk, and the latter asked, "Was this your office in a previous life?" At other times, the situation can be downright maddening, such as when Ellison repeatedly filled up the therapist's voicemail box with angry messages, and frequently brought in various forms that he demanded the therapist complete and sign at his behest, on the spot, no questions asked. As NPD clients typically do not respond to the first few attempts to set limits, therapists have to stand their ground, sometimes in the face of angry assaults. It is imperative for therapists of NPD clients to maintain their accepted clinical and ethical policies, while being as pleasant about the matter as possible, and with a willingness to process the interaction.

Therapists have to walk a fine line between validating the NPD clients' grandiose self-portrayals, and seeming critical by virtue of giving corrective feedback. Therapists must be especially tactful when presenting their conceptualizations to their NPD clients. For example, instead of referring to the clients' sense of specialness and superiority as "entitlement," the therapist might use the term "underdeveloped reciprocity." (This concept has been developed by K. Moras and C. Ratto in a treatment study of medication-resistant depression supported by National Institute of Mental Health grants R21 MH52737 and KO2 MHO1443–03: K. Moras, personal communication.) Since the latter term is less pejorative than entitlement, the clients may be less likely to feel criticized, and, consequently, more likely to accept the feedback.

Another way to navigate this narrow zone is to use the clients' sense of pride to motivate them to tackle difficult therapeutic tasks. For example, we have sometimes elicited a high rate of compliance with homework when we have emphasized that "most clients cannot do such advanced cognitive therapy work so soon in treatment." When put in this manner, homework becomes less of a demand and more of an opportunity to demonstrate prowess. Similarly, when NPD clients steadfastly maintain that their viewpoints are absolutely true and correct, but then evince an exaggerated sense of helplessness and self-reproach in response to stressors, therapists can create therapeutic cognitive dissonance by saying, "It is incomprehensible to me [i.e., I am in a one-down position because I do not know the answer] that someone who is so sure that he is always right can also be so down on himself and helpless!"

Therapists must be secure enough not to get into a competition with the clients, levelheaded enough not to buy into NPD clients' effusive praise or devaluation, benevolent enough to continue to be caring and attentive even in the face of aversive interpersonal behaviors from clients, and self-aware enough to use their internal reactions to guide the process of assessment and intervention. This is a tall order. For example, when Ellison asked for a "better, more senior" therapist, it was explained that he was already seeing the Director of the clinic. The therapist had to steer clear of trying to defend his qualifications, and instead focus on Ellison's sense of helplessness and frustration in treatment. As the therapist said to his client, "By asking for a 'better' therapist, you are suggesting that you believe the advancement of your treatment is completely beyond your personal abilities – you are saying you cannot effect change for yourself, because you need an all-powerful other." Likewise, when Ellison complained that "therapy [wasn't] working," the therapist replied, "Okay, given that 'therapy' is comprised of *you and me*, let's talk about how you and I aren't working." Ellison was caught off guard by this reply, as he had not meant to include himself in the process of assessing how his therapy could be improved.

When NPD clients demonstrate their sense of entitlement in the therapeutic relationship, it sometimes manifests itself in the implicit assumption that the therapist is there to do their personal bidding. The clients may expect that their therapists will advocate for them against others, including public, academic, financial, governmental, and vocational agencies, or at the very least will agree with everything they say. Rayna was very perturbed by her accurate perception that her therapist sometimes disagreed with her. Rayna chastised her therapist for "not supporting" her, whereupon the therapist replied, "If I agree with everything you say, then you have a useless 'yes man' for a therapist, and I think you *deserve better* than to have a lackey for a therapist." Again, this kind of comment creates cognitive dissonance, in that the therapist is showing support, all the while setting firm limits. Likewise, when Tabitha's therapist gave her corrective feedback, she often prefaced her comments by saying, "I *owe* you the truth, even though it may be hard to hear." Again, we're talking about combining positive regard with constructive criticism in a language that NPD clients understand.

Given that working with an NPD client can be quite demanding and disconcerting, therapists are likely to have some strong, negative cognitions and emotions that may hinder the process of therapy (Schultz and Glickauf-Hughes, 1995). It is advisable for therapists who feel this way to examine their own negative thoughts, to find ways to reconstrue the adversity as a learning opportunity, and to seek support and consultations from colleagues. It is at such times that therapists would do well to remind themselves why they went into the mental health field, and to do a mental review of all of the clients who have appreciated their help.

Strategies and techniques

The chapter by Denise Davis in the Beck et al. (1990) volume was one of the first cognitive therapy treatises devoted specifically to NPD. She noted that treatment interventions with this population typically focus on increasing personal responsibility, decreasing cognitive distortions and their concomitant dysfunctional affect, and formulating new attitudes about the self in relation to others. In conjunction with the above list we offer the following categories of goals to pursue with NPD clients:

- an improved ability to self-correct;
- better ability to take perspectives other than one's own (i.e., increase empathy);
- better ability to moderate extreme opinions of self and others;
- improved ability to tolerate limits and frustrations with grace and dignity.

Self-correction skills

One of the most important skills that cognitive therapists teach their clients is the ability to *self-monitor*. Indeed, the entire behavioral and cognitive-behavioral realms of psychotherapy value the importance of self-monitoring as both an assessment methodology and a stimulus for therapeutic change. It is useful for clients to learn to take a perceptual step back, to observe themselves without harsh judgment and as objectively as possible, and to record and understand the "data" of their lives. This enables them to make planned therapeutic changes that can be measured.

For NPD clients, this task is all the more important, and all the more difficult to learn. Because of their difficulties in taking the perspectives of others, their heavy investment in being right and saving face, and their overreactivity to the implication that they are doing something that needs correction, NPD clients do not take kindly to the task of self-correction. One of the hypothesized reasons this is so is that it activates their *defectiveness* schema, which they find most aversive and contrary to the successful image they are trying so hard to project to the world. Nevertheless,

NPD clients can benefit greatly from noticing their mistakes, learning from them, and making positive changes that enable them to adapt more effectively to their work life and relationships.

Given the importance of this psychological skill, and in light of the difficulties in NPD clients accepting its relevance, therapists have to find a way to demonstrate the advantages of self-monitoring to NPD clients. One such way is to look at how it is "smart and advantageous" to be able to self-correct. Far from being a shameful exercise, self-correction is part of evolving as a person, and becoming one of the fittest who survive in a competitive world. Sometimes it is useful to drop the names of famous celebrities, sports figures, or money moguls who rebounded from failures to have highly successful professional lives because they were able to learn from their mistakes. In sum, the purpose of this approach is to help NPD clients make changes while still saving face. In doing so, NPD clients may experience an attenuation of their defectiveness schema, and perhaps a moderation of their unrelenting standards schema as well.

A number of techniques can be used in teaching patients the skill of self-monitoring. Clients can, for example, use standard cognitive therapy forms such as the Daily Activity Schedule (Beck, 1995) to chart the course of their actions during the day. This can help the clients learn to make more effective use of their time, among other benefits. In addition, NPD clients can be taught to use their emotional distress at any given moment as a cue to ask themselves, "Why am I not getting what I want out of this situation right now, and what can I do differently so that the situation can turn around for the better?" For example, the therapist suggested to Ellison that he ask himself the above question each time he felt frustrated by his wife's reaction to his complaints. One goal of this self-monitoring exercise was that Ellison would learn to catch himself when he was expressing "angry helplessness," and instead "rise to the occasion" by talking alternatively about how he would solve his problems.

Clients also can be taught to use the Schema Self-Monitoring Record (SSMR; K. Moras and C. L. Ratto, unpublished data). The SSMR is a modification of the Dysfunctional Thought Record (Beck, 1995) and aims to help clients respond more effectively to their thoughts, thereby reducing negative affect and maladaptive behavior (Figure 8.1). One significant feature of the SSMR is the addition of a "Behavioral Impulse" column. We find that this is an important addition for NPD clients, as their sense of entitlement often makes them vulnerable to acting out their anger without prior reflection. We have found that the SSMR provides clients with an opportunity to slow down so as to think through the activating situation more effectively, with the goal of behaving more adaptively. Figure 8.1 depicts a sample SSMR for Ellison, who tended to behave aggressively in order to get others to meet his demands.

Moras & Ratto NIMH R21-52737
DRD monitse2.wpd 11/2/98

After Ses #:_14
Date: 00/00/00

Ptnt.ID_000_

Complete for: ANGER at SOMEONE   SCHEMA ACTIVATED: Emotional deprivation

SELF-MONITORING RECORD

DATE/ SITUATION	THOUGHTS	FEELINGS	BEHAVIORAL IMPULSES	REFRAME OF THOUGHTS	WHAT YOU ACTUALLY DID
What was going on?	Write down the thoughts that you are having about the situation (e.g., what thoughts are you having about the other person?)	Write down the feelings you have that are associated with each thought	What do you feel like doing when you have the thoughts?	How can you think about the situation differently that will reduce or eliminate your anger at the person?	
Talking to my wife about the idiot mediator. She walked out of the room.	Nobody gives a s — t about me. I have to suffer fools all day and nobody wants to help me.	Angry. Frustrated. Alone.	Chase after my wife and blow my stack because she bailed on me.	She has told me that my anger intimidates her and she can't deal with it. She tried to have a conversation but I got off on an upsetting tangent.	Stayed put and logged on to my computer to distract myself.

Figure 8.1   Sample Schema Self-Monitoring Record.

Taking the perspectives of others/empathy training

One of the skills that clients learn (or enhance) in cognitive therapy is the ability to look at issues and problems from a variety of perspectives. This enables clients to prevent tunnel vision, and to improve their social problem-solving ability. Related to this skill is one's capacity for understanding how someone else is feeling, and ascertaining how that person sees things. These skills have many adaptive functions, including allowing clients to be flexible in their approach to dealing with life's adversities, and relating more compatibly and sympathetically with others. Unfortunately, NPD clients often demonstrate deficiencies in these areas, especially with regard to the ability to take someone else's perspective. It is no wonder then that NPD clients are apt to demonstrate low degrees of empathy. Nevertheless, there are advantages in life in being able to understand the feelings and motivations of others. Cognitive therapists can emphasize these benefits in order to motivate NPD clients to imagine what it must be like to be the other person in a given situation. If NPD clients begin to learn this skill, they will show a lessening in the manifestations of their entitlement and mistrust schemata. There are a number of tacks that therapists can take with regard to the above:

1. When clients complain about important others in their life, or describe conflicts they had with these people, therapists can ask the clients to ponder what the other people may have been thinking or feeling, and to look for supporting evidence.
2. Therapists can initiate discussions about the pros and cons of being able to notice and care about what other people think and feel – especially family members and romantic partners. Similarly, they can focus on the negative consequences of being oblivious to (i.e., acting "thoughtless") or uncaring about others.
3. Therapists can periodically give tactful feedback about what they themselves are thinking and feeling in their problematic interactions with their NPD clients. This cues the NPD clients into the idea that therapists are people too, and serves as a prompt to pay attention to the therapeutic relationship as it is unfolding.
4. Therapists can help NPD clients develop a repertoire of self-statements to prime them to pay better attention to others (e.g., "Listen to her, it's important," or "Give him your undivided attention – it's meaningful").

In order to motivate NPD clients to take part in these interventions, therapists will have to make it clear how it can be *in their best interest* to take the perspective of another person from time to time. Further, therapists can note that this skill is far superior to the simple act of saying, "I know exactly how you feel," which can come across as patronizing, insincere, and "pseudosympathetic." At times, NPD will admit that this is how they perceive the therapist's attempts to demonstrate understanding. The result is a potentially elucidating discussion about "truth in caring," how one provides it, and how to assess it in others.

Moderating extreme opinions of self and others

Instead of being quick to judge people in extreme ways, NPD clients can solidify their self-concept and their rapport with others by taking a moderate approach to evaluating self and others. Otherwise, NPD clients are likely to demonstrate the following problems:

1. Clients oversell themselves to others, leading others to have higher expectations than the NPD clients can fulfill, leading further to avoidance, failure, and shame.
2. Clients denigrate themselves severely for their human foibles, reflecting low self-esteem, helplessness, and hopelessness. This can lead to embarrassing public displays of frustration and anger.
3. Clients make enemies of people whom they label in a gratuitously negative way, an outcome that is especially problematic when the people involved have authority.
4. Clients poison their personal relationships when they expect and demand too much, and then denigrate others for not doing enough.
5. Clients will gain a negative reputation for being insincere, fickle, or manipulative if they praise others excessively in order to gain special favor.

Therapists can serve as effective role models by steering clear of expressing extreme opinions of their own, instead adopting a more accepting attitude toward others, including NPD clients themselves. Using the Socratic, empirical approach for which cognitive therapy is known, therapists should respond to the NPD clients' extreme portrayals of others by asking for the evidence that supports or refutes such characterizations. In like fashion, cognitive therapists can show support for their NPD clients by reviewing data that contradict the latter's patent self-condemnations. The message is clear – it is not useful to judge oneself or others simplistically or harshly – it is far more useful to assess oneself and others based on a balanced review of the facts.

Additionally, NPD clients often are highly aware of how others may be evaluating them. They may seek to win the admiration and adulation of others on the one hand, and be hypervigilant for criticism and disrespect from people on the other hand. The NPD clients' excessive focus on evaluation is often manifest in their need to boast. In its more harmful forms, NPD clients will demonstrate a paranoid-like concern about being disrespected, and will test others in the haughty, manipulative manner of Shakespeare's King Lear ("Which of you, shall we say, doth love us most?"). Therapists can gain some leverage in encouraging NPD clients to relinquish these habits by noting that it may be "beneath them" to go to such extremes, given that the truly competent and loved person does not need repeated validation and proof of his or her worthiness from others.

Tolerating frustration and limits more gracefully

In general, NPD clients desire special treatment, and want to be the beneficiaries of the most favorable outcomes across a wide range of life situations. At one level they believe they deserve this, and they wear their "nothing-but-the-best" motto like a badge of honor. However, this stance also reflects a sense of vulnerability, because they become anxious and distressed if they do *not* have things go their way. The therapist's task is to point out that the ability to tolerate less than ideal situations and circumstances is a mark of strength and valor. To become the person who demonstrates "grace under pressure," or who "keeps his head while others around him are losing theirs" is a more stable, legitimate reason to feel a sense of pride. Adopting and enacting this viewpoint would represent a significant cognitive shift for many NPD clients. The emotional correlate to this change would be an increase in serenity, security, and substantive pride, as well as a concomitant decrease in anger, irritability, and shame.

Unfortunately, clients with NPD who enter therapy experiencing comorbid mood disorders will be especially prone to demonstrating low frustration tolerance. Therefore, they will not be so quick to accept the idea that they should endure the imperfections of life with a smile on their face. Instead, they will want relief from their suffering, and they will not be shy in letting their therapists know about this.

When therapists present the ground rules of therapy, in which NPD clients are told what they can and cannot reasonably expect from therapy, and what they are expected to do as part of the therapy contract, the stage will be set for a power struggle. Therapists will need to respond by maintaining their policies while remaining calm and pleasant, even if the clients escalate in their negative expressed emotion. By doing so, therapists will have a better chance of helping their NPD clients observe proper boundaries, because the foundation for the limits of the therapeutic relationship will have been set at the start. At the same time, therapists will succeed in averting the typical conflicts that NPD clients have come to know in their interactions with others in everyday life. This, in itself, serves as an important corrective cognitive and emotional experience for the NPD clients (Peyton and Safran, 1998), and an important step in moderating their entitlement schema.

Therapists can challenge their NPD clients to "rise to the occasion" in difficult circumstances, and to demonstrate skill and aplomb in navigating unfavorable situations. In other words, therapists should provide their NPD clients with as much positive verbal reinforcement as possible when they succeed in obeying limits, rules, social conventions, and other forms of mature conformity. This approach simultaneously counteracts both their entitlement and emotional deprivation schemata.

Building on an empirical foundation for the future study of NPD

As we have seen, much of the extant research on NPD focuses on the reliability and validity of the diagnosis itself (Ronningstam, 1998b). There is a paucity of empirical data with regard to cognitive-behavioral models, treatment, and outcome (Arntz, 1999). However, to the extent that we may generalize from some data on the treatment of general (or non-NPD) personality disorders, there is some evidence that cognitive therapy can be efficacious in modifying axis II pathology. For example, given the high rates of comorbidity between NPD and BPD, promising data on the treatment of BPD give hope that NPD problems can be addressed successfully as well. The work of Linehan and her associates (1993), along with current studies being conducted on the cognitive therapy of BPD at the University of Pennsylvania, give us reason to be optimistic. As Pretzer and Beck (1996) noted, "the available findings suggest that, for some individuals with an Axis-I disorder and a concurrent Axis-II disorder . . . cognitive-behavioral treatment for the Axis-I disorder not only can be effective . . . for the Axis-I disorder but also can result in overall improvement in the Axis-II disorder as well" (p.95).

Along similar lines, Persons et al. (1988) found that a key variable to the successful treatment of personality disorders is the therapist's ability to keep the client for a full course of treatment, as opposed to having the clients become discouraged and terminate prematurely. Their findings are consistent with unpublished data gathered in the early and mid-1990s at the Center for Cognitive Therapy at the

University of Pennsylvania. In an outcome study of cognitive therapy for avoidant personality disorder (AvPD) and OCPD, those clients who stayed in treatment for the full year improved dramatically. Specifically, 15 out of 22 AvPD clients finished the full course of treatment, at the end of which time only *one* client still met criteria for AvPD when interviewed by blind raters using a structured diagnostic interview. In the OCPD group, nine of 16 clients completed an entire year of cognitive therapy, with blind diagnostic interviews finding that *none* of these remaining clients still met criteria for OCPD. Although we suspect that figures for a similar NPD study would be more modest, these findings suggest that retaining personality-disordered clients for a full, structured, protocol-driven treatment may be a predictor of clinical improvement.

Unfortunately, there are very few empirical studies of the effectiveness of cognitive therapy with NPD per se. Pretzer and Beck's (1996) review noted that only one uncontrolled clinical report and one single-case design had been completed at the time their paper was published. One of the reasons for this dearth of data has to do with the difficulties inherent in designing a randomized clinical trial for NPD. Potential investigators would have to contend with problems related to recruitment of subjects, high rates of comorbidity, frequent protocol violations (which would be likely with clients who feel entitled), and long-term follow-up. The fact that these problems have been addressed by researchers of cognitive-behavioral treatments for BPD (Linehan et al., 1993) gives us hope that it will be feasible to study NPD in the same manner.

An important research direction may be to focus on issues that are relevant to the NPD clients' emotional and interpersonal problems, from a cognitive-behavioral perspective. For example, given the NPD clients' poor interpersonal habits, it may be relevant to examine their beliefs about relationships, including the therapeutic relationship. Such beliefs can be assessed at any point between the pretreatment intake evaluation and the long-term follow-up session. We hypothesize that NPD clients will demonstrate more robust, stable improvements in mood and life satisfaction as they begin to moderate their demands and expectations of others, come to value acts of reciprocity, and improve their interpersonal skills. Similarly, a good outcome would involve their acknowledgment of their role in their own treatment, rather than continuing to believe that "If I don't make improvements in treatment it is certainly due to the fact that my therapist wasn't good enough."

It is also reasonable to posit that the quality of the therapeutic relationship, from the perspectives of *both* participants, would have some predictive value in outcome (Safran and Muran, 2000). The therapeutic relationship is a two-way street, and it is likely that both the NPD client and the therapist have to feel valued, comfortable, and trusting *of each other* in order to facilitate the difficult work of changing ingrained patterns in the client's functioning. We posit that it is not sufficient for NPD clients to learn to feel positively about their therapy. If, by the time termination takes place, the *therapist* still has not felt a sense of attachment to the NPD client – indeed, if the therapist is relieved to be finished with the client – it is unlikely that the client will have long-term success in the world of everyday relationships. Therefore, measurement of the therapeutic alliance must be done from both parties' perspectives.

One such method is the California Psychotherapy Alliance Scale (CALPAS: Gaston and Marmar, 1994), which involves independent ratings done by client and therapist (blind with regard to the other's responses) at the same times during the course of treatment. The use of the CALPAS has proven advantageous in recent outcome trials involving cognitive therapy for personality disorders (unpublished data on the cognitive therapy of AvPD, OCPD, and current pilot work on the cognitive therapy of BPD, University of Pennsylvania), and might be used in future research involving patients with NPD.

The CALPAS can be used along with the other inventories that assess the clients' beliefs and schemata (PBQ: Beck et al. (2001); SQ: Schmidt et al., 1995), with special emphasis placed on examining changes in clients' responses to *interpersonally relevant* beliefs and schemata. We hypothesize that NPD clients who demonstrate a moderation of their beliefs about others, and their own relationships with others, would be more apt to maintain therapeutic gains than NPD clients who simply indicate improved functioning on standard mood inventories. Naturally, it is also necessary to determine at termination whether or not NPD clients still meet diagnostic criteria for NPD. A full, structured, clinical interview for personality disorders (SCID-II: First et al., 1995), conducted by a blind, independent assessment clinician at the end of treatment, as well as at future follow-up points, would be useful in this regard. This measure of outcome should be complemented by an assessment of the NPD clients' general quality of life, which would make for a more complete picture of the clients' posttherapy functioning across many relevant domains (Gladis et al., 1999).

Based on the approach suggested above, we would suggest that NPD is a prime example of a clinical problem that is best studied from a theoretically integrative perspective. Contrasting treatments that have empirical support would be prime candidates to achieve this potentially fruitful hybridization, for example, cognitive-behavioral therapy and interpersonal psychotherapy (Klerman et al., 1984). The goal of finding efficacious treatment for NPD will be advanced if we study the *process* of treatment, including critical moments of high affect, hot cognitions, and hopelessness on the parts of both therapists and clients. The work being done by Safran and colleagues (Safran and Segal, 1990; Safran et al., 1990; Safran and Muran, 1995, 1998, 2000) on the recognition and reparation of ruptures in the therapeutic alliance represents a most fruitful area of inquiry for a population such as NPD, and needs to be better understood and utilized by cognitive-behavioral psychotherapy researchers. Lest we focus only on the problematic aspects of the therapeutic alliance, we should add that a similar benefit would accrue from the study of markers in treatment that indicate a *strengthening* of the therapeutic relationship, and its relationship to outcome.

Conclusion

The last decade has seen the field of cognitive-behavioral therapy turn its attention to the clinical problem of NPD. Many interesting hypotheses have been proffered, and measures have begun to be developed to address beliefs that are pertinent to the full spectrum of axis II disorders, but empirically based recommendations regarding treatment for NPD are in short supply. Although there will be difficulties in producing meaningful data, models of psychotherapy research currently exist that can blaze a path for the elucidation of effective, cognitive-behavioral interventions for NPD. These include outcome studies that already have commenced in the area of cognitive therapy for AvPD, OCPD, and BPD, as well as the study of psychotherapy process, the interpersonal life of the client in treatment, and the therapeutic alliance. Measures such as the CALPAS (Gaston and Marmar, 1994) will assist in this process, as will the further development of inventories such as the PBQ (Beck et al., 2001) and the SQ (Young, 1994). Further advancements are possible if we begin to pay closer attention to the beliefs, attitudes, and emotions of therapists, and how these interact with the treatment of NPD clients.

The treatment of NPD is not a simple, easy enterprise. Therapists who hope to make a significant positive impact on the lives of their NPD clients (and, by extension, the lives of the people who are close to the NPD clients) will need to work to understand themselves, to develop a wide repertoire of therapeutic responses under pressure and distress, and be especially adept at forming attachments with people who have attachment problems in the first place. Such therapists will need to have advanced conceptualization skills, a thorough understanding of the interventions of cognitive therapy, and a working familiarity with the principles of interpersonal psychotherapy, and process research. This is a tall order, but therapists who meet these criteria may prove to have the best chance at affecting meaningful change in a population where it is sorely needed.

REFERENCES

American Psychiatric Association (1980). *Diagnostic and Statistical Manual of Mental Disorders*, 3rd edn. Washington, DC: American Psychiatric Association.

American Psychiatric Association. (1987). *Diagnostic and Statistical Manual of Mental Disorders*, 3rd edn, revised. Washington, DC: American Psychiatric Association.

American Psychiatric Association. (1994). *Diagnostic and Statistical Manual of Mental Disorders*, 4th edn. Washington, DC: American Psychiatric Association.

Arntz, A. (1999). Do personality disorders exist? On the validity of the concept and its cognitive-behavioral formulation and treatment. *Behaviour Research and Therapy*, **37**(suppl. 1), S97–134.

Beck, J. S. (1995). *Cognitive Therapy: Basics and Beyond.* New York: Guilford.

Beck, A. T., Rush, A. J., Shaw, B., and Emery, G. (1979). *Cognitive Therapy of Depression.* New York: Guilford.

Beck, A. T., Freeman, A., and associates (1990). *Cognitive Therapy of Personality Disorders.* New York: Guilford.

Beck, A. T., Butler, A. C., Brown, G. K., Dahlsgaard, K. K., Newman, C. F., and Beck, J. S. (2001). Dysfunctional beliefs discriminate personality disorders, *Behaviour Research and Therapy*, **39**, 1213–25.

Blais, M. A., Hilsenroth, M. J., and Castlebury, F. D. (1997). Content validity of the DSM-IV borderline and narcissistic personality criteria sets. *Comprehensive Psychiatry*, **38**, 31–37.

Bowlby, J. (1973). *Attachment and Loss*, vol. 2. *Separation, Anxiety, and Anger.* New York: Basic Books.

Bushman, B. J. and Baumeister, R. F. (1998). Threatened egotism, narcissism, self-esteem, and direct and displaced aggression: does self-love or self-hate lead to violence? *Journal of Personality and Social Psychology*, **75**(1), 219–29.

Bux, D. A. (1992). Narcissistic personality disorder. In *Comprehensive Casebook of Cognitive Therapy*, ed. A. Freeman and F. M. Dattilio, pp. 223–30. New York: Plenum Press.

Chatham, P. M., Tibbals, C. J., and Harrington, M. E. (1993). The MMPI and MCMI in the evaluation of narcissism in a clinical sample. *Journal of Personality Assessment*, **60**, 239–51.

Clark, L. A., Livesley, W. J., and Morey, L. (1997). Special feature: personality disorder assessment: the challenge of construct validity. *Journal of Personality Disorders*, **11**(3), 205–31.

Curtis, R. C. (1999). The angry client: case and session presentation. *Journal of Psychotherapy Integration*, **9**(2), 133–42.

Davis, D. D. (1990). Narcissistic personality disorder. In *Cognitive Therapy of Personality Disorders*, ed. A. T. Beck, A. Freeman, and associates, pp. 233–56. New York: Guilford.

Emmons, R. A. (1987). Narcissism: theory and measurement. *Journal of Personality and Social Psychology*, **52**(1), 11–17.

Erikson, E. H. (1964). *Childhood and Society*, 2nd edn. New York: W. W. Norton.

First, B., Spitzer, R. L., Gibbon, M., and Williams, J. B. W. (1995). The Structured Clinical Interview for DSM-III-R personality disorders (SCID-II): I. Description. *Journal of Personality Disorders*, **9**(2), 83–91.

Gaston, L. and Marmar, C. R. (1994). The California Psychotherapy Alliance Scales. In *The Working Alliance: Theory, Research, and Practice*, ed. A. O. Horvath and L. S. Greenberg, pp. 85–108. New York: John Wiley.

Gladis, M. M., Gosch, E. A., Dishuk, N. M., and Crits-Christoph, P. (1999). Quality of life: expanding the scope of clinical significance. *Journal of Consulting and Clinical Psychology*, **67**(3), 320–31.

Greenberger, D. and Padesky, C. (1995). *Mind over Mood.* New York: Guilford.

Gunderson, J., Ronningstam, E., and Smith, L. (1991). Narcissistic personality disorder: a review of data on DSM-III-R descriptions. *Journal of Personality Disorders*, **5**, 167–77.

Gunderson, J., Ronningstam, E., and Smith, L. (1995). Narcissistic personality disorder. In *The DSM-IV Personality Disorder Diagnoses*, ed. J. Livesley, pp. 201–12. New York: Guilford.

Hilsenroth, M. J. (1997). *A Multidimensional Assessment of Narcissistic Personality Disorder*. Doctoral dissertation. University of Georgia: Athens, GA.

Holdwick, D. J., Hilsenroth, M. J., Castlebury, F. D., and Blais, M. A. (1998). Identifying the unique and common characteristics among the DSM-IV antisocial, borderline, and narcissistic personality disorders. *Comprehensive Psychiatry*, **39**, 277–86.

Kernberg, O. F. (1975). *Borderline Conditions and Pathological Narcissism*. New York: Jason Aronson.

Kernberg, O. F. (1980). *Internal World and External Reality*. New York: Jason Aronson.

Kernberg, O. F. (1984). *Severe Personality Disorders: Psychotherapeutic Strategies*. New Haven, CT: Yale University Press.

Klerman, G. L., Weissman, M. M., Rounsaville, B. J., and Chevron, E. S. (1984). *Interpersonal Psychotherapy of Depression*. New York: Basic Books.

Kohut, H. (1971). *The Analysis of the Self: A Systematic Approach to the Psychoanalytic Treatment of Narcissistic Personality Disorders*. New York: International Universities Press.

Kruger, J. and Dunning, D. (1999). Unskilled and unaware of it: how difficulties in recognizing one's own incompetence lead to inflated self-assessments. *Journal of Personality and Social Psychology*, **77**(6), 1121–34.

Lasch, C. (1979). *The Culture of Narcissism*. New York: Norton.

Layden, M. A., Newman, C. F., Freeman, A., and Morse, S. B. (1993). *Cognitive Therapy of Borderline Personality Disorder*. Boston, MA: Allyn & Bacon.

Leventhal, S. (1995). The role of empathy in narcissism: an empirical investigation of Heinz Kohut's work. *Dissertation Abstracts*, **55**, 4124.

Linehan, M. M., Heard, H. L., and Armstrong, H. E. (1993). Naturalistic follow-up of a behavioral treatment for chronically parasuicidal borderline clients. *Archives of General Psychiatry*, **50**(12), 971–4.

Lyons, C. M. (1998). *Etiology and Interpersonal Correlates of Narcissistic Personality Traits in Children*. Doctoral dissertation. University of Georgia: Athens, GA.

Maltsberger, J. T. (1998). Pathological narcissism and self-regulatory processes in suicidal states. In *Disorders of Narcissism: Diagnostic, Clinical, and Empirical Implications*, ed. E. Ronningstam, pp. 327–44. Washington, DC: American Psychiatric Press.

Masterson, J. F. (1981). *The Narcissistic and Borderline Disorders*. New York: Brunner/Mazel.

McGlashan, T. and Heinssen, R. (1989). Narcissistic, antisocial, and noncomorbid subgroups of borderline patients. *Psychiatric Clinics of North America*, **12**, 653–71.

Millon, T. (1969). *Modern Psychopathology: A Biosocial Approach to Maladaptive Learning and Functioning*. Philadelphia: Saunders.

Millon, T. (1990). The avoidant personality. In *Handbook of Personality: Theory and Research*, ed. L. A. Pervin, pp. 339–70. New York: Guilford.

Millon, T. and Davis, R. (1996). *Disorders of Personality: DSM-IV and Beyond*, 2nd edn. New York: Wiley.

Morey, L. C. and Jones, J. K. (1998). Empirical studies of the construct validity of narcissistic personality disorder. In *Disorders of Narcissism: Diagnostic, Clinical, and Empirical Implications*, ed. E. F. Ronningstam, pp. 351–73. Washington, DC: American Psychiatric Press.

Newman, C. F. (1997). Maintaining professionalism in the face of emotional abuse from clients. *Cognitive and Behavioral Practice*, **4**, 1–29.

Newman, C. F. (1998). The therapeutic relationship and alliance in short-term cognitive therapy. In *The Therapeutic Alliance in Brief Psychotherapy*, ed. J. D. Safran and J. C. Muran, pp. 95–122. Washington, DC: American Psychological Association.

Perry, C. (1990). Personality disorders, suicide and self-destructive behavior. In *Suicide – Understanding and Responding*, ed. D. Jacobs, H. Brown, and C. T. Madison, pp. 157–69. Madison, CT: International Universities Press.

Persons, J. B., Burns, B. D., and Perloff, J. M. (1988). Predictors of drop-out and outcome in cognitive therapy for depression in a private practice setting. *Cognitive Therapy and Research*, **12**, 557–75.

Peyton, E. and Safran, J. D. (1998). Interpersonal process in the treatment of narcissistic personality disorders. In *Cognitive Psychotherapy of Psychotic and Personality Disorders: Handbook of Theory and Practice*, ed. C. Perris and P. D. McGorry, pp. 379–95. New York: Wiley.

Plakun, E. M. (1990). Empirical overview of narcissistic personality disorder. In *New Perspectives on Narcissism. The Clinical Practice Series*, no. 13, ed. E. M. Plakun, pp. 103–49. Washington, DC: American Psychiatric Press.

Pretzer, J. L. and Beck, A. T. (1996). A cognitive theory of personality disorders. In *Major Theories of Personality Disorder*, ed. J. F. Clarkin and M. F. Lenzenweger, pp. 36–105. New York: Guilford.

Raskin, R. N. and Hall, C. S. (1979). A narcissistic personality inventory. *Psychological Reports*, **45**, 590.

Raskin, R. and Terry, H. (1988). A principal components analysis of the Narcissistic Personality Inventory and further evidence of its construct validity. *Journal of Personality and Social Psychology*, **54**, 890–902.

Reich, J., Yates, W., and Ndvaguba, M. (1989). Prevalence of DSM-III personality disorders in the community. *Social Psychiatry and Psychiatric Epidemiology*, **24**, 12–16.

Reichman, J. and Flaherty, J. (1990). Gender differences in narcissistic styles. In *New Perspective of Narcissism*, ed. E. M. Plakun, pp. 71–100. Washington, DC: American Psychiatric Press.

Ronningstam, E. (1996). Pathological narcissism and narcissistic personality disorder in axis-I disorders. *Harvard Review of Psychiatry*, **3**, 326–40.

Ronningstam, E. F. (1998a). Narcissistic personality disorder and pathological narcissism: long-term stability and presence in Axis-I disorders. In *Disorders of Narcissism: Diagnostic, Clinical, and Empirical Implications*, ed. E. F. Ronningstam, pp. 375–413. Washington, DC: American Psychiatric Press.

Ronningstam, E. F. (1998b). *Disorders of Narcissism: Diagnostic, Clinical, and Empirical Implications*. Washington, DC: American Psychiatric Press.

Ronningstam, E. (1999). Narcissistic personality disorder. In *Oxford Textbook of Psychopathology*, ed. T. Millon, P. H. Blaney, and R. D. Davis, pp. 674–93. New York: Oxford University Press.

Ronningstam, E. F. and Gunderson, J. (1988). Narcissistic traits in psychiatric patients. *Comprehensive Psychiatry*, **29**, 545–9.

Ronningstam, E. F. and Gunderson, J. (1990). Identifying criteria for narcissistic personality disorder. *American Journal of Psychiatry*, **147**, 918–22.

Ronningstam, E. F. and Gunderson, J. (1991). Differentiating borderline personality disorder from narcissistic personality disorder. *Journal of Personality Disorders*, **5**, 225–32.

Rosenfeld, H. (1964). On the psychopathology of narcissism: a clinical approach. *International Journal of Psychoanalysis*, **45**, 332–7.

Ryff, C. D. and Singer, B. H. (1996). Psychological well-being: meaning, measurement, and implications for psychotherapy research. *Psychotherapy and Psychosomatics*, **65**, 14–23.

Ryff, C. D. and Singer, B. H. (1998). The contours of positive human health. *Psychological Inquiry*, **9**, 1–28.

Safran, J. D. and Muran, J. C. (1995). Resolving ruptures in the therapeutic alliance: diversity and integration. *In-Session: Psychotherapy in Practice*, **1**, 81–92.

Safran, J. D. and Muran, J. C. (eds) (1998). *The Therapeutic Alliance in Brief Psychotherapy*. Washington, DC: American Psychological Association.

Safran, J. D. and Muran, J. C. (2000). *Negotiating the Therapeutic Alliance: A Relational Treatment Guide*. New York: Guilford.

Safran, J. D. and Segal, Z. V. (1990). *Interpersonal Process in Cognitive Therapy*. New York: Basic Books.

Safran, J. D., Crocker, P., McMain, S., and Murray, P. (1990). Therapeutic alliance rupture as a therapy event for empirical investigation. *Psychotherapy*, **27**(2), 154–65.

Schmidt, N. B., Joiner, T. E., Jr., Young, J. E., and Telch, M. J. (1995). The Schema Questionnaire: investigation of psychometric properties and the hierarchical structure of a measure of maladaptive schemata. *Cognitive Therapy and Research*, **19**(3), 295–321.

Schultz, R. E. and Glickauf-Hughes, C. (1995). Countertransference in the treatment of pathological narcissism. *Psychotherapy*, **32**(4), 601–7.

Seligman, M. E. P. (1991). *Learned Optimism*. New York: Knopf.

Sperry, L. (1995). *Handbook of Diagnosis and Treatment of DSM-IV Personality Disorders*. New York: Brunner Mazel.

Stone, M. (1989). Long-term follow-up of narcissistic borderline patients. *Psychiatric Clinics of North America*, **12**, 621–42.

Stone, M. (1993). *Abnormalities of Personality: Within and Beyond the Realm of Treatment*. New York: Norton.

Stone, M. H. (1998). Normal narcissism: an etiological and ethological perspective. In *Disorders of Narcissism: Diagnostic, Clinical, and Empirical Implications*, ed. E. F. Ronningstam, pp. 7–28. Washington, DC: American Psychiatric Press.

Tschanz, B. T., Morf, C. C., and Turner, C. W. (1998). Gender differences in the structure of narcissism: a multi-sample analysis of the narcissism personality inventory. *Sex Roles*, **38**, 863–70.

Vaillant, G. and Perry, J. (1985). Personality disorders. In *Comprehensive Textbook of Psychiatry*, vol. I, ed. H. Kaplan and B. Sadock, pp. 1352–87. Baltimore, MD: Williams & Wilkins.

Widiger, T. A. and Rogers, J. H. (1989). Prevalence and comorbidity of personality disorders. *Psychiatric Annals*, **19**, 132–6.

Young, J. E. (1990). *Cognitive Therapy for Personality Disorders: A Schema-focused Approach.* Sarasota, FL: Professional Resource Exchange.

Young, J. E. (1994). *Cognitive Therapy for Personality Disorders: A Schema-focused Approach,* 2nd edn. Sarasota, FL: Professional Resource Exchange.

Young, J. E. (1999). *Cognitive Therapy for Personality Disorders: A Schema-focused Approach,* 3rd edn. Sarasota, FL: Professional Resource Exchange.

Young, J. E. and Flanagan, C. (1998). Schema-focused therapy for narcissistic patients. In *Disorders of Narcissism: Diagnostic, Clinical, and Empirical Implications,* ed. E. F. Ronningstam, pp. 239–62. Washington, DC: American Psychiatric Press.

Zimmerman, M. and Coryell, W. (1990). Diagnosing personality disorders in the community. *Archives of General Psychiatry,* **47**, 527–31.

9

Cognitive therapy and the self

David L. DuBois, Cristy Lopez, and Gilbert R. Parra
University of Missouri, Columbia, MO, USA

Self processes have a prominent role in the conceptual foundations of cognitive therapy. Cognitive therapy is based upon a constructionist viewpoint and assumes that each individual's construal of his or her experiences constitutes a reality of primary importance for that person (Guidano and Liotti, 1985). These perceptions pertain not only to events in the external world, but also to internal attributes of the self (Beck, 1976). Self-referential thought processes accordingly have received significant attention in cognitive theories of psychopathology and treatment (Beck et al., 1990; Freeman et al., 1990; Beck, 1995; Dattilio and Reinecke, 1996; Young, 1999). It has been recommended that assessment of these types of cognitions, as distinct from those with an external orientation, be used to inform treatment planning for individual clients (Beck and Freeman, 1990; Freeman et al., 1990). Furthermore, intervention strategies directed toward changing beliefs about the self play an essential role in cognitive therapy for specific disorders (e.g., depression).

Despite these considerations, theory and research on the self currently exist as an independent literature. Whereas studies in this area have been concerned primarily with the development and testing of general conceptual models, the emphasis in the cognitive therapy literature has been on the role of self factors within an applied context (i.e., psychotherapy). Furthermore, the focus of most self research has been on nonclinical populations. The broader self literature thus constitutes an important frame of reference from which to identify and understand deviations from normal or adaptive self processes among individuals seeking treatment and has the potential to serve as a resource for innovation in assessment and intervention. Contributions of this nature already have been realized in our growing appreciation of the central role of negative views of the self in cognitive models of depression (Beck, 1976), and in cognitive therapy with children (DiGiuseppe, 1989; McCauley et al., 1995). There remains, nevertheless, a need for examination of more recent theory and findings in the self literature with respect to their implications for cognitive therapy.

The major aim of the present chapter is to address this need. Several noteworthy topics currently receiving attention in the self literature are reviewed first. This overview is not intended to be exhaustive, but to be illustrative of the range of potentially relevant areas of inquiry. To facilitate an integrative perspective, a general theme across the areas selected is their relevance to self-esteem as a central organizing feature of the self-system (Harter, 1999). The implications of the self literature for assessment and intervention in cognitive therapy are then examined. Concluding comments include recommendations for research further to enhance integration of self and cognitive therapy literatures.

Self theory and research

Multidimensional, hierarchical models of self-concept

One important topic in the self literature has been the investigation of multidimensional, hierarchical models of self-concept. Findings of this research demonstrate the complex and multidimensional structure of the underlying cognitive organization of the self (for reviews, see Byrne, 1996; Marsh and Hattie, 1996; Harter, 1998). Beginning as early as age 5, children differentiate in how they evaluate themselves across various areas in their lives (Marsh and Hattie, 1996). The number of domains that can be discriminated increases over the course of development (Harter, 1990, 1998), thus providing for distinctive, individualized profiles of self-perceptions that, by adulthood, can be conceptualized as unique to each person (Harré, 1998). Several theorists have proposed hierarchical arrangements or structures for differing dimensions of self views (Byrne, 1996; Marsh and Hattie, 1996). These models propose several levels of self-concept facets that are nested within one another according to varying levels of content specificity, ranging from highly circumscribed views at the lowest levels (e.g., evaluations of behavior in specific situations) to general self-concept or self-esteem at the apex. Views at different levels of these hierarchies are assumed to be causally linked, such that those at any given level directly influence those at the next highest level (Byrne, 1996). To illustrate, children's views of their interactions with different family members, at the lowest level, may serve as the basis for separate facets of self-concept pertaining to relations with parents and siblings, respectively, with these each contributing to a more general family self-concept which, in turn, is influential along with other factors (e.g., peer relations self-concept) in shaping higher-order social and general conceptions of self. Hierarchical, multidimensional models of self-concept have received empirical support through the use of higher-order, confirmatory factor analysis and multitrait–multimethod analyses (Marsh and Hattie, 1996; Byrne, 1996; Harter, 1998). These findings suggest that multiple domains of self views each contribute independently to general self-concept, with those pertaining to certain areas, such as physical appearance, exerting a particularly strong influence (Harter, 1999).

Self-appraisals pertaining to specific domains within hierarchies have been linked to a range of clinically relevant outcomes (DuBois and Tevendale, 1999; Harter, 1999; Rosenberg et al., 1995). Longitudinal studies indicate, for example, that a favorable academic self-concept facilitates better school performance (Marsh and Yeung, 1997) and that a negative body image increases susceptibility to emergence of eating-disorder symptomatology (Attie and Brooks-Gunn, 1989). Profiles of self-evaluation across multiple domains, moreover, have been found to enhance prediction of outcomes beyond that which is possible when considering different domains in isolation or relying solely on global (i.e., undifferentiated) self measures (DuBois and Tevendale, 1999; Harter, 1999). A pervasive pattern of negative views of the self across multiple life domains, for example, has been found to predict greater depressive symptomatology, even after controlling for their association with lower overall feelings of worth.

Individual differences in the underlying structure of multidimensional, hierarchical views of the self may also have clinical implications (Harter, 1998). Showers (1995) reviewed research indicating that some individuals display a tendency to organize self views into categories according to their negative or positive valance (i.e., evaluative compartmentalization) rather than using a content-based approach in which both positive and negative self attributes are grouped together according to domain (i.e., evaluative integration). For those with negative aspects to their self views, the compartmentalized type of structure seems to exacerbate problems with both low self-esteem and negative mood (Showers, 1995). In other research (Linville, 1987), it has been observed that the complexity of hierarchical self-structures that are evident for particular individuals can vary along several dimensions, including the number of levels in the hierarchy, the number of categories, and their degree of differentiation. Interestingly, it also has been suggested that the multiplicity of differing social roles required for successful adaptation in modern society may be so great as to be ill-suited to the construction of a coherent or unified self (Gergen, 1991). There may be significant liabilities associated with this type of proliferation of disparate, multiple selves, including confusion and distress associated with perceived contradictions (Harter, 1998). Of further note is research which suggests that general and less differentiated views about the self may be instrumental in shaping more circumscribed facets of self-perception, in contrast to the more widely posited flow of effects from specific views to more global perceptions (Brown, 1993b).

These issues have only just begun to receive attention in the cognitive therapy literature. Studies suggest, however, that a multidimensional, higher-order structure may be characteristic of clients' maladaptive self schemata (Schmidt et al., 1995) as well as manifest in their ongoing flow of thoughts and beliefs (Cacioppo et al., 1997). This work offers a promising basis for greater integration of a multidimensional, hierarchical perspective on the self-concept into assessment and intervention strategies within cognitive therapy.

Values, standards, and goals

Recent work in the self literature has also addressed the role of values, standards, and goals in self-evaluative processes. Perceived attributes of the self for any given domain, for example, have been hypothesized to influence overall feelings of self-worth (i.e., global or general self-esteem) only to the extent to which the individual attaches personal value or importance to those attributes (Rosenberg, 1979; Harter, 1999). Individuals tend to discount the importance of domains in which they perceive themselves to be less adequate or competent, presumably as a self-protective or self-enhancing strategy (Harter, 1990). This type of strategy, however, is not always effective (Marsh and Hattie, 1996). When areas are widely valued by others within the individual's environment (Harter, 1999), for example this may overshadow any efforts by the individual to afford them less centrality or importance within their own value system (Harter, 1999; Marsh and Hattie, 1996).

Related work highlights the significance of whether perceived self attributes satisfy (or fail to satisfy) the individual's personal standards or ideals (Higgins, 1987; Pelham and Swann, 1989; Marsh, 1999; DuBois et al., 2000). Findings in this area indicate that even when various attributes (e.g., appearance) are described by a given individual in terms that generally would be regarded as favorable or desirable by others, their own self-evaluations none the less may be negative if personal standards for that area are unusually stringent (Harter, 1999). This process may account for linkages observed between excessively high standards or ideals and risk for various types of mental disorder, including depression and anxiety (Higgins, 1987).

Recent research also indicates that, whether standards and goals are derived from internal (i.e., self-oriented) as opposed to external (i.e., socially prescribed) sources may have important implications for mental health outcomes. Self-determination theory (Ryan and Deci, 2000) and its supporting research are particularly noteworthy. This body of work highlights the importance of fostering the expression of individual autonomy and self-direction, and allowing for the formation of standards and goals that are internally derived, as opposed to being based to an unhealthy extent on external criteria or the expectations of others. Of particular note are findings which indicate that success in goal attainment is especially likely to promote overall psychological well-being when goals are personally meaningful and congruent with the individual's personal values and interests (Ryan and Deci, 2000).

These findings indicate an important role for values, standards, and goals within the self-system. As applied to cognitive therapy, factors relating to motivation and personal salience could be conceptualized as mediating the relation of thoughts and beliefs to clients' presenting problems. Accordingly, it may be useful to consider them when selecting treatment strategies.

Perceived self-efficacy

There is an accumulating body of research documenting the role of self-efficacy beliefs in human adaptation. As defined by Bandura (1997), perceived self-efficacy refers to "beliefs in one's capabilities to organize and execute courses of action re- quired to produce given attainments" (p. 2). In as much as self-beliefs vary across settings and activities, Bandura and others adopting his theoretical framework have emphasized their domain-specific nature. Others (e.g., Rutter, 1987), however, have emphasized broader, less task-specific conceptions of self-efficacy that involve a general sense of mastery and ability to influence outcomes in one's environment. Viewed from either perspective, strong efficacy beliefs may offer a variety of benefits, such as encouraging individuals to approach rather than avoid important activi- ties and to exhibit greater persistence in working toward goals (Bandura, 1997). A strong sense of personal efficacy provides an important foundation for feelings of self-worth (Rutter, 1987; Werner and Smith, 1992; DuBois and Tevendale, 1999) and has been indicated to facilitate positive outcomes in a wide range of areas such as health behavior (Bandura, 1997), academic achievement (Zimmerman, 1995), career development (Hackett, 1995), and effective parenting (Elder, 1995). There is also evidence to suggest that efficacy beliefs help protect against the emer- gence of negative patterns of adaptation and disorder (Rutter, 1987; Werner, 1995), ranging from emotional difficulties such as depression and anxiety (Williams, 1992) to behavioral problems such as alcohol and drug abuse (Marlatt et al., 1995).

Self-efficacy theory emphasizes the importance of attending to judgments of per- sonal capability as a specific class of cognitions. In accordance with this view, studies conducted with clinical populations suggest that change in efficacy beliefs may be a common cognitive mechanism helping to account for the impact of a variety of treatment approaches (for a review, see Bandura, 1997). Because of the emphasis accorded not only to a generalized sense of mastery, but also task- and situation- specific beliefs about abilities, self-efficacy theory seems particularly well suited to informing treatment strategies used in cognitive therapy. The manner in which perceived self-efficacy has been incorporated into broader theoretical frameworks

(Bandura, 1997) that address sources of efficacy beliefs (e.g., observational learning) and other related influences on behavior (e.g., outcome expectation) further strengthens possibilities for useful application.

Motivation for self-esteem and self-consistency

Motivational strivings for both self-esteem and self-consistency have received extensive consideration in recent theory and research on the self (Rosenberg, 1979; Blaine and Crocker, 1993; Brown, 1993a; Swann, 1997; Harter, 1998). This work suggests that the desire to acquire and sustain positive feelings of self-worth (i.e., self-esteem) is a universal and fundamental aspect of human functioning (Brown, 1993a). Processes identified as important for achieving this goal include the acquisition of age-appropriate competencies as well as the formation of rewarding relationships with others (Harter, 1999). To a greater or lesser extent, however, all persons also rely on a variety of self-protective–self-enhancing strategies to preserve a favorable sense of self-regard (Rosenberg, 1979; Kaplan, 1986; Blaine and Crocker, 1993; Harter, 1998). As shown in Table 9.1, a range of self-protective responses involving self-referent cognition, personal need-value systems, and personal behavior have been identified (Kaplan, 1986).

There is also considerable research supporting the idea that people actively seek to maintain consistency in how they view themselves (for reviews, see Brown, 1993a, Swann, 1997). Several mechanisms for fulfilling this motive have been discussed, including self-verification (i.e., seeking out feedback from others that is consistent with one's own self-concept; Swann, 1997), self-affirmation (i.e., taking action with the intent of demonstrating to oneself that one's self-concept is accurate; Steele, 1988), and self-regulation (i.e., monitoring current behaviors for discrepancies with the self-concept and acting to reduce any discrepancies by adjusting behavior; Scheier and Carver, 1988). Among individuals with high self-esteem, a desire for self-consistency is likely to be focused on maintaining a positive view of oneself (Rosenberg, 1979). By contrast, among individuals with low self-esteem, motives for esteem-enhancement and self-consistency may be in opposition to one another (Swann, 1997). As Brown (1993a) noted, "For these individuals, the desire to promote a positive self-image conflicts with the need to protect a negative self-view against change" (p. 118).

Implications for persons with low self-esteem

Among individuals with low self-esteem, consistency motivation may contribute to stability (i.e., lack of change) in negative evaluations of the self (Kernis, 1993). Strategies that serve to maintain constancy in self views thus can prove maladaptive when used by those who hold negative views about themselves (Blaine and Crocker, 1993;

Table 9.1 Overview of self-protective–self-enhancing strategies

Self-referent cognition	Personal need-value systems	Personal behavior
Selective interpretation: selective interpretation of observed facts about the self; selective search for reasons, justifications, or excuses, and accounts of one's behavior or its consequences which cast the actions in a favorable light (Rosenberg, 1979)	*Selectivity of values*: attach importance to areas in which self-perceptions are favorable and lack of importance to areas in which views of the self are unfavorable (Rosenberg, 1979; Harter, 1986)	*Selective interaction*: associate with persons or groups who are believed to hold positive views of oneself (Rosenberg, 1979; Faunce, 1984).
Selective attention: selective attention to evidence that leads to positive conclusions about the self and/or overlooking or ignoring facts which do not (Rosenberg, 1979)	*Selective valuation and credulity*: assign greater value and credibility to the views of those who are believed to have a positive view of oneself (Rosenberg, 1979)	*Self-handicapping*: actively arrange circumstances for one's behavior so that, if poor performance occurs, those circumstances can be viewed as the cause rather than a lack of ability or worth (Jones and Berglas, 1978; Berglas, 1985)
Self-serving attributional bias: view self as responsible for successful outcomes and positive behaviors more so than failures and negative actions (Greenwald, 1980)	*Selectivity of standards*: tendency to set personal goals and aspirations for the self that are believed to be within the potential range of one's accomplishments (Rosenberg, 1982)	*Active downward comparison*: derogate others for the purpose of facilitating favorable social comparison (Wills, 1987)
Self-affirmation processes: when perceived integrity or adequacy of the self is threatened, respond with explanation, rationalization, and/or action until positive self-regard is restored (Steele, 1988; see also Aronson et al., 1999)	*Downward comparison*: choose who are less capable or less well-off as standards against which to evaluate oneself (Wills, 1987)	*Situational selectivity*: tendency to seek out environments in which one is likely to be successful and avoid those for which this is not the case (Rosenberg, 1982)
Selective imputation: infer that others view oneself more positively than is actually the case (Wylie, 1979)	*Self-evaluation maintenance*: selectively identify or associate with successful, high-prestige individuals and groups and/or dissociate oneself from relatively unsuccessful, lower-prestige individuals or groups (Tesser and Campbell, 1983)	*Responses to self-devaluing experiences*: cope with self-devaluing experiences by engaging in patterns of avoidance/withdrawal, attacking perceived source of self-rejection, and/or substituting behavior patterns with greater potential for self-enhancement (Kaplan, 1980; see also Baumeister et al., 1996)
Terminological selectivity: apply adjectival terms to self that cast oneself in a positive light (Rosenberg, 1979)	*Defenses*: psychodynamic defense mechanisms used to protect self-esteem (Allport, 1961)	*Efforts to influence conscious awareness*: seek to enhance or protect self-esteem through actions (e.g., meditation, drug use) that increase conscious awareness of positive qualities and/or decrease awareness of personal deficiencies (Baumeister and Boden, 1994; Campbell, 1984)

Note: Several of the self-protective–self-enhancing strategies that are described could be classified into more than one of the indicated categories. Thus, the classifications that are reflected in the table are in some cases somewhat arbitrary.
Source: Adapted from DuBois (2001).

Swann, 1997). Interestingly, there is also research indicating that positive events experienced by persons with low self-esteem can prove threatening to their identity and, as a result, can be stressful for them and even impinge negatively on their health (Brown, 1993a). Moreover, when self-enhancing strategies are engaged in by low-self-esteem individuals, there is no assurance that these will be successful in fostering a more favorable sense of self-regard (Blaine and Crocker, 1993; Brown, 1993a). It will be recalled, for example, that efforts to discount the importance attached to less positive aspects of one's self-concept appear to represent a strategy of only limited effectiveness for maintaining a high level of self-esteem (Marsh and Hattie, 1996). Similar qualifications apply to other self-protective strategies that are depicted in Table 9.1. Illustratively, several strategies involve engaging in negative patterns of interpersonal behavior (e.g., derogating others). Clearly, the consequences of these types of action may be to evoke responses from others that do more to hinder than promote feelings of self-worth (Tennen and Affleck, 1993).

Individuals with high self-esteem

The adaptive implications of the strategies that individuals with high self-esteem engage in to help maintain a positive sense of worth have also received attention in recent research (Harter, 1998). As proposed by Taylor and Brown (1988, 1994), even positive views of the self that are illusory or biased may facilitate enhancements in mood, promote adaptive social behavior (e.g., helping others), and support the use of efficient problem-solving strategies. Self-enhancing responses, furthermore, apparently can be helpful in coping with stressful life events, such as parental divorce (Mazur et al., 1999) and sexual victimization (Taylor and Brown, 1988).

Interestingly, however, there is also increasing evidence linking the use of self-enhancing strategies with poorer mental health and problems in adaptation (Tennen and Affleck, 1993; Colvin and Block, 1994; Harter, 1998). Numerous studies, for example, report less favorable adjustment for individuals who harbor inflated or unrealistically positive views of themselves. Biases of this nature have been implicated in negative patterns of emotional and behavioral functioning both when assessed directly as narcissistic tendencies (Bushman and Baumeister, 1998) and when identified through comparisons against various external criteria such as objective assessments of ability, the views of others who know the person well, or the judgments of experienced mental health professionals (Harter, 1986; Connell and Ilardi, 1987; Shedler et al., 1993; Colvin et al., 1995; Hughes et al., 1997; DuBois et al., 1998). In accordance with these findings, theorists have noted a variety of liabilities that may be associated with positive illusions in self-perceptions, including vulnerability to disconfirmation from others, the pressure of living up to an inflated self-image, limitations in self-understanding, and overconfidence leading to interpersonal difficulties (Blaine and Crocker, 1993; Brown, 1993a; Tennen and

Affleck, 1993; Colvin and Block, 1994; Harter, 1998). Positive illusions about the self may be especially likely to prove problematic when they are extreme (Baumeister, 1989) or when self-protective processes used to support these types of views involve maladaptive behaviors such as aggression or drug use (Kaplan, 1986; Baumeister et al., 1996).

There has been related discussion within the cognitive therapy literature of how cognitive, behavioral, and affective processes may contribute to the formation and maintenance of maladaptive schemata (McGinn and Young, 1996; Young and Gluhoski, 1997; Young and Flanagan, 1998; Young, 1999). Motivational processes within the self-system (i.e., desires for self-consistency and self-esteem) may play a role specifically in the development and maintenance of maladaptive schemata about the self (e.g., dependence/incompetence or entitlement/grandiosity). Research on self-motives in nonclinical populations thus may prove useful in suggesting ways in which self-schemata function in the etiology of different types of disorder (Tennen and Affleck, 1993).

Self-Esteem

For the most part, the self-esteem literature has focused on relatively global and undifferentiated feelings of self-regard as reported directly by the individual from a trait-oriented perspective (Harter, 1998). An important development in recent years, however, has been increased attention to multiple, distinct facets of self-esteem (Byrne, 1996; Harter, 1998, 1999). As can be seen in Table 9.2, these include several aspects of self-evaluation that have not been reflected in prevailing approaches to conceptualizing and assessing self-esteem. Traditional measures (e.g., Rosenberg Self-Esteem Scale) assess overall, trait-oriented aspects of self-evaluation that are explicit and experienced (i.e., those that are consciously accessible and willing to be reported by the individual). They fail, however, to yield information concerning numerous other proposed facets of the construct (e.g., content-specific self-evaluations, separate positive and negative dimensions, short-term stability, feelings about the self that are conveyed implicitly through behavior or conscious awareness, and "true", internally based versus "contingent", externally based feelings of worth).

Studies using statistical procedures such as confirmatory factor analysis and multitrait–multimethod analyses have provided psychometric support for the distinctiveness of multiple facets of self-esteem. As important, however, is a growing body of research in which measures of distinct facets of self-esteem have been found to exhibit theoretically interpretable patterns of association with criterion measures. Results of numerous studies, for example, point toward the adaptive significance of multiple, distinct facets of self-esteem for children and adolescents

Table 9.2 Overview of multiple facets of self-esteem

Facet	Description
Content-specific dimensions (Bracken, 1996; Byrne, 1996; DuBois et al., 1996; Harter, 1998, Harter et al., 1998)	Self-evaluations reflecting feelings about the self in relation to specific roles or contexts (e.g., family) as well as other salient domains of experience (e.g., physical appearance)
Positive and negative dimensions (Brown et al., 1990; Owens, 1994)	Positive: favorable evaluations of the self and feelings of pride Negative: dissatisfaction with the self and feelings of self-derogation/self-depreciation
Experienced and presented (Demo, 1985; Harter, 1999)	Experienced: self as evaluated and reported on by the individual Presented: evaluations of self revealed to others through verbal and nonverbal behavior in social contexts
Trait and stability (Rosenberg, 1985; Kernis, 1993; Roberts and Monroe, 1994)	Trait: individual's characteristic level of self-esteem as it is reflected across time and situations Stability: degree of short-term fluctuation or volatility in feelings of self-worth
Explicit and implicit (Greenwald and Banaji, 1995)	Explicit: aspects of self-evaluation accessible to conscious awareness Implicit: aspects of self-evaluation that are not accessible to conscious awareness
True and contingent (Deci and Ryan, 1995)	True: derived primarily from autonomous actions that involve self-determination based upon internal standards Contingent: based primarily on impression management and living up to externally imposed evaluation criteria

(for reviews, see Harter, 1998, 1999; DuBois and Tevendale, 1999). Cumulatively, these findings indicate that it is not sufficient simply to know that a youth reports feelings good about himself or herself overall as a person (Harter, 1999). Equally important may be whether the child feels satisfied with himself or herself in specific areas such as school, peer relations, and physical appearance, harbors feelings of self-pride (as opposed to merely an absence of feelings of self-dislike), is able to remain in a more or less consistent state of high self-esteem, conveys feelings of self-worth outwardly through behavior, is guided more by "true" self desires rather than the opinions of others, and is free of any feelings of inferiority or self-doubt possibly existing outside personal awareness (DuBois and Tevendale, 1999). Similar results have been obtained in studies conducted with adults. In prospective studies of adult women that assessed positive and negative self-esteem separately, for example, negative self-evaluative tendencies (e.g., feelings of self-derogation), but not the relative absence of positive self-evaluation (e.g., feelings of pride), were indicated to increase risk for depression (Ingham et al., 1987; Brown et al., 1990a). In further analyses, however, high levels of positive self-evaluation were found to protect against the onset of depression in the presence of environmental and psychological risk factors (including high levels of negative self-evaluation) and to facilitate recovery from episodes of both anxiety and depression (Miller et al., 1987; Brown et al., 1990b, 1990c). In other research focusing on self-esteem stability, greater day-to-day fluctuation in feelings of self-worth has been found to be predictive of depression and anger-hostility (Kernis, 1993; Roberts and Monroe, 1994; Baumeister et al., 1996). Scores on indices of self-esteem stability have also been found to interact with more traditional, trait-oriented ratings of self-esteem in the prediction of outcomes (Kernis, 1993). These findings suggest that negative implications of unstable feelings of self-worth are most prominent when found in conjunction with high reported levels of trait self-esteem. At relatively low levels of self-esteem, lack of stability instead may be indicative of adaptive efforts to overcome or interrupt relatively continuous negative self-evaluations (Kernis, 1993).

Recent studies examining multiple, distinct facets of self-esteem have been instrumental in developing a more complex and differentiated understanding of the construct. This work indicates that it may be important to consider the contributions of several different aspects of self-esteem in the etiology and course of different forms of psychopathology. As applied to cognitive therapy, these findings provide a promising basis for a greater understanding of the role of self-referential thoughts, beliefs, and feelings in treatment.

Self in context

A further important theme in recent literature is the need to understand the self in context. Major lines of inquiry in this area center on the role of self as a mediator and a moderator of the effects of environmental events, and on the "degree of fit" between self processes and features of the person's environment.

Self as mediator of contextual influences

Cognitive theories of psychopathology are, at their heart, mediational. They typically take the form of diathesis-stress models and assume an important mediational role for self processes in pathways linking negative environmental events with the emergence of emotional disorders. In a corresponding manner, conceptual frameworks for understanding resilience emphasize the development of self-resources as a means of accounting for the protective effects of favorable life experiences among individuals from high-risk backgrounds (Rutter, 1987; Werner, 1995). Support for views emphasizing a mediational role of self processes has been found in investigations of children and adolescents (Harter, 1998, 1999; DuBois and Tevendale, 1999) as well as college student and adult samples (Ozer, 1995; Waldo et al., 1998). Low feelings of self-worth, for example, appear to mediate the relationship between lack of support from parents and peers and feelings of depression and suicidal ideation among adolescents (Harter, 1999). Likewise, among individuals growing up in high-risk environments, ratings of self-esteem have been found to predict overall quality of adaptation during adulthood (Werner and Smith, 1992).

Self as moderator of environmental risk

A number of studies completed during recent years also implicate self processes as moderators of adjustment in response to stressful life events (Rutter, 1987; Luthar and Zigler, 1991; Hammen, 1992; Werner and Smith, 1992). Feelings of self-worth and perceived self-efficacy can function as protective factors for individuals experiencing stress (Rutter, 1987; Werner, 1995). Conversely, the relative absence of these self-resources appears to intensify vulnerability to emergence of disorder (Kaplan et al., 1983; Miller et al., 1989; Hammen, 1992; Jex and Elacqua, 1999). Higher-order patterns of interaction have also been found. These suggest that the role of self-resources in moderating responses to stressful life events is especially prominent in the context of other manifestations of individual vulnerability or environmental risk, such as negative attributional style (Metalsky et al., 1993; Robinson et al., 1995) or lack of social support (C. A. D'Anna et al., unpublished data).

Of further note are studies indicating that particular types of environmental stress may interact with congruent or matching forms of cognitive vulnerability in placing individuals at risk for emotional distress. Research in this area has been based on predictions by Beck (1983) and Blatt (1995) that excessive concerns about social relatedness (i.e., sociotropy, dependency) and autonomous achievement create vulnerability to depression in response to negative interpersonal and achievement-oriented events, respectively (for reviews, see Robins, 1995; Ingram et al., 1998; Clark et al., 1999). There is also evidence that other forms of matching may be important, such as when stressors and vulnerabilities in self processes both manifest themselves in a particular context of the individual's life (e.g., school; see Metalsky et al., 1993).

Person–environment fit

A related concern receiving attention is the degree of fit or accommodation that is evident between self processes and the individual's environment (Harter, 1998). It appears, for example, that approaches used to acquire and sustain self-esteem may prove adaptive or maladaptive, in part, depending on the adequacy of their fit with relevant features of the person's environment (DuBois and Tevendale, 1999). This perspective provides a plausible framework for interpreting several trends observed in the literature and that has addressed the adaptive implications of self-protective and self-enhancing strategies (D. L. DuBois, unpublished data). These include the tendency for individuals to exhibit problems in adjustment when they hold views of themselves that are unrealistically inflated relative to how they are perceived by others (Harter, 1998).

At the same time, recent research also highlights maladaptive patterns of "over-conforming" to environmental demands in self processes (DuBois and Tevendale, 1999). These include false self behavior (i.e., a tendency to act in ways that do not reflect one's true self; Harter, 1998) as well as the development of externally derived, "contingent" rather than autonomously derived, "true" self-esteem (Deci and Ryan, 1995). It has been found that among adolescents (Harter, 1998), for example, engaging in relatively high levels of false self behavior is predictive of significantly poorer psychological adjustment (e.g., depression).

Overall, recent work reveals dynamic and complex patterns of interrelationship between self and context in processes influencing adaptation and risk for disorder. We now turn to consideration of how these and other areas of self literature can be applied to cognitive therapy.

Applications to cognitive therapy

Recent developments in self theory and research have important implications for both assessment and intervention in cognitive therapy. Within each area, these pertain to the conceptual orientation or focus of the approaches used as well as practical strategies for implementation.

Assessment
Conceptual orientation

One important theme that emerges from the literature is the complex, multifaceted, and interdependent nature of characteristics and processes that comprise the self (Harter, 1998). The self, in short, is not a unitary, stable trait or set of perceptions. Clinically, this suggests a need for approaches to assessment that are broad and process-focused, rather than narrow and static. Components and processes of the self meriting consideration include: (1) multidimensional facets of self-concept at varying levels of specificity and breadth; (2) patterns of values and standards that may be involved in shaping self-beliefs and guiding goal-directed behavior; (3) general as well as situation-specific self-efficacy beliefs; (4) strategies relied on to satisfy motivation for a sense of self-worth and self-consistency; and (5) multiple, distinct facets of self-esteem.

We recommend that assessment in these areas be tailored to the needs of individual patients. Decisions in this regard should be informed by an understanding of the specific self components and processes likely to play a role in the patient's distress, taking into account also the patient's developmental level, demographic variables, and nature and severity of the presenting problems. Consider, for example, an adolescent girl referred for a possible eating disorder. In addition to assessing dimensions of self-concept with established relevance for adolescents (Harter, 1988), several additional targets for assessment would be suggested by the gender and presenting concerns of this patient. These might include issues relating to false self behavior or "contingent" self-esteem commonly observed among adolescent girls (Harter, 1999). It also would be important to assess her personal standards for performance and appearance, as stringent or perfectionistic standards have been implicated in risk for eating disorders (Striegal-Moore et al., 1990). By contrast, the assessment of self processes in an adult male with antisocial tendencies would direct our attention to a differing set of facets of the self-concept (Messer and Harter, 1986). We also might wish to assess deficits in perceived self-efficacy for controlling anger in specific situations as well as outcome expectancies doing so (Bandura, 1997).

There is also a need to consider social and environmental concerns and their relationship to self-oriented assessment data. These include: (1) the extent to which the individual's current life circumstances provide adaptive opportunities for achieving and maintaining a positive sense of self-regard (i.e., competence-building/success experiences and acceptance/validation in relationships with significant others); (2) exposure to stressful life and the availability of social support, including potential interactions with relevant resources and liabilities in self processes; and (3) the degree to which features of the individual's life "fit" with strategies used to acquire and sustain self-esteem and provide sufficient flexibility to accommodate expression of individuality and autonomy.

Instruments and strategies

A range of instruments and strategies have been developed for assessing components and processes within the self-system and associated contextual experiences (a list of these instruments is available from the first author upon request). In several instances, separate forms are available for use with different age groups. Harter and colleagues, for example, have developed a widely used series of age-specific, multidimensional measures of self-concept (Harter, 1999). An emphasis on developmentally sensitive assessment strategies is well-supported by research that has identified age-related shifts in self-structure and processes (Harter, 1999) as well as in pertinent areas of contextual experience (Compas, 1987). Attention has also been given to use of idiographic measures for obtaining information concerning personal goals (Sheldon and Kasser, 1998) and self-efficacy beliefs (Bandura, 1997). These procedures are well-suited to the individualized, phenomenological approach to assessment used in cognitive therapy. A final important feature of assessment strategies used in the self literature is an emerging emphasis on incorporating data from multiple informants, methods, and occasions of measurement. Examples include obtaining ratings from significant others to gauge accuracy of self views (Hughes et al., 1997), use of laboratory tasks to tap into aspects of the self not readily assessed with traditional, paper-and-pencil instruments (e.g., implicit self-esteem; Spalding and Hardin, 1999), and collection of repeated, daily ratings to assess self-esteem stability (Kernis, 1993). This use of multiple informants and methods is quite consistent with cognitive-behavioral assessment practices.

Instruments and strategies already used in cognitive therapy represent a further resource for gathering self-oriented assessment data. These include structured self-report questionnaires, such as the Schema Questionnaire (Young, 1999). Subscale scores on this instrument are well suited to assessing self-related concerns in the areas of self-esteem (e.g., defectiveness/unlovability), perceived self-efficacy (e.g., dependence/incompetence), overly stringent standards for self-evaluation (e.g., unrelenting standards/hypercriticalness), and inflated views of self (e.g., entitlement/grandiosity). Open-ended assessment procedures used in cognitive therapy (e.g., dysfunctional thought record) also may be useful, especially if the data obtained are reviewed with respect to specific areas of concern from a self perspective. Other techniques (e.g., mood monitoring) could readily be modified to allow for direct assessment of self constructs and processes (e.g., self-esteem stability). In pursuing self-oriented assessment with traditional cognitive-behavioral measures and strategies, however, it should be kept in mind that these may not provide either the breadth or refinement of coverage possible with more specialized instruments and procedures available in the self literature.

Intervention

Treatment planning

Similar to assessment, we recommend that treatment planning in cognitive therapy be guided by a consideration of the patient's unique configuration of self components and processes and their relation to presenting problems. Along with remediating weaknesses or deficits in the self that may be contributing to the patient's difficulties, attention should also be given to the development of self-resources that are likely to increase the patient's resilience and overall mental health. For a patient experiencing depression, for example, treatment might entail efforts to bolster specific areas of deficit in self-concept contributing to the individual's sense of dysphoria. Rigid and perfectionistic self-standards might be addressed as well, as might a tendency to overvalue external standards. In pursuing these avenues, the goal could be not only to mitigate feelings of self-derogation (i.e., negative self-esteem), but also to instill a greater sense of pride in self (i.e., positive self-esteem).

As this illustration suggests, it may be necessary to address multiple facets or domains of the self to achieve desired results. Accordingly, when developing a treatment plan, it may be useful, for example, to consider the full, multidimensional, hierarchical structure of the self-concept as well as the multifaceted array of cognitive, behavioral, and affective strategies that have been implicated in motivational processes relating to self-esteem (see Table 9.1). It is worth keeping in mind as well that the self system is just that – a system (Harter, 1998). The degree to which changes in any given area facilitate clinical improvement thus may be influenced by interdependencies across different types of self components and processes. Without addressing personal standards and values, for example, modifications in one or more facets of the self-concept may not translate into desired changes in self-evaluations (i.e., increased satisfaction with those facets) and therefore not be fully effective for improving overall patient feelings of self-worth (i.e., self-esteem) and mood.

In planning self-oriented interventions, the circumstances of the individual's life should also receive careful consideration. This may help, for example, to direct interventions toward self components or processes likely to be of value in protecting the individual from adverse effects of stressful life events. A contextually informed understanding of self processes, furthermore, serves to highlight opportunities to pursue direct change in external conditions. Attempts might be made, for example, to provide experiences that strengthen efficacy beliefs, to increase levels of self-esteem enhancing social support, or to limit the patient's exposure to social and environmental stressors.

Strategies

Cognitive therapy emphasizes patient education, collaborative empiricism, and the assumption that individuals are active interpreters rather than passive recipients of their life experiences (Freeman et al., 1990). Each of these principles is congruent with research on self processes and with efforts to include change in self-beliefs as an explicit focus of treatment. Although many self-related terms (e.g., self-esteem) are familiar to patients, their level of understanding may be insufficient to facilitate effective participation in interventions focused on these areas. It is not uncommon, for example, for terms such as self-concept, self-esteem, and self-efficacy to be used interchangeably in everyday language. Other terms and concepts, such as false self behavior and the idea of motivational strivings for self-consistency and self-esteem, may be unfamiliar to many clients. For these reasons, patient education may be valuable as a means of ensuring that clients understand both structural and process-oriented aspects of the self that will be addressed during therapy. Moreover, individuals tend to believe that beliefs about the self are based on information that is accessible to them and, by contrast, relatively unavailable to others. Self-referential cognitions thus may be among those least amenable to direct disputation by therapists. As a result, it is essential to adopt an attitude of collaborative empiricism and to work together to explore and test the validity of relevant thoughts, beliefs, and assumptions. As noted, cognitive models of psychopathology assume that patients are active interpreters of their experiences. We recognize, then, that interpretive processes may reflect a predisposition toward certain end-states (e.g., schema maintenance; Young, 1999). In accordance with this understanding, when pursuing self-oriented interventions in cognitive therapy specific attention should be given to patients' motivational tendencies toward maintaining both favorable feelings about themselves and consistency in their self views. Useful interventions might include identification of cognitive biases associated with these motivational tendencies and their implications for patients' behaviors and beliefs about themselves.

Standard cognitive interventions (Freeman et al., 1990; Beck, 1995; Young, 1999) are well-suited for addressing self-oriented treatment goals. These include procedures used commonly within sessions to help modify problematic beliefs and reduce cognitive biases, such as techniques for rational restructuring, as well as those used outside treatment, such as self-monitoring and behavioral experiments. Cognitive therapy techniques for challenging automatic thoughts, beliefs, and underlying assumptions could be useful, for example, in attempts to address deficits that are evident within a patient's multidimensional and hierarchically structured self-concept. A range of cognitive procedures could be useful in this regard for modifying beliefs across differing domains and levels of specificity within the patient's self-concept, thereby helping to ensure effective and integrated change in lower-level automatic thoughts, intermediate beliefs, and higher-level core beliefs/schemata.

To produce optimal results, however, it may be necessary to tailor standard cognitive therapy techniques to accommodate empirical findings on the self. The application of rational restructuring procedures to self-referential cognitions, for example, has been limited primarily to modification of beliefs or assumptions that reflect negatively on the client or patient. As we have seen, however, unrealistically inflated views of the self may also represent important targets for change for some clients. As a further illustration, there is reason to expect that it could prove useful to expand standard techniques for reducing cognitive biases to address information-processing tendencies that serve specific functions within the self-system, such as self-protection and self-enhancement (Table 9.1). A unique challenge introduced by adaptations in this area could be the need to find ways to encourage, rather than reduce, reliance on several types of biases (e.g., self-enhancing tendencies), given their potential to serve beneficial functions such as promoting self-esteem and moderating the effects of stressful life events (Taylor and Brown, 1988, 1994). A related concern is the possible need to address resistance of self-referential cognitions to change as a result of motivational processes in the self (e.g., desire for self-consistency). Even powerful, experientially oriented approaches (e.g., behavior experiments) may not be effective unless care is taken to identify obstacles, such as actions the patient might engage in to ensure an outcome in agreement with current self views (Swann, 1997).

Although the strategies described seem promising, they may not be sufficient for achieving treatment goals. Noteworthy characteristics of prevailing models and approaches for conducting cognitive therapy in this regard include: (1) limited attention to modification of certain types of self components and processes that have been associated with psychopathology; and (2) a relative lack of emphasis on environmentally oriented change strategies. Treatment implications and strategies discussed within the self literature may be a valuable resource for addressing concerns in each of these areas (Pope, et al., 1988; Archer, 1994; Brinthaupt and Lipka, 1994; Bednar and Petersen, 1995; Bracken, 1996; Harter, 1999). This literature addresses, for example, techniques that may be helpful for reducing overly stringent standards in self-evaluation and others that may be effective for shifting preoccupation within the self on the expectations and opinions of others to more internally derived goals and perceptions. Contextually, considerable attention has been given to the steps that may be needed to ensure that adaptive sources of self-esteem are available in the patient's environment (Harter, 1999). These include opportunities for acquiring skills and for receiving support and validation from significant others (DuBois, 2001).

Case illustration

The preceding sections provide an overview of how assessment and intervention strategies relating to the self can be incorporated into cognitive therapy. This will now be illustrated through a case example:

Tammy, a 15-year-old Caucasian female, was referred for outpatient therapy due to concerns regarding both behavioral problems (e.g., substance use) and emotional difficulties (e.g., sadness, suicidal ideation) she had begun to exhibit following her parents' divorce. Additional stressors in her life included socioeconomic disadvantage (e.g., low-income neighborhood) as well as academic difficulties that had led her to fail the preceding school year. Moreover, it recently had been determined that Tammy was pregnant and, on this basis her mother had made a decision not to enroll her in school for the current year. Diagnostically, Tammy met DSM-IV criteria for major depressive disorder (American Psychiatric Association, 1994).

Standard cognitive therapy approaches served as a primary focus in assessment and treatment for this case. Innovations consistent with recent self theory and research also received attention.

Assessment

An initial assessment was conducted using both standard methods (e.g., semistructured interviews with the patient and her parents) and procedures specific to cognitive therapy (e.g., monitoring of automatic thoughts). The results provided a wealth of information regarding the possible role of self beliefs and processes in Tammy's presenting problems. This included evidence of overall feelings of low self-worth and inferiority (e.g., "Everything is my fault"). Several factors were identified as contributing to Tammy's low self-esteem. In particular, Tammy's self-concept, when considered from a multidimensional perspective, was found be characterized by a relatively pervasive pattern of negative appraisals across nearly all major domains of her life. These deficits were most severe with respect to family and school. Tammy apparently had begun to devalue in importance of each of these domains as a self-protective strategy. Although her views of her relationships with peers were in many respects positive, these had become a nearly exclusive source of self-esteem for Tammy. This pattern clearly did not constitute an ideal fit with the adaptive demands she was experiencing (e.g., school) or those that she would encounter in the near future (e.g., parenting).

Further assessment revealed that Tammy was closely attached to her mother. This source of approval and support was highly conditional, however, on Tammy's ability to meet excessive and inappropriate expectations that had been established for her in this relationship (e.g., assuming a parental role as a result of psychiatric problems that her mother was experiencing). Tammy also expressed a strong sense of having been abandoned by her father who was not currently involved in her life (e.g., "He took some lady over me"). Juxtaposed against Tammy's focus on interpersonal relations (i.e., family, peers), furthermore, was evidence that she was lacking in both internalized, personally meaningful goals for herself and a sense of individual efficacy (e.g., "Nothing I do is ever right"). The preceding observations suggest several specific concerns pertaining to self components and processes. These include conditions limiting Tammy's potential for personal growth and development, a maladaptive, "contingent" foundation for her feelings of self-worth, and heightened sensitivity to interpersonal rejection or loss.

Instruments and strategies discussed previously that focus specifically on self issues and processes could have been used to advantage as well with this patient. Many of these measures have well-established psychometric properties and produce norm-based scores. As a result, they could provide a stronger basis for conclusions about self-related concerns than the less structured approaches described here.

Most importantly, they would offer the potential for greater depth and refinement in conceptualizing the role of self components and processes (e.g., self-esteem) that are relevant for this youth. This would include, for example, information about several issues pertaining to the self (e.g., separate positive and negative dimensions of self-evaluation) that have been implicated specifically in depressive symptomatology.

Treatment

Based on the preceding case conceptualization, a treatment plan with two major objectives was developed. The first objective was to increase Tammy's opportunities for deriving self-esteem from adaptive and developmentally normative sources (i.e., both competence-building/success experiences and acceptance and validation from significant others). The fact that she was not enrolled in school was a major concern in this regard. This was not only because of the importance of acquiring academic skills, but also because of opportunities that school would provide for establishing supportive ties with teachers and other adults and for becoming involved in age-appropriate extracurricular activities. Because of the special considerations posed by Tammy's pregnancy and recent history of academic failure, arrangements were made to enroll her in an alternative high school that was suited to addressing her needs in these areas.

Further efforts focused on increasing the level of support and validation that Tammy received from her parents through conjoint parent–adolescent therapy. The goals of this aspect of treatment were twofold: to address the tendency for approval and acceptance from her mother to be conditional on Tammy's ability to meet inappropriate expectations in their relationship and to promote more frequent contact with her father. To assist Tammy in developing basic parenting skills, and to provide her with additional sources of support, a referral was made to an education and support group for pregnant teens. The host agency also made an older volunteer mentor available to her, thus providing for the possibility of encouragement and guidance from a special outside adult as a means of esteem-enhancement (Harter, 1999).

The foregoing strategies are consistent with social-contextual approaches to intervention recommended in the self literature. The second major objective of treatment was directly to enhance relevant resources and processes within Tammy's self-system. In doing so, the aim was to foster not only improved self-esteem, but also a sense of self-regard that was based on a stronger, internal foundation (i.e., "true" rather than "contingent" self-esteem; Deci and Ryan, 1995). Standard cognitive therapy techniques were used to modify maladaptive beliefs Tammy expressed about herself. They were also used to address biases (e.g., overgeneralization) that were prominent in her processing of self-relevant information. Strategies for rational responding to automatic thoughts proved useful, for example, in addressing Tammy's doubts concerning her self-sufficiency and efficacy.

Several additional strategies for enhancing self resources and processes derived primarily from the self literature were helpful in developing a more comprehensive treatment approach. These included efforts to promote Tammy's efficacy beliefs for situations and domains with specific relevance for her, such as reentry into school, effective self-care during pregnancy, and assertion of her own needs in interactions with others (e.g., mother). In accordance with the demonstrated role of positive facets of self-esteem in recovery from depressive episodes (Miller et al., 1987; Brown et al., 1990b), further efforts were directed toward fostering Tammy's recognition of her personal strengths and feelings of pride about herself. This objective was pursued, in part, using empirically validated esteem-enhancement strategies for children and adolescents (Haney and Durlak, 1998). Treatment also drew upon intervention strategies to promote identity exploration and development among adolescents (Archer, 1994). These were an important avenue for helping Tammy to clarify her personal values, interests, and goals for the future, thus helping to guard against "a loss of voice" detrimental to her mental health and overall development (Harter, 1999).

From a process-oriented perspective, Tammy was underutilizing self-protective and self-enhancing strategies that could be of help to her in maintaining a high level of self-esteem. Work with Tammy in this area included attributional retraining as a means of curbing her excessive tendencies toward self-blame (Merrell, 2001). She was also instructed in other strategies, such as meditation, to promote more positive forms of self-awareness (Baumeister and Boden, 1994). Along with the environmental intervention components noted earlier, these types of treatment efforts represent a focus on helping patients to establish productive means of acquiring and maintaining self-esteem. If successful, they can be expected to become self-reinforcing and thus sustained independent of treatment (DuBois, 2001).

Conclusions

Self-referential thought processes are an integral component of assessment and intervention in cognitive therapy. Perhaps no other major modality of psychotherapy currently reflects a stronger appreciation of contemporary understanding of the role of self in patterns of adaptation and disorder. Recent trends in theory and research concerning the self, however, are not fully reflected in prevailing models and frameworks for conducting cognitive therapy. Correspondingly, advances in the self literature have not benefited from rigorous examination of their applied utility within the context of treatment. Our discussion illustrates numerous avenues for integration of self-oriented issues into cognitive therapy that could have significant benefits for treatment outcomes.

At present, a comprehensive, theoretically and empirically informed framework is not available for integrating findings on self processes with cognitive theories of psychopathology and treatment. Several issues merit consideration in pursuing this goal. Assessment issues in need of attention include clarification of the degree of overlap between related instruments and concepts in the self and cognitive therapy literatures. This concern pertains to both constructs, such as self-concept and schemata, and processes, such as self-related motivation and cognitive biases. Given the fact that research on the self has been conducted primarily with normal (i.e., community-based) samples, there also needs to be investigation of the extent to which findings such as those described in this chapter generalize to clinical populations. This should include studies of the effects of self variables on risk for disorder both independent of and in interaction with other markers of cognitive and social vulnerability.

Questions might also be raised with regard to treatment outcome and the processes of change in cognitive therapy. Are, for example, changes in self-beliefs associated with more rapid, significant, or stable changes in mood? Might standard cognitive therapy protocols be enhanced by including intervention strategies designed to address self-beliefs and processes that are associated with psychopathology? Investigation of these types of concerns will be necessary to establish empirically informed guidelines for integration of self-oriented interventions into cognitive therapy. An additional goal should be to explore the importance of matching degree and type of emphasis on self issues in treatment to the needs of individual clients. The significance of the self in positive mental health, furthermore, indicates that applications should not be limited solely to the remediation of clinical disorders in treatment. Rather, these concepts may also prove useful in developing programs for preventing mental health problems and for facilitating growth and positive adaptation.

Acknowledgment

The writing of this chapter was supported in part by a grant to the first author from the National Institute of Mental Health (DHHS 5 R29 MH55050).

REFERENCES

Allport, G. W. (1961). *Pattern and Growth in Personality*. New York: Holt, Rinehart and Winston.
American Psychiatric Association (1994). *Diagnostic and Statistical Manual of Mental Disorders* 4th edn. Washington, DC: American Psychiatric Association.
Archer, S. L. (ed.) (1994). *Interventions for Adolescent Identity Development*. Thousand Oaks, CA: Sage.

Aronson, J., Cohen, G., and Nail, P. R. (1999). Self-affirmation theory: an update and appraisal. In *Cognitive Dissonance: Progress on a Pivotal Theory in Social Psychology*, ed. E. Harmon-Jones and J. Mills, pp. 127–47. Washington, DC: American Psychological Association.

Attie, I. and Brooks-Gunn, J. (1989). Development of eating problems in adolescent girls: a longitudinal study. *Developmental Psychology*, **25**, 70–9.

Bandura, A. (1997). *Self-efficacy: The Exercise of Control*. New York: W. H. Freeman.

Barrera, M. (1981). Social support in the adjustment of pregnant adolescents: assessment issues. In *Social Networks and Social Support*, ed. B. H. Gottlieb, pp. 69–96. Beverly Hills: Sage.

Baumeister, R. F. (1989). The optimal margin of illusion. *Journal of Social and Clinical Psychology*, **8**, 176–89.

Baumeister, R. F. and Boden, J. M. (1994). Shrinking the self. In *Changing the Self: Philosophies, Techniques, and Experiences*, ed. T. M. Brinthaupt and R. P. Lipka, pp. 143–73. Albany: State University of New York Press.

Baumeister, R. F., Smart, L., and Boden, J. M. (1996). Relation of threatened egotism to violence and aggression: the dark side of high self-esteem. *Psychological Review*, **103**, 5–33.

Beck, A. T. (1976). *Cognitive Therapy and the Emotional Disorders*. New York: International Universities Press.

Beck, A. T. (1983). Cognitive therapy of depression: new perspectives. In *Treatment of Depression: Old Controversies and New Approaches*, ed. P. J. Clayton and J. E. Barrett, pp. 265–90. New York: Raven Press.

Beck, A. T. (1987). Cognitive models of depression. *Journal of Cognitive Psychotherapy*, **1**, 5–37.

Beck, J. S. (1995). *Cognitive therapy: Basics and Beyond*. New York: Guilford.

Beck, A. T. and Freeman, A. (1990). *Cognitive Therapy of Personality Disorders*. New York: Guilford.

Bednar, R. L. and Peterson, S. R. (1995). *Self-esteem: Paradoxes and Innovations in Clinical Theory and Practice*, 2nd edn. Washington, DC: American Psychological Association.

Berglas, S. (1985). Self-handicapping and self-handicappers: a cognitive/attributional model of interpersonal self-protective behavior. *Perspectives in Psychology*, **1**, 235–70.

Blaine, B. and Crocker, J. (1993). Self-esteem and self-serving biases in reactions to positive and negative events: an integrative review. In *Self-esteem: The Puzzle of Low Self-regard*, ed. R. F. Baumeister, pp. 55–85. New York: Plenum.

Blatt, S. J. (1995). Representational structures in psychopathology. In *Rochester Symposium on Developmental Psychopathology: Emotion, Cognition, and Representation*, vol. 6, ed. D. Cicchetti and S. Toth, pp. 1–34. Rochester, NY: University of Rochester Press.

Bracken, B. A. (1996). Clinical applications of a context-dependent multidimensional model of self-concept. In *Handbook of Self-concept*, ed. B. A. Bracken, pp. 463–503. New York: Wiley.

Brinthaupt, T. M. and Lipka, R. P. (eds) (1994). *Changing the Self: Philosophies, Techniques, and Experiences*. Albany: State University of New York Press.

Brown, J. D. (1993a). Motivational conflict and the self: the double-bind of low self-esteem. In *Self-esteem: The Puzzle of Low Self-regard*, ed. R. F. Baumeister, pp. 117–30. New York: Plenum.

Brown, J. D. (1993b). Self-esteem and self-evaluation: feeling is believing. In *Psychological Perspectives on the Self*, vol. 4, ed. J. Suls, pp. 27–58. Hillsdale, NJ: Erlbaum.

Brown, G. W., Bifulco, A., and Andrews, B. (1990a). Self-esteem and depression: III. Aetiological issues. *Social Psychiatry and Psychiatric Epidemiology*, 25, 235–43.

Brown, G. W., Bifulco, A., and Andrews, B. (1990b). Self-esteem and depression: IV. Effect on course and recovery. *Social Psychiatry and Psychiatric Epidemiology*, 25, 244–9.

Brown, G. W., Andrews, B., Bifulco, A., and Veiel, H. (1990c). Self-esteem and depression: I. Measurement issues and prediction of onset. *Social Psychiatry and Psychiatric Epidemiology*, 25, 200–9.

Bushman, B. J. and Baumeister, R. F. (1998). Threatened egotism, narcissism, self-esteem, and direct and displaced aggression: does self-love or self-hate lead to violence? *Journal of Personality and Social Psychology*, 75, 219–29.

Byrne, B. M. (1996). *Measuring Self-concept across the Life Span*. Washington, DC: American Psychological Association.

Cacioppo, J. T., von Hippel, W., and Ernst, J. M. (1997). Mapping cognitive structures and processes through verbal content: the thought-listing technique. *Journal of Consulting and Clinical Psychology*, 96, 179–83.

Campbell, R. N. (1984). *The New Science: Self-esteem Psychology*. Lanham, MD: University Press of America.

Clark, D. A., Beck, A. T., and Alford, B. A. (1999). *Scientific Foundations of Cognitive Theory and Therapy of Depression*. New York: Wiley.

Colvin, C. R. and Block, J. (1994). Do positive illusions foster mental health? An examination of the Taylor and Brown Formulation. *Psychological Bulletin*, 116, 3–20.

Colvin, C. R., Block, J., and Funder, D. C. (1995). Overly positive self-evaluations and personality: negative implications for mental health. *Journal of Personality and Social Psychology*, 68, 1152–62.

Compas, B. E. (1987). Stress and life events during childhood and adolescence. *Clinical Psychology Review*, 7, 275–302.

Compas, B. E., Davis, G. E., Forsythe, C. J., and Wagner, B. (1987). Assessment of major and daily stressful life events during adolescence: the Adolescent Perceived Events Scale. *Journal of Consulting and Clinical Psychology*, 55, 534–41.

Connell, J. P. and Ilardi, B. C. (1987). Self-system concomitants of discrepancies between children's and teachers' evaluations of academic competence. *Child Development*, 58, 1297–307.

Dattilio, F. D. and Reinecke, M. A. (1996). *Treating Children and Adolescents: A Cognitive-Developmental Approach*. New York: Guilford.

Deci, E., L. and Ryan, R. M. (1995). Human autonomy: the basis for true self-esteem. In *Efficacy, Agency, and Self-esteem*, ed. M. H. Kernis, pp. 31–46. New York: Plenum Press.

Demo, D. H. (1985). The measurement of self-esteem: refining our methods. *Journal of Personality and Social Psychology*, 48, 1490–502.

DiGiuseppe, R. (1989). Cognitive therapy with children. In *Comprehensive Handbook of Cognitive Therapy*, ed. A. Freeman, K. M. Simon, L. E. Beutler, and H. Arkowitz, pp. 515–33. New York: Plenum.

DuBois, D. L. and Tevendale, H. D. (1999). Self-esteem in childhood and adolescence: vaccine or epiphenomenon? *Applied and Preventive Psychology*, 8, 103–17.

DuBois, D. L., Felner, R. D., Brand, S., Phillips, R. S. C., and Lease, A. M. (1996). Early adolescent self-esteem: a developmental-ecological framework and assessment strategy. *Journal of Research on Adolescence*, **6**, 543–79.

DuBois, D. L., Bull, C. A., Sherman, M. D., and Roberts, M. (1998). Self-esteem and adjustment in early adolescence: a social-contextual perspective. *Journal of Youth and Adolescence*, **27**, 557–83.

DuBois, D. L., Tevendale, H. D., Burk-Braxton, C., Swenson, L. P., and Hardesty, J. L. (2000). Self-system influences during early adolescence: investigation of an integrative model. *Journal of Early Adolescence*, **20**, 12–43.

Elder, G. H. (1995). Life trajectories in changing societies. In *Self-efficacy in Changing Societies*, ed. A. Bandura, pp. 46–68. New York: Cambridge University Press.

Faunce, W. A. (1984). School achievement, social status, and self-esteem. *Social Psychology Quarterly*, **47**, 3–14.

Freeman, A., Pretzer, J., Fleming, B., and Simon, K. M. (1990). *Clinical Applications of Cognitive Therapy*. New York: Plenum.

Gergen, K. J. (1991). *The Saturated Self*. New York: Basic Books.

Greenwald, A. G. (1980). The totalitarian ego: fabrication and revision of personal history. *American Psychologist*, **35**, 603–18.

Greenwald, A. G. and Banaji, M. R. (1995). Implicit social cognition: attitudes, self-esteem, and stereotypes. *Psychological Review*, **102**, 4–27.

Guidano, V. F. and Liotti, G. (1985). A constructionist foundation for cognitive therapy. In *Cognition and Psychotherapy*, ed. M. J. Mahoney and A. E. Freeman, pp. 101–42. New York: Plenum.

Hackett, G. (1995). Self-efficacy in career choice and development. In *Self-efficacy in Changing Societies* ed. A. Bandura, pp. 232–58. New York: Cambridge University Press.

Hammen, C. (1992). Life events and depression: the plot thickens. *American Journal of Community Psychology*, **20**, 179–93.

Haney, P. and Durlak, J. A. (1998). Changing self-esteem in children and adolescents: a meta-analytic review. *Journal of Clinical Child Psychology*, **27**, 423–33.

Harré, R. (1998). *The Singular Self*. London: Sage.

Harter, S. (1986). Processes underlying the construction, maintenance and enhancement of the self-concept in children. In *Psychological Perspectives on the Self*, vol. 3, ed. J. Suls and A. Greenwald, pp. 137–81. Hillsdale, NJ: Erlbaum.

Harter, S. (1988). *Manual for the Self-Perception Profile for Adolescents*. Denver, CO: University of Denver.

Harter, S. (1990). Adolescent self and identity development. In *At the Threshold: The Developing Adolescent*, ed. S. S. Feldman and G. R. Eliot, pp. 352–87. Cambridge, MA: Harvard University Press.

Harter, S. (1998). The development of self-representations. In *Handbook of Child Psychology*, vol. 3. *Social, Emotional, and Personality Development*, 5th edn, ed. W. Damon, pp. 553–617. New York: Wiley.

Harter, S. (1999). *The Construction of the Self: A Developmental Perspective*. New York: Guilford.

Harter, S., Waters, P., and Whitesell, N. R. (1998). Relational self-worth: differences in perceived worth as a person across interpersonal contexts. *Child Development*, **69**, 756–66.

Hewitt, P. L., Newton, J., Flett, G. L., and Callander, L. (1997). Perfectionism and suicide ideation in adolescent psychiatric patients. *Journal of Abnormal Child Psychology*, **25**, 95–101.

Higgins, E. T. (1987). Self-discrepancy: a theory relating self and affect. *Psychological Review*, **94**, 319–40.

Hughes, J. N., Cavell, T. A., and Grossman, P. A. (1997). A positive view of self: risk or protection for aggressive children? *Development and Psychopathology*, **9**, 75–94.

Ingham, J. G., Kreitman, N. B., Miller, P. M., Sashidharan, S. P., and Surtees, P. G. (1987). Self-appraisal, anxiety and depression in women: a prospective inquiry. *British Journal of Psychiatry*, **151**, 643–51.

Ingram, R. E., Miranda, J., and Segal, Z. V. (1998). *Cognitive Vulnerability to Depression*. New York: Guilford.

Jex, S. M. and Elacqua, T. C. (1999). Self-esteem as a moderator: a comparison of global and organization-based measures. *Journal of Occupational and Organizational Psychology*, **72**, 71–81.

Jones, E. E. and Berglas, S. (1978). Control of attributions about the self through self-handicapping strategies: the appeal of alcohol and the role of underachievement. *Personality and Social Psychology Bulletin*, **4**, 200–6.

Kaplan, H. B. (1980). *Deviant Behavior in Defense of Self*. New York: Academic Press.

Kaplan, H. B. (1986). *Social Psychology of Self-referent Behavior*. New York: Plenum.

Kaplan, H. B., Robbins, C., and Martin, S. S. (1983). Antecedents of psychological distress in young adults: self-rejection, deprivation of social support, and life events. *Journal of Health and Social Behavior*, **24**, 230–44.

Kernis, M. H. (1993). The roles of stability and level of self-esteem in psychological functioning. In *Self-esteem: The Puzzle of Low Self-regard*, ed. R. Baumeister, pp. 167–82. New York: Plenum.

Linville, P. W. (1987). Self-complexity as a cognitive buffer against stress-related illness and depression. *Journal of Personality and Social Psychology*, **52**, 663–76.

Luthar, S. S. and Zigler, E. (1991). Vulnerability and competence: a review of research on resilience in childhood. *American Journal of Orthopsychiatry*, **61**, 6–22.

Marlatt, G. A., Baer, J. S., and Quigley, L. A. (1995). Self-efficacy and addictive behavior. In *Self-efficacy in Changing Societies*, ed. A. Bandura, pp. 289–315. New York: Cambridge University Press.

Marsh, H. W. (1999). Cognitive discrepancy models: actual, ideal, potential, and future self-perspectives of body image. *Social Cognition*, **17**, 46–75.

Marsh, H. W. and Hattie, J. (1996). Theoretical perspectives on the structure of the self-concept. In *Handbook of Self-concept*, ed. B. A. Bracken, pp. 38–90. New York: Wiley.

Marsh, H. W. and Yeung, A. S. (1997). Causal effects of academic self-concept on academic achievement: structural equation models of longitudinal data. *Journal of Educational Psychology*, **89**, 41–54.

Mazur, E., Wolchik, S. A., Virdin, L., Sandler, I., and West, S. (1999). Cognitive moderators of children's adjustment to stressful divorce events: the role of negative cognitive errors and positive illusions. *Child Development*, **70**, 231–45.

McCauley, E., Kendall, K., and Pavlidis, K. (1995). The development of emotional regulation and emotional response. In *The Depressed Child and Adolescent: Developmental and*

Clinical Perspectives, ed. I. Goodyer, pp. 53–80. Cambridge, England: Cambridge University Press.

McGinn, L. K. and Young, J. E. (1996). Schema-focused therapy. In *Frontiers of Cognitive Therapy*, ed. P. M. Salkovskis, pp. 182–207. New York: Guilford.

Merrell, K. W. (2001). *Helping Students Overcome Depression and Anxiety: A Practical Guide*. New York: Guilford.

Messer, B. and Harter, S. (1986). *Manual for the Adult Self-Perception Profile*. Denver, CO: University of Denver.

Metalsky, G. I., Joiner, T. E., Jr, Hardin, T. S., and Abramson, L. Y. (1993). Depressive reactions to failure in a naturalistic setting: a test of the hopelessness and self-esteem theories of depression. *Journal of Abnormal Psychology*, **102**, 101–9.

Miller, P. M., Ingham, J. G., Kreitman, N. B., Surtees, P. G., and Sashidharan, S. P. (1987). Life events and other factors implicated in onset and in remission of psychiatric illness in women. *Journal of Affective Disorders*, **12**, 73–88.

Miller, P. M., Kreitman, N. B., Ingham, J. G., and Sashidharan, S. P. (1989). Self-esteem, life stress and psychiatric disorder. *Journal of Affective Disorders*, **17**, 65–75.

Owens, T. J. (1994). Two dimensions of self-esteem: reciprocal effects of positive self-worth and self-depreciation on adolescent problems. *American Sociological Review*, **59**, 391–407.

Ozer, E. M. (1995). The impact of childcare responsibility and self-efficacy on the psychological health of professional working mothers. *Psychology of Women Quarterly*, **19**, 315–35.

Pelham, B. W. and Swann, W. B., Jr (1989). From self-conceptions to self-worth: on the sources and structure of global self-esteem. *Journal of Personality and Social Psychology*, **57**, 672–80.

Pope, A. W., McHale, S., and Craighead, W. E. (1988). *Self-esteem Enhancement with Children and Adolescents*. New York: Pergamon.

Roberts, J. E. and Monroe, S. M. (1994). A multidimensional model of self-esteem in depression. *Clinical Psychology Review*, **14**, 161–81.

Robins, C. J. (1995). Personality–event interaction models of depression. *European Journal of Personality*, **9**, 367–78.

Robinson, N. S., Garber, J., and Hilsman, R. (1995). Cognitions and stress: direct and moderating effects on depressive versus externalizing symptoms during the junior high school transition. *Journal of Abnormal Psychology*, **104**, 453–63.

Rosenberg, M. (1979). *Conceiving the Self*. New York: Basic Books.

Rosenberg, M. (1982). Psychological selectivity in self-esteem formation. In *Social Psychology of the Self-concept*, ed. M. Rosenberg and H. B. Kaplan, pp. 535–46. Arlington Heights, IL: Harlan Davidson.

Rosenberg, M. (1985). Self-concept and psychological well-being in adolescence. In *The Development of the Self*, ed. R. L. Leahy, pp. 205–46. Orlando, FL: Academic Press.

Rosenberg, M., Schooler, C., Schoenbach, C., and Rosenberg, F. (1995). Global self-esteem and specific self-esteem: different concepts, different outcomes. *American Sociological Review*, **60**, 141–56.

Rutter, M. (1987). Psychosocial resilience and protective mechanisms. *American Journal of Orthopsychiatry*, **57**, 316–31.

Ryan, R. and Deci, E. (2000). Self-determination theory and the facilitation of intrinsic motivation, social development, and well-being. *American Psychologist*, **55**, 68–78.

Scheier, M. F. and Carver, C. S. (1988). A model of behavioral self-regulation: translating intention into action. In *Advances in Experimental Social Psychology*, vol. 21, ed. L. Berkowitz, pp. 303–46. San Diego: Academic Press.

Schmidt, N. B., Joiner, T. E., Young, J. E., and Telch, M. J. (1995). The Schema Questionnaire: investigation of psychometric properties and the hierarchical structure of a measure of maladaptive schemas. *Cognitive Therapy and Research*, **19**, 295–321.

Shedler, J., Mayman, M., and Manis, M. (1993). The illusion of mental health. *American Psychologist*, **48**, 1117–31.

Sheldon, K. M. and Kasser, T. (1998). Pursuing personal goals: skills enable progress but not all progress is beneficial. *Personality and Social Psychology Bulletin*, **24**, 1319–31.

Showers, C. (1995). The evaluative organization of self-knowledge: origins, process, and implications for self-esteem. In *Efficacy, Agency, and Self-esteem*, ed. M. H. Kernis, pp. 101–22. New York: Plenum Press.

Spalding, L. R. and Hardin, C. D. (1999). Unconscious unease and self-handicapping: behavioral consequences of individual differences in implicit and explicit self-esteem. *Psychological Science*, **10**, 535–9.

Steele, C. M. (1988). The psychology of self-affirmation: sustaining the integrity of the self. In *Advances in Experimental Social Psychology*, vol. 21, ed. L. Berkowitz, pp. 261–302. San Diego: Academic Press.

Striegal-Moore, R. H., Silberstein, L. R., Grunberg, N. E., and Rodin, J. (1990). Competing on all fronts: achievement orientation and disordered eating. *Sex Roles*, **23**, 697–702.

Swann, W. B., Jr (1997). The trouble with change: self-verification and allegiance to the self. *Psychological Science*, **8**, 177–80.

Taylor, S. E. and Brown, J. D. (1988). Illusions and well-being: a social psychological perspective on mental health. *Psychological Bulletin*, **103**, 193–210.

Taylor, S. E. and Brown, J. D. (1994). Positive illusions and well-being revisited: separating fact from fiction. *Psychological Bulletin*, **116**, 21–7.

Tennen, H. and Affleck, G. (1993). The puzzles of self-esteem: a clinical perspective. In *Self-esteem: The Puzzle of Low Self-regard*, ed. R. Baumeister, pp. 241–62. New York: Plenum.

Tesser, A. and Campbell, J. (1983). Self-definition and self-evaluation maintenance. In *Psychological Perspectives on the Self*, vol. 2, ed. J. Suls and A. G. Greenwald, pp. 1–31. Hillsdale, NJ: Lawrence Erlbaum.

Waldo, C. R., Hesson-McInnis, M. S., and D'Augelli, A. R. (1998). Antecedents and consequents of victimization of lesbian, gay, and bisexual young people: a structural model comparing rural university and urban samples. *American Journal of Community Psychology*, **26**, 307–34.

Werner, E. E. (1995). Resilience in development. *Current Directions in Psychological Science*, **4**, 81–5.

Werner, E. E. and Smith, R. S. (1992). *Overcoming the Odds: High Risk Children from Birth to Adulthood*. Ithaca, NY: Cornell University Press.

Williams, S. L. (1992). Perceived self-efficacy and phobic disability. In *Self-efficacy: Thought Control of Action*, ed. R. Schwarzer, pp. 149–76. Washington, DC: Hemisphere.

Wills, T. A. (1987). Downward comparison as a coping mechanism. In *Coping with Negative Life Events: Clinical and Social Psychological Perspectives*, ed. C. R. Snyder and C. Ford, pp. 243–67. New York: Plenum.

Wylie, R. C. (1979). *The Self-concept: Theory and Research on Selected Topics*, vol. 2. Lincoln: University of Nebraska Press.

Young, J. E. (1999). *Cognitive Therapy for Personality Disorders: A Schema-focused Approach*, 3rd edn. Sarasota, FL: Professional Resource Press/Professional Resource Exchange.

Young, J. and Flanagan, C. (1998). Schema-focused therapy for narcissistic patients. In *Disorders of Narcissism: Diagnostic, Clinical, and Empirical Implications*, ed. E. F. Ronningstam, pp. 239–62. Washington DC: American Psychiatric Press.

Young, J. and Gluhoski, V. (1997). A schema-focused perspective on satisfaction in close relationships. In *Satisfaction in Close Relationships*, ed. R. J. Sternberg and M. Hojjat, pp. 356–81. New York: Guilford.

Zimmerman, B. J. (1995). Self-efficacy and educational development. In *Self-efficacy in Changing Societies*, ed. A. Bandura, pp. 202–31. New York: Cambridge University Press.

10

Promoting cognitive change in posttraumatic stress disorder

Elizabeth A. Hembree and Edna B. Foa

University of Pennsylvania School of Medicine, Philadelphia, PA, USA

It has long been observed that traumatic experiences are often followed by a distinct pattern of distressing symptoms. Accounts of such reactions began to appear in the psychiatric literature with greater frequency after the Second World War, resulting in the inclusion of "gross stress reaction" in the first version of the American Psychiatric Association (APA) *Diagnostic and Statistical Manual* (DSM-I) in 1952. Although the DSM-I noted that exposure to extreme stress may trigger great psychological distress, it did not provide diagnostic criteria for the stress reaction. It was not until the third revision of the DSM (DSM-III; APA, 1980) that mental health experts first codified the pattern of posttrauma reactions as a distinct anxiety disorder, termed posttraumatic stress disorder (PTSD), and offered clear and specific diagnostic criteria.

A vast amount of research has been conducted on PTSD since its formal designation over 20 years ago. Although much of this research has been atheoretical, focusing on issues such as phenomenology, prevalence, and comorbidity, theories about the development and maintenance of PTSD have stimulated a number of studies investigating both the psychopathology and the treatment of the disorder. Among the most influential and fruitful models of PTSD are those offered by cognitive or information-processing theory and emotional-processing theory.

In this chapter we first review the diagnosis and prevalence of PTSD. Second, we review the history of the evolution of cognitive models of PTSD. Third, we present a detailed description of emotional-processing theory (Foa and Kozak, 1986; Foa et al., 1989; Foa and Riggs, 1993). Fourth, we describe two treatment interventions that have emerged from the emotional-processing and information-processing models: prolonged exposure therapy (Foa and Rothbaum, 1998) and cognitive processing therapy (CPT) (Resick and Schnicke, 1992). Fifth, we review selected outcome studies that examined the efficacy of cognitive therapy and exposure therapy, as these are the treatments of interest in this chapter. We conclude with a discussion of the existing empirical work, some important questions and issues that remain unanswered, and directions for future research.

PTSD: diagnostic criteria and prevalence

According to the DSM-IV (APA, 1994), PTSD may develop in those who experience or witness with "horror, terror, or helplessness" a traumatic event that involves real or perceived threat to life or physical integrity. The lifetime prevalence of PTSD has been estimated at 24% among trauma survivors and at 9% in the general population (Breslau et al., 1991). The prevalence of current PTSD in trauma survivors varies by type of trauma and by the methods of the various studies (e.g., time elapsing since the investigated trauma had occurred), but has been reported to occur in 12–47% of female assault victims (Rothbaum et al., 1992; Resnick et al., 1993), 15% of Vietnam combat veterans (Kulka et al., 1990), and up to 40% of people surviving serious motor vehicle accidents (Taylor and Koch, 1995). The high prevalence of PTSD renders this disorder a significant public health problem, thus underscoring the need to understand its pathology and treatment.

Three clusters of symptoms characterize PTSD: reexperiencing the trauma (e.g., intrusive and distressing thoughts, flashbacks, nightmares, intense emotional distress, physiological reactions to cues); avoidance behaviors (e.g., avoidance of trauma-related thoughts, feelings, reminders; not remembering important aspects of the trauma, decreased interest, emotional numbing, feeling disconnected from others, sense of foreshortened future); and hyperarousal symptoms (e.g., sleep disturbance, irritability, concentration impairment, hypervigilance, and excessive startle). It is common for traumatized individuals to experience these symptoms shortly after the traumatic event occurs. For most, a process of natural recovery takes place, as reflected in a decline in symptoms. However, some traumatized individuals fail to recover and they develop PTSD and other posttrauma pathology, which becomes chronic and disruptive. The notion that to experience PTSD symptoms immediately following the trauma is a normal reaction is expressed in the duration criterion, which requires at least 1-month symptom duration for the diagnosis of acute PTSD, and at least 3 months' duration for chronic PTSD.

The fact that traumatic events are commonly experienced and that many victims recover from these experiences without developing significant long-term pathology raises the question of what factors determine whether individuals will process a trauma successfully and recover, or whether they will fail to do so and will develop chronic PTSD (Bowman, 1999; Foa and Cahill, 2000). The answer to this question has clear implications for the understanding of the psychopathology of the disorder and its treatment because successful treatment must target the factors that hinder natural recovery.

Evolution of cognitive-behavioral theories of PTSD

When PTSD was designated as an anxiety disorder in the psychiatric nomenclature, cognitive-behavioral scholars initially viewed it as a complex phobia with extensive generalization that produces symptoms that resemble those of generalized anxiety disorder. Accordingly, conceptualizations of the psychopathology of PTSD (and its treatment) were based on prevailing notions of anxiety disorders in the 1960s and 1970s. Thus an early precursor of the information-processing model of PTSD was learning theory.

Learning theory

Mowrer's two-factor theory was highly influential in the conceptualization of pathological anxiety symptoms and in the development of behavioral treatments for these symptoms. Although several theorists and clinical investigators noted the limitations of the two-stage theory in accounting for some clinical phenomena (Rachman, 1980) and became dissatisfied with a nonmediational account of pathological anxiety (Beck, 1976), the first theoretical attempts to account for PTSD relied heavily on Mowrer's theory (Keane et al., 1985; Kilpatrick et al., 1985). According to that theory, the first stage in the development of a phobia is fear acquisition via classical conditioning. When a neutral stimulus (the conditioned stimulus or CS) is paired with a negative or aversive stimulus (the unconditioned stimulus or UCS) the CS will come to elicit a conditioned fear response (the CR). In the context of PTSD, harmless or neutral stimuli that were present at the time of the trauma (e.g., time of day, certain odors, sights) subsequently come to elicit anxiety. Through the processes of generalization and higher-order conditioning, stimuli that are associated with the original stimuli (e.g., strangers, physical attributes of an assailant, crowded places) also come to elicit anxiety.

According to Mowrer's theory, the second stage in the formation of phobia is the establishment of avoidance behavior through the process of operant conditioning. In the adaptation of the theory to PTSD, the PTSD sufferer learns that avoidance and escape from the CS reduce trauma-related anxiety. These behaviors are negatively reinforced by their capacity to reduce or terminate anxiety and fear. However, while avoidance and escape produce temporary relief from anxiety, they prevent learning that the CS has not been followed by the UCS (i.e., that the CS is not actually dangerous), thus maintaining the anxiety symptoms.

Cognitive theory

As noted above, the two-factor theory has been criticized for failing to account for thoughts and appraisals that seem to accompany clinical anxiety. In cognitive theories of PTSD, cognitive mediation factors are viewed as the mechanisms underlying the development and maintenance of the disorder. Cognitive theories of PTSD have been influenced by two branches of psychology: from clinical psychology came a theory rooted in classical cognitive therapy (Beck, 1972; Ellis, 1977; Beck et al., 1979; Beck et al., 1985), and from personality and social psychology emerged theories relating to cognitive schema and structures of meaning (McCann and Pearlman, 1990; Epstein, 1991; Janoff-Bulman, 1992).

Cognitive model of emotional disorders

The theory that has driven cognitive therapy holds that individuals are characterized by the particular ways in which they think about the world, other people, and themselves (Beck, 1972; Beck et al., 1979). These ways of thinking are presumed to influence the manner in which events are interpreted. Furthermore, it is the interpretation of events, rather than the events themselves, which lead to specific emotional responses. As an event can often be interpreted in different ways, a variety of emotional reactions may result. For example, consider a woman driving down a highway who suddenly sees a car containing several men pull alongside her, waving and gesturing to her to stop. If her immediate thought is "oh no, they want to hurt me and steal my car," she is likely to feel afraid and drive faster to escape them. If on the other hand, her immediate thought is "they need help," she might feel concerned, and slow down or pull to the side of the road.

In the first instance, the woman interpreted the behavior of the men as threatening or dangerous, which elicited fear and anxiety. Cognitive theory assumes that different classes of thought are associated with different emotional responses. Thoughts related to loss elicit sadness, thoughts that something is unfair or unjust elicit anger, thoughts about one's own behavior being wrong or unfair elicit guilt, and thoughts about one's self being somehow inadequate or dirty are associated with shame. When benign events are interpreted as somehow threatening, as is common in PTSD as well as other anxiety disorders, pathological or excessive fear and anxiety emerge.

Normal, everyday experiences elicit a range of thoughts and feelings. Pathological emotional responses are distinguished from these by their disruptive intensity, frequency, duration, or incongruity to the situation. Pathological or excessive emotional responses are triggered by distorted or dysfunctional thinking/interpreting of events. Cognitive therapy aims to help people learn to identify such dysfunctional or unhelpful thinking and to modify or correct these thoughts and assumptions. Originally developed to treat depression, cognitive therapy was subsequently extended to encompass the treatment of anxiety disorders (Beck et al., 1985).

According to Beck and colleagues, the primary problem in anxiety disorders is the "overactive cognitive patterns (schemas) relevant to danger that are continually structuring external and/or internal experiences as a sign of danger" (Beck et al., 1985, p. 15). While they did not write extensively about PTSD, Beck et al. did note that patients with traumatic neuroses lose the capacity to determine quickly whether a stimulus signals real danger. Instead, the anxious individual fails to discriminate safe from unsafe and continues to label benign events as danger signals. This view, which is consistent with learning theories of PTSD, continues to be a prominent aspect of current theories of PTSD.

Other schema theories

Theorists of personality and social psychology have also proposed cognitive mediation of posttrauma emotional reactions, emphasizing the role of traumatic experiences in modifying cognitive schemas. Most have suggested that schemata, i.e., central assumptions or beliefs that influence the perception and interpretation of incoming information, must be modified in order for the trauma-related information to be processed. This modification may occur through assimilation of the incoming information to fit preexisting schemata or through accommodation of underlying schemata to allow integration of trauma-related information.

Horowitz (1986) explained posttrauma reactions with concepts borrowed from both psychoanalytic and information-processing theory. He proposed that, when traumatized, individuals must match trauma-related information with their preexisting inner models, and that this process requires revision of both old (prior experience) information and new (trauma) information. This repetitive process (which he termed the "completion tendency") induces the reexperiencing symptoms characteristic of PTSD. Horowitz further proposed that trauma-related information that is congruent with existing inner models will strengthen those models, whereas trauma information that is incongruent with existing models will cause alteration of the preexisting inner model.

Others have specified the internal constructs or beliefs that might be impacted by traumatic events. Epstein (1991) hypothesized that core beliefs changed by traumatic events include the views that the world is benign, the world is meaningful, the self is worthy, and people are trustworthy. Similarly, Janoff-Bulman (1992) suggested that traumatic experiences are incompatible with the basic assumptions held by most people – that the world is benevolent and meaningful and that the self is worthy. McCann and Pearlman (1990) proposed that all individuals develop schemata within certain fundamental psychological needs and that the experience of trauma causes disruption in these schemata. These needs include frame of reference, safety, dependency, trust of self and others, power, esteem, intimacy, and independence.

Early studies conducted by trauma researchers underscored the prominence of cognitive mediation in posttrauma reactions. Frank and Stewart (1984) reported that women who were raped in situations which they believed to be safe had more severe reactions than those who believed the situations to be dangerous. Perloff

(1983) reported that female crime victims who had believed themselves to be invulnerable prior to the event had greater difficulty afterwards as compared to those who believed they were as vulnerable as anyone else.

These findings support the assumption common to most cognitive theories of PTSD, that traumatic experiences disrupt core cognitive constructs and compel the survivor to adapt these constructs. The survivor may adapt by altering her view of the world (e.g., "the world is terribly dangerous and I am not safe in it") or by altering her view of the trauma ("he really wasn't trying to hurt me; he thought I wanted to have sex"). Resick and Schnicke (1992) suggested that assimilation (expressed by the second of these two adaptation responses) is more typical than accommodation, theorizing that it is easier to alter one's view of a single event than one's view of the whole world.

But what happens when the core constructs or pretrauma inner models are not discrepant with incoming information from the traumatic event? What of the individual who has frequently experienced traumatic events and who does not view the world as benevolent and people as trustworthy? Based on these schema models, we would expect that in these individuals trauma information matches internal constructs about the world and about safety such that they will not have a need for accommodation or assimilation. Accordingly, individuals with trauma histories should be expected to recover from a new trauma faster than those without such histories. Inconsistent with this supposition are research findings suggesting that the experience of multiple traumas increases the likelihood of developing PTSD (Burgess and Holstrom, 1978; Resick, 1987; Rothbaum et al., 1992). Thus these early schema models do not fully account for patterns of response known to occur in many individuals.

Emotional-processing theory

Foa and colleagues (Foa et al., 1989; Foa and Riggs, 1993; Foa and Rothbaum, 1998) have advanced a theoretical account of PTSD within the framework of emotional-processing theory (Foa and Kozak, 1985, 1986). This theory integrates concepts derived from the learning, cognitive, and social-personality perspectives described above, and is rooted in Lang's (1977, 1979) bioinformational theory of emotion. According to Lang's theory, fear is a cognitive structure that functions as a program for escape from danger. These fear structures include representations of: (1) feared stimuli; (2) verbal, overt/behavioral, and physiological responses; and (3) the meaning of the stimulus and response elements of the structure.

Pathological fear structures

Foa and Kozak (1985, 1986) noted that fear structures exist in all human beings (hence the ability to recognize and react to realistically dangerous situations), but that the presence of an anxiety disorder reflects a pathological fear structure. They proposed that pathological fear structures are distinguished from normal fear structures in containing excessive response elements (e.g., extensive avoidance, hyperarousal) and in being resistant to modification. This causes the fear experience to be disruptively intense. Furthermore, they proposed that pathological fear structures include erroneous elements: (1) unrealistic stimulus–stimulus associations; (2) strong associations between harmless stimuli and escape/avoidance responses; (3) erroneous associations between stimulus and response representations and meaning representations, including mistaken evaluations or interpretations. The last element includes the beliefs that anxiety will persist indefinitely in the face of feared stimuli unless escape occurs, that the fear response will cause harm (e.g., losing control, "going crazy"), or that very negative consequences will inevitably result from confrontation with the feared stimuli.

The conceptualization of PTSD within emotional-processing theory led Foa and her colleagues to suggest that, like other anxiety disorders, PTSD reflects the presence of a pathological cognitive structure. Foa et al. (1989) suggested that a trauma memory can be conceptualized as a specific fear structure and that a pathological trauma memory is hypothesized to underlie PTSD. This structure is distinguished from a normal trauma memory by the presence of erroneous (unrealistic) stimulus–stimulus associations as well as erroneous evaluations of danger. In contrast, the fear structure associated with a normal or successfully processed trauma memory contains realistic associations and evaluations. Furthermore, they theorized that a pathological trauma memory structure contains an especially large number of stimulus and response representations, rendering the memory highly accessible. The activation of the trauma memory gives rise to PTSD symptoms (e.g., high arousal, flashbacks, and intrusive trauma-related thoughts) that are perceived by the sufferer as extremely aversive and possibly dangerous. Therefore, the individual with PTSD engages extensively in efforts to avoid trauma-related situations that activate the trauma memory.

To illustrate the difference between normal and pathological memory structures, Figures 10.1 and 10.2 depict two schematic models of rape memory structures (taken from Foa and Rothbaum, 1998, pp. 75–76). Figure 10.1 presents a model of a normal trauma memory. This model portrays realistic associations between stimulus and meaning elements. For example, the stimuli "rape," "gun," and "shoot" are all associated with the meaning "dangerous;" the stimuli that represent the general characteristics of the rapist ("man," "tall," and "bald") are not associated with danger. Indeed, all guns are dangerous but not all tall and bald men are rapists. Having the accurate perception that the rapist was a particular person and not that all tall, bald men are dangerous protects the rape survivor from developing the perception that the world is entirely dangerous. Similarly, the response representations present

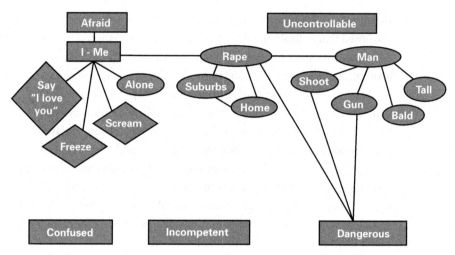

Figure 10.1   Schematic model of normal rape memory.

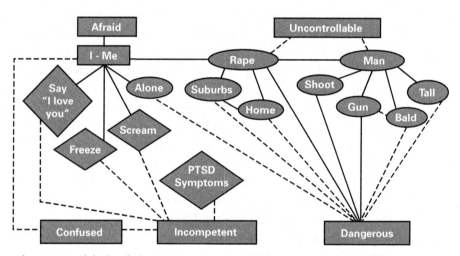

Figure 10.2   Schematic model of pathological rape memory. PTSD, posttraumatic stress disorder.

in the trauma memory ("scream," "afraid," "freeze") accurately represent reality but are not associated with the meaning "incompetent." The experience of being raped is thus not associated with negative self-appraisal.

Figure 10.2 depicts a schematic model of a pathological trauma memory structure that is hypothesized to underlie chronic PTSD. Solid lines depict the realistic associations, and the erroneous, unrealistic associations are depicted by dotted lines. In contrast to the normal trauma memory, this one illustrates: (1) excessive response elements such as avoidance and physiological activity (i.e., PTSD symptoms); (2) erroneous stimulus–stimulus associations that do not accurately represent the world, such as an association between "gun" and "bald;" (3) erroneous associations between objectively safe stimuli such as "tall," "home," "alone," and the meaning "dangerous;" and (4) erroneous associations between harmless stimuli and escape or avoidance responses.

The schematic model in Figure 10.2 also illustrates the erroneous associations between response elements and the meaning "incompetent." The survivor's memory that she complied with the rapist's command to say "I love you" as well as the fact that she froze and screamed are interpreted as signs of inadequacy and incompetence. The presence of the PTSD symptoms themselves is also interpreted by the survivor to mean that she is incompetent.

Core cognitions that maintain PTSD

Foa and colleagues (1989) suggested that the number of stimulus elements in the fear structure underlying PTSD is particularly large. These are erroneously associated with the meaning "danger," leading to the perception of the world as extremely dangerous. As can be inferred from the erroneous associations depicted on the left side of the model, later on Foa and colleagues (Foa and Riggs, 1993; Foa and Rothbaum, 1998; Foa and Jaycox, 1999) suggested that a pathological trauma memory contains elements that lead to the perception of oneself as incompetent (e.g., "having flashbacks and nightmares for such a long time means that I am weak and may lose my mind"). Accordingly, Foa and Riggs (1993) suggested that two major classes of erroneous cognitions characterize individuals with PTSD: (1) the perception of the world as an *extremely dangerous* place; and (2) the conception of oneself as *extremely incompetent.* Common erroneous cognitions underlying PTSD are: the world is extremely dangerous, people are untrustworthy, no place is safe, I am incompetent, PTSD symptoms are a sign of weakness, and PTSD symptoms are dangerous (e.g., signal loss of control).

To examine the PTSD-related cognitions, Foa et al. (1999a) administered a self-report inventory to 392 trauma victims with and without PTSD and compared their responses to those of 209 nontraumatized individuals. They found that the group with current PTSD endorsed significantly more negative thoughts about themselves, the dangerousness of the world, and self-blame. In contrast, there was no difference in the self-reported cognitions among individuals who had experienced trauma but did not have PTSD and those without history of trauma.

Thus, Foa and colleagues (Foa and Rothbaum, 1998) have posited that we will best understand the success of any psychosocial treatment if we construe it as promoting changes in two main erroneous cognitions underlying PTSD: that "the world is extremely dangerous," and "I am extremely incompetent." They argued that successful psychotherapy must access the trauma-related memories, feelings, and thoughts, help organize the traumatic memories, and facilitate the modification of dysfunctional cognitions. Similar conceptualizations have been offered by other experts (Resick and Schnicke, 1992; Ehlers and Clark, 2000) and have fostered the development of cognitive therapy programs for PTSD.

Rigidity and extremity of beliefs

As discussed earlier, some trauma theorists have suggested that posttrauma pathology emerges from the violation of preexisting, positive schemata about the benevolence of the world and the worthiness of the self. These theories come up short in accounting for the empirical finding that multiple traumatic experiences and pretrauma psychological disturbance are associated with increased rates of PTSD (Burgess and Holmstrom, 1978; P. A. Resick, unpublished data; Rothbaum et al., 1992). Indeed, it is reasonable to expect that multiply traumatized individuals would see the world as extremely dangerous and themselves as very incompetent to cope with stress. How does emotional processing theory reconcile or explain these two seemingly contradictory approaches?

Foa and Riggs (1993) accepted the view that a survivor's schemata about the world and self prior to the trauma influence whether he/she will fail to process a trauma successfully and thus contribute to the development of chronic PTSD. However, they argued that what causes an individual to be less adept at successfully processing a traumatic event is not the possession of positive assumptions, but rather the holding of rigid, extreme views. Those who have experienced multiple traumas may also hold rigidly extreme views, but those views are likely negative rather than positive. Other researchers have also stressed that prior beliefs may be either disrupted or confirmed by traumatic events (Resick and Schnicke, 1992, 1993).

According to Foa and colleagues, two types of preexisting schemata may thus hinder successful emotional processing of a trauma. The first type of interference occurs when the trauma violates the individual's preexisting view of him- or herself as *extremely* competent and of the world as *extremely* safe. An example is the woman who had mostly positive experiences throughout her life and in the last years worked in the same office where she felt perfectly safe and content with herself. Her world was shattered by the experience of being robbed at gunpoint while in her office. Not being able to reconcile this extreme event with her pretrauma schemas of safety, security, and self-competence, she came to view the world outside her home as terribly dangerous, as she perceived every strange man to be a potential assailant.

The second type of interference in successful emotional processing occurs when the trauma confirms existing views of oneself as extremely incompetent and of the world as extremely dangerous. If a woman who had already held an extremely negative view of herself is raped, this trauma is taken as conclusive proof that her negative self-perception is correct. An example of this scenario is the woman who presented for treatment for PTSD related to a rape that occurred 1 year prior. After reporting that she had also been raped 10 years before this assault, she said, "I always felt abnormal and ashamed that I was raped back then. But after this, I *know* that something is wrong with me . . . normal women don't get raped." Likewise, a trauma may reinforce previous knowledge that no one can be trusted in this world.

In contrast, Foa and colleagues posit, flexibility in one's rules of interpretation, combined with realistic evaluation of threat, allow finer discriminations of degree of "dangerousness" and "self-competence." Individuals whose life experience has granted them a more flexible and balanced view will be better able to process a trauma as a unique event, one that should not substantially alter their evaluations of themselves and of the world. If the woman in the first example above had such flexible, balanced schemata, she would have regarded the robbery as an extremely frightening, yet extremely infrequent event in her life, and would continue to be a functional human being rather than becoming essentially housebound.

Implications for treatment

Foa and Kozak (1986) proposed that successful treatment for anxiety disorders must correct the pathological elements of the relevant fear cognitive structure (i.e., the memory representation of the trauma in the case of PTSD). Furthermore, they suggested that in order to effect such modification treatment must (1) activate the fear structure and (2) provide information that is incompatible with the pathological elements in the structure, so that they can be corrected. Three factors that we consider critical to the successful processing of traumatic events are emotional engagement with the trauma memory, organization of the trauma narrative, and the correction of dysfunctional cognitions that are common immediately after a traumatic event.

Traditional as well as present-day conceptualizations (Horowitz, 1986) of the psychological effects of trauma and its treatment have postulated that special processing of the traumatic experience needs to take place for recovery to occur. Although trauma theorists generally agree that emotional engagement is a necessary condition for adequate processing of a traumatic event, few studies have directly examined the emotional engagement hypothesis. Two retrospective studies (Bremner et al., 1992; Marmar et al., 1994) and one prospective study (Koopman et al., 1994) provided some support for this hypothesis. Each of these studies found a high correlation between reported dissociation during or immediately after the trauma (i.e., absence of emotional engagement) and subsequent PTSD. In a prospective study of female assault victims, Gilboa-Schechtman and Foa (2001) reasoned that a high level of PTSD symptoms *shortly* after a severe trauma is a normal reaction and therefore can be viewed as reflecting appropriate emotional engagement. Conversely, a low level of PTSD symptoms shortly after the trauma could signal low engagement. Accordingly, Gilboa-Schechtman and Foa predicted that victims whose peak PTSD symptoms occurred shortly after the trauma will show better recovery later on than victims with delayed peak reaction. To test this hypothesis, recent rape victims were divided into two groups: those whose peak PTSD severity occurred within 2 weeks after the trauma and those with peak PTSD between 3 and 6 weeks postrape. Consistent with the prediction, at 14 weeks postassault, victims in the first group exhibited less severe depression and PTSD than did victims in the second group.

Jaycox et al. (1998) examined the effects of emotional engagement on treatment outcome in a group of 37 women with chronic PTSD. Using self-reported distress level during imaginal exposure to the memory of a traumatic event as an index of emotional engagement, Jaycox et al. examined the relationship between changes in the women's distress levels during successive sessions of exposure therapy and treatment outcome. Subjective Units of Discomfort (SUDS) ratings were obtained from the patients every 5 min during each session of imaginal exposure. The average SUDS level was calculated for each session of imaginal exposure, and ratings were compared across successive sessions. Three groups characterized by different response patterns emerged from a cluster analysis of the mean SUDS levels: high initial distress and gradual reduction across sessions, high initial distress and no reduction across sessions, and moderate initial distress (i.e., low engagement) and no reduction. Jaycox et al. reported that the first group – patients who showed high initial distress and gradual habituation across sessions – improved more in treatment as measured by reductions in assessor-rated PTSD severity than those who showed either high or moderate initial distress and no habituation. They concluded that both high engagement and habituation over the course of treatment are clearly important for successful outcome. Thus, the results emerging from several areas of research are supportive of the emotional engagement hypothesis.

The second factor thought to influence recovery is the degree to which the victim is able to organize the trauma narrative. Clinical observations of patients with chronic PTSD suggest that their trauma narratives are characterized by an abundance of speech fillers, repetitions and incomplete sentences and that these narratives often reflect confusion and a discontinuity of time and space. On the basis of studies of trauma narratives during treatment, Foa and Riggs (1993) hypothesized that the natural process of recovery involves organizing and articulating the traumatic memory. Support for this hypothesis comes from the finding that the degree of trauma narrative articulation shortly after the trauma predicted PTSD symptom severity 3 months later (Amir et al., 1998). In this study, Amir et al. subjected a transcription of the patient's trauma narrative, elicited within the first couple of weeks after the trauma, to a computer program that calculated its reading level. Reading level was employed as a measure of articulation, with higher levels indicating better organization and articulation of the traumatic event. Lower level of articulation was associated with higher trauma-related psychopathology at 3-month posttrauma evaluation. Also in support of the narrative organization hypothesis are the findings emerging from a study that analyzed the content of patients' accounts of their assaults in the context of exposure therapy. On the average, the accounts of the last exposure session contained more organized thoughts than those from the first session. Moreover, reduction in the index of fragmentation (e.g., speech fillers, unfinished sentences) was positively related to reduction in PTSD symptoms and increase in organization was negatively related to reduction in depression (Foa et al., 1995).

As discussed earlier in this chapter, the third factor that hinders the processing of a traumatic event is the presence of the dysfunctional cognitions that were found related to PTSD. Accordingly, one goal of treatment for PTSD is to modify these erroneous and destructive cognitions.

Cognitive-behavioral interventions for PTSD

When PTSD was first introduced into the DSM-III as an anxiety disorder, cognitive-behavioral interventions started to be applied systematically to trauma victims and research on treatment efficacy with this population was launched. The conception of PTSD within conditioning theory of fear and phobias led some experts to employ exposure therapy procedures that had been found successful with phobias (Keane et al., 1989). The realization that PTSD sufferers exhibit symptoms of general anxiety led other experts with the same theoretical persuasion to employ anxiety management programs for PTSD (e.g., Stress Inoculation Training; Meichenbaum, 1974; Veronen and Kilpatrick, 1983).

Exposure therapy

The idea that trauma therapy should include some form of exposure to the traumatic event has a long history in psychology and psychiatry, and is central to present-day exposure therapy. Developed to target the mechanisms thought to underlie persistent pathological anxiety, described above, exposure therapy comprises a set of techniques designed to help patients confront their feared objects, situations, memories, and images. Exposure therapy programs vary in degree of contact with the feared object (imaginal versus direct in-vivo exposure), duration of exposure (short versus long), the number of the low-level anxiety situations that precede the introduction of the most fearful situation (gradual versus abrupt), and the arousal level experienced (low versus high). With PTSD, exposure programs often consist of imaginal exposure, i.e., repeated imaginal reliving of the traumatic memory, and in-vivo exposure, i.e., repeated confrontation with trauma-related situations and objects that evoke unrealistic anxiety. Imaginal exposure aims to help the patient to process the trauma emotionally by vividly imagining the traumatic event and describing it aloud, along with the thoughts and feelings that occurred during the event. In-vivo exposure furthers the processing work by encouraging confrontation with external situations, places, or activities that trigger trauma-related fear and anxiety. The patient is instructed to remain in the anxiety-provoking situation until his or her fear declines (i.e., habituates) by a significant amount. Exposure therapy for PTSD is based on the idea that avoidance of trauma-related memories and cues, although an understandable and common response and part of the symptomology of PTSD, interferes with the emotional processing of the traumatic event by maintaining the erroneous cognitions and the resultant unrealistic fear.

An example is a bank teller, who after having been shot during a robbery became extremely fearful of being in public places or any situation in which she had to interact with strangers. She stopped going to work, to stores, and to many other places she used to go freely. This avoidance reduced her distress in the short term, but also maintained her trauma-related symptoms by preventing her from achieving a realistic perspective about her safety in the world and the probability of being shot again. During exposure therapy the woman was asked to recall repeatedly the memory of the robbery as vividly as possible and recount what happened during it. Initially she felt quite anxious and distressed. However, repeatedly reliving the memory of the assault led to a decrease in her anxiety because she learned that it is not dangerous to think or talk about the robbery, that doing so helped her make sense of what happened to her, and that the intense distress it elicited initially subsided with repeated confrontation.

There are several ways that exposure to trauma-related memories and cues leads to improvement in PTSD. First, repeated imaginal reliving of the trauma and in-vivo exposure facilitates habituation or reduction of the anxiety associated with trauma memory. The patient learns that anxiety will decrease without avoidance or escape, thus correcting the erroneous perception that anxiety remains forever unless avoidance or escape is realized. Second, discussing and reliving the trauma with a supportive and empathic therapist helps the patient to realize that thinking about the trauma is not dangerous. Third, focusing on the trauma memory and engaging in in-vivo exposure decreases the generalization of fear by helping the patient to differentiate the traumatic event from other situations. The patient comes to see the trauma as a unique event rather than as representing an extremely "dangerous world." Fourth, confronting rather than avoiding trauma-related fears and memories helps the PTSD sufferer to develop a sense of mastery and competence. Individuals with chronic PTSD commonly view their symptoms as meaning that they are incompetent and weak (Foa et al., 1999a). Exposure counteracts the victim's perception of him-/herself as incompetent.

A case example

"Karen," a 43-year-old woman with severe assault-related PTSD, was treated with prolonged exposure therapy. Karen (some details changed in the interest of confidentiality) had been brutally attacked by an intruder in her home. At one point during this ordeal, she was stabbed in the front of her shoulder. She automatically pressed her hand down over the assailant's, effectively keeping the blade of the knife in her body. Knowing that if he pulled the knife free he would try again to stab her in the chest, Karen retained her grip on the knife, but at the expense of further damage to her body. They struggled like this for some time until she managed to break free and remove the knife herself. This particular aspect of her terrible trauma was one of the most distressing and painful parts of her memory.

Karen accepted the rationale for confronting and processing the traumatic memory, but struggled with fear and avoidance of connecting emotionally with the horror of the assault. In one session, the therapist had Karen focusing in on the "hot spot" of the particular memory described above, going over it repeatedly and encouraging her to relate her feelings (terror, horror) and thoughts ("if I let go he will kill me; if I don't let go, he will destroy my shoulder") as well as what she was feeling in her body (pain, cutting). With the therapist's support and encouragement (given very frequently throughout the session), she tearfully described the horror, the pain, and the terrible choice she had had to make. The therapist responded with strong empathy and agreement that it was indeed a horrible choice and a terrible experience. It was obvious to the therapist that, for the first time, this courageous woman had fully accessed the emotional features of that memory. The therapist commented to Karen that she had survived the attack; she fought for her life and won.

Karen listened to this exposure tape for homework more frequently than she typically listened to her tapes. Imaginal exposure in the following session again focused on that particular memory. She showed habituation of anxiety between sessions and within the next session. This proved to be a turning point in her therapy; her self-reported PTSD symptoms began to decline steadily thereafter and she became more successful at overcoming avoidance.

Components of prolonged exposure therapy

We routinely employ a prolonged exposure treatment program for patients who suffer chronic, assault-related PTSD in the Center for Treatment and Study of Anxiety at the University of Pennsylvania. For a detailed description of the treatment program, see Foa and Rothbaum (1998).

The treatment consists of nine to 12 individual sessions about 90 min in length. The goal of the treatment program is to help the patient acquire and master specific skills that are used to reduce PTSD symptoms. The central components of therapy are education about PTSD symptoms and common reactions to trauma, breathing retraining, in-vivo exposure, and imaginal exposure. Homework, consisting of these skills, is an integral part of the treatment.

Treatment begins with a discussion of the impact of traumatic experiences and the development of PTSD. The patient is presented with the idea that symptoms have persisted because avoidance of thinking about the trauma and avoidance of reminders, although common, have prevented the event from being emotionally processed and integrated. The therapist explains that exposure to the memory (imaginal exposure) and to reminders (in-vivo exposure) blocks avoidance and thus promotes emotional processing of the trauma. This results in increased coherence and organization of the memory, habituation of distress when thinking about the trauma, realization that the memory itself is not dangerous and that anxiety does not last forever, and increased confidence in the patient's competence and coping skills. Breathing retraining is taught as an anxiety management tool.

The therapist provides information about common reactions to trauma, and the patient is encouraged to describe his or her own experience of these reactions. This discussion is intended to help the patient to comprehend that symptoms of PTSD and related problems (e.g., shame, guilt, sadness, and disruptions in relationships, reduced sexual interest) are common reactions to trauma. The goal is to reduce negative appraisal of PTSD symptoms and to set the focus of treatment on PTSD.

In-vivo exposure is introduced in the second treatment session. A hierarchy of objectively safe situations or activities that trigger trauma-related anxiety is constructed. Typical situations may be very specific, such as visiting an area related to the incident or reading about a similar assault in the newspaper, or more general fear-evoking triggers, such as making eye contact with unfamiliar men, being alone, sitting in the dark or standing in line in a crowded store.

Imaginal exposure is introduced in the next treatment session. During imaginal exposure, the patient is instructed to describe aloud what happened during the trauma while visualizing it as vividly as possible. He or she is asked to keep his or her eyes closed and to use the present tense, and also to include the thoughts, emotions, and sensory experiences that occurred during the traumatic event. Immediately following the reliving, the patient and therapist discuss the experience, any new understanding that may have emerged, and patterns of habituation that have occurred both within and between sessions.

Cognitive therapy

The goal of cognitive therapy for PTSD is to teach the patient to identify trauma-related irrational or dysfunctional beliefs that may influence his/her response to a situation and lead to excessive or inappropriate intense negative emotions. In contrast to exposure therapy, in which modification of dysfunctional cognitions is achieved through the introduction of corrective information, cognitive restructuring formally and directly addresses the patient's distorted or unhelpful beliefs about him- or herself and the world by means of verbal discourse. Via the therapist's use of the Socratic method (Beck et al., 1985; Clark, 1986), the patient learns to identify and to challenge these thoughts or beliefs in a logical, evidence-based manner. Relevant facts that support/do not support the belief are examined and alternative ways of interpreting the eliciting situation are considered. The therapist helps the patient to weigh the alternative interpretations and consequently decide whether the belief is helpful and accurately reflects reality, and if not, to replace or modify it.

Cognitive processing therapy

CPT is a treatment program developed by Resick and colleagues at the University of Missouri specifically to address the symptoms and concerns of women with assault-related PTSD. Underlying this approach is the assumption that PTSD symptoms are induced by conflicts between the new information conveyed by a traumatic event and prior schema. Thus the focus of treatment in CPT is on identifying and modifying these conflicts, which are termed "stuck points" (Resick and Schnicke, 1992, 1993). Stuck points or conflicts are hypothesized to be concentrated in particular areas or schemata that are likely to be affected by the trauma of rape. These areas of focus are based on the work of McCann et al. (1988), and include safety, trust, power, esteem, and intimacy. In developing CPT, Resick and Schnicke also considered it important that rape survivors feel the emotions associated with the assault and its aftermath. Therefore, they included a written exposure component designed to encourage expression of affect and to ensure that all the important trauma-related feelings and associated beliefs would be elicited.

Components of cognitive processing therapy

The three primary components of CPT include education about PTSD and information-processing theory, exposure, and cognitive therapy (Resick and Schnicke, 1992, 1993). Treatment consists of 12 sessions of group therapy (six to eight patients per group), each lasting 90 min. Treatment begins with a presentation of an information-processing account of PTSD and group members are asked to write about the meaning of the rape. Next, clients are instructed in identifying and differentiating thoughts and feelings and begin to work toward recognizing connections between them. The next two sessions are devoted to group members writing a detailed account of their assault experiences, including the sensory details, thoughts, and emotions that they experienced. The women are encouraged to experience their emotions fully while writing their rape narratives, which also serve to help identify an individual's "stuck points."

Formal cognitive therapy is initiated after the written exposure component. Patients are taught to identify and challenge faulty or maladaptive beliefs with procedures adapted from Beck et al. (1985). The focus of each cognitive therapy session is determined a priori by the five areas of belief listed above. Patients are also given educational materials to read about each theme that discuss how prior (pretrauma) beliefs might be disrupted or confirmed by the rape. In the final sessions the members again write about the meaning that the rape and its aftermath holds for them.

As in exposure therapy, the practicing of these skills via homework assignments is an integral part of the therapy. Also similar to exposure therapy, in the final session it is emphasized that their work is not done. A central goal of the therapy is to learn the skills they need to continue to challenge and modify their particular maladaptive thinking patterns and beliefs.

Stress inoculation training

Anxiety management approaches were commonly utilized in early studies due to an initial reluctance to use exposure therapy with female sexual assault victims. Although the emphasis in this chapter is on cognitive and exposure-based models of treatment, we will briefly describe anxiety management training as it has been frequently used as a comparison condition in treatment outcome studies of PTSD.

The most commonly employed program is stress inoculation training (SIT; Meichenbaum, 1974), which provides instruction in techniques that the patient can use to manage and reduce anxiety as it occurs. L. J. Veronen and D. G. Kilpatrick (unpublished data) adapted Meichenbaum's SIT for use with rape victims. Their adaptation was specifically designed to teach patients skills they could use to manage and decrease rape-related fear and anxiety. It included education about trauma and PTSD, deep muscle relaxation, breathing exercises, role-playing, covert modeling, thought-stopping, and guided self-dialogue. Patients were explicitly instructed to use these skills when confronted with situations or activities that triggered rape-related anxiety and fear.

Outcome studies

In this section we review results from selected treatment outcome studies. For more comprehensive reviews, see Foa and Rothbaum (1998) or Rothbaum et al. (2000). Our selection of studies was guided by two factors: one, we restrict our selection to well-controlled, comparative treatment outcome studies. Second, we present studies that investigated the efficacy of exposure therapy, cognitive therapy (including cognitive restructuring and CPT), or combinations of these interventions, with special emphasis on those studies that directly compared exposure and cognitive treatments.

Many well-controlled studies have found exposure therapy to be an effective treatment in reducing PTSD and related pathology, such as depression and anxiety. Keane et al. (1989) and Cooper and Clum (1989) found that veterans with PTSD treated with imaginal exposure (which they termed "imaginal flooding") improved relative to waitlist control and standard treatment, respectively, but the improvement was moderate. Exposure treatment of rape-related PTSD has also been found quite effective. Foa et al. (1991) treated female rape victims with chronic PTSD with nine sessions of either prolonged (imaginal and in-vivo) exposure (PE), SIT, or supportive counseling (SC), and compared the outcome of these treatments to a waitlist control group. At the end of treatment, exposure and SIT, and to a lesser extent, supportive counseling, significantly improved from pretreatment, whereas the waitlist group did not improve. The SIT group showed the most improvement on PTSD symptoms. By the 3-month follow-up, the PE group appeared superior to the other groups in PTSD symptoms, depression, and anxiety, although differences were not significant.

Foa et al. (1999b) replicated and extended these findings. Reasoning on the basis of the previous study that the combination of PE and SIT might be most effective at promoting emotional processing of the trauma and reducing anxiety, they compared the outcome of women randomized to PE alone, SIT alone, the combination PE/SIT, and waitlist control. They found that female rape and nonsexual assault victims in all active treatments showed significant and fairly equivalent reduction in PTSD severity and depression, whereas the waitlist control group did not show any improvement. Contrary to expectations, exposure alone (PE) was superior to SIT and PE/SIT on several indices of treatment outcome. Treatment gains were maintained at 6-month and 12-month follow-up evaluations.

Foa et al. (1999b) reasoned that the failure to find superiority of PE/SIT might have been due to the problems inherent in squeezing two multicomponent treatment programs into the space more typically allotted to each of them individually. Further reasoning that cognitive restructuring was likely to be the most potent ingredient of SIT, we designed a third treatment study that compared the outcome of PTSD patients either treated with PE alone, PE combined with cognitive restructuring (PE/CR), or assigned to a waitlist. This study is nearing completion. Preliminary results indicate that nine or 12 sessions (determined by rate of improvement in self-reported PTSD symptoms) of exposure alone and exposure with cognitive restructuring effected large and equal improvement in PTSD and depression symptoms, with improvements maintained over follow-up.

Interestingly, based on the 145 women assault victims who completed treatment in this study, exposure alone seems to be a more efficient program compared to exposure plus cognitive restructuring: 51% of women in the exposure alone condition have been able to end therapy at nine sessions by meeting the success criterion of at least 70% improvement in PTSD symptoms; in contrast, only 30% in the combined group met this criterion after nine sessions.

Resick and Schnicke (1992) used group CPT to treat symptoms of PTSD and depression in female victims of rape. They reported significantly greater reduction in PTSD symptoms and in depression following CPT compared to a naturally occurring waitlist control group. At both posttreatment and 6-month follow-up evaluations, none of the 19 women treated with CPT met diagnostic criteria for PTSD. Although these results suggested that CPT was a promising treatment for chronic posttraumatic stress, Resick and Schnicke acknowledged that the study design did not allow investigation of the relative importance of the cognitive therapy and (written) exposure components.

In effort to address this question, Resick and colleagues recently completed a study that compared the efficacy of 12 sessions of individually administered CPT to nine sessions of Foa et al.'s exposure therapy (alone) for rape victims with PTSD. Results generally indicated that both treatments are highly and equally effective at reducing PTSD, with treatment gains maintained through a 9-month follow-up (Resick et al., 2002).

The studies described above included women whose PTSD resulted from an assault. Several investigations of PTSD treatment have been conducted with individuals whose PTSD resulted from a variety of traumatic events, including assault, motor vehicle accidents, disasters, and childhood sexual abuse. Most of these have produced findings similar to those found in female assault victims.

Marks et al. (1998) treated patients with chronic PTSD resulting from mixed trauma with either exposure alone (PE), cognitive restructuring alone (CR), combined exposure and cognitive restructuring, or relaxation training. They found that PE, CR, and the combination of PE and CR were highly and equally effective and were superior to relaxation. Results of evaluations conducted 3 and 6 months after treatment showed that the PTSD symptoms of patients treated with exposure, either alone or in combination with cognitive restructuring, continued to decrease over time at a greater rate than those treated only with cognitive restructuring. The latter group showed a decrease in symptoms from post- to 3-month evaluations, followed by a slight increase at 6 months. On the basis of the finding that at 6 months patients in the exposure group showed significantly greater improvement than the cognitive restructuring group on 14 outcome measures, it seemed that the groups that received exposure fared better over time than those who received cognitive therapy alone.

Tarrier et al. (1999) conducted a study that aimed to compare the relative efficacy of "pure" cognitive therapy and "pure" exposure therapy. The exposure condition consisted of only imaginal exposure (i.e., no in-vivo). The chronic PTSD of patients in this study resulted mostly from criminal victimization and motor vehicle accidents. Overall, exposure (IE) and cognitive (CT) therapies were found to be significantly and equally effective at ameliorating PTSD severity. Tarrier et al. also claimed that, according to the independent assessor, a significantly greater number of the patients who showed worsening symptoms from pre- to posttreatment were in the IE condition (nine out of 12). This difference disappeared at 6-month follow-up, however. Interestingly, on other measures of clinical improvement (e.g., percentage with PTSD diagnosis, absence of clinical problem, and return to work), no significant differences among groups were obtained and more patients in the IE condition tended to show improvement compared to CT. Of note, in a subsequently published report on the subjective (self-rated) improvements of patients in this sample, Tarrier and Humphreys (2000) reported that when patients who failed to respond to treatment were excluded, patients who received IE showed significantly greater improvement than those receiving CT.

The failure to define "worsening" and the absence of an adequate method for evaluating treatment integrity render the Tarrier et al's findings uninterpretable (for a discussion, see Devilly and Foa, 2001). As noted by Devilly and Foa, the effects of both treatments in the Tarrier et al. study were considerably more modest than those reported in previous studies, raising questions about the manner in which those interventions were delivered. The exclusion of in-vivo exposure from the typical program of exposure-based treatment and the brevity of session length are particularly troublesome.

Summary of outcome studies

Taken together, the treatment outcome research indicates that exposure therapy and cognitive therapy are effective at ameliorating symptoms of chronic PTSD as well as depression and anxiety. Importantly, these results have been obtained in a variety of PTSD treatment centers and with patients experiencing a range of traumas. In addition, most comparative studies have found that patients treated with cognitive therapy and exposure therapy have equivalent outcome, although exposure may be more efficient, more durable, and, for treatment responders, more effective.

A greater number of studies demonstrating the efficacy of exposure therapy have been published relative to cognitive therapy. This has resulted in its current distinction as the most efficacious treatment for chronic PTSD and as the psychosocial treatment recommended as the first-line intervention by expert consensus (Foa et al., 1999c). More studies of cognitive therapy are clearly needed. Furthermore, three studies – by Marks et al. (1998), Tarrier et al. (1999), and Resick et al. (2002) – are to date the only published studies that have directly compared cognitive therapy with exposure therapy.

Summary and conclusion

There is some agreement among leading researchers in cognitive-behavioral therapy for PTSD about which factors are crucial for successful outcome. As noted earlier, emotional-processing theory (Foa and Kozak, 1986) explicitly specifies that, in order for treatment to reduce anxiety disorder symptoms, it needs to correct the pathological elements of the target fear structure. Foa and Kozak (1986) further noted that this corrective process is the essence of "emotional processing" which the therapy aims to achieve. Moreover, successful emotional processing requires both the accessing of the fear structure (indicated by fear activation) and the introduction of corrective information that is incompatible with the pathological aspects of the structure. The idea that fear activation is essential to the success of exposure therapy has been noted by exposure researchers all along (e.g., Lang, 1977; Borkovec and Sides, 1979). Accordingly, the central feature of exposure therapy for PTSD is the promotion of emotional engagement with the trauma memory via reliving of the memory (imaginal exposure), or via direct contact with external situations and activities that will trigger it (in-vivo exposure). While the role of fear activation has been less central to theories about mechanisms of change in cognitive therapy for anxiety disorders (Beck et al., 1985), activation of affect has been traditionally seen as playing a critical role in promoting change in psychotherapy. In the treatment of PTSD, current models of cognitive therapy recognize that it is important for patients to connect emotionally with the traumatic memory, but primarily in the service of facilitating the access to distorted cognitions thought to be relevant to PTSD (Resick and Schnicke, 1993; Ehlers and Clark, 2000).

The importance of introducing corrective information to modify erroneous or distorted cognitions is underscored by both emotional-processing theory of exposure therapy (Foa and Kozak, 1986) and by proponents of cognitive therapy. However, the method by which this process is achieved varies in the types of treatments. In exposure therapy, erroneous cognitions are corrected via the experiences of the patient during exposure, when these experiences disconfirm the erroneous cognitions. Cognitive therapists, on the other hand, utilize verbal discourse to help the patient directly to identify the distorted cognitions, challenge their validity, and replace them with more rational, functional cognitions. Indeed, Resick and Schnicke (1992) posited that because CPT "*directly* confronts conflicts and maladaptive beliefs [it] might be more effective than prolonged exposure alone. Prolonged exposure activates the memory structure but does not provide direct corrective information regarding misattributions or other maladaptive beliefs" (p. 749). As discussed earlier, CPT is not more effective than exposure therapy and the results of numerous studies have demonstrated the efficacy of exposure therapy alone in reducing PTSD.

Does the similar efficacy of exposure therapy and cognitive therapy reflect similar mechanisms? Those who suggest that the primary mechanism underlying exposure therapy is habituation (and therefore prolonged exposures are more effective than short ones) advocate different mechanisms. For example, according to Marks et al. (1998), "exposure gradually alters behavior, physiology, and cognition by habituation" (p. 324) but cognitive therapy changes perspectives irrespective of whether or not habituation occurs. In contrast, when discussing mechanisms of exposure for PTSD, Ehlers and Clark (2000) deemphasize the role of habituation while focusing entirely on the process of modifying appraisals of the trauma and the trauma sequelae. Exposure, according to Ehlers and Clark, serves only as a vehicle for modifying cognition. Foa and Kozak (1986) take an integrative stance in proposing that exposure modifies cognitive structures and that habituation (change in stimulus–response associations) is one type of such modification, the other being change in appraisals, evaluation, and beliefs.

Another mechanism of exposure therapy for PTSD emerging from emotional-processing theory is the elaboration and organization of the trauma narratives. As discussed earlier, Foa et al. (1995) reported that increase in organization from first to last exposure sessions was highly correlated with improvement. A similar position has been taken by Ehlers and Clark (2000) in explaining the role of reliving (imaginal exposure) in the treatment of PTSD. They proposed that trauma memory is poorly elaborated and inadequately integrated with other experiences and that reliving combined with cognitive therapy enhances elaboration and integration.

In summary, current cognitive theories of treatment of PTSD differ substantially from the traditional view of exposure therapy, but are quite similar to the views emerging from emotional-processing theory. They all agree that emotional engagement with the traumatic memories and modification of pathological cognitions are necessary for the success of the treatment. Which methods best achieve these goals is still a controversial issue that requires further study.

While current cognitive-behavioral treatments have been found to be effective for many individuals with chronic PTSD, there is a sizable minority of patients who do not respond to these treatments (Hembree et al., 2001). There is a dearth of knowledge on predictors of response to treatment. We know little about whether different treatments are differentially effective at changing particular symptoms or symptom clusters. More research is needed to expand our knowledge of: (1) mechanisms of change; (2) how individual differences in patient characteristics such as schemata, prior trauma history, cognitive flexibility and rigidity, and resilience are associated with treatment response; (3) what symptoms respond best to particular interventions; and (4) effective matching of patients with specific treatment modalities. Knowledge emerging from studies about these issues will hopefully guide us in developing interventions that will be effective with our treatment failures.

REFERENCES

American Psychiatric Association. (1952). *Diagnostic and Statistical Manual of Mental Disorders.* Washington, DC: American Psychiatric Association.

American Psychiatric Association. (1980). *Diagnostic and Statistical Manual of Mental Disorders,* 2nd edn. Washington, DC: American Psychiatric Association.

American Psychiatric Association. (1994). *Diagnostic and Statistical Manual of Mental Disorders,* 4th edn. Washington, DC: American Psychiatric Association.

Amir, N., Stafford, J., Freshman, M., and Foa, E. B. (1998). Relationship between trauma narratives and trauma pathology. *Journal of Traumatic Stress,* 11(2), 385–92.

Beck, A. T. (1972). *Depression: Causes and Treatment.* Philadelphia: University of Pennsylvania Press.

Beck, A. T. (1976). *Cognitive Therapy and the Emotional Disorders.* New York: International University Press.

Beck, A. T., Rush, A. J., Shaw, B. F., and Emery, G. (1979). *Cognitive Therapy of Depression.* New York: Guilford Press.

Beck, A. T., Emery, G., and Greenberg, R. L. (1985). *Anxiety Disorders and Phobias: A Cognitive Perspective.* New York: Basic Books.

Borkovec, T. D., and Sides, J. K. (1979). The contribution of relaxation and expectancy to fear reduction via graded, imaginal exposure to feared stimuli. *Behaviour Research and Therapy,* 17(6), 529–40.

Bowman, M. L. (1999). Individual differences in posttraumatic distress: problems with the DSM-IV model. *Canadian Journal of Psychiatry,* 44, 21–33.

Bremner, J. D., Southwick, S., Brett, E., et al. (1992). Dissociation and posttraumatic stress disorder in Vietnam combat veterans. *American Journal of Psychiatry,* 149, 328–32.

Breslau, N., Davis, G.C., Andreski, P., and Peterson, E. (1991). Traumatic events and posttraumatic stress disorder in an urban population of young adults. *Archives General Psychiatry,* 48, 218–28.

Burgess, A. W. and Holmstrom, L. L. (1978). Recovery from rape and prior life stress. *Research in Nursing and Health,* 1, 165–74.

Clark, D. M. (1986). A cognitive approach to panic. *Behaviour Research and Therapy,* 24, 461–70.

Cooper, N. A. and Clum, G. A. (1989). Imaginal flooding as a supplementary treatment for PTSD in combat veterans: a controlled study. *Behavior Therapy,* 20, 381–91.

Devilly, G. J. and Foa, E. B. (2001). The investigation of exposure and cognitive therapy: comment on Tarrier et al. (1999). *Journal of Consulting and Clinical Psychology,* 69(1), 114–16.

Ehlers, A. and Clark, D. M. (2000). A cognitive model of persistent posttraumatic stress disorder. *Behavior Research and Therapy,* 38(4), 319–45.

Ellis, A. (1977). The basic clinical theory and rational-emotive therapy. In *Handbook of Rational-emotive Therapy,* ed. A. Ellis and R. Grieger, pp. 3–34. New York: Springer.

Epstein, S. (1991). The self-concept, traumatic neurosis, and the structure of personality. In *Perspectives on Personality,* vol. 3, ed. D. Ozer, J. M. Healy, Jr, and A. J. Stewart, pp. 63–98. London: Jessica Kingsley.

Foa E. B. and Cahill, S. (2000). Specialized treatment for PTSD: matching survivors to the appropriate modality. In *Treating Trauma Survivors with PTSD: Bridging the Gap Between Intervention Research and Practice*, ed. R. Yehuda, pp. 43–62. Washington, DC: American Psychiatric Press.

Foa, E. B. and Jaycox, L. H. (1999). Cognitive-behavioral theory and treatment of post traumatic stress disorder. In *Efficacy and Cost-effectiveness of Psychotherapy*, ed. D. Spiegel, pp. 23–61. Washington, DC: American Psychiatric Press.

Foa, E. B. and Kozak, M. J. (1985). Treatment of anxiety disorders: implications for psychopathology. In *Anxiety and the Anxiety Disorders*, ed. A. H. Tuma and J. D. Maser, pp. 421–52. Hillsdale, NY: Lawrence Erlbaum.

Foa, E. B. and Kozak, M. J. (1986). Emotional processing of fear: exposure to corrective information. *Psychological Bulletin*, **99**, 20–35.

Foa, E. B. and Meadows, E. A. (1997). Psychosocial treatments for post traumatic stress disorder: a critical review. In *Annual Review of Psychology*, ed. J. Spence, J. M. Darley and D. J. Foss, vol. 48, pp. 449–80. Palo Alto, CA: Annual Reviews.

Foa, E. B. and Riggs, D. S. (1993). Post traumatic stress disorder in rape victims. In *American Psychiatric Press Review of Psychiatry*, vol. 12, ed. J. Oldham, M. B. Riba, and A. Tasman, pp. 273–303. Washington, DC: American Psychiatric Press.

Foa, E. B. and Rothbaum, B. O. (1998). *Treating the Trauma of Rape*. New York: Guilford.

Foa, E. B., Steketee, G., and Rothbaum, B. (1989). Behavioral/cognitive conceptualizations of post-traumatic stress disorder. *Behavior Therapy*, **20**, 155–76.

Foa, E. B., Rothbaum, B. O., Riggs, D. S., and Murdock, T. (1991). Treatment of post traumatic stress disorder in rape victims: a comparison between cognitive-behavioral procedures and counseling. *Journal of Consulting and Clinical Psychology*, **59**, 715–23.

Foa, E. B., Molnar, C., and Cashman, L. (1995). Change in rape narratives during exposure therapy for PTSD. *Journal of Traumatic Stress*, **8**(4), 675–90.

Foa, E. B., Ehlers, A., Clark, D., Tolin, D., and Orsillo, S. (1999a). The posttraumatic cognitions inventory (PTCI): development and validation. *Psychological Assessment*, **11**(3), 303–14.

Foa, E. B., Dancu, C. V., Hembree, E. A., et al. (1999b). The efficacy of exposure therapy, stress inoculation training and their combination in ameliorating PTSD for female victims of assault. *Journal of Consulting and Clinical Psychology*, **67**, 194–200.

Foa, E. B., Davidson, J. R. T., and Frances, A. (1999c). The Expert Consensus Guidelines series: treatment of posttraumatic stress disorder. *Journal of Clinical Psychiatry*, **60**(16), 4–76.

Frank, E. and Stewart, B. D. (1984). Depressive symptoms in rape victims. *Journal of Affective Disorders*, **1**, 269–77.

Gilboa-Schechtman, E. and Foa, E. B. (2001). Patterns of recovery after trauma: the use of intraindividual analysis. *Journal of Abnormal Psychology*, **110**(3), 392–400.

Hembree, E. A., Fitzgibbons, L., Marshall, R. D., and Foa, E. B. (2001). The difficult to treat PTSD patient. In *The Difficult to Treat Psychiatric Patient*, ed. M. Dewan, pp. 149–78. New York: APA Press.

Horowitz, M. J. (1986). *Stress Response Syndromes*, 2nd edn. Northvale, NJ: Jason Aronson.

Janoff-Bulman, R. (1992). *Shattered Assumptions: Towards a New Psychology of Trauma*. New York: The Free Press.

Jaycox, L. H., Foa, E. B., Morral, A. R., et al. (1998). The influence of emotional engagement and habituation on exposure therapy for PTSD. *Journal of Consulting and Clinical Psychology*, **66**(1), 185–92.

Keane, T. M., Fairbank, J. A., Caddell, J. M., Zimering, R. T., and Bender, M. E. (1985). A behavioral approach to assessing and treating post traumatic stress disorder in Vietnam veterans. In *Trauma and its Wake*, ed. C. R. Figley, pp. 225–94. New York: Brunner/Mazel.

Keane, T. M., Fairbank, J. A., Caddell, J. M., and Zimering, R. T. (1989). Implosive (flooding) therapy reduces symptoms of PTSD in Vietnam combat veterans. *Behavior Therapy*, **20**, 245–60.

Kilpatrick, D. G., Best, C. L., Veronen, L. J., et al. (1985). Mental health correlates of criminal victimization: a random community survey. *Journal of Consulting and Clinical Psychology*, **53**, 866–73.

Koopman, C., Classen, C., and Spiegel, D. A. (1994). Predictors of posttraumatic stress symptoms among survivors of the Oakland/Berkeley, California, firestorm. *American Journal of Psychiatry*, **151**, 888–94.

Kulka, R. A., Schlenger, W. E., Fairbank, J. A., et al. (1990). *Trauma and the Vietnam War Generation*. New York, NY: Brunner/Mazel.

Lang, P. J. (1977). Imagery in therapy: an information processing analysis of fear. *Behavior Therapy*, **8**, 862–86.

Lang, P. J. (1979). A bio-informational theory of emotional imagery. *Psychophysiology*, **6**, 495–511.

Marks, I., Lovell, K., Noshirvani, H., Livanou, M., and Thrasher, S. (1998). Treatment of posttraumatic stress disorder by exposure and/or cognitive restructuring. *Archives of General Psychiatry*, **55**, 317–25.

Marmar, C. R., Weiss, D. S., Schlenger, W. E., et al. (1994). Peritraumatic dissociation and posttraumatic stress in male Vietnam theater veterans. *American Journal of Psychiatry*, **151**, 902–7.

McCann, I. L. and Pearlman, L. A. (1990). *Psychological Trauma and the Adult Survivor: Theory, Therapy and Transformation*. New York: Brunner/Mazel.

McCann, I. L., Sakheim, D. K., and Abrahamson, D. J. (1988). Trauma and victimization: a model of psychological adaptation. *Counseling Psychologist*, **16**, 531–94.

Meichenbaum, D. (1974). *Cognitive Behavior Modification*. Morristown, NJ: General Learning Press.

Mikulincer, M. and Solomon, Z. (1988). Attributional style and related posttraumatic stress disorder. *Journal of Abnormal Psychology*, **97**, 308–13.

Perloff, L. S. (1983). Perceptions of vulnerability to victimization. *Journal of Social Issues*, **39**, 41–61.

Rachman, S. (1980). Emotional processing. *Behaviour Research and Therapy*, **18**, 51–60.

Resick, P. A. (1987). The impact of rape on psychological functioning. Unpublished manuscript, University of Missouri-St. Louis.

Resick, P. A. and Schnicke, M. K. (1992). Cognitive processing therapy for sexual assault victims. *Journal of Consulting and Clinical Psychology*, **60**, 748–56.

Resick, P. A. and Schnicke, M. K. (1993). *Cognitive Processing Therapy for Rape Victims: A Treatment Manual*. Thousand Oaks, CA: US: Sage.

Resick, P. A., Nishith, P., Weaver, T. L., Astin, M. C., and Feuer, C. A. (2002). A comparison of cognitive processing therapy, prolonged exposure, and a waiting condition for the treatment of posttraumatic stress disorder in female rape victims. *Journal of Consulting and Clinical Psychology*, **70**(4), 867–79.

Resnick, H. S., Kilpatrick, D. G., Dansky, B. S., Saunders, B. E., and Best, C. L. (1993). Prevalence of civilian trauma and posttraumatic stress disorder in a representative national sample of women. *Journal of Consulting and Clinical Psychology*, **61**(6), 984–91.

Rothbaum, B. O., Foa, E. B., Riggs, D. S., Murdock, T., and Walsh, W. (1992). A prospective examination of post traumatic stress disorder in rape victims. *Journal of Traumatic Stress*, **5**, 455–75.

Rothbaum, B. O., Meadows, E. A., Resick, P., and Foy, D. W. (2000). Cognitive-behavioral therapy. In *Effective Treatments for PTSD: Practice Guidelines from the International Society for Traumatic Stress Studies*, ed. E. B. Foa, T. M. Keane, and M. Friedman, pp. 60–83. New York, NY: Guilford Press.

Tarrier, N. and Humphreys, L. (2000). Subjective improvement in PTSD patients with treatment by imaginal exposure or cognitive therapy: session by session changes. *British Journal of Clinical Psychology*, **39**, 27–34.

Tarrier, N., Pilgrim, H., Sommerfield, C., et al. (1999). A randomized trial of cognitive therapy and imaginal exposure in the treatment of chronic posttraumatic stress disorder. *Journal of Consulting and Clinical Psychology*, **67**, 8–13.

Taylor, S. and Koch, W. J. (1995). Anxiety disorders due to motor vehicle accidents: nature and treatment. *Clinical Psychology Review*, **15**(8), 721–38.

Veronen, L. J. and Kilpatrick, D. G. (1993). Stress management for rape victims. In *Stress Reduction and Prevention*, ed. D. Meichenbaum and M. E. Jaremko, pp. 341–74. Boulder, CO: Perseus.

11

Cognitive theory and therapy of social phobia

Judith K. Wilson and Ronald M. Rapee

Macquarie University, Sydney, NSW, Australia

Introduction

Social phobia (social anxiety disorder) is defined in the *Diagnostic and Statistical Manual of Mental Disorders*, – fourth edition (DSM-IV; American Psychiatric Association, 1994) as "a marked and persistent fear of one or more social or performance situations in which the person is exposed to unfamiliar people or to possible scrutiny by others. The individual fears that he or she will act in a way (or show anxiety symptoms) that will be humiliating or embarrassing" (p. 416). Situations which people with social phobia commonly fear include public speaking, interacting with unfamiliar people, social gatherings such as parties, meetings, speaking to authority figures and situations requiring assertive behavior (Rapee, 1995). Fears may encompass most social situations (generalized social phobia), or may be restricted to one or a few social or performance situations (nongeneralized social phobia) (American Psychiatric Association, 1994). Regardless of the range of feared situations, social phobia is only diagnosed when fears result in significant functional impairment or marked distress (American Psychiatric Association, 1994).

Research indicates that the onset of social phobia frequently occurs during childhood or adolescence (Schneier et al., 1992), and suggests that the disorder tends to follow a chronic, stable course (Solyom et al., 1986). The anxiety and avoidance associated with social phobia can lead to considerable impairment in many aspects of life functioning, including education, employment, interpersonal relationships, and recreational interests (Schneier et al., 1994). Furthermore, research indicates that social phobia is associated with an increased risk of developing comorbid psychiatric disorders, particularly other anxiety disorders, mood disorders such as major depression, and substance use disorders (Schneier et al., 1992; Magee et al., 1996; Regier et al., 1998; Kessler et al., 1999). In view of epidemiological evidence from the USA which indicates that the lifetime prevalence of social phobia in the population may be as high as 13.3% (Kessler et al., 1994), it is evident that the nature and treatment of the disorder are issues of considerable concern.

The research literature regarding social phobia has indeed facilitated a greater understanding of the disorder, leading to significant advances in theory and treatment. Evidence concerning symptomatology indicates that actual or anticipated entry into feared social situations may elicit considerable anxious affect in people with social phobia, including physiological symptoms such as sweating, trembling, blushing, heart palpitations, and nausea (Amies et al., 1983). The typical behavioral manifestation of social phobia is avoidance, which may range from subtle strategies designed to prevent attention being drawn to oneself during social encounters (such as reduced verbal output or avoiding eye contact during interactions), to avoiding feared social situations altogether (Rapee and Heimberg, 1997). Cognitive features of social phobia include a high frequency of negative self-evaluative thoughts during social situations (Stopa and Clark, 1993). The specific fears associated with social situations vary between individuals, with typical examples including fears of blushing or shaking in front of other people, being unable to think of anything interesting to say, or making a mistake (Heckelman and Schneier, 1995). However, such specific fears are thought to represent a general underlying fear considered to be a central feature of social phobia: namely, a fear of being evaluated negatively by other people (Butler, 1985).

Fear of negative evaluation by other people essentially represents a cognitive construct, as it is assumed to reflect the thoughts and beliefs which people with social phobia hold in relation to social situations (Elting and Hope, 1995). Although the specific genetic and/or environmental origins of the types of thoughts and beliefs that underlie the disorder may vary between individuals (see Hudson and Rapee, 2000 for a recent review of etiological factors), cognitive theory and research provide a unifying framework for the understanding and treatment of social phobia. The aim of the present chapter is to examine the status of current knowledge regarding the cognitive aspects of social phobia, by reviewing contemporary cognitive models, their contribution to current clinical practice, and relevant empirical evidence concerning the nature and treatment of social phobia.

History of cognitive models

Social phobia was first included as a separate diagnostic category in the third edition of the *Diagnostic and Statistical Manual of Mental Disorders* in 1980 (DSM-III; American Psychiatric Association, 1980). Therefore, research regarding the disorder as defined by these specific diagnostic criteria did not commence until after this time. Theoretical conceptualizations of social phobia have thus been informed to a large extent by research regarding related constructs such as shyness, heterosocial anxiety, communication apprehension, stage fright, speech anxiety, and subclinical social anxiety (Leary and Kowalski, 1995a). Such constructs are generally considered to be qualitatively similar to social phobia, differing primarily in severity and the extent of associated impairment (Rapee, 1995). Around the time that social phobia was introduced into the DSM-III, prevailing theoretical perspectives regarding the source and treatment of social anxiety reflected: (1) a classical conditioning approach, which proposed that social anxiety may develop as a result of a traumatic conditioning episode in which social stimuli were associated with an aversive event; (2) a social skills deficit approach, which suggested that social anxiety was a consequence of undesirable social experiences resulting from an inadequate repertoire of social skills; or (3) a cognitive approach, which assumed that dysfunctional beliefs and maladaptive thought processes mediated social anxiety (Leary, 1983). Treatment approaches suggested by these different models ranged from relaxation and systematic desensitization (based on the classical conditioning perspective) to social skills training (based on the skills deficit view) and modification of cognitive distortions (based on the cognitive approach) (Leary, 1983).

Although evidence at the time suggested that each of the three treatment approaches may be effective in reducing social anxiety (Leary, 1983), cognitive theories seemed to provide a more comprehensive account of social anxiety than did the classical conditioning or skills deficit approaches. As Leary (1983) asserts, both the classical conditioning and skills deficit models may be accounted for by the cognitive approach, by assuming that cognitive factors mediate the development of social anxiety through classical conditioning episodes or skills deficits, as well as the gains achieved through treatment based on these models. Moreover, research has indicated that neither classical conditioning episodes nor a lack of social skills seem to be necessary or sufficient factors in accounting for the development of excessive social anxiety (Leary, 1983; Stemberger et al., 1995). Cognitive theories have thus gained prominence in terms of understanding the nature and treatment of social phobia, and have generated a burgeoning research literature in the area.

Current cognitive models of social phobia

One of the most prominent and enduring cognitive models of social anxiety is the "self-presentation" theory, proposed by Schlenker and Leary (1982). According to this view, social anxiety will be experienced when an individual is: (1) motivated to make a particular impression on other people; and (2) doubts that he or she will be successful in making this impression. Prior to this model, cognitive views had emphasized the role of specific factors such as negative self-evaluations, irrational beliefs regarding the importance of gaining approval from others, or excessively high standards for social performance in producing social anxiety (Leary, 1983). Such views did not, however, provide an adequate explanation of why such factors should produce anxiety in social situations (Leary, 1983; Leary and Kowalski, 1995b). By emphasizing the role of performance expectancies *in relation to* interpersonal goals, the self-presentation approach provides a more comprehensive understanding of the factors which underlie social anxiety.

Other contemporary cognitive models of social phobia draw from and expand upon the self-presentation approach, as well as more general cognitive theories of anxiety (Beck et al., 1985; Carver and Scheier, 1988). One model proposed by Clark and Wells (1995) provides a comprehensive account of the cognitive processes which serve to produce and maintain anxiety in social situations. According to this theory, individuals with social phobia hold a number of maladaptive assumptions regarding themselves and their social world (presumably developed through learning experiences and genetic factors), which are activated when social situations are encountered. These assumptions may include excessively high standards for evaluating one's social performance, "conditional beliefs" regarding social evaluation (e.g., the belief that making a mistake will result in rejection by others), and/or negative global beliefs about oneself (e.g., the belief that one is inadequate). Activation of these assumptions results in a perception of danger in social situations, with this perceived danger relating to the possibility of behaving in an incompetent or unacceptable manner, and the belief that serious interpersonal consequences will ensue from such behavior. In the Clark and Wells (1995) model, this appraisal of danger automatically triggers the cognitive, affective, somatic, and behavioral manifestations of an "anxiety program." These symptoms are interpreted as further sources of danger, and thus serve to maintain or exacerbate anxiety in a social situation.

The model proposed by Clark and Wells (1995) places particular emphasis on the role of several processes which maintain social anxiety by preventing the disconfirmation of negative beliefs held by individuals with social phobia regarding the probability and cost of negative evaluation by other people. For instance, they suggest that the appraisal of danger in social situations results in individuals shifting attentional focus toward themselves, becoming preoccupied with the physical sensations associated with anxiety and negative social-evaluative thoughts. This self-focus heightens awareness of interoceptive information, which is then used by the individual to construct an impression of how he or she is perceived by others. Furthermore, excessive self-focus is assumed to impede the ability to process cues in the external social environment, such that objective evidence which is inconsistent with the negative impressions of performance based on interoceptive cues is not considered. In addition, Clark and Wells (1995) propose that "in-situation safety behaviors," or actions aimed toward decreasing the likelihood of feared social outcomes (e.g., gripping one's drinking glass tightly so trembling will not be evident to others), may contribute to the maintenance of social anxiety in several ways: (1) by exacerbating symptoms (e.g., a tight grip on one's glass may increase trembling); (2) by interfering with effective social performance (e.g., one may seem to behave in a less sociable manner due to avoiding self-disclosure or eye contact), which may, in turn, elicit less positive reactions from other people; and (3) nonoccurrence of the feared outcome may be attributed to the use of the safety behavior, thus preventing disconfirmation of unhelpful beliefs concerning negative evaluation. Finally, Clark and Wells (1995) suggest that individuals with social phobia tend to engage in detailed reviews or "postmortems" following social events. Because extensive processing of negative self-images during social encounters may result in such images being strongly encoded in memory, such "postmortems" are likely to be dominated by negative self-evaluations, thus consolidating negative beliefs and contributing to the maintenance of anxiety.

A further cognitive theory of social phobia proposed in recent years by Rapee and Heimberg (1997) emphasizes similar mechanisms to those included in the Clark and Wells (1995) model. According to this model, the perception of an audience during real or anticipated interpersonal encounters activates two simultaneous processes in socially anxious individuals: first, the formation of a mental representation of how they believe they appear to the audience; and second, the preferential allocation of attentional resources to this mental representation, as well as to perceived indicators of negative evaluation in the external social environment. The notion that attention is directed toward an image of how one is viewed by others *as well as* to threat-related cues in the external environment is a distinguishing feature of the Rapee and Heimberg (1997) model, given that other theories (Clark and Wells, 1995) have primarily emphasized the role of self-directed attention in generating and maintaining social anxiety (see below for further discussion of this issue). According to the Rapee and Heimberg (1997) model, the mental representation of one's external appearance is based on a number of sources of information (e.g., images in long-term memory from photographs and mirrors, interoceptive cues, and external feedback), and may vary during the course of the social encounter according to which inputs are most salient at a given time. The subjective nature of these mental representations of the self as seen by the audience makes them prone to distortion, and, given the presumed tendency for socially anxious individuals to focus their attention toward potential indicators of threat, it is likely that the image such individuals construct is negatively biased.

In addition to forming the "mental representation of self" described above, Rapee and Heimberg (1997) suggest that individuals make a judgment concerning the standard of performance expected by the audience in social situations. A crucial aspect of the model involves a comparison by the individual between the mental representation of external appearance and behavior with the appraisal of the standard of performance expected by the audience. The outcome of this comparison is presumed to lead to judgments concerning the probability and consequences of negative evaluation from the audience. Thus, the greater the discrepancy between the individual's mental image of performance and the estimated standards of the audience, the greater the perceived likelihood of negative evaluation from the audience, and the greater the consideration of the social consequences of this anticipated unfavorable evaluation. In this way, the model is a direct extension of self-presentation theory. The expectation of being negatively evaluated, in turn, is proposed to lead to the behavioral, cognitive, and physical components of anxiety. These manifestations of anxiety are assumed to feed back into the individual's mental representation of performance, adversely affecting this internal image and renewing the cycle of anxiety. In a similar fashion to the model of Clark and Wells (1995), Rapee and Heimberg (1997) suggest that the behavioral manifestations of social anxiety will include subtle avoidance (the type of "safety behaviors" described previously) that may be interpreted by an audience as a lack of social skills, thus potentially eliciting negative feedback and further contributing to the maintenance and possible intensification of anxiety.

Summary of main features of current cognitive models of social phobia

Consideration of current cognitive theories regarding social phobia indicates that there are a number of primary cognitive features thought to be associated with the development and maintenance of anxiety in social situations. First, a common feature of current conceptualizations of social phobia is the notion that, in anticipated or actual interpersonal situations, socially anxious individuals construct a negatively biased image of how they assume other people see them. Second, cognitive models generally assume that socially anxious individuals selectively orient their attention toward the concepts of danger or threat in a social situation. In particular, it is assumed that this attentional bias involves excessive focus on the self, as socially anxious individuals tend to monitor closely aspects of themselves which may impede social performance and hence elicit negative evaluation. The issue of whether this preferential attentional allocation also applies to external threat cues in the social situation (as proposed in the Rapee and Heimberg (1997) model) is a source of debate, with some authors (e.g., Clark and Wells, 1995) suggesting that social anxiety may be characterized by a nonselective impairment in processing of cues in the external social environment. The third important feature of current cognitive models is the notion that social phobia involves a discrepancy between a standard appraised as being necessary for one's social performance to be judged as adequate by other people, and one's perceived ability to meet that standard, resulting in increased estimates of the probability of negative evaluation from others.

Fourth, it is assumed that social anxiety is associated with a strong motivation for one's social performance to be perceived favorably by others, and hence involves overestimations of the cost of negative evaluation by other people. Finally, cognitive theories assume that social anxiety becomes a negative self-perpetuating cycle, in which physiological, cognitive, and behavioral symptoms are given processing priority and interpreted as further indications of inadequate social performance, thus contributing to the maintenance or exacerbation of anxiety in social situations. Further, the information-processing mechanisms discussed here are thought to be protected by behavioral manifestations of social anxiety, hence maintaining the cycle. The empirical evidence for each of these elements of cognitive theories of social anxiety is considered below.

Empirical evidence

Mental representation of self

The notion that people with social phobia form an impression or image of themselves as they believe they appear to others in social situations has been supported by a number of recent studies. Hackmann et al. (1998), for instance, found that social phobics, when asked to rate retrospectively anxiety-provoking social situations, reported a greater frequency of images than did nonpatient controls, and furthermore, differed from controls in terms of the perspective from which the image was viewed. Specifically, it was found that social phobics were significantly more likely to report viewing images from an "observer perspective" (observing oneself as if from an external point of view) than controls, with the latter group tending to view images more from a "field perspective" (as if looking out through one's own eyes). A similar study by Wells and Papageorgiou (1999) found that social phobics reported experiencing images in anxiety-provoking social situations from an observer perspective to a significantly greater degree than did blood-injury phobics, agoraphobics, and nonpatient controls. Moreover, research suggests that the tendency of people with social phobia to view images from an observer perspective is specific to social situations, with two studies finding that social phobics were just as likely as nonpatient controls to report experiencing images from a field perspective during neutral (nonsocial) situations (Wells et al., 1998; Wells and Papageorgiou, 1999).

Research regarding the content of social phobics' impressions of themselves as seen by others supports the notion that such impressions are negatively biased. Hackmann et al. (1998), for example, found that the images and impressions experienced by social phobics during anxiety-provoking social interactions were more negative than those of nonpatient controls. In addition, a number of studies have shown that independent observers rate social phobics' performance in social situations significantly more favorably than social phobics rate their own performance, and the tendency to underestimate markedly their social performance differentiates social phobics from both nonclinical controls and patients with other anxiety disorders (Rapee and Lim, 1992; Stopa and Clark, 1993). Furthermore, evidence indicating that socially anxious individuals underestimate their physical attractiveness relative to judges' ratings (R. M. Rapee and K. J. Young, unpublished data), and appraise their personal attributes in a more negative manner than do nonanxious individuals (Mansell and Clark, 1999), suggests that an underlying global negative self-image may contribute to unfavorable perceptions relating to how they are seen by others. Taken in combination, these studies support the view that negatively biased representations regarding how one is seen by others may be an important factor in social phobia.

Attention

There exists a growing body of evidence indicating that social anxiety is associated with maladaptive attentional processes. In particular, empirical research suggests that excessive self-focused attention may be an important factor in social anxiety. A number of studies, for instance, have shown that higher scores on self-reported measures of self-focused attention during a social interaction are associated with more negative biases in self versus observer ratings of behavior (Mellings and Alden, 2000), as well as increased levels of social anxiety (Melchior and Cheek, 1990; Hope et al., 1990a). In addition, research (Hope and Heimberg, 1988) has shown that trait social anxiety correlates positively with public self-consciousness (dispositional awareness of oneself as a social object; see Fenigstein et al., 1975), and that social phobics obtain significantly higher scores on a measure of public self-consciousness than do other clinical groups or nonpatient controls (Jostes et al., 1999). Evidence concerning the relationship between social anxiety and private self-consciousness (general awareness of inner thoughts and feelings) has been less consistent, suggesting that this construct may be of less importance in the understanding of social phobia (Hope and Heimberg, 1988). Furthermore, although several mood induction studies suggest that negative affect in general may induce a state of self-focus (Wood et al., 1990; Salovey, 1992), a causal role of increased self-focused attention in exacerbating social anxiety has also been demonstrated empirically (Woody, 1996). According to the theories of social anxiety described above, a primary mechanism by which increased self-directed attention may contribute to anxiety in social situations is via a heightened focus upon a negative mental representation of the self as seen by others, thus contributing to unfavorable views of one's performance and increasing the perceived likelihood of failing to meet the audience's expected standard (Rapee and Heimberg, 1997). Increased self-focused attention may further contribute to negative mental representations of performance and consequent increases in anxiety due to reduced attentional resources being available for information relevant to successful task execution, thus leading to actual performance deficits (Rapee and Heimberg, 1997). Consistent with these theoretical views is evidence suggesting that increased self-focused attention contributes to an increase in negative thoughts, and a decrease in positive thoughts associated with social interactions (Burgio et al., 1986), as well as evidence showing that increased self-focus may, in some cases, lead to performance deficits in evaluative situations (Wine, 1971; Liebling and Shaver, 1973). Taken in combination, therefore, these results are consistent with the idea that the allocation of attentional resources toward the self, particularly as the individual believes he or she is being perceived by others, is an important factor in the maintenance of social anxiety.

As noted previously, the question of whether increased self-directed attention in socially anxious individuals is accompanied by excessive monitoring of threat cues in the external social environment, or nonselective impairment of processing of environmental stimuli, is a source of debate. Numerous research paradigms have been employed in an attempt to answer this question. One such paradigm is the modified Stroop task, in which subjects are presented with words printed in different colors, and are required to name the color in which the word is printed as quickly and accurately as possible, whilst ignoring the word's meaning (Stroop, 1935). Longer response latencies in naming the color in which words are printed is generally thought to reflect greater difficulty in directing attention away from the semantic content of the word. A number of studies using this methodology have demonstrated that social phobics differ from nonpatient controls and panic disorder patients by exhibiting greater interference in color-naming words denoting social-evaluative threat (e.g., foolish) versus words denoting physical threat or neutral concepts (Hope et al., 1990b; Mattia et al., 1993; McNeil et al., 1995; Lundh and Ost, 1996; Maidenberg et al., 1996). Comparable results have also been obtained in a study by Asmundson and Stein (1994) using a visual dot probe paradigm. In this study, neutral words and words denoting either physical or social threat were briefly presented (500 ms) in pairs on a computer screen, followed by a small dot in the location of one of the words. Subjects were required to read whichever word appeared in the uppermost position, and then to respond to the dot probe as quickly as possible by pressing a button. Results showed that social phobics were faster to respond to dot probes following social threat words than to probes following physical threat or neutral words, when attention had been initially directed toward the words (by the subject reading them aloud). Nonpatient controls showed no difference in response latencies to probes following the three different stimulus types. These results, in conjunction with the aforementioned evidence from modified Stroop tasks, have generally been interpreted as an indication that social phobics allocate greater attentional resources to information related to social threat than individuals without the disorder.

A number of recent studies, however, suggest that the interpretation of such results is less than conclusive. In particular, the interpretation of studies such as those cited above has been questioned due to the use of verbal stimuli to represent social threat, rather than stimuli which may be more directly relevant in social-evaluative settings, such as facial expressions. As Clark and Wells (1995) assert, it may be that an attentional bias towards social-threat words in socially anxious individuals may reflect a preoccupation with negative self-evaluative thoughts, rather than hypervigilance for potentially threatening cues in the external social environment. Investigations that have employed more realistic social-threat stimuli in order to examine attention to external cues in socially anxious individuals have produced discrepant results. One study employing reaction times to visual dot probes following pictures of faces depicting different emotional expressions, for instance, found no difference between high and low socially anxious subjects in attention for emotional (happy or aggressive) versus neutral faces (Bradley et al., 1997), while another found that subjects high in fear of negative evaluation acutally directed attention away from negative faces relative to neutral faces, while subjects low in fear of negative evaluation did not show this effect (Yuen, 1994, cited in Mansell et al., 1999). A similar recent study by Mansell et al. (1999) suggests that these discrepant results may be explained by an important methodological difference – namely, state anxiety being induced prior to the experimental task by the threat of an upcoming social-evaluative situation in the latter study, but not in the former. In the Mansell et al. (1999) study (which also employed visual dot probes following pictures of faces), high socially anxious subjects demonstrated an attentional bias away from faces depicting either positive or negative expressions compared to low socially anxious subjects, although this effect only occurred when anxiety was induced by telling subjects that they would have to give a speech. However, given preliminary evidence from another study that socially anxious individuals may be characterized by automatic hypervigilance for information relevant to social-threat at short stimulus durations, followed by strategic avoidance of such information at longer durations (Amir et al., 1998a), conclusive evidence of reduced attention toward external social-evaluative cues in socially anxious individuals would require studies employing shorter stimulus durations than have been used in the studies reported above (Mansell et al., 1999).

Although it is not clear as to whether social anxiety is characterized by the spontaneous allocation of attentional resources to external threat cues, a recent study by Veljaca and Rapee (1998) indicates that when socially anxious individuals' attention is specifically directed toward others' reactions, it is likely to be directed toward the detection of negative evaluative cues. In this study, subjects were required to give a speech in front of a small audience, and to indicate when they detected positive or negative audience reactions. Results indicated that high socially anxious subjects detected significantly more negative reactions and significantly fewer positive reactions that did subjects low in social anxiety. In addition, the Veljaca and Rapee (1998) study, in combination with a number of other investigations (Winton et al., 1995; Amir et al., 1998b; Constans et al., 1999; Stopa and Clark, 2000), suggests that socially anxious individuals are characterized by a tendency to interpret social information in a more negative manner than nonanxious individuals or patients with other anxiety disorders. Thus, overall, the evidence supports the view that social anxiety may involve maladaptive processing in relation to the external environment.

Performance-standard discrepancies and estimates regarding the probability of negative evaluation

As noted above, a central feature of many cognitive models of social anxiety is the idea that the degree of anxiety experienced in a social situation is positively related to the extent to which individuals perceive their actual or anticipated performance to fall short of a performance standard they believe is required in order to make a desired impression on other people. Thus, it is assumed that anxiety arises when one believes that other people's performance expectations exceed one's performance ability in social encounters. Evidence in support of this notion includes a study by Baumgardner and Brownlee (1987), who found in an unselected sample that subjects' anxiety levels were more pronounced when they believed that other people held high expectations of them in a social-evaluative situation, as compared to when they believed others' expectations were low, but this difference only held when they were not confident of their ability to meet these high expectations. Similarly, Maddux et al. (1988) found that social anxiety correlated positively with the extent to which individuals doubted their ability to perform specific interpersonal behaviors required in problematic social situations. Research comparing clinical and subclinical socially anxious populations with nonanxious controls has yielded comparable results, showing that socially anxious individuals' estimations of the standard expected of them by other people in social situations significantly exceed their ratings of their own social performance abilities, whereas nonanxious control subjects judge their social ability to be equivalent to others' expectations (Wallace and Alden, 1991, 1997). The notion that the critical factor underlying social anxiety is a perceived inability to meet other people's standards for performance, rather than one's own standards, is also supported by the finding that socially anxious individuals' ratings of their social abilities do not differ significantly from their ratings of personal standards for performance (Strauman, 1989; Wallace and Alden, 1991).

Research concerning the source of the perceived discrepancy between social performance ability and others' standards in socially anxious individuals suggests that this discrepancy may arise primarily from negative self-judgments regarding competence levels, rather than from excessively high estimates of other people's performance expectations. For instance, several studies have shown that ratings of personal social capabilities are significantly lower in socially anxious populations compared to nonanxious controls, while these groups do not differ in their predictions of the performance standard expected by other people in a social interaction (Wallace and Alden, 1991, 1997; Alden et al., 1994). Notwithstanding these results, it is possible that overestimations of others' social performance standards may contribute to anxiety in a subset of individuals with social phobia (Bieling and Alden, 1997). It is also interesting to note that positive feedback from other people during social interactions does not appear to influence socially anxious individuals' judgments of their social ability, but instead seems to be interpreted as an indication that others will have higher expectations of them during future interactions (Wallace and Alden, 1995, 1997). Given that this occurrence has been found to increase the perceived discrepancy between performance ability and others' expectations (Wallace and Alden, 1997), it is perhaps not surprising to find evidence indicating that when socially anxious individuals perceive others' performance expectations to be high, they may engage in strategic attempts to lower these expectations at the outset of social interactions when further evaluation is anticipated (Baumgardner and Brownlee, 1987).

It seems logical to assume that a perceived inability to convey an impression in social situations which meets others' performance standards may contribute to social anxiety by increasing individuals' estimations of the probability of negative evaluation by other people. Indeed, there are several studies which show that socially anxious individuals estimate the occurrence of negative social events to be more likely than do nonanxious controls, whereas both groups give similar ratings regarding the probability of negative nonsocial events (Teglasi and Fagin, 1984; Lucock and Salkovskis, 1988; Foa et al., 1996). Furthermore, Smari et al. (1998) found a significant negative correlation between self-reported social skills and the expectancy of negative social events, consistent with the notion that unfavorable judgments concerning one's social abilities may at least partially underlie increased estimates of the likelihood of negative social outcomes in individuals who are socially anxious.

Appraisals of the consequences of negative evaluation

A critical assumption of cognitive models of social anxiety is that a high estimation of the likelihood of negative evaluation by others will only produce anxiety in social encounters to the extent that it is accompanied by a strong motivation to convey more favorable impressions to other people. It is therefore presumed that socially anxious individuals attach considerable importance to being evaluated in a positive manner by other people (or at least, to avoiding negative evaluation by others). Indeed, research has consistently demonstrated a strong positive association between social anxiety and fear of negative evaluation (Watson and Friend, 1969; Jones et al., 1986), and furthermore, a decrease in fear of negative evaluation has been found to be a primary mediator of treatment-related improvements in social phobia (Mattick and Peters, 1988; Mattick et al., 1989). Similarly, research has shown that social anxiety is positively associated with estimates of the cost of negative social occurrences (the degree to which such events are considered aversive) (Smari et al., 1998), and has also demonstrated that social phobics judge the occurrence of negative social events to be significantly more costly than do nonanxious controls (Foa et al., 1996). This type of judgmental bias does not apply to nonsocial events (Foa et al., 1996). Moreover, the Foa et al. (1996) study found that decreases in social anxiety following treatment were mediated by reductions in estimates of the cost, rather than the probability, of negative social events, thus providing further evidence that judgmental biases regarding the consequences of negative social events are central to the understanding of social phobia.

Despite the widespread recognition that fear of negative evaluation is central to the understanding of social phobia, the question of why socially anxious individuals attach greater importance to others' evaluations of them has remained largely unanswered. There have been very few investigations concerning either the factors which contribute to exaggerated estimates of the cost of negative evaluation by others in socially anxious individuals, or the specific nature of the consequences which they attach to negative evaluation. Evidence which is available regarding the meaning which individuals attribute to negative evaluation, however, suggests that socially anxious individuals tend to interpret negative social occurrences in a catastrophic fashion. A recent study by Stopa and Clark (2000), for instance, compared social phobics with nonpatient controls and patients with other anxiety disorders in terms of their interpretations of mildly negative social events (e.g., "You've been talking to someone for a while and it becomes clear that they're not really interested in what you're saying"). Their results indicated that social phobics were significantly more likely than the other groups to interpret such events as an indication of negative self-characteristics (e.g., I was boring) and/or as having adverse implications for their future (e.g., I will lose all my friends). This is consistent with evidence from attributional studies, which have shown that social anxiety is associated with a reversal of the "self-serving bias" in terms of the way that individuals account for success or failure in various situations (Hope et al., 1989). Thus, while nonanxious individuals tend to explain success in terms of internal characteristics and blame failure on external factors, socially anxious individuals tend to show the reverse pattern of attributions. It is important to note, however, that the attributional style shown by socially anxious individuals is associated with a range of other forms of psychopathology (most notably depression; Seligman et al., 1979), such that the degree to which social phobics' interpretations of negative evaluation by others are specific to the disorder is difficult to ascertain.

The factors which may contribute to socially anxious individuals' tendency to overestimate the cost associated with negative evaluation by others remain largely conjectural at this stage, given the paucity of research relating to this issue. However, there are several findings documented in the empirical literature that may be potentially relevant. One such finding is that people in general, regardless of dispositional levels of social anxiety, are more likely to experience anxiety in social-evaluative situations in which the other people present are regarded as attractive, competent, or powerful (Leary and Kowalski, 1995a). This is presumed to occur for two primary reasons: (1) because people generally attach greater value to the evaluations of high-status individuals, and perceive them as mediating access to both positive and negative outcomes, thus resulting in greater motivation to make a positive impression on such individuals; and (2) because high-status individuals may be perceived as holding higher standards for social performance, resulting in less confidence in one's ability to impress them (Leary and Kowalski, 1995a). In other words, an individual's estimates of both the cost and probability of negative evaluation are presumed to increase as the perceived status of other people in a social situation increases. One question which may arise from this finding is whether individuals high in trait social anxiety tend to focus to a greater degree than nonanxious individuals on the attributes of other people (particularly potential evaluators) which are indicative of expertise or social power. Given the aforementioned evidence that socially anxious individuals do not differ from nonanxious individuals in their judgments concerning others' performance standards, it is possible that such an information-processing bias in relation to other people may contribute to overestimations of the cost of negative evaluation. Indeed, there is some evidence to suggest that, in comparison to nonanxious individuals, socially anxious individuals may appraise other people in social situations in a more positive manner (Alden and Wallace, 1995), and tend to focus more on high-status members of an audience (Seta and Seta, 1996). However, given that other studies have shown no difference between individuals with social phobia and nonclinical controls in terms of their appraisals of other people (Rapee and Lim, 1992; Stopa and Clark, 1993), an alternative possibility is that the size of the perceived discrepancy between others' versus one's own status or expertise may be an important factor underlying increased estimates of the cost of negative evaluation in socially anxious individuals. Thus, if socially anxious individuals are more likely than nonanxious individuals to perceive other people's opinions as having greater validity or authority than their own, they may be more vulnerable to interpreting negative evaluation by others as being a "true" or "correct" assessment of the self, and thus incorporate such adverse information into the self-concept. Similarly, if socially anxious individuals are more likely than nonanxious individuals to perceive other people's power to be greater than their own in terms of the ability to mediate access to both positive and negative outcomes, negative evaluation by others may be interpreted as having more adverse implications for the future, as valued outcomes will be seen as less accessible, and unfavorable outcomes as being more likely. Indeed, research using Levenson's (1973) Locus of Control Scale has shown that social phobics tend to attribute control over events less to internal resources, and more to "powerful others" than do nonanxious subjects (Cloitre et al., 1992; Leung and Heimberg, 1996). However, the relevance of such findings to estimations of the cost of negative evaluation in socially anxious individuals is yet to be demonstrated.

Symptoms of social anxiety

The perception that negative evaluation by other people is likely, and may have serious consequences, is generally thought to underlie a state of anxiety in social situations. As noted above, anxiety is comprised of cognitive components (e.g., negative thoughts concerning one's performance), subtle avoidance or "safety" behaviors (e.g., avoiding eye contact with others), and physiological/affective symptoms (e.g., blushing, trembling, sweating, increased heart rate, subjective feelings of discomfort), all of which are assumed to maintain and potentially exacerbate anxiety in social situations by serving as further direct or indirect sources of negative input into one's mental representation of the image one is conveying to other people.

The self-perpetuating nature of social anxiety is supported by research examining the contribution of physiological sensations and safety behaviors to negative self-images and appraisals of danger in social situations. Arntz et al. (1995), for instance, found that social phobics (as well as patients with other anxiety disorders) were influenced by objective danger information as well as by information concerning personal anxiety response when rating the degree of danger associated with a situation, whereas nonpatient controls were influenced only by objective danger information. In addition, McEwan and Devins (1983) found that high socially anxious individuals who experienced elevated somatic symptoms overestimated their behavioral signs of anxiety when self-ratings were compared to ratings of subjects made by peers, whereas low socially anxious individuals showed no such overestimation. Similarly, a recent study by Mulkens et al. (1999) found that women with a high fear of blushing gave higher ratings than women low in fear of blushing to their blush intensity when exposed to a social stressor, despite physiological measures showing no differences between the groups in physiological measures of blushing (cheek coloration and temperature) or general arousal level (skin conductance). Furthermore, Mansell and Clark (1999) reported that increases in perceived bodily sensations while giving a speech were associated with more negative self-ratings of appearance in high socially anxious subjects, but not low socially anxious subjects. Perceptions of bodily sensations were not associated with ratings of appearance made by observers for either group. In combination, these results are consistent with the notion that socially anxious individuals overestimate the extent to which somatic sensations are visible to others, and thus appraise such sensations as further sources of threat to effective social performance.

There is also some evidence to support the idea that safety behaviors may interfere with effective social performance and consequently elicit less positive reactions from other people. Although research has yielded mixed results regarding whether or not socially anxious individuals perform in a less capable manner in social situations than do nonanxious individuals (Strahan and Conger, 1999), there is some evidence to suggest that social anxiety is associated with a "protective" self-presentation style in situations which are appraised as threatening. This style is characterized by behaviors designed to avoid social disapproval (e.g., the type of subtle avoidance or "safety" behaviors described previously), contrasting with the "acquisitive" self-presentation style generally adopted by nonanxious subjects, which involves active attempts to gain approval (Arkin et al., 1986). Research by Alden and Bieling (1998) suggests that such safety behaviors are strategically adopted by socially anxious subjects when situations are appraised as threatening, rather than simply being the result of social skills deficits or anxiety-mediated inhibition. Furthermore, evidence has demonstrated that such behaviors may indeed elicit negative responses from other people (Alden and Bieling, 1998; Creed and Funder, 1998), which may potentially provide negative input into socially anxious individuals' perceptions regarding how well they are coming across to others, and consequently contribute to the maintenance of social anxiety.

Additional cognitive factors in social anxiety

Additional factors considered to be important in contemporary cognitive models of social phobia are anticipatory and postevent processing. Rapee and Heimberg (1997), for instance, suggest that the processes which generate and maintain anxiety during social encounters may also occur during anticipation of future encounters, as well as retrospective "brooding over" previous social situations. In the model of Clark and Wells (1995), it is assumed that when anticipating a social event, socially anxious individuals tend to recall selectively negative images concerning their previous social performances, thus contributing to unfavorable predictions concerning social outcomes. Evidence in support of the notion that socially anxious individuals selectively retrieve and dwell on negative information regarding how they believe others perceive them was obtained in a recent study by Mansell and Clark (1999). These researchers investigated the effects of social threat (anticipation of giving a speech) on memory for trait words which subjects had encoded prior to threat by rating the extent to which the words were either self-descriptive (private self-referent), descriptive of how they thought other people viewed them (public self-referent), or descriptive of their neighbor (other-referent). It was found that socially anxious subjects recalled fewer positive trait adjectives than control subjects only for words encoded in a public self-referent manner, and only when both groups anticipated giving a speech. However, a further study by Mellings and Alden (2000) found that the retrieval of information regarding a specific previous social event did not differ for socially anxious subjects who were anticipating a further interaction versus those who were not. These latter results, in conjunction with additional studies which have failed to demonstrate memory biases in social phobia (Rapee et al., 1994), suggest that further research is needed in order to clarify the role of memory in the maintenance of social phobia.

In addition, as noted previously, Clark and Wells (1995) assume that postevent processing in socially anxious individuals may involve a detailed "postmortem" of social events, in which negative self-evaluations will receive further processing after social situations and hence reinforce unfavorable judgments regarding social performance. This idea was also examined in the study by Mellings and Alden (2000), with their results indicating that socially anxious subjects engaged in postevent rumination to a greater extent than nonanxious subjects in the day following a social interaction. As well, there was a significant positive association between the frequency of postevent processing and subjects' recall of negative self-related information. Their results are therefore consistent with the view that postevent processing may be an important factor in the maintenance of social anxiety.

Etiological factors

Before proceeding to a discussion regarding treatment implications for social phobia, it is worthwhile briefly considering factors that may be involved in the etiology of the disorder. Although a comprehensive discussion of etiological factors is beyond the scope of this chapter (see Hudson and Rapee, 2000 for a review), the origins of the types of dysfunctional cognitions that appear to mediate social phobia are of considerable interest. Overall, research in this area indicates that an interaction of both genetic and environmental factors contributes to the development of social phobia. Family studies, which confound both factors, have found higher rates of social phobia amongst relatives of people with social phobia compared to relatives of panic disorder subjects, and relatives of nonclinical controls (Reich and Yates, 1988; Fyer et al., 1993). However, the majority of evidence from twin studies suggests that the primary genetic component of social phobia may consist of a predisposition to general neurosis (Andrews et al., 1990; Andrews, 1996), although evidence of a specific genetic contribution to the development of social-evaluative concerns has also been obtained (Kendler et al., 1992). Further support for a generalized genetic tendency to the development of anxiety disorders has been derived from research demonstrating a link between behavioral inhibition in children (an aspect of temperament characterized by fear and withdrawal in unfamiliar situations (Garcia-Coll et al., 1984; Kagan et al., 1984), and an increased risk of the development of anxiety disorders (Biederman et al., 1993; Turner et al., 1996a). These data are thus consistent with theoretical conceptualizations of social phobia which assume that a biological vulnerability to anxious apprehension is involved in the etiology of the disorder (Barlow, 1988).

Research regarding the contribution of environmental variables to the development of social phobia suggests that a genetic predisposition to anxiety in general may be expressed specifically as social-evaluative concerns as a result of learning experiences (Hudson and Rapee, 2000). While there is research suggesting that, in some cases, social fears may arise from traumatic conditioning experiences in which social stimuli are paired with an aversive event, such as being criticized (Ost and Hugdahl, 1981; Stemberger et al., 1995), experiences within the family environment appear to be particularly important. For instance, evidence has shown that social phobics perceive one or both parents as having been more fearful and avoidant of social situations, as well as having overemphasized others' opinions, isolated them from social experiences, deemphasized family sociability, and employed shame as a disciplinary tactic to a greater extent than nonclinical or agoraphobic populations (Bruch et al., 1989; Bruch and Heimberg, 1994). Several authors (Hudson and Rapee, 2000) postulate that such parental characteristics may contribute to the development of social phobia via observational learning or modeling of social fear and avoidance, and restricted opportunities to learn effective interaction due to reduced exposure to social situations. In addition, parental overprotection has been associated with anxiety disorders in general (Rapee, 1997), and social phobia in particular (Parker, 1979), leading to the suggestion that overprotection may contribute to anxiety by promoting in the child a notion that the world is threatening, and the sense that he or she is not capable of coping with this danger (Hudson and Rapee, 2000). Moreover, the implication that one's parents view one as not competent may adversely affect the mental representation of how one is viewed by others (Rapee and Heimberg, 1997).

Further evidence suggests that additional environmental factors, such as negative peer relationships, may also play a role in the development of social anxiety. For instance, a prospective study by Vernberg et al. (1992) indicated that increases in social anxiety in adolescents resulted from lower levels of companionship and intimacy in friendships, as well as more frequent rejection experiences, although their results suggest a reciprocal causal relationship operates between social anxiety and peer relationships. It is possible that negative peer experiences may contribute to the cognitive factors involved in social anxiety, perhaps by adversely affecting perceptions of social competence (Hudson and Rapee, 2000).

On the basis of research concerning the origins of social phobia, Rapee and colleagues (Rapee and Heimberg, 1997; Hudson and Rapee, 2000) have suggested that a general tendency to direct attention toward threat-related cues may be genetically mediated, whereas environmental factors may be at least partially responsible for channeling this attentional bias specifically toward cues relating to social threat. Evidence such as that outlined above also provides insight into environmental factors that may contribute to the underlying negative beliefs or schema related to the self and the social world that may place an individual at risk for developing social phobia (e.g., negative beliefs about one's social competence). However, the specific content of such underlying assumptions has not been clearly delineated in the empirical literature, and hence is an issue that requires further research before the precise nature of the genetic and environmental contributions to such belief systems can be further specified.

Treatment considerations

Theory and research regarding the role of maladaptive cognitions in the development and maintenance of social phobia have provided the basis for significant developments in the treatment of the disorder. In particular, the literature considered above implies that the effectiveness of interventions will be based, to a large degree, on their success in modifying dysfunctional beliefs and thought processes. Cognitive-behavioral interventions, which aim to achieve such cognitive modification through techniques such as education regarding the role of thoughts and behaviors in producing and maintaining anxiety, cognitive restructuring (i.e., teaching clients to identify, analyze, and challenge cognitive distortions), and gradually exposing clients to feared situations have become widely used methods in the treatment of social phobia (Heimberg and Juster, 1994; Chambless and Hope, 1996; Merluzzi, 1996). Numerous empirical investigations have demonstrated the efficacy of this type of treatment in decreasing social anxiety, showing its effects to be superior to those achieved in waiting-list and supportive-educational therapy conditions (Heimberg et al., 1990; Chambless and Gillis, 1993; Heimberg and Juster, 1994), and approximately equivalent to ongoing pharmacological treatment (at least in terms of overall response rate) (Gould et al., 1997; Heimberg et al., 1998). Moreover, evidence suggests that gains achieved through cognitive-behavioral treatment of social phobia are maintained in the long term, and symptoms may show continued improvement after the cessation of treatment (Heimberg et al., 1993; Hunt and Andrews, 1998). Indeed, there is some evidence to suggest that cognitive-behavioral therapy may be associated with a lower rate of relapse following treatment discontinuation than pharmacological interventions (Liebowitz et al., 1999), with one study finding that 88% of individuals who responded to prolonged treatment with moclobemide deteriorated when treatment was withdrawn (Versiani et al., 1997). In addition, group cognitive-behavioral therapy for social phobia appears to have the advantage of being more cost-effective than pharmacological treatments (Gould et al., 1997).

Much of the research to date concerning the effective components in the treatment of social phobia has focused primarily on the relative contributions of direct cognitive restructuring techniques versus behavioral interventions, such as exposure to feared social situations. While evidence suggests that cognitive interventions and exposure may both result in reductions in social anxiety (see Heimberg and Juster, 1995; Juster and Heimberg, 1995 for reviews), research addressing the question of whether direct cognitive restructuring is a necessary adjunct to behavioral interventions has yielded few firm conclusions. Although several studies have found that a combination of direct cognitive restructuring plus exposure resulted in more positive treatment outcomes in individuals with social phobia than exposure only (Mattick and Peters, 1988; Mattick et al., 1989; Taylor, 1996), other researchers have failed to find benefits of cognitive restructuring over and above what is achieved through exposure alone (Feske and Chambless, 1995; Hope et al., 1995). These results, however, are not inconsistent with cognitive theories of social phobia, as the success of behavioral interventions in reducing social anxiety may vary according to the extent to which they are effective in facilitating changes in the cognitive variables associated with anxiety in social situations (Butler, 1985; Chambless and Gillis, 1993).

The notion that cognitive change may underlie treatment efficacy in social phobia is also consistent with studies demonstrating a positive effect of other behavioral treatments such as social skills training (see Taylor, 1996, for a metaanalysis). As noted previously, research findings have been inconsistent with regard to whether or not socially anxious individuals demonstrate inferior social performance relative to controls, and, furthermore, have failed to demonstrate that any observed performance deficits are due to the absence of social skills, rather than anxiety-related inhibition of skills (Rapee, 1995). Furthermore, evidence indicating that people with specific versus generalized subtypes of social phobia may differ in symptom severity, but do not differ in terms of social skills (Turner et al., 1992), raises doubts as to whether social skills deficits are implicated in the level of impairment experienced by people with social phobia. Nevertheless, social skills training may be of benefit in the treatment of social phobia by improving individuals' perceptions regarding their social abilities, thus enhancing the mental representation of the self in social situations (Hofmann, 2000). Furthermore the possibility that a proportion of social phobics may benefit from an improved repertoire of social skills cannot be dismissed (Ost et al., 1981). Thus, although there is little empirical evidence to suggest that treatment programs incorporating social skills training are more effective than other forms of therapy (Mersch, 1995; Taylor, 1996), a number of contemporary treatment programs have included a social skills component in addition to other cognitive-behavioral techniques (Turner et al., 1994; Rapee and Sanderson, 1998).

While the broad cognitive and behavioral interventions described may result in significant and lasting reductions in social anxiety, it is important to note that a proportion of individuals fail to make significant gains, and, of those that do, improvement is often moderate (Chambless and Gillis, 1993). A metaanalysis of controlled treatment outcome studies for social phobia (Gould et al., 1997) indicated that the mean effect size for cognitive-behavioral treatment of social anxiety is in the moderate but significant range (0.80 for cognitive restructuring plus exposure). In addition, Feske and Chambless (1995) reported that estimates of the proportion of individuals achieving clinically significant change or high end-state functioning following cognitive-behavioral treatment for social phobia varied between studies from 22% to 95%. To date, there have been few data that elucidate the characteristics of people with social phobia who fail to benefit from treatment. Those research findings that have been reported suggest that subtype of social phobia and symptom severity at pretreatment are not predictive of the degree of improvement achieved by treatment, although social phobics with the generalized subtype (and hence more severe symptoms prior to treatment) remain more impaired following treatment (Brown et al., 1995; Turner et al., 1996b). Similar results have been found for social phobics with axis I or II comorbidity versus those without (Hofmann et al., 1995; Turner et al., 1996b), although Chambless et al. (1997) reported that higher initial levels of depression were predictive of less favorable responses to cognitive-behavioral treatment for social phobia. Chambless et al. (1997) further found that expectancies regarding treatment were predictive of outcome, with clients who reported more positive expectancies regarding improvement at the beginning of treatment showing greater gains following group cognitive-behavioral therapy than those with lower expectations. Such findings provide useful information concerning additional components of treatment that may be required for people who manifest symptoms that are resistant to cognitive-behavioral treatment for social phobia.

Developments in cognitive theory and research regarding social phobia in recent years have generated ideas for ways in which cognitive-behavioral treatment of the disorder may be improved. Although empirical testing of comprehensive treatment models based on the theories of Clark and Wells (1995) and Rapee and Heimberg (1997) is still in progress at the present time, a number of studies have been reported investigating the efficacy of specific therapeutic techniques targeting factors which current models of social phobia suggest are instrumental in the development and maintenance of the disorder. For instance, based on the suggestion that negatively biased mental representations of the self as seen by others may contribute to anxiety in social situations, Rapee and Hayman (1996) examined the question of whether video feedback regarding social performance may assist socially anxious subjects to evaluate their performance more objectively, and consequently reduce anxiety. Although standard cognitive-behavioral treatment programs for social phobia usually address self-appraisals via cognitive restructuring and verbal feedback from others regarding individuals' social performance, Rapee and Hayman (1996) hypothesized that video feedback may address distorted self-evaluations more directly. Indeed, these researchers found that socially anxious subjects' ratings of their own speech performance were more consistent with ratings given by independent observers after subjects viewed a video recording of their performance, as compared to self-ratings made prior to video feedback. Moreover, self-ratings of a second speech performance continued to be more concordant with objective observer ratings for subjects who had seen a video recording of their first speech, compared to those who had not. It should be noted, however, that all subjects showed similar reductions in self-rated anxiety during the second speech as compared to the first, regardless of whether or not video feedback had been provided. Thus, it may be that habituation to anxiety achieved through exposure outweighs the effects of providing objective information on performance via video feedback, such that additional feedback techniques may be required in order to demonstrate an effect on anxiety levels (Rapee and Hayman, 1996). Indeed, evidence from a recent study showed that increases in self-ratings of speech performance following video feedback were more pronounced for individuals who received "cognitive preparation" (techniques designed to highlight the differences between self and video images) prior to viewing the video compared to those who did not (Harvey et al., 2000). Unfortunately, this study did not examine the question of whether the beneficial effects of cognitive preparation on self-ratings of performance following video feedback manifested in reduced anxiety levels. Research that incorporates this technique into standard cognitive-behavioral programs is necessary in order to determine whether it adds to such programs in terms of reducing social anxiety.

Additional research has examined the effect of interventions designed to decrease self-focused attention, and increase attention to nonthreatening factors in the external environment as well as to the task at hand (Rapee, 1998; Rapee and Sanderson, 1998). Results from initial studies support the idea that interventions addressing maladaptive attentional factors may be beneficial in the treatment of social phobia. For instance, Bogels et al. (1997) reported that attentional training resulted in reductions in fear, negative beliefs, and avoidance in several case studies of social phobia involving primary fears of blushing, although efficacy was enhanced by providing a rationale and instructions for exposure (Mulkens et al., 1999a). A recent empirical study by these researchers, in which the effects of attentional training versus exposure were compared in the treatment of social phobics with a predominant fear of blushing, found that attentional training tended to produce greater reductions in fear of blushing than did exposure immediately following treatment, although there was no difference between the two interventions at 1-year follow-up on measures of fear of blushing, negative cognitions, or anxiety (Mulkens et al., 2001). Wells and Papageorgiou (1998) also demonstrated positive effects of an attentional intervention in the treatment of eight individuals with social phobia. These authors found that providing a rationale and instructions for directing attention away from the self and toward the external social environment during one session of brief exposure to a feared situation was significantly more effective in reducing anxiety and belief in feared outcomes than exposure which did not include these instructions. Furthermore, the inclusion of the attentional intervention resulted in a perspective shift in individuals' images of feared situations from one in which they saw themselves as if from an external point of view to one in which they viewed the situation from inside their own body looking outwards. Finally, Woody et al. (1997) found that social phobics' self-focused attention during interpersonal situations significantly decreased over the course of a cognitive-behavioral treatment program which included an intervention designed to encourage participants to focus their attention on external stimuli during social encounters, and furthermore found that reductions in self-focused attention were associated with treatment gains on several outcome measures. It is interesting to note, however, that in this study, reductions in self-focus during treatment were not accompanied by a corresponding increase in attention to external events during social encounters. This finding suggests that interventions leading to decreases in social phobics' self-focused attention will not necessarily be sufficient in terms of increasing their attention to information in the external environment which is incompatible with their fears.

Further research by Wells and colleagues (1995) investigated the question of whether interventions emphasizing the curtailment of subtle avoidance or "safety behaviors" during social situations would be of benefit in the treatment of social phobia. In a single case series of eight individuals with social phobia, Wells et al. (1995) found that a rationale and instructions for intentionally decreasing safety behaviors during one session of exposure to a feared social situation produced greater reductions in subjects' anxiety and belief in feared outcomes than did one session of exposure accompanied only by an extinction rationale. Thus, this study suggests that the identification and elimination of safety behaviors during social situations is an important component of treatment for social phobia.

Finally, there is preliminary evidence suggesting that a combination of treatment interventions based on recent cognitive models of social phobia may be particularly effective in reducing negative social cognitions and concomitant anxiety in social situations. This evidence is reported in a single case study by Bates and Clark (1998), who successfully treated an adult female with social phobia by means of: eliminating her safety behaviors during exposure to feared social situations; providing verbal and video feedback regarding her performance; instructing her to focus her attention on the external environment rather than internal sensations; encouraging her to risk new behaviors and to evaluate others' reactions; deconstructing and modifying her underlying dysfunctional assumptions; ensuring that she had achieved a clear understanding of the cognitive-behavioral factors underlying her social anxiety; and consolidating alternative and more adaptive self-appraisals and assumptions concerning others' evaluations. The client showed substantial gains on measures of cognition and affect, including a change on the fear of negative evaluation scale from the maximum score (30) to a score below the general population mean (9) from pre- to posttreatment. Although these results are yet to be empirically validated, and it is yet to be demonstrated whether such a treatment provides greater benefits than do traditional treatment programs for social phobia, the study by Bates and Clark (1998) suggests that recent developments in the understanding and treatment of social phobia may hold considerable promise for the future.

Summary and directions for future research

Theory and research regarding the cognitive factors that underlie anxiety in social situations have resulted in considerable progress in understanding of the development and maintenance of social phobia, thus contributing to significant advances in the treatment of this debilitating disorder. In particular, recent cognitive models of social phobia imply that important treatment components may include interventions designed to: (1) promote individuals' awareness and understanding of the ways in which cognitive and behavioral factors contribute to social anxiety; (2) modify individuals' negatively biased perceptions regarding the way they are viewed by others during social situations (e.g., through methods such as verbal and video feedback); (3) redirect attention from internal factors such as negative self-evaluative thoughts and somatic sensations, and from external negative evaluative cues to the task at hand and to neutral or positive feedback cues; (4) modify underlying assumptions (e.g., negative beliefs about the self, or about the meaning of being negatively evaluated by others) which may contribute to increased estimates regarding the probability and cost of negative social outcomes; and (5) decrease the use of subtle avoidance ("safety behaviors") during exposure to feared social situations. Although research investigating the use of such techniques is at an early stage, initial results have been encouraging.

Notwithstanding the progress that has been made in understanding and treating social phobia, additional research is required in relation to a number of issues. For instance, research findings are inconclusive with regard to whether socially anxious individuals spontaneously allocate attention to threat cues in the external social environment, or whether attention to situational cues is impaired in a non-selective manner. There is some evidence to suggest, however, that when attention is explicitly directed toward the external environment, socially anxious individuals tend to focus on cues associated with negative evaluation. Moreover, there is evidence suggesting that even when positive cues from other people in a social situation are noticed, they may be interpreted by socially anxious individuals as an indication of others having higher expectations for their performance in future interactions, rather than as an indication of adequate social ability. This may have important implications for treatment strategies which aim to increase attention to stimuli in the external environment. Specifically, it suggests that interventions designed to increase the attention directed by socially anxious individuals towards positive evaluative cues from others may require supplemental strategies to ensure that individuals process the information in a manner which increases confidence in their own social competence (Wallace and Alden, 1997). Alternatively, it may be the case that socially anxious individuals will derive more benefit from strategies designed to increase attention towards the task at hand as well as to external factors which are not related to others' evaluations of the self (Hartman, 1983; Rapee and Sanderson, 1998), particularly if the aim of treatment is to enable socially anxious individuals to become less sensitive to the way in which others evaluate them. Future research is thus required in order to address the following questions: (1) Do socially anxious individuals preferentially allocate attentional resources to negative cues in the external social environment? (2) What are the relative benefits of decreasing self-focused attention versus increasing externally focused attention, given evidence that these two factors may be at least partially independent (Woody et al., 1997)? (3) What are the effects of increased attention to external cues associated with evaluation of oneself by others versus increased attention to external factors that do not relate to the self? It is evident that with regard to the first question, research strategies are required which measure spontaneous direction of attention in a naturalistic social-evaluative task. Research addressing the second and third questions will be required to employ measures which separate internal from external attention, and which separate external attention related to others' evaluation of the self versus external attention which is not related to others' opinions of the self.

A second major topic for future research relates to socially anxious individuals' estimates of the cost of negative evaluation by others. As noted above, recent research suggests that socially anxious individuals may interpret negative evaluation from others as an indication of negative self-characteristics, and as having adverse implications for their future. However, the factors that may contribute to the perception that negative evaluation will result in serious consequences have received little attention in the literature. Whether this perception merely reflects underlying negative assumptions concerning the self, standards for performance, or the meaning of negative evaluation by others (Clark and Wells, 1995), or whether additional processes are involved has not been established. Further research regarding the content of any underlying assumptions or schema that may contribute to exaggerated cost estimates of negative social events in social phobia, as well as the nature of the genetic and/or environmental influences which may be responsible for the development of such schema, is therefore necessary. A further potential line of enquiry may relate to the manner in which socially anxious individuals evaluate the status, competency, and power of other people, particularly in relation to their perceptions of their own personal qualities. Given evidence indicating that decreases in fear of negative evaluation and in estimates of the cost of negative social occurrences are significant mediators of treatment outcome in social phobia, factors associated with the consequences attached to negative evaluation represent an important area for future research.

Finally, the specificity of cognitive factors in social phobia is an issue that requires further research, particularly in terms of identifying the features that differentiate social anxiety and depression. Research has indicated that depression and social anxiety are positively related (Bruch et al., 1993), and has further indicated similarities in the cognitive factors associated with both conditions, including more negative self-evaluative cognitions relative to people without anxiety or depression (Alden et al., 1995), maladaptive attributional styles (Anderson and Arnoult, 1985), and an increase in self-focused attention (Ingram, 1990). Research that teases apart the cognitive factors which underlie the two conditions may provide valuable information regarding treatment, particularly in terms of whether different interventions are required for social phobics with, versus without, comorbid depression. Furthermore, the similarities between the two conditions highlight the need for future research to control for the effects of depression when investigating cognition in social phobia (Ingram, 1989; Johnson et al., 1992; Sanz and Avia, 1994).

In conclusion, it is evident that cognitive theory and research have greatly facilitated the understanding of social phobia, thus providing a conceptual framework upon which increasingly effective treatments are being built. Although there is considerable work yet to be done, the past decade, in particular, has seen a substantial increase in the literature relating to the area. If theory and research continue to progress at the current rate, there is a promising outlook for the future for those people whose lives are affected by social phobia.

REFERENCES

Alden, L. E. and Bieling, P. (1998). Interpersonal consequences of the pursuit of safety. *Behaviour Research and Therapy*, **36**, 53–64.

Alden, L. E. and Wallace, S. T. (1995). Social phobia and social appraisal in successful and unsuccessful social interactions. *Behaviour Research and Therapy*, **33**, 497–505.

Alden, L. E., Bieling, P. J., and Wallace, S. T. (1994). Perfectionism in an interpersonal context: a self-regulation analysis of dysphoria and social anxiety. *Cognitive Therapy and Research*, **18**, 297–316.

Alden, L. E., Bieling, P. J., and Meleshko, K. G. A. (1995). An interpersonal comparison of depression and social anxiety. In *Anxiety and Depression in Adults and Children*, ed. K. D. Craig and K. S. Dobson, pp. 57–81. Thousand Oaks, CA: Sage Publications.

American Psychiatric Association. (1980). *Diagnostic and Statistical Manual of Mental Disorders*, 3rd edn. Washington, DC: American Psychiatric Association.

American Psychiatric Association. (1994). *Diagnostic and Statistical Manual of Mental Disorders*, 4th edn. Washington, DC: American Psychiatric Association.

Amies, P. L., Gelder, M. G., and Shaw, P. M. (1983). Social phobia: a comparative clinical study. *British Journal of Psychiatry*, **142**, 174–9.

Amir, N., Foa, E. B., and Coles, M. E. (1998a). Automatic activation and strategic avoidance of threat-relevant information in social phobia. *Journal of Abnormal Psychology*, **107**, 285–90.

Amir, N., Foa, E. B., and Coles, M. E. (1998b). Negative interpretation bias in social phobia. *Behaviour Research and Therapy*, **36**, 945–57.

Anderson, C. A. and Arnoult, L. H. (1985). Attributional style and everyday problems in living: depression, loneliness, and shyness. *Social Cognition*, **3**, 16–35.

Andrews, G. (1996). Comorbidity in neurotic disorders: the similarities are more important than the differences. In *Current Controversies in the Anxiety Disorders*, ed. R. M. Rapee, pp. 3–20. New York: Guilford Press.

Andrews, G., Stewart, G., Allen, R., and Henderson, A. S. (1990). The genetics of six neurotic disorders: a twin study. *Journal of Affective Disorders*, **19**, 23–9.

Arkin, R. M., Lake, E. A., and Baumgardner, A. H. (1986). Shyness and self presentation. In *Shyness: Perspectives on Research and Treatment*, ed. W. H. Jones, J. M. Cheek, and S. R. Briggs, pp. 189–203. New York: Plenum Press.

Arntz, A., Rauner, M., and van den Hout, M. (1995). "If I feel anxious, there must be danger": *Ex-consequentia* reasoning in inferring danger in anxiety disorders. *Behaviour Research and Therapy*, **33**, 917–25.

Asmundson, G. J. G., and Stein, M. B. (1994). Selective processing of social threat in patients with generalized social phobia: evaluation using a dot-probe paradigm. *Journal of Anxiety Disorders*, **8**, 107–17.

Barlow, D. H. (1988). *Anxiety and its Disorders: The Nature and Treatment of Anxiety and Panic*. New York: Guilford Press.

Bates, A. and Clark, D. M. (1998). A new cognitive treatment for social phobia: a single-case study. *Journal of Cognitive Psychotherapy: An International Quarterly*, **12**, 289–302.

Baumgardner, A. H. and Brownlee, E. A. (1987). Strategic failure in social interaction: evidence for expectancy disconfirmation processes. *Journal of Personality and Social Psychology*, **52**, 525–35.

Beck, A. T., Emery, G., and Greenberg, R. L. (1985). *Anxiety Disorders and Phobias: A Cognitive Perspective*. New York: Basic Books.

Biederman, J., Rosenbaum, J. F., Bolduc-Murphy, E. A., et al. (1993). A 3-year follow-up of children with and without behavioral inhibition. *Journal of the American Academy of Child and Adolescent Psychiatry*, **32**, 814–21.

Bieling, P. J. and Alden, L. E. (1997). The consequences of perfectionism for patients with social phobia. *British Journal of Clinical Psychology*, **36**, 387–95.

Bogels, S. M., Mulkens, S., and De Jong, P. J. (1997). Task concentration training and fear of blushing. *Clinical Psychology and Psychotherapy*, **4**, 251–8.

Bradley, B. P., Mogg, K., Millar, N., et al. (1997). Attentional biases for emotional faces. *Cognition and Emotion*, **11**, 25–42.

Brown, E. J., Heimberg, R. G., and Juster, H. R. (1995). Social phobia subtype and avoidant personality disorder: effect on severity of social phobia, impairment, and outcome of cognitive behavioral treatment. *Behavior Therapy*, **26**, 467–86.

Bruch, M. A. and Heimberg, R. G. (1994). Differences in perceptions of parental and personal characteristics between generalized and nongeneralized social phobics. *Journal of Anxiety Disorders*, **8**, 155–68.

Bruch, M. A., Heimberg, R. G., Berger, P., and Collins, T. M. (1989). Social phobia and perceptions of early parental and personal characteristics. *Anxiety Research*, **2**, 57–65.

Bruch, M. A., Mattia, J. I., Heimberg, R. G., and Holt, C. S. (1993). Cognitive specificity in social anxiety and depression: supporting evidence and qualifications due to affective confounding. *Cognitive Therapy and Research*, **17**, 1–21.

Burgio, K. L., Merluzzi, T. V., and Pryor, J. B. (1986). Effects of performance expectancy and self-focused attention on social interaction. *Journal of Personality and Social Psychology*, **50**, 1216–21.

Butler, G. (1985). Exposure as a treatment for social phobia: some instructive difficulties. *Behaviour Research and Therapy*, **23**, 651–7.

Carver, C. S. and Scheier, M. F. (1988). A control-process perspective on anxiety. *Anxiety Research*, **1**, 17–22.

Chambless, D. L. and Gillis, M. M. (1993). Cognitive therapy of anxiety disorders. *Journal of Consulting and Clinical Psychology*, **61**, 248–60.

Chambless, D. L. and Hope, D. A. (1996). Cognitive approaches to the psychopathology and treatment of social phobia. In *Frontiers of Cognitive Therapy*, ed. P. M. Salkovskis, pp. 345–82. New York: Guilford Press.

Chambless, D. L., Tran, G. Q., and Glass, C. R. (1997). Predictors of response to cognitive-behavioral group therapy for social phobia. *Journal of Anxiety Disorders*, **11**, 221–40.

Clark, D. M. and Wells, A. (1995). A cognitive model of social phobia. In *Social Phobia: Diagnosis, Assessment, and Treatment*, ed. R. G. Heimberg, M. R. Liebowitz, D. A. Hope, and F. R. Schneier, pp. 69–93. New York: Guilford Press.

Cloitre, M., Heimberg, R. G., Liebowitz, M. R., and Gitow, A. (1992). Perceptions of control in panic disorder and social phobia. *Cognitive Therapy and Research*, **16**, 569–77.

Constans, J. I., Penn, D. L., Ihen, G. H., and Hope, D. A. (1999). Interpretive biases for ambiguous stimuli in social anxiety. *Behaviour Research and Therapy*, **37**, 643–51.

Creed, A. T. and Funder, D. C. (1998). Social anxiety: from the inside and outside. *Personality and Individual Differences*, **25**, 19–33.

Elting, D. T. and Hope, D. A. (1995). Cognitive assessment. In *Social Phobia: Diagnosis, Assessment, and Treatment*, ed. R. G. Heimberg, M. R. Liebowitz, D. A. Hope, and F. R. Schneier, pp. 232–58. New York: Guilford Press.

Fenigstein, A., Scheier, M. F., and Buss, A. H. (1975). Public and private self-consciousness: assessment and theory. *Journal of Consulting and Clinical Psychology*, **43**, 522–7.

Feske, U. and Chambless, D. L. (1995). Cognitive behavioral versus exposure only treatment for social phobia: a meta-analysis. *Behavior Therapy*, **26**, 695–720.

Foa, E. B., Franklin, M. E., Perry, K. J., and Herbert, J. D. (1996). Cognitive biases in generalized social phobia. *Journal of Abnormal Psychology*, **105**, 433–9.

Fyer, A. J., Mannuzza, S., Chapman, T. F., Liebowitz, M. R., and Klein, D. F. (1993). A direct interview family study of social phobia. *Archives of General Psychiatry*, **50**, 286–93.

Garcia-Coll, C., Kagan, J., and Reznick, J. S. (1984). Behavioral inhibition in young children. *Child Development*, **55**, 1005–19.

Gould, R. A., Buckminster, S., Pollack, M. H., Otto, M. W., and Yap, L. (1997). Cognitive-behavioral and pharmacological treatment for social phobia: a meta-analysis. *Clinical Psychology – Science and Practice*, **4**, 291–306.

Hackmann, A., Surawy, C., and Clark, D. M. (1998). Seeing yourself through others' eyes: a study of spontaneously occurring images in social phobia. *Behavioural and Cognitive Psychotherapy*, **26**, 3–12.

Hartman, L. M. (1983). A metacognitive model of social anxiety: implications for treatment. *Clinical Psychology Review*, **3**, 435–56.

Harvey, A. G., Clark, D. M., Ehlers, A., and Rapee, R. M. (2000). Social anxiety and self-impression: cognitive preparation enhances the beneficial effects of video feedback following a stressful social task. *Behaviour Research and Therapy*, **38**, 1183–92.

Heckelman, L. R. and Schneier, F. R. (1995). Diagnostic issues. In *Social Phobia: Diagnosis, Assessment, and Treatment*, ed. R. G. Heimberg, M. R. Liebowitz, D. A. Hope, and F. R. Schneier, pp. 3–20. New York: Guilford Press.

Heimberg, R. G. and Juster, H. R. (1994). Treatment of social phobia in cognitive-behavioral groups. *Journal of Clinical Psychiatry*, **55** (6, suppl.), 38–46.

Heimberg, R. G. and Juster, H. R. (1995). Cognitive-behavioral treatments: literature review. In *Social Phobia: Diagnosis, Assessment, and Treatment*, ed. R. G. Heimberg, M. R. Liebowitz, D. A. Hope, and F. R. Schneier, pp. 261–309. New York: Guilford Press.

Heimberg, R. G., Dodge, C. S., Hope, D. A., et al. (1990). Cognitive behavioural group treatment for social phobia: comparison with a credible placebo control. *Cognitive Therapy and Research*, **14**, 1–23.

Heimberg, R. G., Salzman, D. G., Holt, C. S., and Blendell, K. A. (1993). Cognitive-behavioral group treatment for social phobia: effectiveness at five-year followup. *Cognitive Therapy and Research*, **17**, 325–39.

Heimberg, R. G., Liebowitz, M. R., Hope, D. A., et al. (1998). Cognitive behavioral group therapy vs phenelzine therapy for social phobia – 12-week outcome. *Archives of General Psychiatry*, **55**, 1133–41.

Hofmann, S. G. (2000). Treatment of social phobia: potential mediators and moderators. *Clinical Psychology: Science and Practice*, **7**, 3–16.

Hofmann, S. G., Newman, M. G., Becker, E., Taylor, C. B., and Roth, W. T. (1995). Social phobia with and without avoidant personality disorder: preliminary behavior therapy outcome findings. *Journal of Anxiety Disorders*, **9**, 427–38.

Hope, D. A. and Heimberg, R. G. (1988). Public and private self-consciousness and social phobia. *Journal of Personality Assessment*, **52**, 626–39.

Hope, D. A., Gansler, D. A., and Heimberg, R. G. (1989). Attentional focus and causal attributions in social phobia: implications from social psychology. *Clinical Psychology Review*, **9**, 49–60.

Hope, D. A., Heimberg, R. G., and Klein, J. F. (1990a). Social anxiety and the recall of interpersonal information. *Journal of Cognitive Psychotherapy*, **4**, 185–95.

Hope, D. A., Rapee, R. M., Heimberg, R. G., and Dombeck, M. J. (1990b). Representations of the self in social phobia: vulnerability to social threat. *Cognitive Therapy and Research*, **14**, 177–89.

Hope, D. A., Heimberg, R. G., and Bruch, M. A. (1995). Dismantling cognitive-behavioral group therapy for social phobia. *Behaviour Research and Therapy*, **33**, 637–50.

Hudson, J. L. and Rapee, R. M. (2000). The origins of social phobia. *Behavior Modification*, **24**, 102–29.

Hunt, C. and Andrews, G. (1998). Long-term outcome of panic disorder and social phobia. *Journal of Anxiety Disorders*, **12**, 395–406.

Ingram, R. E. (1989). Unique and shared cognitive factors in social anxiety and depression: automatic thinking and self-appraisal. *Journal of Social and Clinical Psychology*, **8**, 198–208.

Ingram, R. E. (1990). Self-focused attention in clinical disorders: review and a conceptual model. *Psychological Bulletin*, **107**, 156–76.

Johnson, K. A., Johnson, J. E., and Petzel, T. P. (1992). Social anxiety, depression, and distorted cognitions in college students. *Journal of Social and Clinical Psychology*, **11**, 181–95.

Jones, W. H., Briggs, S. R., and Smith, T. G. (1986). Shyness: conceptualization and measurement. *Journal of Personality and Social Psychology*, **51**, 629–39.

Jostes, A., Pook, M., and Florin, I. (1999). Public and private self-consciousness as specific psychopathological features. *Personality and Individual Differences*, **27**, 1285–95.

Juster, H. R. and Heimberg, R. G. (1995). Social phobia: longitudinal course and long-term outcome of cognitive-behavioral treatment. *Psychiatric Clinics of North America*, **18**, 821–42.

Kagan, J., Reznick, J. S., Clarke, C., Snidman, N., and Garcia-Coll, C. (1984). Behavioral inhibition to the unfamiliar. *Child Development*, **55**, 2212–25.

Kendler, K. S., Neale, M. C., Kessler, R. C., Heath, A. C., and Eaves, L. J. (1992). The genetic epidemiology of phobias in women: the interrelationship of agoraphobia, social phobia, situational phobia, and simple phobia. *Archives of General Psychiatry*, **49**, 273–81.

Kessler, R. C., McGonagle, K. A., Zhao, S., et al. (1994). Lifetime and 12-month prevalence of DSM-III-R psychiatric disorders in the United States: results from the National Comorbidity Survey. *Archives of General Psychiatry*, **51**, 8–19.

Kessler, R. C., Stang, P., Wittchen, H. U., Stein, M., and Walters, E. E. (1999). Lifetime comorbidities between social phobia and mood disorders in the US National Comorbidity Survey. *Psychological Medicine*, **29**, 555–67.

Leary, M. R. (1983). *Understanding Social Anxiety: Social, Personality, and Clinical Perspectives.* Beverly Hills: Sage Publications.

Leary, M. R. and Kowalski, R. M. (1995a). *Social Anxiety.* New York: Guilford Press.

Leary, M. R. and Kowalski, R. M. (1995b). The self-presentation model of social phobia. In *Social Phobia: Diagnosis, Assessment, and Treatment*, ed. R. G. Heimberg, M. R. Liebowitz, D. A. Hope, and F. R. Schneier, pp. 94–112. New York: Guilford Press.

Leung, A. W. and Heimberg, R. G. (1996). Homework compliance, perceptions of control, and outcome of cognitive-behavioral treatment of social phobia. *Behaviour Research and Therapy*, **34**, 423–32.

Levenson, H. (1973). Multidimensional locus of control in psychiatric patients. *Journal of Consulting and Clinical Psychology*, **41**, 397–404.

Liebling, B. A. and Shaver, P. (1973). Evaluation, self-awareness, and task performance. *Journal of Experimental Social Psychology*, **9**, 297–306.

Liebowitz, M. R., Heimberg, R. G., Schneier, F. R., et al. (1999). Cognitive-behavioral group therapy versus phenelzine in social phobia: long term outcome. *Depression and Anxiety*, **10**, 89–98.

Lucock, M. P. and Salkovskis, P. M. (1988). Cognitive factors in social anxiety and its treatment. *Behaviour Research and Therapy*, **26**, 297–302.

Lundh, L. G. and Ost, L. G. (1996). Stroop interference, self-focus and perfectionism in social phobics. *Personality and Individual Differences*, **20**, 725–31.

Maddux, J. E., Norton, L. W., and Leary, M. R. (1988). Cognitive components of social anxiety: an investigation of the integration of self-presentation theory and self-efficacy theory. *Journal of Social and Clinical Psychology*, **6**, 180–90.

Magee, W. J., Eaton, W. W., Wittchen, H. U., McGonagle, K. A., and Kessler, R. C. (1996). Agoraphobia, simple phobia, and social phobia in the National Comorbidity Survey. *Archives of General Psychiatry*, **53**, 159–68.

Maidenberg, E., Chen, E., Craske, M., Bohn, P., and Bystritsky, A. (1996). Specificity of attentional bias in panic disorder and social phobia. *Journal of Anxiety Disorders*, **10**, 529–41.

Mansell, W. and Clark, D. M. (1999). How do I appear to others? Social anxiety and processing of the observable self. *Behaviour Research and Therapy*, **37**, 419–34.

Mansell, W., Clark, D. M., Ehlers, A., and Chen, Y. P. (1999). Social anxiety and attention away from emotional faces. *Cognition and Emotion*, **13**, 673–90.

Mattia, J. I., Heimberg, R. G., and Hope, D. A. (1993). The revised Stroop color-naming task in social phobics. *Behaviour Research and Therapy*, **31**, 305–13.

Mattick, R. P. and Peters, L. (1988). Treatment of severe social phobia: effects of guided exposure with and without cognitive restructuring. *Journal of Consulting and Clinical Psychology*, **56**, 251–60.

Mattick, R. P., Peters, L., and Clarke, J. C. (1989). Exposure and cognitive restructuring for social phobia: a controlled study. *Behavior Therapy*, **20**, 3–23.

McEwan, K. L. and Devins, G. M. (1983). Is increased arousal in social anxiety noticed by others? *Journal of Abnormal Psychology*, **92**, 417–21.

McNeil, D. W., Ries, B. J., Taylor, L. J., et al. (1995). Comparison of social phobia subtypes using Stroop tests. *Journal of Anxiety Disorders*, **9**, 47–57.

Melchior, L. A. and Cheek, J. M. (1990). Shyness and anxious self-preoccupation during a social interaction. *Journal of Social Behavior and Personality*, **5**, 117–30.

Mellings, T. M. B. and Alden, L. E. (2000). Cognitive processes in social anxiety: the effects of self-focus, rumination and anticipatory processing. *Behaviour Research and Therapy*, **38**, 243–57.

Merluzzi, T. V. (1996). Cognitive assessment and treatment of social phobia. In *Cognitive Rehabilitation for Neuropsychiatric Disorders*, ed. P. W. Corrigan, and S. C. Yudofsky, pp. 167–90. Washington, DC: American Psychiatric Press.

Mersch, P. P. A. (1995). The treatment of social phobia: the differential effectiveness of exposure in vivo and an integration of exposure in vivo, rational emotive therapy and social skills training. *Behaviour Research and Therapy*, **33**, 259–69.

Mulkens, S., Bogels, S. M., and de Jong, P. J. (1999a). Attentional focus and fear of blushing: a case study. *Behavioural and Cognitive Psychotherapy*, **27**, 153–64.

Mulkens, S., de Jong, P. J., Dobbelaar, A., and Bogels, S. M. (1999b). Fear of blushing: fearful preoccupation irrespective of facial coloration. *Behaviour Research and Therapy*, **37**, 1119–28.

Mulkens, S., Bogels, S. M., de Jong, P. J., and Louwers, J. (2001). Fear of blushing: effects of tasks concentration training versus exposure in vivo on fear and physiology. *Journal of Anxiety Disorders*, **15**, 413–32.

Ost, L. G. and Hugdahl, K. (1981). Acquisition of phobias and anxiety response patterns in clinical patients. *Behaviour Research and Therapy*, **19**, 439–47.

Ost, L. G., Jerremalm, A., and Johansson, J. (1981). Individual response patterns and the effects of different behavioral methods in the treatment of social phobia. *Behaviour Research and Therapy*, **19**, 1–16.

Parker, G. (1979). Reported parental characteristics of agoraphobics and social phobics. *British Journal of Psychiatry*, **135**, 555–60.

Rapee, R. M. (1995). Descriptive psychopathology of social phobia. In *Social Phobia: Diagnosis, Assessment, and Treatment*, ed. R. G. Heimberg, M. R. Liebowitz, D. A. Hope, and F. R. Schneier, pp. 41–66. New York: Guilford Press.

Rapee, R. M. (1997). Potential role of childrearing practices in the development of anxiety and depression. *Clinical Psychology Review*, **17**, 47–67.

Rapee, R. M. (1998). *Overcoming Shyness and Social Phobia: A Step-by-step Guide*. Killara, Australia: Lifestyle Press.

Rapee. R. M. and Hayman, K. (1996). The effects of video feedback on the self-evaluation of performance in socially anxious subjects. *Behaviour Research and Therapy*, **34**, 315–22.

Rapee, R. M. and Heimberg, R. G. (1997). A cognitive-behavioral model of anxiety in social phobia. *Behaviour Research and Therapy*, **35**, 741–56.

Rapee, R. M. and Lim, L. (1992). Discrepancy between self- and observer ratings of performance in social phobics. *Journal of Abnormal Psychology*, **101**, 728–31.

Rapee, R. M. and Sanderson, W. C. (1998). *Social Phobia: Clinical Application of Evidence-based Psychotherapy*. Northvale, NJ: Jason Aronson.

Rapee, R. M., McCallum, S. L., Melville, L. F., Ravenscroft, H., and Rodney, J. M. (1994). Memory bias in social phobia. *Behaviour Research and Therapy*, **32**, 89–99.

Regier, D. A., Rae, D. S., Narrow, W. E., Kaelber, C. T., and Schatzberg, A. F. (1998). Prevalence of anxiety disorders and their comorbidity with mood and addictive disorders. *British Journal of Psychiatry*, **173** (suppl. 34), 24–8.

Reich, J. and Yates, W. (1988). Family history of psychiatric disorders in social phobia. *Comprehensive Psychiatry*, **29**, 72–5.

Salovey, P. (1992). Mood-induced self-focused attention. *Journal of Personality and Social Psychology*, **62**, 699–707.

Sanz, J. and Avia, M. D. (1994). Cognitive specificity in social anxiety and depression: self-statements, self-focused attention, and dysfunctional attitudes. *Journal of Social and Clinical Psychology*, **13**, 105–37.

Schlenker, B. R. and Leary, M. R. (1982). Social anxiety and self-presentation: a conceptualisation and model. *Psychological Bulletin*, **92**, 641–69.

Schneier, F. R., Johnson, J., Hornig, C. D., Liebowitz, M. R., and Weissman, M. M. (1992). Social phobia: comorbidity and morbidity in an epidemiologic sample. *Archives of General Psychiatry*, **49**, 282–8.

Schneier, F. R., Heckelman, L. R., Garfinkel, R., et al. (1994). Functional impairment in social phobia. *Journal of Clinical Psychiatry*, **55**, 322–31.

Seligman, M. E., Abramson, L. Y., Semmel, A., and von Baeyer, C. (1979). Depressive attributional style. *Journal of Abnormal Psychology*, **88**, 242–7.

Seta, C. E. and Seta, J. J. (1996). When more is less: an averaging/summation analysis of social anxiety. *Journal of Research in Personality*, **30**, 496–509.

Smari, J., Bjarnadottir, A., and Bragadottir, B. (1998). Social anxiety, social skills and expectancy/cost of negative social events. *Scandinavian Journal of Behaviour Therapy*, **27**, 149–55.

Solyom, L., Ledwidge, B., and Solyom, C. (1986). Delineating social phobia. *British Journal of Psychiatry*, **149**, 464–70.

Stemberger, R. T., Turner, S. M., Beidel, D. C., and Calhoun, K. S. (1995). Social phobia: an analysis of possible developmental factors. *Journal of Abnormal Psychology*, **104**, 526–31.

Stopa, L. and Clark D. M. (1993). Cognitive processes in social phobia. *Behaviour Research and Therapy*, **31**, 255–67.

Stopa, L. and Clark, D. M. (2000). Social phobia and interpretation of social events. *Behaviour Research and Therapy*, **38**, 273–83.

Strahan, E. Y. and Conger, A. J. (1999). Social anxiety and social performance: why don't we see more catastrophes? *Journal of Anxiety Disorders*, **13**, 399–416.

Strauman, T. J. (1989). Self-discrepancies in clinical depression and social phobia: cognitive structures that underlie emotional disorders? *Journal of Abnormal Psychology*, **98**, 14–22.

Stroop, J. R. (1935). Studies of interference in serial verbal reactions. *Journal of Experimental Psychology*, **18**, 643–62.

Taylor, S. (1996). Meta-analysis of cognitive-behavioral treatments for social phobia. *Journal of Behavior Therapy and Experimental Psychiatry*, **27**, 1–9.

Teglasi, H. and Fagin, S. S. (1984). Social anxiety and self-other biases in causal attribution. *Journal of Research in Personality*, **18**, 64–80.

Turner, S. M., Beidel, D. C., and Townsley, R. M. (1992). Social phobia: a comparison of specific and generalized subtypes and avoidant personality disorder. *Journal of Abnormal Psychology*, **101**, 326–31.

Turner, S. M., Beidel, D. C., Cooley, M. R., and Woody, S. R. (1994). A multicomponent behavioral treatment for social phobia: social effectiveness therapy. *Behaviour Research and Therapy*, **32**, 381–90.

Turner, S. M., Beidel, D. C., and Wolff, P. L. (1996a). Is behavioral inhibition related to the anxiety disorders? *Clinical Psychology Review*, **16**, 157–72.

Turner, S. M., Beidel, D. C., Wolff, P. L., Spaulding, S., and Jacob, R. G. (1996b). Clinical features affecting treatment outcome in social phobia. *Behaviour Research and Therapy*, **34**, 795–804.

Veljaca, K. A. and Rapee, R. M. (1998). Detection of negative and positive audience behaviours by socially anxious subjects. *Behaviour Research and Therapy*, **36**, 311–21.

Vernberg, E. M., Abwender, D. A., Ewell, K. K., and Beery, S. H. (1992). Social anxiety and peer relationships in early adolescence: a prospective analysis. *Journal of Clinical Child Psychology*, **21**, 189–96.

Versiani, M., Amrein, R., and Montgomery, S. A. (1997). Social phobia: long-term treatment outcome and prediction of response – a moclobemide study. *International Clinical Psychopharmacology*, **12**, 329–44.

Wallace, S. T. and Alden, L. E. (1991). A comparison of social standards and perceived ability in anxious and nonanxious men. *Cognitive Therapy and Research*, **15**, 237–54.

Wallace, S. T. and Alden, L. E. (1995). Social anxiety and standard setting following social success or failure. *Cognitive Therapy and Research*, **19**, 613–31.

Wallace, S. T. and Alden, L. E. (1997). Social phobia and positive social events: the price of success. *Journal of Abnormal Psychology*, **106**, 416–24.

Watson, D. and Friend, R. (1969). Measurement of social-evaluative anxiety. *Journal of Consulting and Clinical Psychology*, **33**, 448–57.

Wells, A. and Papageorgiou, C. (1998). Social phobia: effects of external attention on anxiety, negative beliefs, and perspective taking. *Behavior Therapy*, **29**, 357–70.

Wells, A. and Papageorgiou, C. (1999). The observer perspective: biased imagery in social phobia, agoraphobia, and blood/injury phobia. *Behaviour Research and Therapy*, **37**, 653–8.

Wells, A., Clark, D. M., Salkovskis, P., et al. (1995). Social phobia: the role of in-situation safety behaviours in maintaining anxiety and negative beliefs. *Behavior Therapy*, **26**, 153–61.

Wells, A., Clark, D. M., and Ahmad, S. (1998). How do I look with my mind's eye? Perspective taking in social phobia imagery. *Behaviour Research and Therapy*, **36**, 631–4.

Wine, J. (1971). Test anxiety and direction of attention. *Psychological Bulletin*, **76**, 92–104.

Winton, E. C., Clark, D. M., and Edelmann, R. J. (1995). Social anxiety, fear of negative evaluation and the detection of negative emotion in others. *Behaviour Research and Therapy*, **33**, 193–6.

Wood, J. V., Saltzberg, J. A., and Goldsamt, L. A. (1990). Does affect induce self-focused attention? *Journal of Personality and Social Psychology*, **58**, 899–908.

Woody, S. R. (1996). Effects of focus of attention on anxiety levels and social performance of individuals with social phobia. *Journal of Abnormal Psychology*, **105**, 61–9.

Woody, S. R., Chambless, D. L., and Glass, C. R. (1997). Self-focused attention in the treatment of social phobia. *Behaviour Research and Therapy*, **35**, 117–29.

12

The cognitive model of bulimia nervosa

Daniel le Grange

University of Chicago, Chicago, IL, USA

Introduction

Bulimia nervosa is a highly prevalent eating disorder that has a profound impact on the lives of many women and their families. In the first clinical account, Russell (1979) described bulimia nervosa as a separate eating disorder with key features of binge eating, accompanied by feelings of loss of control during such eating episodes, followed by guilt and remorse. A fear of fatness leads to repeated attempts to lose weight through dieting and/or inappropriate compensatory purging behaviors, e.g., self-induced vomiting, laxative or diuretic abuse, and excessive exercise. Bulimia nervosa usually arises in adolescence with peak onset at 18 years, and affects as many as 2% of young women (Mitchell et al., 1987a).

Bulimia nervosa is a major source of psychiatric morbidity and leads to impairments in several areas of physiological and psychological functioning. Clinical features include high rates of depression and anxiety, personality disorders, disturbances in social functioning, alcohol and drug abuse, and suicide attempts (Fahy and Russell, 1993). Rates of sexual abuse appear to be higher in bulimia nervosa than in other psychiatric groups (Waller, 1991), although this issue has not been sufficiently explored. Adolescents with bulimia nervosa often experience significantly lower self-esteem than those without an eating disorder (Crowther and Chernyk, 1986); they also report significantly more suicidal ideation and suicide attempts than other adolescents (H. M. Hoberman et al., unpublished data). Beyond psychiatric morbidity, preoccupation with food and body weight can impair social, school, and work functioning.

Although bulimia nervosa is a psychiatric condition, it is also associated with significant medical complications, morbidity, and mortality (Fisher, 1992). As many as one-quarter of patients may require hospitalization for medical reasons (Kreipe et al., 1995). Moreover, the physiological effects of recurrent binge eating and vomiting create a mortality risk, as does the potential medical instability of these patients. This is exacerbated by their tendency to deny the severity of their condition (Altshuler et al., 1990).

Hypokalemia is common, while hypocalcemia, hypomagnesemia, hypophosphatemia, esophageal irritation and bleeding, Mallory–Weiss tears, gastric rupture, and large-bowel abnormalities have all been noted (Mitchell et al., 1987b). The use of ipecac to induce vomiting can cause emetine cardiomyopathy, hepatic toxicity, or peripheral myopathy (Palmer and Guay, 1985). Body weight for most individuals with bulimia nervosa is usually within normal range. Dental caries, periodontal disease, and menstrual irregularities are common, while approximately 25% of cases present with secondary amenorrhea and 33% present with irregular menses (Mitchell, 1995).

Hoek (1991) found the incidence of bulimia nervosa to be 11.4 per 100 000 population per year between the years 1985 and 1989. He warns that this may underestimate actual rates as we lack community-based studies, and detection of cases is complicated due to the secrecy that surrounds bulimia nervosa. In a later study, Hoek (1995) found that little over one-tenth of the potential cases of bulimia nervosa in the community are detected. Only half of these persons are referred for treatment.

North American studies have found between 4% (Stangler and Printz, 1980) and 13% (Halmi et al., 1981) of college students experience symptoms of bulimia nervosa. There is evidence to suggest that disordered eating in males may be similar to that observed in females (Whitaker et al., 1990; Keel and Mitchell, 1997). Bulimia nervosa may be as prevalent among nonwestern and ethnic-minority females as it is among Caucasian adolescents (Szabo and Tury, 1991; Story et al., 1994).

An increase in the prevalence of bulimia nervosa among adolescents and preadolescents has also been noted. Community samples have shown that a wide range (10–50%) of adolescent girls and boys frequently engage in binge-eating behavior (Johnson et al., 1984; Pope et al., 1984; Crowther et al., 1985; Killen et al., 1987). Applying stringent diagnostic criteria, studies have found 2–5% of adolescent girls surveyed qualify for a diagnosis of bulimia nervosa (Ledoux et al., 1991). Several recent reports have described even higher numbers of adolescents presenting with bulimia nervosa (Remschmidt and Herpertz-Dahlmann, 1990; Woodside and Garfinkel, 1992; Schmidt et al., 1995; Stein et al., 1998).

Clearly, bulimia nervosa is a highly prevalent and serious health concern that affects adolescents and young adults across diverse ethnic groups. As a result, much attention has been given to the evaluation of a variety of treatments for bulimia nervosa. Cognitive-behavioral therapy (CBT) has received most of the research and clinical attention.

The aim of this chapter is to discuss the cognitive model for the maintenance of bulimia nervosa and to summarize the treatment that arises from this model.

The efficacy and shortcomings of this therapy will also be reviewed. Christopher Fairburn's approach forms the basis of this chapter. Fairburn's work and that of several collaborators is the extant cognitive model of bulimia nervosa and its associated treatment strategies. Despite criticism, this is the prevailing cognitive explanation for the maintenance and treatment of bulimia nervosa. The origins of this model, its treatment strategies, and a critical review of research evidence in support of this approach toward bulimia nervosa will be presented. Finally, some limitations of the cognitive model and directions for future research will be considered.

Description of the cognitive model for bulimia nervosa

The etiology of bulimia nervosa is poorly understood. None the less, there is a consensus that the causes are multifactorial and that it arises from an interaction between neurobiological, psychological, familial, and sociocultural factors. In terms of neurobiological factors, it is possible that a tendency toward eating disorders may be due to heritable factors. This notion is supported in part by family and twin studies (Kendler, 1991; Strober, 1995; Strober et al., 2001). The exact manner in which genes might contribute to the familial aggregation of eating disorders remains unclear and is the subject of current investigation (W. Kaye, personal communication). Certain psychological characteristics appear to increase the propensity to develop an eating disorder. For instance, low self-esteem, a profound sense of ineffectiveness, and perfectionism have all been said to play a role in the origins of eating disorders (Vitousek and Hollon, 1990). Bulimia nervosa remains more prevalent in certain cultural environments and almost exclusively in women. It is therefore quite possible that social factors may play a predisposing role in the development of this disorder (Vandereycken and Hoek, 1992). Finally, bulimia nervosa has been attributed to disturbed family interaction, high levels of criticism from parents toward their bulimic offspring, or to early traumatic life events (Vandereycken, 1995). The role of the psychosocial and neurobiological factors in the etiology of bulimia nervosa remains largely speculative and outside the scope of this chapter.

The most influential model of bulimia nervosa is that of Fairburn (1981). His cognitive model focuses almost exclusively on psychological/personality factors and how these pertain to the *maintenance* as opposed to the *etiology* of symptomatic behavior. Although this model pays only scant attention to the origins of the disorder, it has given rise to the influential CBT for bulimia nervosa. CBT for bulimia nervosa grew out of Beck et al.'s (1979) original work on depression, as well as Mahoney and Mahoney's (1976) behavioral treatment of obesity. Fairburn's (1981) cognitive model is essentially an amalgam of these two approaches. The publication of Fairburn's (1985) detailed manual greatly facilitated the development of CBT for bulimia nervosa. The aim of these interventions is systematically to target each of

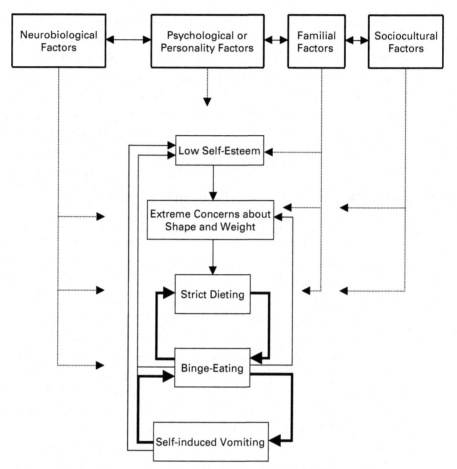

Figure 12.1   The cognitive view of the maintenance of bulimia nervosa. Thickness of lines = strength of evidence supporting relationship; broken lines = etiological additions to Fairburn's original maintenance model. Adapted from C. G. Fairburn, M. D. Marcus, and G. T. Wilson Cognitive-behavioral therapy for binge eating and bulimia nervosa: a comprehensive treatment manual (Chapter 16, p. 369). In Christopher G. Fairburn and G. Terence Wilson, eds, *Binge Eating. Nature, Assessment and Treatment*, New York: Guilford Press, 1993. Reprinted with permission.

the primary maintaining factors of bulimia nervosa as identified in the cognitive theory. More recently, Fairburn et al. (1993b) published an expanded version of this manual to include adaptations for binge-eating disorder and anorexia nervosa.

The most recent version of the original model of bulimia nervosa, unchanged since 1993, is presented schematically in Figure 12.1. The present author has added possible predisposing and precipitating factors to this equation. Fairburn's model focuses on symptom development in an individual with undue low self-esteem, and the maintenance of these symptomatic behaviors due to overvalued ideals of weight and body shape. These overvalued ideals are usually accompanied by problematic and inaccurate beliefs and thoughts that are concentrated in three core domains: (1) unrealistic expectations for body weight and shape; (2) the belief that desirable outcomes such as enhanced self-worth will follow if this idealized body weight and shape are obtained; and (3) inaccurate beliefs about food, food consumption, and how eating influences weight.

Dysfunctional beliefs about food and about one's body usually result in extreme dissatisfaction with shape and weight. This, in turn, gives rise to the development of a rigid and restrictive eating pattern that is designed to control and alter weight and shape. The result of dysfunctional beliefs is that eating becomes regulated by a set of self-generated rules and regulations instead of regular internal signals of hunger and satiety. These rules include what kind of food is eaten, how much food is eaten during any specific meal, and how often food is eaten.

It is usually taxing to remain on a restrictive diet and, consequently, physiological and psychological deprivation develops, e.g., extreme hunger and/or social isolation. The consequences of this deprivation includes strong urges to eat, an excessive focus on food, and eventual loss of control over eating, i.e., bingeing. Even though the binge itself may sometimes be experienced as pleasurable, more often than not it is followed by anxiety about weight gain and self-deprecating thoughts. These, in turn, reinforce the restrictive behavior.

Bulimic individuals engage in purging behaviors in an attempt to compensate for the consumption of calories, to reduce concerns about weight gain, and to regain self-control. Self-induced vomiting is the most common form of inappropriate compensatory behaviors, although laxative and diuretic abuse, and excessive exercise are also used as methods of purging. Purging helps maintain binge eating by reducing the individual's anxiety about potential weight gain, and by disrupting learned satiety signals that usually regulate food intake. Purging is also followed by a rededication to a strict dietary regimen.

Finally, feelings of guilt, self-disgust, and a sense of failure because of bingeing and purging strengthen the desire to regain control and esteem via attainment of the idealized body weight and shape. In other words, the physiological sequelae of this pathological behavior serve to sustain the disordered beliefs (Vitousek, 1996). Following on from this cognitive model, Fairburn (1985) has articulated a clear treatment plan for bulimia nervosa, which is presented in the following section of this chapter.

Overview of treatment plan

Since Fairburn's first description of CBT for bulimia nervosa in 1981, this therapy has been further developed at several research centers in both the USA and western Europe (Agras et al., 1989; Mitchell et al., 1990; Fairburn et al., 1991; Walsh et al.,

1997). This treatment model has also been articulated in several therapist guides and patient self-help manuals (Cooper, 1995; Agras and Apple, 1997).

CBT does not aim to bring about a sophisticated psychological understanding of the origins of this disorder. Instead, treatment addresses the presenting behaviors of binge eating and purging. Most important, dietary restraint must be replaced with regular and healthy eating, while dysfunctional thoughts and beliefs about the personal significance of weight and shape should be addressed and altered. Treatment is typically time-limited and involves three main phases: (1) establishing regular eating patterns; (2) evaluating and changing cognitions about weight and shape; and (3) relapse prevention.

In the first phase of treatment, the primary aim is to establish a regular eating pattern. Interventions are aimed at regulating the chronic dieting that is believed to be the cause of binge eating. The focus here is on helping clients to eat regular meals at regular times, i.e., three meals and two snacks per day. Phase 1 begins with a simplified explanation of the cognitive model of the maintenance of bulimia nervosa. This includes discussions about overvalued ideas of slenderness that give rise to dietary restriction, how this leads to bingeing and purging which, in turn, reinforce the overvalued ideas of slenderness. Particular emphasis is placed on reducing dietary restriction and on normalizing food intake. It is hypothesized that this will lead to a reduction in bingeing and purging.

The second phase of treatment focuses on the identification of and change in problematic beliefs and thoughts about shape and weight. This is accomplished through cognitive restructuring. Examples of such thoughts and beliefs are: "Because I gained 2 pounds (1 kg) this week, this must mean that I will continue to gain weight," or "Everyone ignored me at the meeting, so it must mean that they think I'm fat and ugly." The cognitive model for bulimia nervosa assumes that it is these thoughts and beliefs that contribute to body dissatisfaction and dietary restriction.

At this point in the treatment process, most clients have established a fairly regular eating pattern, and made significant improvements in terms of bingeing and purging. Broadening the usually narrow range of "permissible" foods is one of the central aims of this phase of treatment. Additional binge triggers such as overvalued ideas of thinness are addressed.

The final focus for this phase of the treatment is training in problem-solving techniques. These are aimed at teaching clients healthier ways to deal with situations that usually lead to binge eating. These skills are included in the treatment package because some clients resort to bingeing and purging in order to cope with stressful situations.

The final phase, or relapse prevention, serves to clarify the changes the client has already made, and prepares the client for residual problems that may be found once treatment has been terminated. The therapist reviews with the client the progress made during treatment; this includes the identification of specific actions and thoughts associated with treatment setbacks and gains. A relapse plan is developed that includes the identification of warning signs of relapse, specific plans to be used in response to these signs, and encouragement to use the strategies that have been found to be useful in the past.

Evidence for the cognitive model

The cognitive model does not address, nor is there much evidence for, the *etiology* of bulimia nervosa in terms of an interaction between neurobiological, personality, family, and cultural factors on the individual. Support for the cognitive view of the *maintenance* of bulimia nervosa, however, has been sizeable, albeit largely indirect. For instance, Mizes and Christiano (1995) provide evidence of the cognitive characteristics of bulimia nervosa patients. The link between dieting, binge eating and purging has also received research support in several laboratory studies (Blundell and Hill, 1993; Polivy and Herman, 1993). These authors have shown that a self-sustaining feedback loop develops, where restricting intake (regulation) leads to episodes of bingeing and purging (dysregulation); the dysregulation, in turn, reinforces regulation.

According to Fairburn (1997), the large body of research indicating that CBT has a major and lasting impact on the disorder provides the strongest support for the cognitive view of bulimia nervosa. The most important of this support comes from patients who have recovered in behavioral terms. For these patients, the severity of their concerns about shape and weight at the end of treatment was directly related to the likelihood of relapse (Fairburn et al., 1993a). Additional support comes from dismantling studies in which interventions designed to produce cognitive change have been removed. Fairburn claims that in such instances the effects of CBT are attenuated, leaving patients markedly prone to relapse.

Taken together, the cognitive model for bulimia nervosa is relatively well developed, especially in terms of a specific treatment approach which is derived from this model. The most important limitations, though, are the lack of attention to the etiology of bulimia nervosa, and the fact that evidence for the cognitive model of the maintenance of bulimia nervosa is largely indirect. In the following section, a critical review of the treatment evidence in support of the cognitive model of bulimia nervosa is presented in more detail.

Critical status of cognitive therapy for bulimia nervosa

Bulimia nervosa seriously affects physical, emotional, and social development, and it often follows a chronic and severe course (Maddocks et al., 1992; Keel and Mitchell,

1997; Herzog et al., 1999). It is therefore not surprising that much attention has been given to the evaluation of treatments for patients with bulimia nervosa. CBT for adults with bulimia nervosa has received more attention from investigators than any other treatment modality. Treatment is complex and requires attention to broad psychiatric, medical, and nutritional aspects of the disease (Yager et al., 1993). Reports comparing psychosocial and pharmacological therapies have come to dominate research in the field.

Well over 20 controlled studies have been conducted during the past 15 years, with the majority attesting to the effectiveness of CBT for bulimia nervosa (see Table 12.1 for a summary of these studies). Many of these randomized studies have demonstrated that CBT produces a mean reduction in binge eating and purging approaching 80%, and a mean abstinence rate approaching 55% (Fairburn et al., 1992; Wilson and Fairburn, 1998). Dietary restraint is also significantly lessened, and the disturbed attitudes to body weight and shape are greatly reduced (Fairburn et al., 1991; Garner et al., 1993). Several studies have shown good maintenance of change at follow-up ranging from 6 months to 5.8 years (Fairburn et al., 1993a, 1995; Agras et al., 1994). CBT has also been found to be superior to most other treatments with which it had been compared. In a review of controlled trials of pharmacological and psychological treatments for bulimia nervosa, Mitchell et al. (1993) demonstrated that CBT is consistently superior to waiting-list control conditions. Most recently, Whittal et al. (1999) conducted a metaanalysis of psychosocial and pharmacological treatments of bulimia nervosa and confirmed that CBT is the treatment of choice for this disorder. For instance, for 26 CBT trials pooled effect size scores for binge and purge frequency were 1.28 and 1.22 respectively.

CBT compared with other psychotherapies

As mentioned above, in most controlled studies CBT has proven to be significantly more effective than any psychological treatment with which it has been compared. For instance, CBT was more effective than supportive psychotherapy at the end of treatment and at 1-year follow-up (Agras et al., 1989). Garner et al. (1993) found CBT to be superior to supportive-expressive therapy in decreasing purging, lessening dietary restraint, and modifying dysfunctional attitudes to shape and weight. CBT has also been compared to behavior therapy and interpersonal therapy (IPT) (Fairburn et al., 1991). In this study, IPT focused on interpersonal difficulties, and omitted the cognitive and behavioral interventions that are part of CBT. At the end of treatment, CBT and IPT were similar in percent reductions in objective bulimic episodes. There was also no significant difference in those who abstained from objective bulimic episodes. Both conditions were equally effective in terms of a reduction in depression, general psychopathology, and improvements in social functioning. However, CBT was significantly more effective than IPT in reducing purging, dietary restraint, and attitudes to shape and weight. It was also superior

Table 12.1 Controlled psychotherapy trials for bulimia nervosa since 1990[1]

Authors	Treatment format	n	Reduction in binge and/or purge frequency (%)	Abstinence at end of treatment (%)
Mitchell et al. (1990)	Group CBT and Placebo	34	89	45
	Group CBT and Imipramine	52	92	56
	Imipramine	54	49	16
	Placebo	31	–	–
Fairburn et al. (1991)	Individual CBT	25	97	71
	Individual behavior therapy	25	91	62
	Individual interpersonal therapy	25	89	62
Fairburn et al. (1995)	Individual CBT	25	–	50
(5.8-year follow-up)	Individual behavior therapy	25	–	18
	Individual interpersonal therapy	25	–	52
Wilson et al. (1991)	CBT with exposure and response prevention		78	55
	CBT		75	64
Agras et al. (1989)	Self-monitor	19	63	24
	Group CBT	22	75	56
	Group CBT and exposure and response prevention	17	52	31
	Waitlist	18	–	–
Agras et al. (1992)	Individual desipramine (16 weeks)	12	13 (increase)	35
	Individual desipramine (24 weeks)	12	44	42
	Individual CBT and desipramine (16 weeks)	12	57	65
	Individual CBT and desipramine (24 weeks)	12	89	70
	Individual CBT	23	71	55
Agras et al. (1994)	Individual desipramine (16 weeks)	12	–	16
(1-year follow-up)	Individual desipramine (24 weeks)	12	–	67
	Individual CBT and desipramine (16 weeks)	57	–	40
	Individual CBT and desipramine (24 weeks)	89	–	78
	Individual CBT	23	–	54
Mitchell et al. (1993)	Group CBT (high emphasis on abstinence/high intensity)	33	77	70
	High/low	41	78	73
	Low/high	35	88	71
	Low/low	34	62	32

(cont.)

Table 12.1 (*cont.*)

Authors	Treatment format	*n*	Reduction in binge and/or purge frequency (%)	Abstinence at end of treatment (%)
Wolf and Crowther	Group behavioral	15	68	–
(1992)	Group CBT	15	33	–
	Waitlist	11	10 (increase)	–
Garner et al. (1993)	Individual psychodynamic	30	62	12
	Individual CBT	30	82	36
Goldbloom et al. (1997)	Fluoxetine	23	70	17
	Individual CBT	24	80	43
	Individual CBT + fluoxetine	29	87	25
Walsh et al. (1997)	Individual CBT + placebo	25	19	–
	Individual supportive therapy + placebo	22	12	–
	Individual CBT and medication	23	50	–
	Individual supportive therapy and medication	22	18	–
	Medication only	28	25	–
Agras et al. (2000)[2]				
(end treatment)	Individual CBT	110	–	29
(1 year follow-up)	Individual interpersonal therapy	110	–	6
	Individual CBT	–		28
	Individual interpersonal therapy	–		17

[1] Only randomized controlled studies that investigated the efficacy of cognitive-behavioral therapy (CBT) for bulimia nervosa were selected for inclusion in this table. The majority of these controlled studies include Caucasian female participants in their mid-20s who were recruited from clinic populations.
[2] Intent-to-treat analysis.
– Not reported.

to behavior therapy in relation to dietary restraint and attitudes to body shape and weight. At a closed 1-year follow-up (Fairburn et al., 1993a) CBT and IPT were clearly superior to behavior therapy. Results for IPT were similar to CBT in that both treatments produced significant but equivalent reductions in bulimic episodes. Both treatments were also equally effective in improvements in secondary measures such as general psychiatric symptoms, depression, self-esteem, and attitude towards weight and body shape.

Taken together, CBT's superiority to other credible psychotherapies – with the possible exception of IPT – is indisputable. Fairburn et al.'s (1993a) finding that IPT is as effective as CBT was unexpected. The reduction in cognitive distortions in both treatments was especially noteworthy, as IPT does not target these symptoms. In two subsequent publications (Fairburn et al., 1995; Agras et al., 2000) the comparable effects of CBT and IPT were again demonstrated. Although these studies suggest that IPT may be as effective as CBT, findings from the large multicenter study of Agras et al. indicated CBT's significantly swifter ability to engender improvements in bulimic symptoms. These authors conclude that CBT should be considered the psychotherapeutic treatment of choice for bulimia nervosa.

Arnow (1998), in a comprehensive review of psychotherapeutic treatments for eating disorders, proposed that *common* factors, which have been hypothesized as curative in all psychotherapies (Goldfried, 1980), are responsible for the positive effects of both CBT and IPT. However, Fairburn et al.'s (1993a) position is that *specific* factors distinguish CBT from other treatments. First, CBT was superior to behavior therapy in follow-up data gathered from their 1991 cohort. Second, CBT was found to be superior to self-monitoring (Agras et al., 1989). Third, transitory differences in the treatment response pattern for individuals receiving CBT or interpersonal psychotherapy suggest specific, albeit different mechanisms of change. CBT is likely to operate directly on eating behavior and cognitions, while IPT operates directly via gradual changes in interpersonal patterns. It is possible that, in CBT, a correction of eating behavior leads to improved interpersonal functioning while, in IPT, an improvement in social relations leads to improvements in eating habits (Agras, 1993). This remains an empirical and conceptual question.

CBT's underlying conceptualization emphasizes restrained eating and disturbed attitudes toward weight and shape. Arnow (1998) argues that a shortcoming of CBT is its failure to address issues of affective instability and deficits in emotion self-regulation. Both these shortcomings have been noted in the empirical literature (Lingswiler et al., 1989) and identified by bulimic clients (Arnow, 1996; Le Grange and Gelman, 1998). Arnow suggests that it is possible that IPT, as opposed to CBT, has a health-promoting effect upon affect self-regulation. The specific mechanisms of change, however, are not well understood. The possibility that IPT may have significant benefits and that both CBT and IPT may have specific effects, mediated through different mechanisms, requires empirical verification.

CBT and antidepressant medication

In addition to CBT, antidepressant medications in the treatment of bulimia nervosa have received intense research attention. Investigations into antidepressant medications were prompted by observations that there is an increased frequency of mood disturbance associated with bulimia nervosa. About one-third of those with this disorder have experienced an episode of depression prior to the onset of their eating disorder. Depression is also common among the relatives of bulimia nervosa patients (Kendler et al., 1991). One mechanism that might account for the link between affective disorder and vulnerability to an eating disorder is an abnormality in serotonin (5-HT) functioning. Low levels of serotonin have been implicated in both affective disorder and bulimia nervosa (Kaye, 1992). These observations have led to a series of double-blind, placebo-controlled trials of antidepressants among adults with bulimia nervosa (Fichter et al., 1991; Agras et al., 1992). Several classes of antidepressant medication have been examined, including the tricyclics, monoamine oxidase inhibitors, selective seretonin reuptake inhibitors (SSRIs), and atypical antidepressants such as amfebutamone and trazodone. In almost all the controlled trials, both tricyclics and one SSRI (fluoxetine) have proven superior to placebo in reducing binge frequency. Generally, mood disturbance and preoccupation with shape and weight also show greater improvement with medication than with placebo (Mitchell and deZwaan, 1993).

Several controlled studies have directly evaluated the relative and combined effectiveness of CBT and antidepressant drug treatment (Mitchell et al., 1990; Fichter et al., 1991; Agras et al., 1992; Leitenberg et al., 1994; Walsh et al., 1997). Taken together, these studies indicate that CBT is superior to medication on its own, and that combining CBT with medication is significantly more effective than medication alone. However, this combination provides only modest incremental benefits over CBT alone. Further support for CBT comes from the findings that it is more acceptable to patients, and results in fewer dropouts during treatment (Wilson and Fairburn, 1998). In contrasting CBT and medication, perhaps the most important finding is that there is little evidence to support the long-term effectiveness of pharmacological treatment. There has been one exception in terms of the durability of drug treatment: Agras and colleagues (1994) have shown that 6 months of treatment with desipramine produced lasting improvement even after the medication was withdrawn.

It is difficult to challenge the superiority of CBT as the treatment of choice for bulimia nervosa. Consequently, recent debate has focused on how this treatment can be further refined, its abstinence rates improved, how best to treat nonresponders, and whether the effective components of CBT can be delineated. In the following section of this chapter, the last of these four questions is addressed through a discussion of dismantling studies.

Effective components of CBT for bulimia nervosa

In an attempt to learn more about the effective components of CBT, Kirkley et al. (1985) allocated bulimic females to either a self-monitoring group combined with nondirective therapy, or to CBT. Results indicated a significant advantage for CBT in reducing binge and purge frequency. However, in terms of secondary measures such as depression and anxiety, posttreatment results yielded no differences between the two groups. This study showed that the behavior change procedures associated with CBT may be important, although it did not shed light on which specific interventions were associated with an improvement in symptoms.

Freeman et al. (1988), in a study examining the relative contribution of cognitive and behavioral procedures, randomly assigned bulimic women to CBT, behavior therapy, group therapy, or a waitlist control group. The major difference between the CBT and behavior therapy groups was that the latter did not contain cognitive procedures aimed at altering dysfunctional thoughts. Contrary to expectations, results at the end of treatment revealed no significant differences among the active groups. This led the authors to conclude that there were no added advantages to these specific cognitive procedures in CBT. The absence of follow-up data for this study, however, renders their findings inconclusive. Wilson and Fairburn (1993) remind us that the cognitive model predicts that CBT will compare most favorably with comparison treatments during follow-up – an opportunity not afforded by the design of the Freeman et al. (1988) study.

On the same topic, Wolf and Crowther (1992) assigned bulimic women to CBT, behavior therapy, or a waitlist group to investigate whether cognitive interventions add to the efficacy of behavioral tasks in CBT. Both active treatments were superior to the control treatment in terms of a reduction in binge eating at posttreatment. Contrary to Wilson and Fairburn's (1993) prediction, at 3-month follow-up, patients in the behavior therapy group continued to improve in terms of binge eating. Those in CBT showed a modest trend toward relapse, although they demonstrated a greater reduction in preoccupation with dieting and lower levels of general psychopathology compared to the behavior therapy condition. Arnow (1998) is of the opinion that the brevity of treatment as well as the relatively short follow-up may have reduced the effectiveness of CBT.

Fairburn and his colleagues (1991, 1993, 1995) conducted a series of studies comparing CBT and behavior therapy. Overall, results were mixed with respect to the active ingredients of CBT. There were no significant differences between CBT and behavior therapy at posttreatment in relation to those who abstained from objective bulimic episodes or self-induced vomiting. CBT was, however, more effective in reducing dietary restraint and body shape concerns. Arnow (1998) concludes that the debate about the active ingredients of CBT is far from settled. Whereas behavior change interventions associated with CBT clearly appear to be effective, the added benefit of cognitive interventions remains uncertain.

In the final section of this chapter the benefits of CBT in the treatment of bulimia nervosa will be summarized. This is followed by a discussion of areas where the application of the cognitive model and subsequent manualized treatment for bulimia nervosa may be problematic, and indications for future research efforts.

Discussion and future research directions

There is considerable evidence attesting to the effectiveness of CBT for bulimia nervosa. As noted, over 20 controlled studies have evaluated the effectiveness of CBT for bulimia nervosa. Most of these studies have shown that CBT is more effective than no treatment, nondirective psychotherapy, manual-based psychodynamic psychotherapy, stress management, and antidepressant medication (Mitchell et al., 1990; Agras et al., 1992; Fairburn et al., 1993a; Garner et al., 1993). Research has shown that about half of clients exposed to CBT stop binge eating and purging by the completion of treatment. Moreover, attitudes regarding weight and body shape also improve. Improvements continue after treatment, leading to a symptom-free rate of around 65% at 6–12-month follow-up (Agras et al., 1994). Long-term outcome results are also encouraging. More than 80% of patients report full or partial recovery at 7–10-year follow-up (Collings and King, 1994; Herzog et al., 1999).

Despite these optimistic findings, a significant number of bulimic patients do not respond favorably to CBT (Agras, 1993). The reasons for this mixed response are unclear. One possible explanation concerns the inherent limitations of manualized treatment, especially for bulimic patients with comorbid psychopathology. Many therapists might argue that CBT, which stipulates a lock-step approach to treatment, renders it unsuitable for clients with a complicated presentation. Carrying out a more idiographic assessment, and drawing on a wider range of cognitive and behavioral strategies, allows therapists to tailor therapy toward the needs of the individual client. Wilson and Fairburn (1993) agree that this is a clinically appealing proposal, though they question whether the greater range and flexibility of an idiographic implementation of CBT would be beneficial (Wilson, 1996; Wilson et al., 1997). They argue that personal biases undermine the utility of an idiographic approach. Weighing up the wealth of research evidence in support of manualized CBT against the perceived influences of such biases, Wilson and his colleagues (1997) conclude that an idiographic approach does not increase effectiveness of treatment techniques, and if CBT does not provide the desired effect, the therapist ought to progress on to another empirically validated approach.

Given the paucity of other empirically validated treatments of bulimia nervosa, the clinician's only option is, in fact, IPT. Johnson and his colleagues (1990) would argue that psychodynamic psychotherapy provides another option. The findings of their study suggest that when psychodynamic psychotherapy is added to CBT, a significant number of bulimic patients with a personality disorder improve (Johnson et al., 1990); however, patients required an average of 100 treatment sessions over 1 year, substantially more than the 20 sessions advocated for CBT. Tobin (1993), espousing a psychodynamic model in the etiology and treatment of bulimia nervosa, concedes that it may be easier to shift from a cognitive-behavioral approach to a psychodynamic one, as opposed to the other way round. The status of our current knowledge, however, does not enable us to match a client with one treatment as opposed to another. This, too, remains an important empirical question.

A second issue concerns the optimal strategy for implementing core cognitive approaches in CBT for bulimia nervosa (Wilson et al., 1997). Hollon and Beck (1994) suggest that the use of cognitive restructuring, a complex cognitive technique, has been less than optimal. Wilson et al. (1997) admit that CBT for bulimia nervosa describes a basic version of cognitive restructuring, while more elaborate versions of this technique have been put forward for the treatment of anorexia nervosa (Garner and Bemis, 1985), and for depression and anxiety disorders (Clark, 1989; Fennell, 1989). Wilson and colleagues (1997) justify their use of a simplified version of cognitive restructuring on the grounds that this technique is difficult to master and that a more complex form would be formidable. They express concern that cognitive restructuring, as a technique, may not be "exportable." That is to say, it may be difficult to apply this strategy with the same ease across different diagnoses. In defending the existing CBT manual, Wilson et al. (1997) state that there is no evidence from work with other disorders that added emphasis on cognitive restructuring would produce better results. They do, however, concede that there may be situations where a more extensive model of cognitive restructuring is required, e.g., bulimia nervosa patients who fail to respond to regular CBT, or more difficult to treat anorexic patients. Whether expanded cognitive restructuring techniques will improve the outcome in nonresponders is an important question that has not been tested empirically.

A third issue of concern is that CBT focuses on changing overvalued ideas about body weight and shape (Fairburn et al., 1998), but does not directly address interpersonal concerns or deficits in affect regulation. This is best demonstrated by treatment studies showing that IPT, a treatment that does not focus on the eating disorder per se, might be a viable alternative to CBT. By conducting a comprehensive enquiry into the client's history, IPT seeks to identify underlying interpersonal problem areas. The rationale for IPT for bulimia nervosa suggests that those who develop the disorder exhibit interpersonal problems of which they are unaware (Apple, 1999). Addressing these key areas in therapy can lead to improved interpersonal functioning and, consequently, improved eating habits and thinking about weight and body shape issues.

The marked success of IPT is noteworthy. In CBT, patients may improve because a decrease in bulimic symptoms leads to an improvement in interpersonal functioning (Agras, 1993). IPT, on the other hand, leads to improved interpersonal relations which, in turn, may bring about a decrease in bulimic symptoms. The success of IPT begs consideration of the cognitive model's explanation of factors that precipitate and perpetuate bulimia nervosa. As pointed out earlier in this chapter, identifying which clients are more likely to benefit from a primarily cognitive approach as opposed to an interpersonal approach remains a key question. Comparing CBT and IPT will reveal the respective effective components of these treatments. Given the conceptual and procedural differences between CBT and IPT, it seems likely that these treatments might have different effects on different subgroups of bulimia nervosa patients.

In terms of future research directions, at least six areas of inquiry merit consideration: (1) the etiology of bulimia nervosa is poorly understood, both in a general sense as well as from a cognitive perspective; (2) the application of CBT for adult anorexia nervosa and its utilization for adolescent bulimia nervosa deserve further investigation; (3) CBT protocols should formally examine the inclusion of an affect regulation component; (4) the application of CBT to treatment nonresponders needs further investigation; (5) the processes of change in both CBT and IPT are poorly understood; and (6) the basic tenets of the cognitive model of bulimia nervosa have not been subjected to systematic evaluation.

Concluding remarks

Despite the appeal of the cognitive model of bulimia nervosa, as well as the successes reported in treatment studies examining CBT, limitations in its conceptualization and applicability continue. This model does not shed much light on the origins of this disorder and may, as a result, not pay sufficient attention to the impact of factors other than self-esteem, weight, and body shape concerns. Also, about 40% of those receiving CBT do not respond favorably, and long-term outcomes for this treatment remain unclear. The treatment of CBT nonresponders should be a priority.

An important development arising from research over the past decade is the clinical appeal of IPT. Because of its focus on interpersonal problems, this treatment may be particularly well suited to clients with bulimia nervosa. Interpersonal difficulties are a common feature of bulimia nervosa and have been implicated in the etiology of this disorder (Striegel-Moore et al., 1986). A treatment that focuses on interpersonal difficulties should be effective in improving self-esteem and self-acceptance, thereby removing one of the primary reasons for excessive concern with weight, which results in dieting, bingeing, and purging. CBT, by contrast, directly treats maladaptive eating habits and underlying problematic thoughts and beliefs. If eating is normalized and excessive weight and body shape concerns dissipate, self-esteem and self-efficacy may improve. This in turn could lead to improved interpersonal functioning, thus demonstrating a different mode of action from IPT. Matching clients with different needs to treatments with different modes of action is clearly the next step in research efforts.

The fact that a significant number of persons with bulimia nervosa respond favorably to IPT as opposed to CBT is a theoretically and clinically significant finding. It demonstrates that the applicability of the cognitive model of bulimia nervosa and CBT may have limitations. Although CBT is regarded as the gold-standard treatment for bulimia nervosa, and for now should be regarded as the treatment of choice for this clinical population, it does not appear to be a universal remedy for bulimia nervosa.

REFERENCES

Agras, W. S. (1992). *Cognitive-behavioral therapy and interpersonal therapy for bulimia nervosa.* Unpublished manuscript, Stanford University, California.

Agras, W. S. (1993). Short-term psychological treatments for binge eating. In *Binge Eating: Nature, Assessment, and treatment*, ed. C. G. Fairburn and G.T. Wilson, pp. 270–86. New York: Guilford Press.

Agras, W. S. and Apple, R. F. (1997). *Overcoming Eating Disorders. Therapist Guide.* San Antonio: The Psychological Corporation.

Agras, W. S., Schneider, J. A., Arnow, B., Raeburn, S. D., and Telch, C. F. (1989). Cognitive-behavioral and response-prevention treatments for bulimia nervosa. *Journal of Consulting and Clinical Psychology*, **57**, 215–21.

Agras, W. S., Rossiter, E. M., Arnow, B., et al. (1992). Pharmacologic and cognitive- behavioral treatment for bulimia nervosa: a controlled comparison. *American Journal of Psychiatry*, **149**, 82–7.

Agras, W. S., Rossiter, E. M., Arnow, B., et al. (1994). One-year follow-up of psychosocial and pharmacologic treatments for bulimia nervosa. *Journal of Clinical Psychiatry*, **55**, 179–83.

Agras, W. S., Walsh, B. T., Fairburn, C. G., Wilson, G. T., and Kraemer, H. C. (2000). A multicenter comparison of cognitive-behavioral therapy and interpersonal psychotherapy for bulimia nervosa. *Archives of General Psychiatry*, **57**, 459–66.

Altshuler, B. D., Dechow, P. C., Waller, D. A., and Hardy B. (1990). An investigation of the oral pathologies occurring in bulimia nervosa. *International Journal of Eating Disorders*, **9**, 191–9.

American Psychiatric Association. (1980). *Diagnostic and Statistical Manual of Mental Disorders*, 3rd edn (DSM-III). Washington, DC: American Psychiatric Press.

Apple, R. F. (1999). Interpersonal therapy for bulimia nervosa. *Journal of Clinical Psychology*, **55**, 715–26.

Arnow, B. (1996). Cognitive-behavioral therapy for bulimia nervosa. In *Treating Eating Disorders*, ed. J. Werne, pp. 101–41. San Francisco: Jossey-Bass.

Arnow, B. (1998). Psychotherapy of anorexia and bulimia nervosa. In *Baillière's Clinical Psychiatry: Eating Disorders*, ed. D. Jimmerson and W. Kaye, pp. 235–57. London: W. B. Saunders.

Beck, A. T., Rush, A. J., Shaw, B. J., and Emery, G. (1979). *Cognitive Therapy for Depression.* New York: Guilford Press.

Blundell, J. E. and Hill, A. J. (1993). Binge eating: psychobiological mechanisms. In *Binge Eating. Nature, Assessment, and Treatment*, ed. C. G. Fairburn and G. T. Wilson, pp. 206–26. New York: Guilford Press.

Clark, D. M. (1989). Anxiety states: panic and generalized anxiety. In *Cognitive Behavior Therapy for Psychiatric Problems*, ed. K. Hawton, P. M. Salkovskis, J. Kirk and D. M. Clark, pp. 52–96. New York: Oxford University Press.

Collings, S. and King, M. (1994). Ten-year follow-up of 50 patients with bulimia nervosa. *British Journal of Psychiatry*, **164**, 80–7.

Cooper, P. J. (1995). *Bulimia Nervosa and Binge-eating. A Guide to Recovery*. London: Robinson.

Crowther, J. H. and Chernyk, B. (1986). Bulimia and binge eating in adolescent females: a comparison. *Addictive Behaviors*, **11**, 415–24.

Crowther, J. H., Post, G., and Zaynor, L. (1985). The prevalence of bulimia and binge eating in adolescent girls. *International Journal of Eating Disorders*, **4**, 29–42.

Fahy, T. A. and Russell, G. F. M. (1993). Outcome and prognostic variables in bulimia nervosa. *International Journal of Eating Disorders*, **14**, 135–46.

Fairburn, C. G. (1981). A cognitive-behavioral approach to the management of bulimia. *Psychological Medicine*, **11**, 707–11.

Fairburn, C. G. (1985). Cognitive-behavioral treatment for bulimia. In *Handbook of Psychotherapy for Anorexia Nervosa and Bulimia*, ed. D. M. Garner and P. E Garfinkel, pp. 160–92. New York: Guilford Press.

Fairburn, C. G. (1997). Interpersonal therapy for bulimia nervosa. In *Handbook of Treatment for Eating Disorders*, ed. D. M. Garner and P. E. Garfinkel, pp. 67–93. New York: Guilford Press.

Fairburn, C. G., Jones, R., Peveler, R. C., et al. (1991). Three psychological treatments for bulimia nervosa. *Archives of General Psychiatry*, **48**, 463–9.

Fairburn, C. G., Agras, W. S., and Wilson, G.T. (1992). The research on the treatment of bulimia nervosa: Practical and theoretical implications. In *The Biology of Feast and Famine: Relevance to Eating Disorders*, ed G. H. Anderson and S. H. Kennedy, pp. 318–40. New York: Academic Press.

Fairburn, C. G., Jones, R., Peveler, R. C., Hope, R. A., and O'Connor, M. (1993a). Psychotherapy and bulimia nervosa: the longer term effects of interpersonal psychotherapy, behavior therapy and cognitive-behavior therapy. *Archives of General Psychiatry*, **50**, 419–28.

Fairburn, C. G., Marcus, M. D., and Wilson, G.T. (1993b). Cognitive-behavioral therapy for binge eating and bulimia nervosa: a comprehensive treatment manual. In *Binge Eating: Nature, Assessment and Treatment*, ed. C. G. Fairburn and G.T. Wilson, pp. 361–404. New York: Guilford Press.

Fairburn, C. G., Norman, P. A., Welch, S. L., et al. (1995). A prospective study of outcome in bulimia nervosa and the long-term effects of three psychological treatments. *Archives of General Psychiatry*, **52**, 304–12.

Fairburn, C. G., Shafran, R., and Cooper, Z. (1998). A cognitive behavioural theory of anorexia nervosa. *Behaviour Research and Therapy*, **37**, 1–13.

Fennell, M. (1989). Depression. In *Cognitive Behavior Therapy for Psychiatric Problems*, ed. K. Hawton, P. M. Salkovskis, J. Kirk, and D. M. Clark, pp. 169–234. New York: Oxford University Press.

Fichter, M. M., Leibl, K., Rief, W., et al. (1991). Fluoxetine versus placebo: a double-blind study with bulimic inpatients undergoing intensive psychotherapy. *Pharmacopsychiatry*, **24**, 1–7.

Fisher, M. (1992). Medical complications of anorexia and bulimia nervosa. *Adolescent Medicine: State of the Art Reviews*, **3**, 481–502.

Freeman, C. P. L., Barry, F., Dunkeld-Turnbull, J., and Henderson, A. (1988). Controlled trial of psychotherapy for bulimia nervosa. *British Medical Journal*, **296**, 521–5.

Garner, D. M. and Bemis, K.M. (1982). A cognitive-behavioral approach to anorexia nervosa. *Cognitive Therapy and Research*, **6**, 123–50.

Garner, D. M. and Bemis, K.M. (1985). Cognitive therapy for anorexia nervosa. In *Handbook of Psychotherapy for Anorexia Nervosa and Bulimia*, ed. D. M. Garner and P. E. Garfinkel, pp. 107–46. New York: Guilford Press.

Garner, D. M., Garfinkel, P. E., and Bemis, K. M. (1982). A multidimensional psychotherapy for anorexia nervosa. *International Journal of Eating Disorders*, **1**, 3–46.

Garner, D. M., Rockert, W., Davis, R., et al. (1993). A comparison between cognitive-behavioral and supportive-expressive therapy for bulimia nervosa. *American Journal of Psychiatry*, **150**, 37–46.

Garner, D. M., Vitousek, K. M., and Pike, K. M. (1997). Cognitive-behavioral therapy for anorexia nervosa. In *Handbook of Treatment for Eating Disorders*, ed. D. M. Garner and P. E. Garfinkel, pp. 94–144. New York: Guilford Press.

Goldbloom, D. S., Olmsted, M., Davis, R., et al. (1997). A randomized controlled trial of fluoxetine and cognitive-behavioral therapy for bulimia nervosa: short-term outcome. *Behavior Research and Therapy*, **35**, 803–11.

Goldfried, M. R. (1980). Toward the delineation of therapeutic change principles. *American Psychologist*, **35**, 991–9.

Halmi, K. A., Falk, J. R., and Schwartz, E. (1981). Binge-eating and vomiting: a survey of a college population. *Psychological Medicine*, **11**, 697–706.

Herzog, D. B., Dorer, D. J., Keel, P. K., et al. (1999). Recovery and relapse in anorexia and bulimia nervosa: a 7.5-year follow-up study. *Journal of the American Acadamy of Child and Adolescent Psychiatry*, **38**, 829–37.

Hoek, H. W. (1991). The incidence and prevalence of anorexia nervosa and bulimia nervosa in primary care. *Psychological Medicine*, **21**, 455–60.

Hoek, H. W. (1993). Review of the epidemiological studies of the eating disorders. *International Journal of Eating Disorders*, **5**, 61–74.

Hoek, H.W. (1995). The distribution of eating disorders. In *Eating Disorders and Obesity: A Comprehensive Handbook*, ed. K. D. Brownell and C. G. Fairburn, pp. 207–11. New York: Guilford Press.

Hollon, S. D. and Beck, A. T. (1994). Cognitive and cognitive-behavioral therapies. In *Handbook of Psychotherapy and Behavior Change: An Empirical Analysis*, 4th edn, ed. S. L. Garfield and A. E. Bergin, pp. 428–66. New York: Wiley.

Johnson, C., Lewis, C., Love, S., et al. (1984). Incidence and correlates of bulimic behavior in a female high school population. *Journal of Youth and Adolescence*, **13**, 15–27.

Johnson, C., Tobin, D. L., and Dennis, A. (1990). Differences in treatment outcome between borderline and non-borderline bulimics at one-year follow-up. *International Journal of Eating Disorders*, **9**, 617–27.

Kaye, W. H. (1992). Neuropeptide abnormalities. In *Psychobiology and Treatment of Anorexia Nervosa and Bulimia Nervosa*, ed. K. A. Halmi, pp. 169–91. Washington, DC: American Psychiatric Press.

Keel, P. K. and Mitchell, J. E. (1997). Outcome in bulimia nervosa. *American Journal of Psychiatry*, **154**, 313–21.

Kendler, K. S., MacLean, C., Neale, M., et al. (1991). The genetic epidemiology of bulimia nervosa. *American Journal of Psychiatry*, **148**, 1627–37.

Killen, J. D., Taylor, C. B., Telch, M. J., et al. (1987). Depressive symptoms and substance use among adolescent binge eaters and purgers: a defined population study. *American Journal of Public Health*, **77**, 1539–41.

Kirkley, B. G., Schneider, J. A., Agras, W. S., and Bachman, J. A. (1985). Comparison of two group treatments for bulimia. *Journal of Consulting and Clinical Psychology*, **53**, 43–8.

Kreipe, R. E., Golden, N. H., Katzman, D. K., et al. (1995). Eating disorders in adolescents: a position paper for the Society of Adolescent Medicine. *Journal of Adolescent Health*, **16**, 476–9.

Ledoux, S., Choquet, M., and Flament, M. (1991). Eating disorders among adolescents in an unselected French population. *International Journal of Eating Disorders*, **10**, 1–89.

Le Grange, D. and Gelman, T. (1998). Patients' perspective of treatment in eating disorders: a preliminary study. *South African Journal of Psychology*, **28**, 182–6.

Leitenberg, H., Rosen, J. C., Wolf, J., et al. (1994). Comparison of cognitive-behavior therapy and desipramine in the treatment of bulimia nervosa. *Behaviour Therapy and Research*, **32**, 37–46.

Lingswiler, V. M., Crowther, J. H., and Stephens, M. A. P. (1989). Affective and cognitive antecedents to eating episodes in bulimia and binge eating. *International Journal of Eating Disorders*, **8**, 533–9.

Maddocks, S. E., Kaplan, A. S., Woodside, D. B., Langdon, L., and Piran, N. (1992). Two year follow-up of bulimia nervosa: the importance of abstinence as the criterion of outcome. *International Journal of Eating Disorders*, **12**, 133–41.

Mahoney, M. H. and Mahoney, K. (1976). *Permanent Weight Control*. New York: Norton.

Mitchell, J. E. (1995). Medical complications of bulimia nervosa. In *Eating Disorders and Obesity. A Comprehensive Handbook*, ed. K. D. Brownell and C. G. Fairburn, pp. 271–7. New York: Guilford Press.

Mitchell, J. E. and deZwaan, M. (1993). Pharmacological treatments of binge eating. In *Binge Eating: Nature, Assessment and Treatment*, ed. C. G . Fairburn and G. T. Wilson, pp. 250–69. New York: Guilford Press.

Mitchell, J. E., Hatsukami, D., Pyle, R. L., Eckert, E. D., and Soll, E. (1987a). Late onset bulimia. *Comprehensive Psychiatry*, **28**, 323–8.

Mitchell, J. E., Seim, H. C., Colon, E., and Pomeroy, C. (1987b). Medical complications and medical management of bulimia nervosa. *Annals of Internal Medicine*, **107**, 71–7.

Mitchell, J. E., Pyle, R. L., Eckert, E. D., et al. (1990). A comparison study of antidepressants and structured intensive group psychotherapy in the treatment of bulimia nervosa. *Archives of General Psychiatry*, **47**, 149–57.

Mitchell, J. E., Raymond, N., and Specker, S. (1993). A review of the controlled trials of pharmacotherapy and psychotherapy in the treatment of bulimia nervosa. *International Journal of Eating Disorders*, **14**, 229–48.

Mizes, J. S. and Christiano, B. A. (1995). Assessment of cognitive variable relevant to cognitive behavioral perspectives on anorexia nervosa and bulimia nervosa. *Behaviour Research and Therapy*, **33**, 95–105.

Palmer, E. P. and Guay, A. T. (1985). Reversible myopathy secondary to abuse of Ipecac in patients with major eating disorders. *New England Journal of Medicine*, **313**, 1457–9.

Polivy, J. and Herman, C. P. (1993). Etiology of binge eating: psychological mechanisms. In *Binge Eating: Nature, Assessment and Treatment*, ed. C. G. Fairburn and G. T. Wilson, pp. 173–205. New York: Guilford Press.

Pope, H. G., Hudson, J. I., Yurgelon-Todd, D., and Hudson, M. S. (1984). Prevalence of anorexia nervosa and bulimia in three student populations. *International Journal of Eating Disorders*, **3**, 45–51.

Remschmidt, H. and Herpertz-Dahlmann, B. (1990). Bulimia in children and adolescents. In *Bulimia Nervosa. Basic Research, Diagnosis and Therapy*, ed. M. Fichter, pp. 84–98. Chichester: John Wiley.

Russell, G. F. M. (1979). Bulimia nervosa: an ominous variant of anorexia nervosa. *Psychological Medicine*, **9**, 429–48.

Schmidt, U., Tiller, J., Hodes, M., and Treasure, J. (1995). Risk factors for the development of early onset bulimia nervosa. In *Eating Disorders in Adolescence: Anorexia and Bulimia Nervosa*, ed. H. C. Steinhausen, pp. 83–93. New York: Walter de Gruyter.

Stangler, R. S. and Printz, A. M. (1980). DSM-III: psychiatric diagnosis in a university population. *American Journal of Psychiatry*, **137**, 937–40.

Stein, S., Chalhoub, N., and Hodes, M. (1998). Very early onset bulimia nervosa: report of two cases. *International Journal of Eating Disorders*, **24**, 323–7.

Story, M., Hauck, F. R., Broussard, B. A., et al. (1994). Weight perceptions and weight control practices in American Indian and Alaska Native adolescents. *Archives of Pediatric and Adolescent Medicine*, **148**, 567–71.

Striegel-Moore, R. H., Silberstein, L. R., and Rodin, J. (1986). Toward an understanding of risk factors for bulimia. *American Psychologist*, **41**, 246–63.

Strober, M. (1995). Family-genetic perspectives on anorexia nervosa and bulimia Nervosa. In *Eating Disorders and Obesity. A Comprehensive Handbook*, ed. K. D. Brownell and C. G. Fairburn, pp. 212–18. New York: Guilford Press.

Strober, M., Freeman, R., Lampert, C., Diamond, J., and Kaye, W. (2001). Males with anorexia nervosa: a controlled study of eating disorders in first-degree relatives. *International Journal of Eating Disorders*, **29**, 263–9.

Szabo, P. and Tury, F. (1991). The prevalence of bulimia nervosa in a Hungarian college and secondary school population. *Psychotherapy and Psychosomatics*, **56**, 43–7.

Tobin, D. L. (1993). Psychodynamic psychotherapy and binge eating. In *Binge Eating, Nature, Assessment, and Treatment*, ed. C. G. Fairburn and G. T. Wilson, pp. 287–316. New York: Guilford Press.

Vandereycken, W. (1995). The families of patients with an eating disorder. In *Eating Disorders and Obesity. A Comprehensive Handbook*, ed. K. D. Brownell and C. G. Fairburn, pp. 219–23. New York: Guilford Press.

Vandereycken, W. and Hoek, H. W. (1992). Are eating disorders culture-bound syndromes? In *Psychobiology and Treatment of Anorexia Nervosa and Bulimia Nervosa*, ed. K. A. Halmi, pp. 19–36. Washington, DC: American Psychiatric Press.

Vitousek, K. B. (1996). The current status of cognitive-behavioral models of anorexia nervosa and bulimia nervosa. In *Frontiers of Cognitive Therapy*, ed. P. Salkovskis, pp. 383–418. New York: Guilford Press.

Vitousek, K. B. and Hollon, K. B. (1990). The investigation of schematic content and processing in eating disorders. *Cognitive Therapy and Research*, **14**, 191–214.

Waller, G. (1991). Sexual abuse as a factor in eating disorders. *British Journal of Psychiatry*, **159**, 664–71.

Walsh, B. T., Wilson, G. T., Loeb, K. L., et al. (1997). Medication and psychotherapy in the treatment of bulimia nervosa. *American Journal of Psychiatry*, **154**, 523–31.

Whitaker, A., Johnson, J., Shaffer, D., et al. (1990). Uncommon troubles in young people: prevalence estimates of selected psychiatric disorders in a nonreferred adolescent population. *Archives of General Psychiatry*, **47**, 487–96.

Whittal, M. L., Agras, W. S., and Gould, R. A. (1999). Bulimia nervosa: a meta-analysis of psychosocial and pharmacological treatments. *Behavior Therapy*, **30**, 117–35.

Wilson, G. T. (1996). Treatment of bulimia nervosa: when CBT fails. *Behaviour Research and Therapy*, **34**, 197–212.

Wilson, G. T. and Fairburn, C. G. (1993). Cognitive treatments for eating disorders. *Journal of Consulting and Clinical Psychology*, **61**, 261–9.

Wilson, G. T. and Fairburn, C. G. (1998). Treatment of eating disorders. In *Psychotherapies and Drugs that Work: A Review of the Outcome Studies*. ed. P. E. Nathan and J. M. Gorman, pp. 501–30. New York: Oxford University Press.

Wilson, G. T., Fairburn, C. G., and Agras, W. S. (1997). Cognitive- behavioral therapy for bulimia nervosa. In *Handbook of Treatment for Eating Disorders*, ed. D. M. Garner and P. E. Garfinkel, pp. 67–93. New York: Guilford Press.

Wolf, E. M. and Crowther, J. H. (1992). An evaluation of behavioral and cognitive-behavioral group intervention for the treatment of bulimia nervosa in women. *International Journal of Eating Disorders*, **11**, 3–16.

Woodside, D. B. and Garfinkel, P. E. (1992). Age of onset in eating disorders. *International Journal of Eating Disorders*, **12**, 31–6.

Yager, J., Andersen, A., Devlin, M., et al. (1993). American Psychiatric Association practice guidelines for eating disorders. *American Journal of Psychiatry*, **150**, 201–28.

13

Cognitive therapy and schizophrenia

Patrick W. Corrigan and Joseph D. Calabrese

University of Chicago, Tinley Park, IL, USA

Aaron Beck and his contemporaries developed cognitive therapy for the treatment of major depression several decades ago. Barlow, Clark, and others soon applied these models to other clinical conditions, including obsessive-compulsive disorder and panic disorder. Compared to these efforts, cognitive therapy for schizophrenia is a relatively new enterprise. In some ways, the idea of applying cognitive therapy in the treatment of schizophrenia seems to exceed the relatively clear and bounded constructs developed in research on cognitive therapy for depression and anxiety. Nevertheless, cognitive models are by no means novel for understanding the disorder. From its earliest formulations by Bleuler and Kraepelin, schizophrenia was described as a thought disorder. Since then, a variety of rehabilitation treatments have been proposed as adjuncts to psychotropic medications for treating the cognitive deficits of schizophrenia (Corrigan and Yudofsky, 1996). Still, one might think there are significant differences between cognitive deficits in schizophrenia (Steffy, 1993) and those associated with depression and anxiety (Clark et al., 1999). The former, for example, is typically viewed as representing a neurodevelopmental deficit that arises prodromally during childhood and manifests acutely with psychotic symptoms during later adolescence and early adulthood. In contrast, the cognitive deficits of depression and anxiety represent self- and world-conceptualizations that affect one's mood and consequent behavior. Hence, one might reasonably ask, does schizophrenia belong in a book on cognitive therapy? In answering this question, we begin the chapter by considering the similarities and differences between constructs used in understanding cognitive deficits associated with schizophrenia, depression, and anxiety disorders. Results of this review not only demonstrate the centrality of cognition and cognitive therapy in understanding schizophrenia, they remind us that the research literature on cognition and schizophrenia is old, distinguished, and well developed. Rather than offer a comprehensive review, which has been done well elsewhere (Green, 1998; Spaulding et al., 1999), we briefly summarize the literature as it relates to key cognitive processes and therapies related to schizophrenia.

We follow this summary with a discussion of three issues that need to be considered in future research on cognitive therapy for persons with schizophrenia.

Cognition in schizophrenia, depression, and anxiety

There is a fairly well-developed literature examining cognitive deficits in schizophrenia (Steffy, 1993; Green, 1998, 1999). Schizophrenia is seen as a neurodevelopmental disorder stemming from genetic or in-utero insult. Neurochemical abnormalities are believed to serve as a foundation for observed cognitive deficits and for diminished cognitive performance. These models are process-oriented, and are rooted in information-processing paradigms that divide the complex phenomena of human cognition into discrete processes and interacting systems (Corrigan and Stephenson, 1994). What impact has this paradigm had on understanding cognitive deficits in schizophrenia?

Researchers first looked for unique processes that were deficient in schizophrenia, what one researcher called the "holy grail of cognitive psychopathology" (Cromwell, 1984). Unfortunately, this line of research failed to yield the one or two unique process deficits one might expect. Rather, research has indicated that almost all discrete intellectual functions (e.g., attention, short-term memory, recognition, consolidation, long-term memory, decision-making) are diminished in schizophrenia. As a consequence, investigators turned their attention toward identifying processes that might explain the range of observed deficits. Nuechterlein and Dawson (1984), for example, proposed a limited-capacity model postulating that the cognitive demands of some attention and memory tasks overwhelm the limited capacity of persons with schizophrenia.

These models represent a linear view of information processing; i.e., a step-by-step operation in which information is attended to, encoded, consolidated, and recalled in fixed order. In response to the limits of these models, more recent approaches have used parallel distributed processing (PDP) paradigms (Cohen et al., 1992). PDP models represent the complex event of human cognition as concurrent, and sometimes independent, processes. Researchers have applied PDP models for understanding cognitive deficits associated with schizophrenia (Cohen and Servan-Schreiber, 1992). Other recent conceptualizations have framed cognitive deficits in schizophrenia as reflecting a failure of cognitive systems to process data in an integrated fashion (Green and Nuechterlein, 1999; Spaulding and Poland, 2001).

These process models of cognitive deficits in schizophrenia share a number of assumptions. All assume that: (1) information-processing deficits stem from discrete neurophysiological abnormalities that result from the disease (Green, 1998) and can be localized biologically; and (2) information-processing deficits can be assessed by neuropsychological tasks. In practice, it is assumed that information-processing capacities can be represented by performance-based tasks. The models further assume that: (3) cognitive deficits are considered primary dysfunctions of schizophrenia and indirectly lead to the more molar disabilities associated with the disease (Green, 1999). Subtle cognitive deficits are present at an early age, even though the onset of frank symptoms of schizophrenia typically occurs during young adulthood. These deficits undermine the acquisition of basic social and coping skills that people use to accomplish their goals and to deal with life's inevitable problems (Corrigan et al., 1992). Persons without these skills, tend, when exposed to stressful events, to develop psychiatric symptoms. Cognitive deficits further exacerbate psychiatric symptoms because persons lack basic skills needed to make sense of social situations (Penn et al., 1997). Moreover, the absence of these skills and basic social understanding lead to the emergence of "macrodisabilities" which plague persons with schizophrenia. These disabilities include an inability to live independently, as well as difficulties developing close relationships and obtaining competitive work with a good income.

These basic assumptions differ in important ways from those which serve as the conceptual foundation of traditional cognitive-behavioral models for depression and anxiety. Cognitive therapy for these disorders rests largely on content-oriented models (Barlow, 1997; Clark et al., 1999). Inaccurate or maladaptive representations of one's self, world, and future are viewed as root cognitive deficits. These representations are believed to be psychological in origin, having developed from key learning events during important developmental stages. Moreover, the pernicious effects of these deficits seem to be more direct. That is to say, negative representations of the self and the world are typically seen as proximal causes of depressed or anxious mood. These moods, in turn, lead to a loss in interpersonal functioning. At first glance, then, cognitive models for schizophrenia are biologically based, process-oriented, and relatively indirect. Cognitive models for depression and anxiety disorders, in contrast, are psychologically based, content-oriented, and fairly direct.

Similarities in models

A closer review of extant research, however, suggests that cognitive models of schizophrenia and mood/anxiety disorders are similar in important ways. Consider, for example, the ostensible difference between process and content-based models. As several authors have noted, clinical depression is associated with changes in both cognitive contents and processes (Engel and DeRubeis, 1993; Clark et al., 1999). Moreover, recent attempts by depression and anxiety researchers to answer the question "Why do some persons develop negative images of their world such that they are repeatedly hampered by depression or anxiety?" have led to the development of information-processing paradigms using concepts such as automatic and effortful processing. They have speculated that interference in effortful processing and dominance of negative automatic thoughts are associated with depression (Hartlage et al., 1993). They have also focused upon mood-dependent changes in information encoding and retrieval – suggesting that persons with depression generate negative attributions because attention, encoding, and retrieval processes are dominated by negative information (Bootzin and McKnight, 1998; Gotlib and Krasnoperova, 1998). Moreover, researchers have proposed that relationships may exist between cognitive deficits in depression and specific biological dysfunctions (Frith, 1999).

Nor are content-based models irrelevant for understanding disabilities in schizophrenia. Research suggests that depression is an important experience for understanding the course and disabilities of schizophrenia (DeLisi, 1990; Siris, 1995). Depending on the stage of the illness, 25–80% of individuals with schizophrenia also meet diagnostic criteria for major depression (Hirsch et al., 1989; Leff et al., 1990). This makes sense – persons who struggle with severe forms of psychopathology, such as schizophrenia, are likely to experience feelings of hopelessness, loss, and dysphoria. One of the important unanswered questions in this area is whether relapse of the positive symptoms of schizophrenia leads to depression or whether depressive episodes elicit the acute symptoms of schizophrenia. This literature reminds us that depression (and, no doubt, anxiety) are relevant disorders for understanding schizophrenia. As a result, cognitive models that have been developed to understand vulnerability for depression and anxiety may also prove useful in understanding the course of schizophrenia.

To summarize, although research describing cognitive deficits in schizophrenia and depression/anxiety developed independently and may incorporate concepts and methods that seem to be mutually exclusive, evidence suggests a commonality in perspectives. The assumptions of cognitive therapy may be relevant to understanding some of the life problems of persons with this disease. Moreover, cognitive therapy interventions may prove useful for developing treatments for these problems.

Applications of cognitive psychotherapy to schizophrenia

Although interventions aimed at the cognitive deficits of schizophrenia are based primarily on information-processing perspectives, content-oriented cognitive psychotherapy has been applied to schizophrenia almost from its genesis (Beck, 1952). This approach targets distressing psychotic symptoms and maladaptive understandings of mental illness using a collaborative empirical framework. The therapist explores the distressing cognitions with the person, attempting to reframe them as beliefs rather than facts, empathically discussing how one might arrive at such beliefs (but also recognizing their emotional costs), reviewing evidence for and against the beliefs, and trying to find less distressing alternative interpretations (Chadwick et al., 1996; Garety et al., 2000).

Several early studies examined implications of this model for treating patients suffering from schizophrenia. Using Brehm's concept of "psychological reactance," Watts et al. (1973) argued that a confrontational approach would more likely strengthen than weaken a delusional belief. This view was supported by Milton and colleagues (1978), who compared a group of patients treated with a confrontational approach to a group treated in a nonconfrontational manner. They found that conviction in the beliefs initially decreased for both groups but that, after 6 weeks, the confrontation group's conviction had increased to above pretreatment levels, whereas the nonconfrontation group remained at posttreatment levels. The authors suggested that therapists can minimize psychological reactance by beginning with weakly held beliefs and working towards more strongly held beliefs, not requiring patients to change beliefs but simply discussing them, focusing on the evidence for various beliefs rather than their truth, and encouraging the patient (rather than the therapist) to voice arguments against beliefs.

In recent years, cognitive therapy for psychotic symptoms has been studied most in the UK (Chadwick and Lowe, 1990; Tarrier et al., 1993; Drury et al., 1996; Kuipers et al., 1997). In a randomized controlled trial of cognitive therapy for acute psychosis, patients receiving cognitive-behavioral therapy (CBT) showed a more marked decline in positive symptoms at posttest. Moreover, at 9-month follow-up 5% of the cognitive therapy group showed moderate to severe residual symptoms compared to more than half the control group (Drury et al., 1996).

In a similar manner, Kingdon and Turkington (1991) found that CBT was effective in reducing patients' catastrophic interpretations of their symptoms and the stigma attached to mental illness generally. The authors attempted to normalize the symptoms by comparing their beliefs to normal experiences. More recently, Garety and colleagues (2000) used CBT techniques to promote social functioning and to prevent relapse.

Although these initial findings have been promising, much research is needed on cognitive therapy for schizophrenia. A recent review and effect-size analysis, for example, identified only seven controlled outcome studies (Gould et al., 2001). One could argue that four of these studies were inadequate in that the treatment groups combined cognitive and behavioral techniques, creating a confound. Few dismantling studies have been completed to determine the effects of cognitive interventions alone (Drury et al., 1996, is an exception). Studies generally include cognitive therapy as a component of a comprehensive treatment program that also includes such things as training in social and coping skills (Tarrier et al., 1993, 1998; Garety et al., 1994; Kuipers et al., 1997), relaxation techniques (Tarrier et al.,

1993; Kuipers et al., 1997), increasing social interaction (Tarrier et al., 1993), or key-person counseling (Buchkremer et al., 1997; Klingberg et al., 1999). Moreover, most of these studies have used control groups in which patients receive supportive therapy or structured leisure time, rather than another credible therapeutic intervention. As such, there is no way to determine which specific components of the treatment program were associated with improvement. Nevertheless, preliminary research shows that cognitive interventions for schizophrenia, in conjunction with other interventions, may be of some value. Additional controlled-outcome research, in conjunction with dismantling studies and research into processes of change in psychotherapy, is needed.

Three directions for future research

The remainder of this chapter addresses three issues for future research. As discussed, much of the existing research has focused on information-processing deficits demonstrated by patients with schizophrenia. However, *social* cognitive paradigms may yield different heuristics for developing a cognitive therapy of schizophrenia (Penn et al., 1997). Our understanding of deficits which characterize schizophrenia may change when we adopt a social cognitive model, rather than an information-processing paradigm.

Second, cognitive-behavioral approaches for treating schizophrenia assume that changing discrete deficits in information processing and developing knowledge structures will effect more molar domains of functioning. Future research needs to examine this assumption directly. For example, does improvement in the way in which persons with schizophrenia attend to and understand their world affect their ability to live independently or to keep a competitive job?

Third, much of the research on the neurocognitive deficits of schizophrenia is based on the assumption that these deficits are neurodevelopmental in origin. In other words, they arise as a result of the primary biologic dysfunctions that represent the disease of schizophrenia. Claude Steele (1997) has argued that many of the cognitive deficits of other groups arise from stereotype threat. The possibility exists that many of the deficits targeted in CBT arise from social factors. This kind of finding would have significant implications for treatment of this disorder.

Information processing versus social cognition deficits

As noted, many current approaches to understanding cognitive deficits in schizophrenia are based upon information-processing paradigms (Green, 1998, 1999). These models dominate cognitive rehabilitation approaches to schizophrenia (Corrigan and Yudofsky, 1996). Information-processing models have evolved from relatively simple linear models, searching for a single process that might account for the range of cognitive deficits, to parallel processing and interacting system theories. Research should continue in this vein as research indicates that associations may exist between measures of cognitive performance (e.g., selective attention, verbal memory, and executive functioning) and social functioning. Research has found that deficits in attention, memory, and executive functioning may be related to performance in four important social domains. It has been found that information-processing deficits are associated with:

1. *Program behavior.* Persons with information-processing deficits show fewer interpersonal skills and greater behavior problems within treatment programs (Dickerson et al., 1991; Penn et al., 1996).
2. *Community outcome.* Persons report a better quality of life and higher occupational functioning when they demonstrate more competent information processes (Johnstone et al., 1990; Wykes et al., 1990; Jaeger and Douglas, 1992; Wykes and Dunn, 1992; Goldman et al., 1993; Buchanan et al., 1994; Lysaker et al., 1995; Addington and Addington, 1999).
3. *Problem solving.* Persons are better able to understand and resolve interpersonal problems when they have fewer information-processing deficits (Penn et al., 1993, 1995; Bellack et al., 1994; Bowen et al., 1994; Corrigan and Toomey, 1995; Addington and Addington, 1999).
4. *Skill learning.* Persons are better able to learn social and coping skills when they demonstrate fewer processing deficits (Mueser et al., 1991; Kern et al., 1992; Bowen et al., 1994; Corrigan et al., 1994; Lysaker et al., 1995).

These observations are important in that they guide the development of cognitive rehabilitation and therapy programs. They suggest what cognitive rehabilitation strategy may best improve community outcome and may facilitate skill learning and problem solving.

Limits to information-processing models

Although information-processing models have contributed to our understanding of schizophrenia, they are not without limits. First, the correlations observed between measures of information processing and social functioning are generally modest (Green, 1996; Penn et al., 1997; Corrigan and Penn, 2001). This suggests that a significant amount of the variance in social outcome (e.g., social skill, community functioning) may be accounted for by other variables. Similarly, the search for the "primary processing" deficit of schizophrenia has not proven successful (Spaulding, 1997; Spaulding and Poland, 2001). Thus, other domains of functioning, in addition to cognitive factors, need to be considered.

A second limitation of cognitive models of schizophrenia is that focusing on cognitive processes without attending to social context leads to models of functioning that are incomplete (Corrigan and Penn, 2001). In other words, social behavior, whether demonstrated by someone with schizophrenia or by a person without a psychiatric disorder, is likely a function of numerous factors, which include, but are not limited to, information processes. Forming an impression of someone, for example, depends on the ability to "perceive" that individual accurately. However, impression formation may also be influenced by the perceiver's history with that person, whether the individual's behavior is constrained by the situation, and attributions the perceiver makes about the person's behavior (Gilbert, 1995). Thus, observing that someone is ill-tempered may not necessarily lead to the impression that she is "cantankerous" if you find out that she was recently robbed. Our initial impression may be corrected based upon situational factors.

Social cognition defined

A new generation of processing models has attempted to integrate findings on comprehension of nonsocial stimuli, as characterizes contemporary information-processing paradigms, with findings from research on social cognition (Knight and Silverstein, 1998; Silverstein et al., 1998). Social cognition differs from nonsocial cognition in a number of ways, the most salient being the target of information processing. Unlike nonsocial stimuli (e.g., letters, numbers, and inanimate objects), social stimuli tend to be mutable over time, personally relevant, and act as their own causal agents (Fiske and Taylor, 1991; Fiske, 1995). Furthermore, humans tend to be more concerned with the unobservable characteristics of social, compared to nonsocial, stimuli, leading us to search for the causes behind others' behavior (e.g., forming attributions) (Fiske, 1995). Finally, relationships between perceiver and social object tend to be bidirectional; the object can think about the perceiver, which in turn, can influence the perceiver's impression of the social object. This process, described by Fiske (1995) as "mutual perception," is less likely to occur in the processing of nonsocial stimuli.

In addition to differences between the types of processed stimuli, cognition and social cognition differ with respect to how performance is evaluated. For example, performance on nonsocial cognitive tasks among persons with schizophrenia is typically indexed in terms of "deficits." Thus, a group with schizophrenia will be compared to a control sample (or, less frequently, normative data) on a task (e.g., Wisconsin Card Sorting Task; Span of Apprehension) and their relative performance assessed. In this sense, the person with schizophrenia either does or does not have a particular skill. This approach clearly has a number of advantages, including the ability to compute subjects' accuracy across a range of tests. However, the emphasis on accuracy and deficits tends to be at the cost of examining other indices of performance, such as biases, that may be of greater interest to social cognition researchers.

As discussed by Penn et al. (1997), biases refer to a characteristic response style that does not necessarily indicate impaired performance. For example, a recent study showed that undergraduate students high in social anxiety were more likely to interpret an ambiguous passage about a blind date in a negative manner compared to research participants low in social anxiety (Constans et al., 1999). Although the response style of socially anxious research participants may be maladaptive in terms of their characteristic way of approaching the social environment, it is not necessarily deficient or incorrect. In fact, interpreting an ambiguous situation negatively may be a conservative, yet beneficial, behavioral strategy (e.g., deciding not to walk down a particular street in which a group of youths have congregated). In a similar manner, focusing on biases in schizophrenia may lead to a better understanding of a characteristic response style, the adaptiveness of which may only be understood in reference to the context in which it occurs.

The distinction between social and nonsocial cognition has been made in other areas of inquiry, including clinical neurology, evolutionary biology, primate behavior, and developmental psychology (Ostrom, 1984; Penn et al., 1997; Silverstein, 1997). Data indicate, for example, that dissociations between disorders of face recognition and object recognition imply some (but not complete) specialization of functioning for interpersonal stimuli (Farah, 1992). In the area of evolutionary biology, it has been suggested that natural selection has influenced how individuals reason, and that reasoning for adaptive problems involves specific cognitive mechanisms (Cosmides, 1989; Cosmides and Tooby, 1989, 1994). In other words, cognitive processes are not "content-free" but are tied to specific social and adaptive functions (Cosmides and Tooby, 1994). Similarly, Brothers (1990a, 1990b) argued that certain behaviors, such as primates trying to deceive or comfort other members of their group, may reflect an ability to make inferences regarding the disposition of others – a social-cognitive ability. Finally, Ostrom (1984) reviews evidence suggesting that children may understand causality for social events before physical events, and that person permanence may develop before object permanence. Thus, an argument can be made that social cognition represents a construct that is not redundant with nonsocial cognition. The degree of overlap between these domains, especially as applied to the study of schizophrenia, is not clear and is worthy of further study (Silverstein, 1997).

Cognitive deficits versus role functioning

As noted, research in the fields of cognitive therapy and cognitive rehabilitation indicates that cognitive and behavioral interventions can be helpful for patients with schizophrenia. These interventions have led to changes in a person's experience with delusions and hallucinations (Tarrier et al., 1988; Garety et al., 1997; Kuipers et al., 1997) as well as improvements in discrete information-processing deficits, e.g., attention and recall memory (see Corrigan and Storzbach, 1993; Storzbach and Corrigan, 1996 for literature reviews). It is postulated that changes in primary cognitive deficits will be associated with improvements in social functioning.

Preliminary findings are positive in that these gains are associated with enhanced vocational and independent living skills (Spaulding et al., 1999).

Others, however, have taken a dim view of these results (Bellack et al., 1999). Although acknowledging these gains, Bellack and colleagues argue that the essential disabilities that define schizophrenia – the discomfort of recurring symptoms, inability to live independently, and inability to maintain competitive work – remain relatively unchanged after participating in cognitive therapies and cognitive rehabilitation. They are recapitulating a salient point made by neuropsychologists:

Consistent with human information processing theory, the attainment of skill and expertise appears to entail only the acquisition of domain-specific knowledge and pattern–action connections without changing basic processes and information-processing capacity limits (Bellack et al., 1999, p. 48).

Might it be that changes in cognitive functioning have little or no effect on the more prominent disabilities of schizophrenia?

Bellack and colleagues (1992, 1999) raised three questions which must be addressed if cognitive therapy and cognitive rehabilitation are to stand as important treatments for schizophrenia: (1) Do cognitive impairments play a central role in the social disability and other problems experienced by persons with schizophrenia? (2) Must these impairments be remediated to achieve effective rehabilitation? (3) Is the prognosis for rehabilitation as positive as that suggested in preliminary investigations?

The responses of Bellack et al. to these questions have been, on the whole, negative. Although there is evidence that relationships may exist between measures of cognitive and social cognitive skills and deficits and performance on measures of daily living, the correlations are modest and issues of causality have not been resolved. Moreover, even if cognitive and social cognitive deficits were shown to cause poor interpersonal functioning, there is no clear evidence that remediating these cognitive deficits will lead to improved adaptive functioning and attainment of life goals. Bellack et al. (1999), as such, are sanguine regarding the usefulness of cognitive therapy and cognitive rehabilitation as currently conceived.

These conclusions are similar to those made in the 1970s by Strauss and Carpenter (1972, 1974, 1977). They characterized domains of functioning (e.g., need for hospitalization, social contact, employment) as "open-linked systems." Although small to moderate correlations across systems have been reported, functioning in specific domains is largely independent of other domains. As a consequence, researchers need to examine the quality of functioning in specific domains of interest. Moreover, clinicians need to develop intervention packages that are specific to the exigencies of each functional domain. These assertions now need to be applied to research on cognitive therapy and cognitive rehabilitation.

Cognitive therapy and stereotype threat

As discussed earlier, most researchers assume that the cognitive and social deficits related to the disabilities of schizophrenia are neurobiologically based. For example, a 1999 issue of *Schizophrenia Bulletin* championed the term "neurocognitive processes," equating cognitive deficits with the neurodevelopmental dysfunctions that caused them (Green, 1999). It is commonly assumed that cognitive deficits are caused by neurophysiological or structural dysfunctions that arise developmentally and account for the primary symptoms and disabilities of the illness.

We would suggest, however, that focusing on putative neurobiological substrates of deficits in cognition may not provide a complete picture (Corrigan and Holtzman, 2001). Schizophrenia strikes with a two-edged sword: it is a *disease*, which leads to symptoms and dysfunctions that interfere with a quality life, and it results in *discrimination*, which further exacerbates handicaps and impedes opportunities (Corrigan and Penn, 1997). For example, a person with schizophrenia may not obtain a job because of negative symptoms (a result of biological disease) that interfere with the social interactions and sense of industriousness needed to impress employers during a job interview. Alternatively, persons labeled "mentally ill" may not be hired because of stereotypes held by the employer. The possibility exists that persons with schizophrenia may be less able to work, earn a reasonable income, live independently, and start a family, at least in part, due to social stigma.

Stereotype threat

Steele (1997) proposed a model for understanding the effects of social stigma on cognitive performance. He argued that negative stereotypes undermine a person's identification with a specific domain (e.g., school, work, social interactions) and lessen the person's motivation to achieve in that domain. He coined the term "stereotype threat" to describe this phenomena. Stereotype threat occurs when members of a stereotyped group (e.g., persons with schizophrenia) find themselves in a situation specific to a domain for which a negative stereotype applies.

Steele (1997) described several characteristics of stereotype threat. He suggested that stereotype threat is not tied to the psychology of particular stigmatized groups. Rather, it can affect any group about whom there are widely held negative stereotypes (e.g., persons with mental illness are confused and cannot understand the subtleties of interpersonal situations). Moreover, there may be a concurrence between stereotypes and situations that initiate stereotype threat. Rather than being an omnipresent phenomenon, stereotype threats are most acutely felt when persons find themselves in situations about which stereotypes occur. Finally, it is worth noting that one need not believe a stereotype to experience stereotype threat (Aronson et al., 1999). Persons with mental illness need not believe that all persons with schizophrenia are confused and incapable of independent decisions to worry that the average citizen might endorse this view about them. Recognition of this belief can lead persons into worrying about whether others will accept this notion ("my boss thinks I'm inept because I had a psychiatric relapse"), thereby experiencing the threat of this stereotype.

What accounts for the effects of stereotype threat? Persons who occasionally experience the emotional distress that results from stereotype stress may *disengage* from the situations in which this stress occurs (Crocker et al., 1998; Major et al., 1998). Alternatively, people who experience stereotype threat and emotional distress over a prolonged time may *disidentify* with the domain and task altogether (Steele, 1997). Disengaging from and disidentifying with performance undermine achievement motivation for tasks in that domain and interfere with cognitive performance.

Changing stereotype threat to improve cognitive performance

Studies suggest that one way to improve cognitive performance is to diminish stereotype threat. Hence, strategies aimed at these social factors may help individuals cope with the emotional distress and reduce their tendency to disengage or disidentify with the tasks. If a model of stereotype threat applies to the social cognitive deficits of schizophrenia, it suggests that another way to remediate these cognitive deficits is through changing the person's social environment. The strength of this effect was shown in several studies where cognitive performance was improved after exposing outgroup members to positive stereotypes (Levy, 1999; Shih et al., 1999). For example, performance on memory tests improved after elderly subjects were exposed to positive stereotypes about the aged (Levy, 1999). This approach differs radically from remedial programs based upon the prevailing view that poor performance stems from internal processes ranging from genes to internalized deficits (Steele, 1997). It is worth acknowledging that the impact of stereotype threat has not yet been demonstrated among persons with schizophrenia. It is clear, however, that schizophrenia is a stigmatizing disease. As such, the possibility exists that attempts to alleviate social stigma and to reduce stereotype threat will have effects on the social cognitive deficits and adaptive functioning of persons with schizophrenia. As we have seen, existing cognitive therapy and cognitive rehabilitation programs are inadequate for addressing the full range of deficits which characterize the disorder of schizophrenia. A broader conceptual paradigm, which incorporates strategies for reducing stereotype threat, may prove useful in addressing the social cognitive deficits of schizophrenia.

Summary

Although cognitive approaches to depression and anxiety may appear, at first reading, to be conceptually and methodologically distinct from research on schizophrenia, we present evidence in this chapter that there is a significant rapprochement in perspectives. Many persons with schizophrenia also suffer from depression or anxiety, and content-focused cognitive therapies have been used in conceptualizing and treating positive symptoms of schizophrenia. We then examined three issues that need to be addressed in future research on cognitive therapy and schizophrenia: (1) How do social cognitive models advance our knowledge about cognitive deficits in schizophrenia? (2) How do we span the bridge between the discrete cognitive deficits of schizophrenia and the more molar disabilities that undermine their quality of life (e.g., recurring symptoms, inability to live independently, inability to attain competitive work? (3) What are the relative effects of neurodevelopmental and social (stereotype-based) etiologies on the cognitive deficits of schizophrenia? What implications do these different models have for designing effective therapies for schizophrenia?

Our review suggests that research on schizophrenia has advanced from psychotic symptomatology and microlevel analysis of underlying cognitions to understanding the macrolevels of social functioning, social cognition, and social stigma. A promising path for understanding the link between the most macrosocial cognitions (culturally embedded stereotypes) and the most micropsychological cognitions (i.e., performance on cognitive tests) is Steele's concept of "stereotype threat." Research in this area may advance our understanding of cognitive deficits which characterize schizophrenia and support the development of more effective treatments.

REFERENCES

Addington, J. and Addington, D. (1999). Neurocognitive and social functioning in schizophrenia. *Schizophrenia Bulletin*, **25**, 173–82.

Aronson, J., Lustina, M. J., Good, C., et al. (1999). When white men can't do math: necessary and sufficient factors in stereotype threat. *Journal of Experimental Social Psychology*, **35**, 29–46.

Barlow, D. H. (1997). Cognitive-behavioral therapy for panic disorder: current status. *Journal of Clinical Psychiatry*, **58** (suppl. 2), 32–7.

Beck, A. T. (1952). Successful outpatient psychotherapy of a chronic schizophrenic with a delusion based on borrowed guilt. *Psychiatry*, 15, 305–12.

Bellack, A. S., Mueser, K. T., Wade, J., Sayers, S., and Morrison, R. (1992). The ability of schizophrenics to perceive and cope with negative affect. *British Journal of Psychiatry*, **160**, 473–80.

Bellack, A. S., Sayers, S., Mueser, K. T., and Bennett, M. (1994). Evaluation of social problem solving in schizophrenia. *Journal of Abnormal Psychology*, **103**, 371–8.

Bellack, A. S., Gold, J. M., and Buchanan, R. W. (1999). Cognitive rehabilitation for schizophrenia: problems, prospects, and strategies. *Schizophrenia Bulletin*, **25**, 257–74.

Bootzin, R. R. and McKnight, K. M. (1998). The role of deficited information processing in depression: evaluation and implications for treatment. *Behavior Therapy*, **29**, 619–30.

Bowen, L., Wallace, C. J., Glynn, S. M., et al. (1994). Schizophrenic individuals–cognitive functioning and performance in interpersonal interactions and skills training procedures. *Journal of Psychiatric Research*, **28**, 289–301.

Brothers, L. (1990a). The neural basis of primate social communication. *Motivation and Emotion*, **14**, 81–91.

Brothers, L. (1990b). The social brain: a project for integrating primate behavior and neurophysiology in a new domain. *Concepts in Neuroscience*, **1**, 27–61.

Buchanan, R. W., Strauss, M. E., Kirkpatrick, B., et al. (1994). Neuropsychological impairments in deficit versus nondeficit forms of schizophrenia. *Archives of General Psychiatry*, **51**, 804–11.

Buchkremer, G., Klingberg, S., Holle, R., Shulze Monking, H., and Hornung, W. P. (1997). Psychoeducational psychotherapy for schizophrenic patients and their key relatives or caregivers: results of a 2-year follow-up. *Acta Psychiatrica Scandinavica*, **96**, 483–91.

Chadwick, P. D. J. and Lowe, C. F. (1990). Measurement and modification of delusional beliefs. *Journal of Consulting and Clinical Psychology*, **58**, 225–32.

Chadwick, P. D. J., Birchwood, M., and Trower, P. (1996). *Cognitive Therapy for Delusions, Voices and Paranoia*. Chichester, England: John Wiley.

Clark, D. A., Beck, A. T., and Alford, B. A. (1999). *Scientific Foundations of Cognitive Theory and Therapy of Depression*. New York: John Wiley.

Cohen, J. D. and Servan-Schreiber, D. (1992). A neural network model of disturbances in the processing of context in schizophrenia. *Psychiatric Annals*, **22**, 131–6.

Cohen, J. D., Servan-Schreiber, D., and McClelland, J. (1992). A parallel distributed processing model of automaticity. *American Journal of Psychology*, **105**, 239–69.

Constans, J., Penn, D. L., Ihnen, G., and Hope, D. A. (1999). Interpretation deficites in social anxiety. *Behaviour Research and Therapy*, **37**, 643–651.

Corrigan, P. W. and Holtzman, K. (2001). Do stereotype threats influence social cognitive deficits in schizophrenia? In *Social Cognition and Schizophrenia*, ed. P. W. Corrigan and D. L. Penn, pp. 175–94. Washington, DC: APA Press.

Corrigan, P. W. and Penn, D. L. (1997). Disease and discrimination: two paradigms that describe severe mental illness. *Journal of Mental Health* , **6**, 355–66.

Corrigan, P. W. and Penn, D. L. (eds) (2001). *Social Cognition and Schizophrenia*. Washington, DC: American Psychological Association Press.

Corrigan, P. W. and Stephenson, J. A. (1994). Information processing and clinical psychology. In *Encyclopedia of Human Behavior*, vol. 2, ed. V. S. Ramachandran, pp. 645–654. Orlando, FL: Academic Press.

Corrigan, P. W. and Storzbach, D. M. (1993). The ecological validity of cognitive rehabilitation for schizophrenia. *Journal of Cognitive Rehabilitation*, **11**, 14–21.

Corrigan, P. W. and Toomey, R. (1995). Interpersonal problem solving and information processing in schizophrenia. *Schizophrenia Bulletin*, **21**, 395–404.

Corrigan, P. W. and Yudofsky, S. C. (eds) (1996). *Cognitive Rehabilitation for Neuropsychiatric Disorders*. Washington, DC: American Psychiatric Press.

Corrigan, P. W., Schade, M., and Liberman, R. P. (1992). Social skills training. In *Handbook of Psychiatric Rehabilitation*, ed. R. P. Liberman, pp. 95–126. New York: Macmillan.

Corrigan, P. W., Wallace, C. J., Schade, M. L., and Green, M. F. (1994). Learning medication self-management skills in schizophrenia: relationships with cognitive deficits and psychiatric symptoms. *Behavior Therapy*, **25**, 5–15.

Cosmides, L. (1989). The logic of social exchange: has natural selection shaped how humans reason? Studies with the Wason selection task. *Cognition*, **31**, 187–276.

Cosmides, L. and Tooby, J. (1989). Evolutionary psychology and the generation of culture, Part II. Case study: a computational theory of social exchange. *Ethology and Sociobiology*, **10**, 51–97.

Cosmides, L. and Tooby, J. (1994). Beyond intuition and instinct blindness: toward an evolutionarily rigorous cognitive science. *Cognition*, **50**, 41–77.

Crocker, J., Major, B., and Steele, C. M. (1998). Social stigma. In *The Handbook of Social Psychology*, 4th edn, vol. 2, ed. D. Gilbert, S. T. Fiske, and G. Lindzey, pp. 504–53. New York: McGraw-Hill.

Cromwell, R. L. (1984). Preemptive thinking and schizophrenia research. In *Theories of Schizophrenia and Psychosis*, ed. W. D. Spaulding and J. K. Cole, pp. 1–46. Lincoln: University of Nebraska Press.

DeLisi, L. E. (1990). *Depression in Schizophrenia*. Washington, DC: American Psychiatric Press.

Dickerson, R. B., Ringel, N. B., and Boronow, J. J. (1991). Neuropsychological deficits in chronic schizophrenics: relationship with symptoms and behavior. *Journal of Nervous and Mental Disease*, **179**, 744–9.

Drury, V., Birchwood, M., Cochrane, R., and Macmillan, F. (1996). Cognitive therapy and recovery from acute psychosis: a controlled trial I. Impact on psychotic symptoms. *British Journal of Psychiatry*, **169**, 593–601.

Engel, R. and DeRubeis, R. (1993). The role of cognition in depression. In *Psychopathology and Cognition*, ed. K. Dobson and P. Kendall, pp. 339–56. San Diego: Academic Press.

Farah, M. J. (1992). Is an object an object and object? Cognitive and neuropsychological investigations of domain specificity in visual object recognition. *Current Directions in Psychological Science*, **1**, 164–9.

Fiske, S. T. (1995). Social cognition. In *Advanced Social Psychology*, ed. A. Tesser, pp. 149–93. New York: McGraw-Hill.

Fiske, S. T. and Taylor, S. E. (1991). *Social Cognition*, 2nd edn. New York: McGraw-Hill.

Frith, U. (1999). Cognitive development and cognitive deficit. In *The Blackwell Reader in Development Psychology*, ed. A. Slater and D. Muir, pp. 509–22. Malden, MA: Blackwell.

Garety, P. A., Kuipers, L., Fowler, D., Chamberlain, F., and Dunn, G. (1994). Cognitive behavioural therapy for drug-resistant psychosis. *British Journal of Medical Psychology*, **67**, 259–71.

Garety, P., Fowler, D., Kuipers, E., et al. (1997). London–East Anglia randomised controlled trial of cognitive-behavioural therapy for psychosis. *British Journal of Psychiatry*, **171**, 420–6.

Garety, P., Fowler, D., and Kuipers, E. (2000). Cognitive-behavioral therapy for medication-resistant symptoms. *Schizophrenia Bulletin*, **26**, 73–86.

Gilbert, D. T. (1995). Attribution and interpersonal perception. In *Advanced Social Psychology*, ed. A. Tesser, pp. 99–147. New York: McGraw-Hill.

Goldman, R. S., Axelrod, B. N., Tandon, R., et al. (1993). Neuropsychological prediction of treatment efficacy and one-year outcome in schizophrenia. *Psychopathology*, **126**, 122–6.

Gotlib, I. H. and Krasnoperova, E. (1998). Deficited information processing as a vulnerability factor for depression. *Behavior Therapy*, **29**, 603–17.

Gould, R. A., Mueser, K. T., Bolton, E., Mays, V., and Goff, D. (2001). Cognitive therapy for psychosis in schizophrenia: an effect size analysis. *Schizophrenia Research*, **48**, 335–42.

Green, M. F. (1996). What are the functional consequences of neurocognitive deficits in schizophrenia? *American Journal of Psychiatry*, **153**, 321–30.

Green, M. F. (1998). *Schizophrenia from a Neurocognitive Perspective: Probing the Impenetrable Darkness*. Boston: Allyn and Bacon.

Green, M. F. (1999). Interventions for neurocognitive deficits. *Schizophrenia Bulletin*, **25**, 197–200.

Green, M. and Nuechterlein, K. (1999). Should schizophrenia be treated as a neurocognitive disorder? *Schizophrenia Bulletin*, **25**, 309–20.

Hartlage, S., Alloy, L. B., Vazquez, C., and Dykman, B. (1993). Automatic and effortful processing in depression. *Psychological Bulletin*, **113**, 247–78.

Hirsch, S. R., Jolley, A. G., Barnes, T. R., and Liddie, P. F. (1989). Dysphoric and depressive symptoms in chronic schizophrenia. *Schizophrenia Research*, **2**, 259–64.

Jaeger, J. and Douglas, E. (1992). Adjunctive neuropsychological remediation in psychiatric rehabilitation: program description and preliminary data. *Schizophrenia Research*, **4**, 304–5.

Johnstone, E. C., Macmillan, J. F., Frith, C. D., Benn, D. K., and Crow, T. J. (1990). Further investigation of the predictors of outcome following first schizophrenic episodes. *British Journal of Psychiatry*, **157**, 182–9.

Kern, R. S., Green, M. F., and Satz, P. (1992). Neuropsychological predictors of skills training for chronic psychiatric patients. *Journal of Psychiatric Research*, **43**, 223–30.

Kingdon, D. G. and Turkington, D. (1991). The use of cognitive behavior therapy with a normalizing rationale in schizophrenia. *Journal of Nervous and Mental Disease*, **179**, 207–11.

Klingberg, S., Buckremer, G., Holle, R., Monking, H., and Hornung, W. (1999). Differential therapy effects of psychoeducational psychotherapy for schizophrenic patients – results of a 2-year follow-up. *European Archives of Psychiatry and Clinical Neuroscience*, **249**, 66–72.

Knight, R. A. and Silverstein, S. M. (1998). The role of cognitive psychology in guiding research on cognitive deficits in schizophrenia. In *Origins and Development of Schizophrenia: Advances in Experimental Psychopathology*, ed. M. Lenzenweger and R. H. Dworkin, pp. 247–95. Washington, DC: APA Press.

Kuipers, E., Garety, P., Fowler, D., et al. (1997). The London–East Anglia randomised controlled trial of cognitive-behavioural therapy for psychosis. I: Effects of the treatment phase. *British Journal of Psychiatry*, **171**, 319–27.

Leff, J. P., Berkowitz, R., Shavit, A., et al. (1990). A trial of family therapy v. relatives–groups for schizophrenia: two year follow up. *British Journal of Psychiatry*, **157**, 571–7.

Levy, B. R. (1999). The inner self of the Japanese elderly: a defense against negative stereotypes of aging. *International Journal of Aging and Human Development*, **48**, 131–44.

Lysaker, P., Bell, M., and Beam-Goulet, J. (1995). Wisconsin card sorting test and work performance in schizophrenia. *Schizophrenia Research*, **56**, 45–51.

Major, B., Spencer, S., Schmader, T., Wolfe, C., and Crocker, J. (1998). Coping with negative stereotypes about intellectual performance: the role of psychological disengagement. *Personality and Social Psychology Bulletin*, **24**, 34–50.

Milton, F., Patwa, K., and Hafner, R. J. (1978). Confrontation vs. belief modification in persistently deluded patients. *British Journal of Medical Psychology*, **51**, 127–30.

Mueser, K. T., Bellack, A. S., Douglas, M. S., and Wade, J. H. (1991). Prediction of social skill acquisition in schizophrenic and major affective disorder patients from memory and symptomatology. *Psychiatry Research*, **37**, 281–96.

Nuechterlein, K. H. and Dawson, M. E. (1984). Vulnerability and stress factors in the developmental course of schizophrenic disorders. *Schizophrenia Bulletin*, **10**, 158–9.

Ostrom, T. M. (1984). The sovereignty of social cognition. In *Handbook of Social Cognition*, vol. 1, ed. R. S. Wyer and T. K. Srul, pp. 1–37. Hillsdale, NJ: Erlbaum.

Penn, D. L., Van Der Does, A. J. W., Spaulding, W. D., et al. (1993). Information processing and social cognitive problem solving in schizophrenia: assessment of interrelationships and changes over time. *Journal of Nervous and Mental Disease*, **181**, 13–20.

Penn, D. L., Mueser, K. T., Spaulding, W., et al. (1995). Information processing and social competence in chronic schizophrenia. *Schizophrenia Bulletin*, **21**, 269–281.

Penn, D. L., Spaulding, W. D., Reed, D., and Sullivan, M. (1996). The relationship of social cognition to ward behavior in chronic schizophrenia. *Schizophrenia Research*, **20**, 327–35.

Penn, D. L., Corrigan, P. W., Bentall, R., Racenstein, M., and Newman, L. (1997). Social cognition in schizophrenia. *Psychological Bulletin*, **121**, 114–32.

Shih, M., Pittinsky, T. L., and Ambady, N. (1999). Stereotype susceptibility: identity salience and shifts in quantitative performance. *Psychological Science*, **10**, 80–3.

Silverstein, S. M. (1997). Information processing, social cognition, and psychiatric rehabilitation in schizophrenia. *Psychiatry*, **60**, 327–40.

Silverstein, S. M., Bakshi, S., Chapman, R. M., and Nowlis, G. (1998). Perceptual organization of configural and nonconfigural visual patterns in schizophrenia: effects of repeated exposure. *Cognitive Neuropsychiatry*, **3**, 209–23.

Siris, S. G. (1995). Depression in schizophrenia. In *Contemporary Issues in the Treatment of Schizophrenia*, ed. C. L. Shriqui and H. A. Nasrallah, pp. 155–66. Washington, DC: American Psychiatric Press.

Spaulding, W. D. (1997). Cognitive models in a fuller understanding of schizophrenia. *Psychiatry*, **60**, 341–6.

Spaulding, W. D. and Poland, J. S. (2001). Cognitive rehabilitation for schizophrenia: enhancing social cognition by strengthening neurocognitive functioning. In *Social Cognition and Schizophrenia*, ed. P. W. Corrigan and D. L. Penn, pp. 217–47. Washington, DC: APA Press.

Spaulding, W., Fleming, S. D. R., Sullivan, M., Storzbach, D., and Lam, M. (1999). Cognitive functioning in schizophrenia: implications for psychiatric rehabilitation. *Schizophrenia Bulletin*, **25**, 275–89.

Steele, S. (1990). *The Content of our Character*. New York: St Martin's Press.

Steele, C. M. (1997). A threat in the air: how stereotypes shape intellectual identity and performance. *American Psychologist*, **52**, 613–29.

Steffy, R. (1993). Cognitive deficits in schizophrenia. In *Psychopathology and Cognition*, ed. K. Dobson and P. Kendall, pp. 622–34. San Diego: Academic Press.

Storzbach, D. M. and Corrigan, P. W. (1996). Cognitive rehabilitation for schizophrenia. In *Cognitive Rehabilitation for Neuropsychiatric Disorders*, ed. P. W. Corrigan and S. C. Yudofsky, pp. 299–328. Washington, DC: American Psychiatric Press.

Strauss, J. S. and Carpenter, W. T. (1972). The prediction of outcome in schizophrenia: I. Characteristics of outcome. *Archives of General Psychiatry*, **27**, 739–46.

Strauss, J. S. and Carpenter, W. T. (1974). The prediction of outcome in schizophrenia: II. Relationships between predictor and outcome variables: a report from the WHO International Pilot Study of Schizophrenia. *Archives of General Psychiatry*, **31**, 37–42.

Strauss, J. S. and Carpenter, W. T. (1977). Prediction of outcome in schizophrenia: III. Five year outcome and its predictors. *Archives of General Psychiatry*, **34**, 159–63.

Tarrier, N., Barrowclough, C., Vaughn, C. E., et al. (1988). The community management of schizophrenia: a controlled trial of a behavioral intervention with families to reduce relapse. *British Journal of Psychiatry*, **153**, 532–42.

Tarrier, N., Beckett, R., Harwood, S., et al. (1993). A trial of two cognitive-behavioural methods of treating drug-resistant residual psychotic symptoms in schizophrenic patients: I. Outcome. *British Journal of Psychiatry*, **162**, 524–32.

Tarrier, N., Yusupoff, L., Kinney, C., McCarthy, E., and Gledhill, A. (1998). Randomised controlled trial of intensive cognitive behaviour therapy for patients with chronic schizophrenia. *British Medical Journal*, **317**, 303–7.

Watts, F. N., Powell, E. G., and Austin, S. V. (1973). The modification of abnormal beliefs. *British Journal of Medical Psychology*, **46**, 359–63.

Wykes, T. and Dunn, G. (1992). Cognitive deficit and the prediction of rehabilitation success in a chronic psychiatric group. *Psychological Medicine*, **22**, 389–98.

Wykes, T., Sturt, E., and Katz, R. (1990). The prediction of rehabilitative success after three years: the use of social, symptom and cognitive variables. *British Journal of Psychiatry*, **157**, 865–70.

14

Cognitive-behavioral interventions for alcohol abuse and dependence

Helen S. Raytek,[1] Thomas J. Morgan,[2] and Nicola M. Chung,[2]

[1] National Council on Alcoholism and Drug Dependence, Newark, NJ, USA
[2] Rutgers, the State University of New Jersey, Piscataway, NJ, USA

In the last several decades, a great deal of empirical work in the addiction field has focused on cognitive-behavioral therapy (CBT) for alcohol abuse and dependence. This chapter will review the history of cognitive-behavioral models for treating alcohol problems, describe the extent and impact of alcohol problems, describe current cognitive-behavioral models and empirical support for them, identify unresolved issues and areas most in need of investigation, and suggest strategies to address these issues.

History of classification of alcohol-use disorders

In the nineteenth century, medical writers began discussing alcohol problems in a way that emphasized the concept of addiction or dependence and led to the development of the disease concept of alcoholism (Grant and Dawson, 1999). Kraeplin (1909–15) continued in this approach with his emphasis on organic disorders associated with alcoholism. Jellinek (1960) elaborated the disease model with the focus on the atypical physiological response to alcohol that leads to involuntary loss of control over drinking behavior and an inability to return to normal drinking. The disease model views alcoholism as a progressive syndrome that cannot be cured but can be managed by treatment that helps the alcoholic maintain abstinence. According to Jellinek, an alcoholic progresses through several stages: symptomatic, prodromal, crucial, and chronic phases. The chronic phase is characterized by physical and behavioral deterioration and leads to disability or death unless the alcoholic receives treatment. In addition, Jellinek was the first prominent theorist to discuss alcohol-use disorders that did not involve dependence (his alpha, beta, and epsilon types), which he differentiated from types that involve dependence (gamma and delta types).

Edwards and Gross (1976) developed the concept of the alcohol dependence syndrome (ADS) which moved even further from the idea of a disease model and described alcohol dependence as a learned behavior which existed on a continuum of severity and included tolerance and withdrawal symptoms and salience of drink-seeking behavior. The American Psychiatric Association (APA) was influenced by the ADS concept and first included nondependent substance-use disorders (substance "abuse" as opposed to "dependence") in the third edition of the *Diagnostic and Statistical Manual of Mental Disorders* (DSM-III; APA, 1980). DSM-IV (APA, 1994) symptoms of alcohol dependence include tolerance, withdrawal, impaired control, neglect of activities, great deal of time spent using alcohol, and continued use despite problems. DSM-IV symptoms of alcohol abuse include failure to fulfill major role obligations, use in physically hazardous situations, alcohol-related legal problems, and continued use despite problems.

Prevalence of alcohol-use disorders

The most recent community survey of alcohol use in the USA is the National Longitudinal Alcohol Epidemiologic Survey (NLAES) with more than 40 000 respondents, 18 years of age and older (Grant et al., 1994). Lifetime estimates are 13.3% for dependence and 4.9% for abuse. Past-year estimates are 4.4% for dependence and 3.0% for abuse. An estimated 18 million adults age 18 years or older currently experience problems that arise from alcohol abuse or dependence (Rua, 1990).

Pathological effects of alcohol use

Excessive alcohol use can be toxic to the central nervous system, the gastrointestinal system, and the cardiovascular system (Moak and Anton, 1999). It can result in cognitive deficits such as difficulties with abstraction and problem solving. Symptoms of depression and anxiety are common in heavy drinkers, although these symptoms are often alleviated with abstinence (Moak and Anton, 1999). Alcoholics are also at higher risk for suicide attempts (Hesselbrock et al., 1988). Social effects of excessive alcohol use include poor interpersonal functioning and domestic violence, poor occupational functioning, increased incidence of motor vehicle accidents, burn injuries, and violent crimes (Moak and Anton, 1999). In 1990, the estimated total cost of alcohol-use disorders (including medical expenses, loss of productivity, and costs related to crime) was $98.6 billion (Institute for Health Policy, Brandeis University, 1993).

Etiology of alcohol-use disorders

People with alcohol-use disorders are a widely varying group with different patterns of onset and a number of etiological factors (biological, psychological, and environmental). Overall, a person who develops an alcohol-use disorder initially finds alcohol use rewarding (Rotgers, 1996). Peer group influence and modeling may be particularly powerful in initiating alcohol use in adolescence. From an operant conditioning framework, alcohol may provide positive effects (for example, relaxation) and remove negative effects (for example, alleviate a negative mood or withdrawal symptoms). These reinforcing properties of alcohol play an important role in the development of an alcohol-use disorder (Carroll, 1999). Classical conditioning plays a role in conditioned craving and withdrawal and in environmental cues that lead to alcohol use. These same processes are involved in the maintenance of alcohol-use disorders. In addition, as a person turns to alcohol for its rewarding properties, he or she will not look as much to other ways to feel rewarded and will not develop as many constructive coping approaches for daily problems. Our etiological models lack explicit research on developmental psychopathological processes. We are more at a point of identifying various risk factors (biological, psychological, and environmental) as all contributing.

History of cognitive-behavioral treatments for alcohol-use disorders

Most early treatments for alcohol problems developed specifically within the addiction field and were based on a disease model. Inpatient and outpatient treatment approaches based on the 12-step philosophy of Alcoholics Anonymous (such as the Minnesota Model) continue to be used widely today (Longabaugh and Morgenstern, 1999). However, over time, developments in learning theory began to have an impact on the treatment of many emotional and behavioral disorders. For example, Eysenck (1959) expressed the hope that behavior therapy, with its basis in learning theory and scientific methods, would challenge the psychoanalytic model of treatment which was then dominant in the treatment of most emotional and behavioral disorders other than alcohol abuse. Classical behavioral theory (Watson, 1919; Pavlov, 1927), operant conditioning (Skinner, 1953), and social learning theory (Bandura, 1977) have been central to the development of cognitive-behavioral treatments.

Rotgers (1996) describes how these developments in learning theory led to specific treatments for alcohol problems. Classical conditioning theory (pairing a previously neutral stimulus repeatedly with an unconditioned stimulus to elicit a conditioned response) led to the development of several treatments for alcohol abuse and dependence. Cue exposure approaches focus on exposing the client to environmental triggers that lead to urges. Since clients no longer drink in those situations, they habituate to the environmental cues and eventually stop having urges to drink in those situations (Childress et al., 1993). Stimulus control techniques encourage the client to remove or rearrange items that are associated with drinking (bottles of alcohol, furniture associated with drinking, etc.) (Bickel and

Kelly, 1988). Relaxation training teaches clients alternate means of relaxing (Monti et al., 1989). Covert sensitization and other aversion therapy techniques help clients develop negative reactions to thoughts or sight of alcohol (Rimmele et al., 1989).

Operant conditioning (increasing the frequency of behaviors through reinforcement and decreasing them through punishment) led to the development of several treatments. The community reinforcement approach focuses on having significant others in the client's life (family members, coworkers, etc.) reward the client for abstinence (Azrin et al., 1982). Behavioral marital therapy for alcohol dependence involves the spouse of the client in the treatment in order to build motivation and coping skills for abstinence (McCrady and Epstein, 1996). Network therapy emphasizes involvement of people close to the client to provide ongoing support and promote attitude and behavior change (Galanter, 1997). Modeling theory led to the development of a social skills training approach for treating alcohol problems (Monti et al., 1989). Several theorists began to focus on the cognitive mediation of behavior and its relevance to treatment of various emotional and behavioral disorders (Ellis et al., 1988; Beck et al., 1993). These approaches focused on identifying and changing maladaptive thoughts that can lead to negative emotional states and alcohol use.

Other approaches used a social learning theory framework (Bandura, 1977) which views human behavior and cognition as products of classical conditioning, operant conditioning, and modeling and posits that cognitive processes can mediate behavioral change. For example, Marlatt and Gordon (1985) integrated cognitive and behavioral techniques and developed a relapse prevention approach that focused on identifying and coping with high-risk situations, dealing with cravings, coping with lapses, and developing a more balanced lifestyle. Most subsequent research on CBT for alcohol-use disorders has been based on Marlatt and Gordon's (1985) relapse prevention approach (Longabaugh and Morgenstern, 1999). Alcohol treatment approaches using CBT were among the first to receive empirical support (Chaney et al., 1978; Oei and Jackson, 1980). Since then, many other studies have continued to provide empirical evidence for the clinical and cost-effectiveness of CBT (Finney and Monahan, 1996; Longabaugh and Morgenstern, 1999).

Currently, CBT for alcohol-use disorders targets cognitive and behavioral skills with the goal of changing drinking behavior (Longabaugh and Morgenstern, 1999). Some of the treatment approaches described above continue to be a main focus of current treatment and research programs (for example, behavioral marital therapy, social skills training, and network therapy). Other approaches (such as stimulus control techniques) have been integrated into more comprehensive treatment approaches such as relapse prevention (Marlatt and Gordon, 1985). A few techniques are rarely used due to lack of empirical support or lack of compliance by clients (for example, aversion therapy techniques). Various CBT techniques are similar in being based on social learning theory (Bandura, 1977), emphasizing coping skills, and use of instruction, modeling, role play, and behavioral rehearsal (Longabaugh and Morgenstern, 1999) but differ in duration, modality (group, individual, couples) content, and treatment setting (inpatient or outpatient) (Miller et al., 1995).

Current cognitive-behavioral models

Cognitive-behavioral treatments for alcohol abuse and dependence include a broad range of approaches that may emphasize behavioral interventions (Bickel and Kelly, 1988; Childress et al., 1993), cognitive interventions (Ellis et al., 1988; Beck et al., 1993), or an integration of behavioral principles with cognitive mediation (Marlatt and Gordon, 1985). Some approaches (Bickel and Kelly, 1988; Childress et al., 1993) focus more specifically on alcohol use while other approaches also address other problem areas that may be associated with alcohol use (Monti et al., 1989). All of these treatment models are based on learning principles. They posit that much of human behavior (including alcohol abuse) is learned and that learning principles can suggest ways to change behavior. Rotgers (1996) outlined the basic assumptions of these approaches:

1. Human behavior is largely learned rather than being determined by genetic factors.
2. The same learning processes that create problem behaviors can be used to change them.
3. Behavior is largely determined by contextual and environmental factors.
4. Covert behaviors such as thoughts and feelings are subject to change through the application of learning principles.
5. Actually engaging in new behaviors in the contexts in which they are to be performed is a critical part of behavior change.
6. Each client is unique and must be assessed as an individual in a particular context.
7. The cornerstone of adequate treatment is a thorough behavioral assessment.

These principles play an important role in cognitive-behavioral treatments and will be referred to in upcoming sections of this chapter. The next section discusses basic tasks for any cognitive-behavioral treatment of alcohol-use disorders.

Motivation to change

Clients come to alcohol treatment with various levels of motivation to change. One framework for categorizing clients is the stages-of-change model (Prochaska et al., 1992). Individuals pass through five stages as they initiate and maintain change of any behavior: (1) precontemplation – not believing one has a problem that needs changing; (2) contemplation – beginning to think that one has a problem but being ambivalent about trying to change; (3) preparation – realizing that one does have a problem and preparing to make a change; (4) action – making specific behavior changes; and (5) maintenance – doing what is necessary to maintain the changes. It is important to know what stage of change a client is in order to provide appropriate interventions. For example, if a client has been coerced into alcohol treatment by a spouse and is in the precontemplation stage, the therapist would focus on discussing issues with the client that will help him or her begin to see that he or she has a problem that should be addressed.

Miller and Rollnick (1991) have developed motivational interviewing, a treatment approach in which the therapist facilitates the type of environment that will enhance the client's internal motivation to change. The therapist acknowledges the client's ambivalence about changing, reviews the positive and negative consequences of making changes, and adds support to the positive things that may happen for the client as a result of making the changes. Motivational enhancement therapy (MET) provides objective feedback to the individual, develops the discrepancy between the ideal self and substance-using self, and fosters a therapeutic relationship that will encourage an individual's commitment to change. Providing options, encouraging personal responsibility for decisions, and facilitating self-efficacy are important factors in motivational enhancement. In addition, informational input, cognitive appraisal (weighing the pros and cons of change), and self-evaluation are important elements of the self-regulation model proposed by Miller and Brown (1991), as well as common to the motivational enhancement intervention.

Although the therapist will try to help the client increase his or her motivation for change, the stage of readiness to change at which the client starts treatment strongly influences the process of treatment participation and commitment (Prochaska et al., 1992) and a readiness-to-change score has been found to be the strongest predictor of clients' rating of the therapeutic alliance (Connors et al., 2000). Miller et al.'s (1995) metaanalysis of 211 outcome studies of various treatment approaches shows MET to be one of the most effective CBT treatments.

Developing a therapeutic relationship

As a client enters cognitive-behavioral treatment for an alcohol-use disorder, he or she begins to interact with the therapist. Throughout the treatment, the discussions the client has and the techniques and coping skills he or she learns will occur within the context of the relationship with the therapist. The therapy relationship and treatment techniques are integrated aspects of a single process. The therapeutic relationship is therefore a central contextual factor that will influence the client's behavior. Alcohol treatment research has found that a confrontational therapist style is associated with poorer treatment outcomes (Miller et al., 1993). In Project MATCH, better working alliance scores were associated with improved alcohol outcomes across treatment conditions and modalities (Connors et al., 1997).

Follette et al. (1996) proposed specific mechanisms of the therapeutic relationship that may be responsible for mediating change in the client. They see the therapist as a provider of two kinds of social reinforcement to the client. "General contingent reinforcement" refers to the general expressions of support the therapist provides to the client for simply being in treatment to deal with difficult problems and allows the therapist to begin to exert social influence. The therapist begins general contingent reinforcement from the start of the first session to reward the client for making the effort to be in therapy. The therapist then begins to use "specific contingent reinforcement" to shape effective client behaviors. Follette et al. (1996) feel that general contingent reinforcement should be a constant background throughout treatment independent of initial progress toward treatment goals, since it helps clients stay in therapy, which is a necessary condition for positive treatment outcome.

Completing a comprehensive functional analysis

Since people with alcohol-use disorders are heterogeneous in terms of what factors initiated and maintain alcohol use and in terms of areas in their lives that may be affected by alcohol use, an important initial treatment intervention is analyzing the antecedent environmental and psychological triggers for alcohol use as well as the positive and negative consequences that follow. A DSM-IV diagnosis places a client in a certain substance-use disorder category. A functional analysis of alcohol use utilizes a learning theory framework and emphasizes environmental, affective, and cognitive antecedents to drinking and on reinforcing consequences of drinking. A functional analysis goes further than a diagnosis by providing detailed information on the client's alcohol-use patterns and life problems (including interpersonal, emotional, physical, occupational, financial, and legal) associated with use. This information enables the therapist to formulate a plan for what factors in the client's life need to be modified in order to avoid alcohol use and what other life areas are in need of improvement.

Specific elements of a functional analysis include the identification of high-risk situations. These situations are external factors such as people, places, and things that trigger alcohol usage. Once these high-risk situations are identified, an individual may choose to avoid the situation or develop a plan to cope with it. Another element of the functional analysis is the identification of irrational or "risky" thoughts. These thoughts tend to justify alcohol use (Marlatt and Gordon, 1985; Beck et al., 1993). Many of these risky thoughts are related to the individual's positive expectancies of alcohol use. Interventions at the cognitive level of the functional analysis include developing more negative expectancies of using alcohol and increasing positive expectancies of abstinence. Also, interventions focus on developing and enhancing an individual's self-efficacy, particularly as he or she begins to cope more effectively with risky situations.

Developing treatment goals

Abstinence is the ideal risk-reduction goal in that it allows a client to avoid harm from excessive alcohol use. As the classification of alcohol-use disorders broadened in the last several decades to conceptualize problems on a continuum that includes abuse as well as dependence, the setting of treatment goals with a client has become a more flexible and collaborative process. Clients have been found to be more motivated for and committed to treatment when they select their goals (Marlatt et al., 1993). Although abstinence may be the ideal goal for a person dependent on alcohol, if a client does not want to have abstinence as a goal, the therapist may agree to work initially towards a reduction in drinking and harm related to alcohol use, partly as a way to keep the client engaged in treatment (Miller and Page, 1991). In addition, controlled drinking may be a workable goal for clients who are experiencing negative consequences to use (alcohol abusers) but are not dependent on alcohol. However, this area continues to be highly controversial (Marlatt et al., 1993). If the therapist determines that the client is engaged in a level of use that is potentially life-threatening, the client may be referred to a detoxification program to achieve at least temporary abstinence.

Developing coping skills

Abuse of alcohol may be viewed as a maladaptive way of coping with negative affect, interpersonal conflict, or peer pressure. However, alcohol can lead to feelings of sadness even if the person expects it to elevate mood (Schuckit and Monteiro, 1988). In addition, the majority of relapse episodes after treatment occur during situations involving negative emotional states (Miller et al., 1996). A task of treatment is to assist the individual in learning new strategies to cope with urges and high-risk situations. In addition, symptoms of depression and anxiety in problem drinkers may arise partly from the effects of alcohol and are often alleviated with abstinence (Moak and Anton, 1999). Research has shown active coping is more effective than avoidance or passive coping (Annis and Davis, 1989; Moos et al., 1990). The importance of engendering effective coping strategies is apparent in studies that show higher abstinence rates are associated with use of a greater number of coping strategies (Litman et al., 1979; Moser and Annis, 1996).

Preventing relapse

Once an individual has sustained abstinence for a period of time, the task in treatment shifts to preventing relapse. Cummings et al. (1980) described a number of situations that are most frequently related to relapse, across a number of addictive behaviors: (1) negative emotional states; (2) social pressure to use; (3) interpersonal conflicts; and (4) urges and temptations. Other factors related to relapse include decreased commitment to abstinence (Hall et al., 1990), lowered cognitive vigilance (Litman et al., 1983), and low self-efficacy (Burling et al., 1989; Soloman and Annis, 1990; McKay et al., 1993).

Specific treatment approaches

In this section we will provide a more detailed description of one broad treatment approach that integrates cognitive and behavioral interventions (Marlatt and Gordon's relapse prevention (RP) model) and two approaches that focus more specifically on cognitive techniques (rational emotive behavior therapy (REBT) and Beck's cognitive therapy).

Relapse prevention

Although the phrase used to describe this approach developed by Marlatt and Gordon (1985) focuses on maintaining change in the future, it actually provides a comprehensive approach for understanding and treating substance abuse that is helpful for most clients who present for alcohol treatment. In the RP framework, the person with an alcohol-use disorder is viewed as focused on the expectation of positive effects from alcohol use and has decreased self-efficacy regarding his or her ability to avoid alcohol use. Basic treatment techniques in the RP approach include self-monitoring and functional analysis of alcohol use, identification and avoidance of high-risk situations, developing strategies for recognizing and coping with urges to drink, developing alternative coping approaches for high-risk situations, exploration of the decision chains leading to alcohol use (including seemingly irrelevant decisions), learning from slips in order to prevent future relapses, and addressing lifestyle balance.

Marlatt and Gordon define a high-risk situation as any circumstance that threatens a person's sense of control and increases the risk of relapse. The most common high-risk situations are negative emotional states, interpersonal conflicts, and social pressure to drink. Clients who develop effective means of coping with high-risk situations will become more confident about their ability to avoid alcohol, which will decrease their likelihood of relapse. Another important treatment tool in the RP approach is teaching clients about the abstinence violation effect (AVE). The AVE happens as a result of the conflict a client feels if he or she has made a commitment to avoid alcohol but experiences a slip. The client feels guilty and a loss of control and is in danger of giving up on abstinence and going on to a full relapse of alcohol use. If a client is aware of the AVE, he or she is more able to minimize the length and intensity of the slip. Interested readers are referred to Larimer et al. (1999) for a concise summary of the RP model.

Ellis's rational emotive behavior therapy of substance abuse

Rational emotive behavior therapy (REBT) views behavior as a chain of events, A–B–C, where A is the external event to which the individual is exposed, B is the belief the individual has about A, and C is the emotion or behavior that results from B. Thus, the emotional or behavioral response to an external event is due to beliefs about that event rather than to the event itself (Ellis et al., 1988). Clients are taught that it is the irrational beliefs they have that lead to dysfunctional emotional and behavioral consequences rather than the activating events. In therapy, two more events, D–E, are added to the A–B–C chain. D is the therapist's attempt to alter the client's irrational beliefs and E is the alternative thoughts and beliefs that result from D. In this model, it is necessary for clients initially to identify and acknowledge unhealthy negative feelings and self-defeating behaviors that arise from alcohol use. REBT for alcohol-use disorders targets irrational beliefs that support using alcohol as a way of coping with negative emotions. The therapist helps the client in the process of rational disputation of the irrational beliefs that directly or indirectly lead to alcohol use and assists the client in building tolerance for negative emotional states. Common themes that are addressed in REBT for alcohol problems are denial of alcohol-related problems, use of alcohol as a way of coping with emotional problems, demandingness (believing that the world should be a certain way because one desires that it be so), low frustration tolerance, needs for high levels of stimulation and excitement, avoidance of all negative emotions, shame for being an alcoholic, and beliefs that change is too difficult.

Beck's cognitive therapy of substance abuse

Beck developed his general cognitive approach when he was investigating the thoughts of depressed individuals and discovered a basic negative bias. He identified three levels of cognition that are part of the depressive experience: automatic thoughts, schemata, and cognitive biases (Beck, 1967), and developed cognitive therapy for depression based on that framework. Later, Beck and colleagues applied cognitive techniques to the treatment of substance abuse (Beck et al., 1993). They view alcohol use as involving many complex behaviors driven by alcohol-related beliefs, automatic thoughts, and facilitating beliefs. Alcohol-related beliefs involve positive expectancies about the effects of substance use such as "A drink will help me relax." Automatic thoughts are brief, spontaneous thoughts and images (similar to the B component of the A–B–C model of Ellis et al.) that individuals may not even notice unless they consciously try to monitor them. Automatic thoughts reflect the person's appraisal of a situation rather than the objective reality and lead directly to his or her emotional and behavioral responses. Examples of automatic thoughts are "It's party time" and "Who cares, just do it." Facilitating beliefs involve permission to use alcohol in contrast to a prior commitment to abstinence.

According to this model, alcohol use is triggered by "activating stimuli" (the same as Marlatt and Gordon's "high-risk situations"), which are external or internal cues for drinking. External cues include being offered a drink, seeing other people drinking, occupational problems, and experiencing interpersonal conflict. Internal cues include cravings, and positive and negative emotional states. In response to these external or internal cues, a person may begin to think that alcohol will increase positive feelings or decrease negative feelings. These expectations lead to automatic thoughts that lead to craving alcohol. Facilitating beliefs may then give the person permission to drink.

Treatment with Beck's approach focuses on teaching the client to identify and challenge two kinds of thoughts: thoughts that directly involve positive expectancies of alcohol use and thoughts that are associated with negative emotional states such as anxiety, depression, and anger that may indirectly lead to alcohol use. The therapist then helps the client replace those thoughts with more adaptive cognitions. Other areas of therapeutic work include learning life skills to achieve more satisfaction and confidence about handling life without alcohol and addressing the cognitive triad (negative views of oneself, the world, and the future) so that clients have more self-esteem, feel less helpless, and are more hopeful.

Comparison of RP, REBT, and Beck's models

These three models are all based on the learning principles described earlier in this chapter. They can also be classified as "broad spectrum treatment approaches" (Longabaugh and Morgenstern, 1999) in that they do not address only drinking problems but target other life problems that can lead to drinking. For example, since failures in coping may lead to negative emotional states which in turn can lead to drinking, these three models help clients identify situations that arouse sad, angry, and anxious feelings and develop coping skills to deal with those situations more constructively.

The RP model presents a broad framework for understanding the initiation, maintenance, and treatment of alcohol-use disorders. It provides an integrated cognitive-behavioral model of alcohol-use disorders and offers a broad range of interventions in both behavioral and cognitive spheres and has guided much of the research on CBT treatment for alcohol problems (Longabaugh and Morgenstern, 1999). The RP framework incorporates aspects of the cognitive approaches by accepting the importance of the cognitive mediation of behavior – alcohol-related thoughts are contributory causes of drinking and behavioral interventions in the RP model and are seen as exerting their effect through changes in cognitive structures. However, it does not view cognitive change as sufficient for maintaining abstinence from alcohol. Rather, it views the cognitive and behavioral aspects of experience as exerting influence on each other.

REBT and Beck's model focus more specifically than does RP on identifying and modifying maladaptive cognitions related to alcohol use since a person's thoughts and expectancies are viewed as mediating behavior. REBT and Beck's approach are not etiologic models. Cognitions are not viewed as initiating alcohol use, since the etiology of alcohol use is multiply determined by biological, psychological, and social factors. However, the more cognitive models of treatment (REBT and Beck's) do provide a framework for understanding the maintenance of alcohol use and the process of relapse to use. In addition, the cognitive models suggest various points of intervention–cognitions that can be addressed in treatment to attain and maintain abstinence or reduced use. Clients learn to identify maladaptive cognitions that lead to drinking, to anticipate negative consequences of drinking, and to develop alternative cognitive coping strategies. Addressing alcohol-related cognitions is a necessary part of treatment and abstinence will be maintained only if the underlying alcohol-related thoughts and beliefs are changed. However, REBT and Beck's model also address behavioral issues and utilize some behavioral techniques since cognitive therapy interventions for alcohol-use disorders that do not include a behavioral component have not been as effective as cognitive-behavioral treatments (Holder et al., 1991). Therefore, the therapist using REBT or Beck's model monitors client changes in affective and behavioral realms in addition to cognitive changes.

Unlike RP, REBT and Beck's models have not been the focus of much research when used for alcohol problems (Miller et al., 1995). In addition, they have not achieved the prominence of distinct cognitive models of depression and anxiety disorders. REBT and Beck's model are similar in that they both address irrational beliefs specifically tied to alcohol and the general irrational beliefs that lead to negative emotional states that may indirectly lead to alcohol use. The more general areas of therapeutic work differ in these two approaches in that REBT targets demandingness cognitions and low frustration tolerance and Beck's model targets the cognitive triad (negative views of oneself, the world, and the future).

Cognitive processes in the initiation and maintenance of alcohol-use disorders

Individuals can take many different paths in developing an alcohol-use disorder. Learning principles of classical and operant conditioning and modeling can be used to explain these various pathways. In addition, cognitive processes mediate these experiences, are changed by these experiences, and are a contributing factor to future behaviors. A typical course of development could involve a person being exposed to peers and/or family members who use alcohol excessively. A person exposed to these social influences may begin to think about alcohol as a normal and positive part of life. The person may then find first experiences with alcohol to be rewarding in terms of the feeling of intoxication and relief from upsetting emotions. These rewarding aspects of alcohol may well be internalized in the person's cognitions. The person may begin to think about alcohol as a means of coping with stress and may become inhibited in the development of more constructive ways of coping. In Beck's model, facilitating beliefs give permission to the person to use alcohol as a way to deal with stress and are thus proximal causes to alcohol use. Distal causes to alcohol use include alcohol-related thoughts activated by high-risk situations. Some of the cognitions that contribute to alcohol use may be nonconscious or preconscious. The term "seemingly irrelevant decisions" (SIDs) refers to the small decisions that a person may make that seem to have nothing to do with alcohol use but can culminate in exposure to a high-risk situation. The SIDs framework assumes that a person trying to be abstinent from alcohol use may still feel ambivalent about abstaining. That person is at risk for having the positive expectancies of alcohol use exerting their influence and leading the person to placing himself or herself in a situation in which they may be more likely to use alcohol.

People who do not develop alcohol-use disorders may be protected in several ways. They may not be exposed to anyone who uses alcohol excessively or they may have negative reactions to someone who uses it excessively. They may already have a broad range of activities that provide them gratification and a good set of coping skills to utilize for everyday stress. They may realize that excessive alcohol use would be detrimental for achieving valued personal goals. They may try alcohol but not like the taste or may not like the feeling of being intoxicated.

Mechanism of change in therapy

The same learning processes that led to the development of a client's alcohol-use disorder are utilized in therapy to help him or her attain and maintain abstinence. Factors common to most therapies (such as expectations of improvement and a good therapeutic alliance) contribute to treatment outcome (Carroll, 1999). Throughout therapy, the therapist provides general contingent reinforcement to the client for being in therapy and specific contingent reinforcement as the client attains and maintains abstinence and develops the coping skills to manage trigger situations without alcohol.

Unique, active ingredients of these treatment approaches are also assumed to play a role in treatment outcome. The relapse prevention approach emphasizes the acquisition and implementation of skills such as the ability to identify and avoid high-risk situations, strategies for identifying and coping with craving, alcohol refusal skills, tools for minimizing the harm from a slip, and improved lifestyle balance (Carroll, 1999). RP, REBT, and Beck's model all posit the cognitive mediation of behavior and view behavioral interventions as exerting their effect through changes in cognitive structures. Behavioral, cognitive, and emotional processes are seem as integrally related in all human experiences, including the development of or recovery from an alcohol-use disorder. The client must move from expecting alcohol use to be rewarding to expecting abstinence to be more rewarding. Changing maladaptive cognitions that play a role in maintaining alcohol use is necessary for the maintenance of abstinence. Most clients enter therapy already aware of some of the negative consequences of alcohol use. The therapist reinforces those perceptions and tries to expand the client's awareness to include other negative consequences of use. The therapist helps the client identify the positive consequences that come from abstinence in order to increase the client's motivation to remain abstinent. These positive consequences of abstinence become salient reinforcers for the client and begin to replace the reinforcement associated with alcohol use. The therapist also helps the client develop meaningful reinforcers other than alcohol (activities and relationships) to help maintain abstinence (Carroll, 1999).

Predictors of treatment response

The main factors associated with relapse are lack of social support, presence of negative emotional states, social pressures to drink, skill deficits, negative life events, and concomitant psychiatric disorders (Larimer et al., 1999). Clients with higher levels of commitment to abstinence and greater intentions to avoid high-risk situations have been found to be at lower risk for relapse (Morgenstern et al., 1996). Clients who do experience a slip but have learned about the AVE may be in less danger of giving up on abstinence and plunging into a full relapse of alcohol use. If a client is aware of the AVE, he or she is better able to minimize the length and intensity of the slip.

Critical review of empirical evidence in support of these models

Over the past few years several reviews have been undertaken to evaluate the evidence for the efficacy of cognitive-behavioral treatment for alcohol problems. Since the late 1970s, Miller and his colleagues have been reviewing alcohol treatment studies. In their latest review, Miller et al. (1995) completed a metaanalysis that took into account the methodological quality of 211 outcome studies on 43 different treatment approaches used with a variety of clients with alcohol-use disorders. The treatment approaches with the top five cumulative evidence scores (CES) use CBT strategies based on learning principles to improve cognitive and behavioral skills: (1) brief interventions; (2) social skills training; (3) motivational enhancement; (4) community reinforcement approach; and (5) behavioral contracting. Although relapse prevention, behavioral marital therapy, and cognitive therapy were lower on the list, these interventions also showed a positive CES.

Carroll (1996) reviewed 26 studies across a number of addictive behaviors. The Carroll review included studies that: (1) were randomized controlled trials;

(2) utilized a treatment approach defined as relapse prevention or coping skills training that explicitly invoked the work of Marlatt; and (3) evaluated and reported on substance use as a primary outcome variable. Although hundreds of alcohol treatment studies have been conducted, only six met the criteria for inclusion in the Carroll review. Of these studies, three reported significant main effects for the superiority of cognitive-behavioral treatment when compared to other treatments. Carroll also reviewed interaction effects – did certain kinds of clients do better in certain kinds of treatments ("matching effects")? Several studies did report matching effects with CBT. In an article by Kadden et al. (1989), clients higher on measures of sociopathy and psychopathology had better drinking outcomes in CBT treatments than in treatment approaches aimed at improving interpersonal relationships. Clients higher on neuropsychological impairment had better outcomes when treated with the interpersonal approach than with CBT. However, recent results from Project MATCH failed to replicate these previous matching effects.

Irvin et al. (1999) conducted a metaanalysis to evaluate the efficacy of relapse prevention treatment. To be included in the metaanalysis, a study had to: (1) identify the treatment as relapse prevention or be clearly consistent with Marlatt and Gordon's approach; (2) report tests of statistical significance when determining the effectiveness of relapse prevention; and (3) use relapse prevention techniques as a specific treatment, rather than as a component in a broader treatment approach. Results from this metaanalysis suggested that relapse prevention treatment effects were strong and reliable for alcohol use and for polysubstance use. The modality (individual, group, or couples therapy) in which relapse prevention was delivered was not shown to moderate its effectiveness. Also, medications to treat alcoholism (e.g., disulfiram or naltrexone) may contribute substantially to enhancing treatment effectiveness. In addition to reducing alcohol use, results suggested relapse prevention also improved psychosocial adjustment. The authors caution that the studies in the metaanalysis did not have long-term follow-ups, so duration of effects could not be addressed.

Project MATCH (Project MATCH Research Group, 1997) has begun to publish results from the largest treatment research study ever conducted in the alcoholism field. The purpose was to determine whether different kinds of patients respond best to specific forms of treatment for alcoholism (patient by treatment "matching effects"). The treatments that were tested were: (1) MET; (2) CBT; and (3) twelve-step facilitation (TSF). Overall results indicated that all three treatment conditions were equally effective in terms of significant and sustained improvements in drinking outcomes for all kinds of clients and that there was little evidence for a treatment matching effect (certain kinds of clients did not respond better to one of the three treatment conditions). However, Project MATCH did find that patients with fewer symptoms of alcohol dependence had better drinking outcomes when treated with

CBT rather than TSF in an *aftercare* setting (a setting in which they received out-patient therapy after being in an inpatient setting).

There has been little recent empirical work directly addressing cognitive therapy approaches (REBT and Beck's model) for alcohol problems (Miller et al., 1995) since most researchers have focused on the comprehensive cognitive-behavioral relapse prevention framework of Marlatt and Gordon (1985). Several studies have compared Ellis's general rational emotive therapy approach to a relapse prevention approach (Rosenberg and Brian, 1986) or to insight therapy (Brandsma, 1980) and found all approaches to be equally effective in reducing drinking. Several other studies compared general cognitive approaches (replacing cognitions that produce negative affect and desires to drink) to social skills and communication training. Again, the researchers concluded that all of the approaches were effective in reducing drinking (Jackson and Oei, 1978; Brandsma, 1980; Oei and Jackson, 1982; Monti et al., 1990).

There has been some recent research on "outcome expectancies" (cognitions concerning the anticipated effects of alcohol), a factor that is analogous to "maladaptive cognitions" related to alcohol and a central part of the cognitive therapy models. For example, among college students, those with higher expectations regarding the positive effects of alcohol ("outcome expectancies") tend to drink more (Carey, 1995). They also tend to focus on the immediate positive effects and minimize the potential negative consequences of heavy drinking. Finney et al. (1998) have found that alcohol treatment with either CBT or TSF approaches leads to a reduction in positive substance-use expectancies and an increase in positive expectancies regarding desirable consequences of quitting substance use. Expectancies about the negative effects of alcohol may increase motivation for abstinence (Jones and McMahon, 1994).

Evidence regarding mediators of change

An important issue when looking at the effectiveness of various treatment approaches is identifying the mechanisms of action (mediators of change) that lead to improvements in drinking behavior. Longabaugh and Morgenstern (1999) reviewed nine well-controlled CBT studies that tried to identify the factors responsible for treatment effectiveness. To be considered a mediator of change, Longabaugh and Morgenstern (1999) posited three factors that had to be demonstrated:

At least part of the observed effectiveness of the treatment had to be attributable to an increase in the mediator variable ... a correlation had to exist between the patient's posttreatment status with respect to the mediator variable ... and drinking outcome, and statistical analyses had to demonstrate that when the effect of the mediating variable was selectively eliminated, overall treatment effectiveness declined (p. 80).

Only one of the nine studies identified a factor (social skills) that could be considered a mediator of change under Longabaugh and Morgenstern's definition, and that factor reached only marginal significance. The authors describe the other eight studies:

Either coping skills that increased through CBST [cognitive-behavioral coping skills therapy] were unrelated to drinking outcomes, or coping skills related to drinking outcome were not increased to a greater extent with CBST than with the comparison treatment. Furthermore, several studies did not determine whether CBST increased a particular coping skill more than did the comparison treatment and whether that same skill was related to improved drinking outcome … Although the review of the nine clinical trials indicated that better coping skills generally were associated with better drinking outcomes, it allowed no conclusions regarding the active ingredients of CBST. The studies demonstrated neither that CBST led to increases in specific coping skills that resulted in better drinking outcomes nor that CBST's greater effectiveness was attributable to better coping skills. Thus, researchers do not yet know how CBST works to improve drinking outcome (p. 80).

Longabaugh and Morgenstern's (1999) review suggests that we do not know what factors mediate change in substance abuse treatment and that we do not know whether the hypothesized active ingredients are actually responsible for treatment outcome.

Conclusions about the effectiveness of CBT

CBT is a theoretically coherent and empirically supported treatment for alcohol-use disorders. CBT has equal effectiveness when compared to other theoretically coherent approaches such as TSF therapy (Finney et al., 1998) or supportive group therapy plus naltrexone (O'Malley et al., 1992). It has been shown to have superior effectiveness when delivered as part of a comprehensive treatment program such as inpatient treatment for alcoholism (Longabaugh and Morgenstern, 1999) and to specific client subgroups (clients with less severe alcohol dependence in an aftercare setting). One could argue that CBT has lost ground since the initial clinical trials done in the 1980s when it was among the first alcoholism treatments shown to be effective. However, it seems more likely that comparison treatments have become more effective and have integrated many of the active elements that mediate change in CBT. Clinicians may choose to use CBT with clients who do not want to pursue alternative effective therapies (for example, TSF therapy or pharmacotherapy) or with clients who have characteristics that would likely make CBT a more effective approach (for example, clients in an aftercare setting with less severe drinking problems). One serious gap in the research is the failure to identify specific mediators of change such as changes in alcohol-related beliefs or coping strategies that could account for the effectiveness of CBT for alcohol problems.

We also lack information on what client characteristics are associated with various treatment outcomes, long-term follow-up studies, and research in community settings.

Priorities for future research

Treatment process analyses and identification of mediators of change

Little is known about what specific aspects of treatment for alcohol-use disorders mediate change in clients. Even monitoring and categorizing what happens moment-to-moment in various treatments remains largely unexplored. Developing precise specification of treatments is necessary before mechanisms of change can begin to be identified so that we can know more about how mediating processes are linked to outcome and what skills clients are applying in real-life situations. In addition, many studies on the effectiveness of CBT may not have been entirely faithful to the CBT approach or had treatment of sufficient duration for positive outcomes (Longabaugh and Morgenstern, 1999).

Although conceptually distinct, different treatments for alcohol-use disorders may not be all that different in practice and may exert their effect on outcome through common factors (Morgenstern et al., 1996) or through equivalent interventions. Treatment variables shared by various approaches to therapy include the therapeutic relationship, a therapeutic rationale, education about the nature of the disorder, and expectation of improvement. Active ingredients of an approach have been viewed as the unique interventions in that approach not shared with other treatment approaches that contribute to helping clients change. For example, in the RP approach, active ingredients include learning how to avoid or cope with high-risk situations, learning from slips to prevent future relapses, and addressing lifestyle imbalances. In REBT and Beck's cognitive therapy model, active ingredients include the identification and challenging of irrational thoughts. The relative contribution of common versus specific factors to treatment outcome has rarely been examined in cognitive-behavioral treatment for alcohol-use disorders (Carroll, 1999). If a client attains and maintains abstinence during and after treatment delivered in the RP framework, are these changes due to having learned to avoid or cope with high-risk situations and from changing lifestyle imbalances? Could much of the change in the client come from wanting to gain positive reinforcement from the therapist for abstinence? In addition, approaches other than CBT treatments, such as TSF therapy, often help clients improve in factors previously viewed as specific to CBT such as self-efficacy and coping skills and therefore may have interventions equivalent to CBT approaches. For example, coping skills are developed, confidence and feelings of efficacy are enhanced, and new skills are practiced in other treatments such as TSF treatments (Finney et al., 1998). What previously have been viewed as "unique" active ingredients may be shared by other treatment models.

CBT approaches assume that clients learn skills during treatment and apply the skills in real-life situations. However, such demonstrations have not generally been a part of research studies (Longabaugh and Morgenstern, 1999). Researchers need to explore this issue by assessing whether clients have learned and are exercising skills during and after treatment. Morgenstern et al. (1996) used this approach and found that clients with higher levels of commitment to abstinence and greater intention to avoid high-risk situations were at lower risk for relapse. One tool for assessing alcohol-related coping skills is the Situational Competency Test (Chaney et al., 1978) that utilizes a role-playing approach. Another tool is the Coping Responses Inventory (Moos, 1993) that assesses coping skills in stressful situations. These instruments could be used to determine whether clients acquire new coping skills as a result of treatment for alcohol-use disorders.

One way to explore whether cognitive processes targeted in therapy lead to abstinence is to use the Articulated Thoughts in Simulated Situations (ATSS) paradigm (Davison et al., 1983), which is a methodology to assess naturalistic and representative online cognitive activity that occurs during emotion activation. The ATSS paradigm provides open-ended verbal reporting of thoughts as they are experienced during an emotional reaction. In the ATSS method, participants listen to an audiotaped scenario and imagine that they are an active part of the interaction. After a brief segment of the tape is played, they are asked to articulate their thoughts for 30 s. Eckhardt et al. (1998) applied the ATSS paradigm to study maritally violent men during anger arousal. The ATSS approach could be used to explore the cognitions of clients with a history of alcohol-use disorders in various alcohol-related scenarios.

Another way to generate information about the important elements in the therapy process is to take the approach advocated by Fishman (1999): begin with the client and the situation (alcohol-use disorder treatment) and build a record, case by case, of intervention strategies. Follette et al. (1996) suggest a method of assessing treatment effectiveness as a function of the client–therapist relationship by coding client behavior and therapist contingent responding. A cumulative record could be used to show that clients' effective behaviors are increasing over time and less effective behaviors are decreasing. A lag sequential approach could be used to test whether the probability of a client response changed given a therapist's contingent reinforcement. Multiple baseline approaches could be used to demonstrate that targeted problem behaviors improve while untargeted problem behaviors remain at baseline level. Either lag sequential analyses or multiple baseline approaches could be used to show that the client–therapist relationship is a mechanism of change through in-session differential reinforcement.

Broad-spectrum CBT

Since many different approaches to substance abuse treatment have been found to be effective, the effectiveness of CBT may be enhanced by incorporating elements from those treatments such as self-help groups, involving significant others in the treatment, motivational enhancement, and pharmacotherapies (Longabaugh and Morgenstern, 1999). Guidelines could be developed to help clinicians decide what specific treatment elements could be provided to each client based on assessed needs and client preferences. Research would then focus on the efficacy of the decision guidelines that help the clinician decide what treatment elements to offer a specific client. Though the focus of evaluation would be on underlying treatment principles, researchers could also collect data that would help delineate the effective components of treatment and identify how these mediators of change exert their effects in various treatment packages.

Clients who present for treatment of alcohol-use disorders are a heterogeneous group. While there is some evidence that CBT is more effective with certain kinds of clients, results have been mixed and at times contradictory, and effects sizes are small (Longabaugh and Morgenstern, 1999). It is important that research studies continue to try to determine which treatment approaches are most effective for various clients. The ultimate goal of matching research is to develop guidelines for providing treatments that are more responsive to the needs of the particular client (Mattson and Allen, 1991). Matching studies have to be guided by a theory that specifies how mediating processes are linked to outcome (Morgenstern et al., 1996).

When investigating client–treatment interactions, one of the most difficult steps is conceptualizing the dimensions of client variables that may have important implications for selecting treatment approaches (Mattson and Allen, 1991). Four classes of client variables have been explored: demographics, drinking behaviors, psychopathology, and social/personal characteristics. Other important client variables to explore are motivation for treatment, stage of change, and level of social skill assets and deficits. Membership in a "special population" (minorities, women, adolescents, elderly) may affect treatment outcome. It is important to identify how these client variables interact with therapy components. Clients who vary in these ways may have different needs in terms of the intensity and staging of treatment (using different treatments in different settings at different phases of the disorder). Researchers could help clinicians develop a menu of effective treatment options and a system for deciding which treatment elements are likely to be most effective for each client at different points of treatment.

Conclusion

CBT offers a theoretically coherent and empirically supported treatment approach for alcohol abuse and dependence. In addition, Marlatt and Gordon's (1985) RP framework provides a systematic and empirically supported integration of various cognitive and behavioral interventions. Many elements of cognitive-behavioral treatments for alcohol abuse and dependence have been integrated into other treatment approaches, such as TSF therapy. For clients who may not want to engage in other effective treatments (such as taking medication to block urges for alcohol or TSF), CBT offers a comprehensive and effective set of treatment interventions. CBT is possibly superior to other approaches under certain circumstances, but we need more research to provide support for that possibility and identify the circumstances in which CBT would be the preferred treatment approach. We need to understand more about the treatment factors that mediate change in CBT for alcohol-use disorders and to develop guidelines for choosing from among a menu of effective treatment options to offer each particular client the most beneficial treatment.

REFERENCES

American Psychiatric Association. (1980). *Diagnostic and Statistical Manual of Mental Disorders*, 3rd edn. Washington, DC: APA.

American Psychiatric Association. (1994). *Diagnostic and Statistical Manual of Mental Disorders*, 4th edn. Washington, DC: APA.

Annis, H. M. and Davis, C. S. (1989). Relapse prevention. In *Handbook of Alcoholism Treatment Approaches*, ed. R. K. Hester and W. R. Miller, pp. 170–82. New York: Pergamon Press.

Azrin, N. H., Sisson, R. W., Meyers, R., and Godley, M. (1982). Alcoholism treatment by disulfiram and community reinforcement therapy. *Journal of Behavior Therapy and Experimental Psychiatry*, **13**, 105–12.

Bandura, A. (1977). *Social Learning Theory.* Englewood Cliffs, NJ: Prentice Hall.

Beck, A. T. (1967). *Depression: Clinical, Experimental, and Theoretical Aspects.* New York: Harper & Row.

Beck, A. T., Wright, F. D., Newman, C. F., and Liese, C. F. (1993). *Cognitive Therapy of Substance Abuse.* New York: Guilford Press.

Bickel, W. K. and Kelly, T. H. (1988). The relationship of stimulus control to the treatment of substance abuse. In *Learning Factors in Substance Abuse.* NIDA Research Monograph 84, ed. B. A. Ray, pp. 122–40. Washington, DC: US Government Printing Office.

Brandsma, J. M. (1980). *The Outpatient Treatment of Alcoholism: A Review and Comparative Study.* Baltimore, MD: University Park Press.

Burling, T. A., Reilly, P. M., Moltzen, J. O., and Ziff, D. C. (1989). Self-efficacy and relapse among inpatient drug and alcohol abusers: a predictor of outcome. *Journal of Studies on Alcohol*, **50**, 354–60.

Carey, K. B. (1995). Alcohol-related expectancies predict quantity and frequency of heavy drinking among college students. *Psychology of Addictive Behaviors*, **9**, 236–41.

Carroll, K. M. (1996). Relapse prevention as a psychosocial treatment: a review of controlled clinical trials. *Experimental and Clinical Psychopharmacology*, **4**, 46–54.

Carroll, K. M. (1999). Behavioral and cognitive behavioral treatments. In *Addictions: A Comprehensive Guidebook*, ed. B. S. McCrady and E. E. Epstein, pp. 250–67. New York: Oxford University Press.

Chaney, E. F., O'Leary, M. R., and Marlatt, G. A. (1978). Skill training with alcoholics. *Journal of Consulting and Clinical Psychology*, **46**, 1092–104.

Childress, A. R., Hole, A. V., Ehrman, R. N., et al. (1993). Cue reactivity and cue reactivity interventions in drug dependence. In *Behavioral Treatments for Drug Abuse and Dependence*. NIDA Research Monograph 137, ed. L. S. Onken, J. D. Blaine, and J. J. Boren, pp. 73–95. Washington, DC: US Government Printing Office.

Connors, G., Carrol, K. M., DiClemente, C. C., Longabaugh, R., and Donovan, D. (1997). The therapeutic alliance and its relationship to alcoholism treatment participation and outcome. *Journal of Consulting and Clinical Psychology*, **65**, 588–98.

Connors, G. J., DiClemente, C. C., Derman, K. H., et al. (2000). Predicting the therapeutic alliance in alcoholism treatment. *Journal of Studies on Alcohol*, **61**, 139–49.

Cummings, C., Gordon, J. R., and Marlatt, G. A. (1980). Relapse: strategies of prevention and prediction. In *The Addictive Behaviors*, ed. W. R. Miller, pp. 291–321. Oxford, England: Pergamon Press.

Davison, G. C., Robins, C., and Johnson, M. K. (1983). Articulated thoughts during simulated situations: a paradigm for studying cognition in emotion and behavior. *Cognitive Therapy and Research*, **7**, 17–40.

Eckhardt, C. I., Barbour, K. A., and Davison, G. C. (1998). Articulated thoughts of maritally violent and nonviolent men during anger arousal. *Journal of Consulting and Clinical Psychology*, **66**, 259–69.

Edwards, G. and Gross, M. M. (1976). Alcohol dependence: provisional description of a clinical syndrome. *British Medical Journal*, **1**, 1058–61.

Ellis, A., McInerney, J. F., DiGiuseppe, R., and Yeager, R. J. (1988). *Rational-emotive Therapy with Alcoholics and Substance Abusers*. New York: Pergamon Press.

Eysenck, H. J. (1959). Learning theory and behaviour therapy. *British Journal of Medical Science*, **105**, 61–75.

Finney, J. W. and Monahan, S. C. (1996). The cost-effectiveness of treatment for alcoholism: a second approximation. *Journal of Studies on Alcohol*, **57**, 229–43.

Finney, J. W., Noyes, C. A., Coutts, A. I., and Moos, R. (1998). Evaluating substance abuse treatment process models: I. Changes on proximal outcome variables during 12-step and cognitive-behavioral treatment. *Journal of Studies on Alcohol*, **59**, 371–80.

Fishman, D. B. (1999). *The Case for Pragmatic Psychology*. New York: New York University Press.

Follette, W. C., Nagle, A. E., and Callaghan, G. M. (1996). A radical behavioral understanding of the therapeutic relationship in effecting change. *Behavior Therapy*, **27**, 623–41.

Galanter, M. (1997). Network therapy. In *Substance Abuse: A Comprehensive Textbook*, 3rd edn, ed. J. H. Lowinson, P. Ruiz, R. B. Millman, and J. G. Langrod, pp. 478–84. Baltimore: Williams & Wilkins.

Grant, B. F. and Dawson, D. A. (1999). Alcohol and drug use, abuse, and dependence: classification, prevalence, and comorbidity. In *Addictions: A Comprehensive Guidebook*, ed. B. S. McCrady and E. E. Epstein, pp. 9–29. New York: Oxford University Press.

Grant, B. F., Harford, T. C., Dawson, D. A., et al. (1994). Prevalence of DSM-IV alcohol abuse and dependence: United States, 1992. *Alcohol, Health, and Research World*, **18**, 243–7.

Hall, S. M., Havassy, B. E., and Wasserman, D. A. (1990). Commitment to abstinence and acute stress in relapse to alcohol, opiates, and nicotine. *Journal of Consulting and Clinical Psychology*, **58**, 175–81.

Hesselbrock, M., Hesselbrock, V., Syzmanski, K., and Weidenman, M. (1988). Suicide attempts and alcoholism. *Journal of Studies on Alcohol*, **49**, 436–42.

Holder, H. D., Longabaugh, R., Miller, W. R., and Rubonis, A. V. (1991). The cost effectiveness of treatment for alcohol problems: a first approximation. *Journal of Studies on Alcohol*, **52**, 517–40.

Institute for Health Policy, Brandeis University. (1993). *Substance Abuse: The Nation's Number One Health Problem: Key Indicators for Policy*. Princeton, NJ: Robert Wood Johnson Foundation.

Irvin, J. E., Bowers, C. A., Dunn, M. E., and Wang, M. C. (1999). Efficacy of relapse prevention: a meta-analytic review. *Journal of Consulting and Clinical Psychology*, **67**, 563–70.

Jackson, P. and Oei, T. P. S. (1978). Social skills training and cognitive restructuring with alcoholics. *Drug and Alcohol Dependence*, **3**, 369–74.

Jellinek, E. M. (1960). *The Disease Concept of Alcoholism*. New Haven, CT: College and University Press.

Jones, B. T. and McMahon, J. (1994). Negative alcohol expectancy predicts post-treatment abstinence survivorship: the whether, when, and why of relapse to a first drink. *Addiction*, **89**, 1653–65.

Kadden, R. M., Cooney, N. L., Getter, H., and Litt, M. D. (1989). Matching alcoholics to coping skills or interact ional therapies: posttreatment results. *Journal of Consulting and Clinical Psychology*, **57**, 698–704.

Kraeplin, E. (1909-15). *Psychiatric ein Lehrbuch*, 8th edn, vols 1–4. Leipzig, Germany: J. A. Barth.

Larimer, M. E., Palmer, R. S., and Marlatt, G. A. (1999). Relapse prevention: an overview of Marlatt's cognitive-behavioral model. *Alcohol Research and Health*, **23**, 151–60.

Lazarus, A. A. (1994). Archives. *Behavior Therapist*, **17**, 16.

Litman, G. K., Eiser, J. R., Rawson, N., and Oppenheim, A. N. (1979). Differences in relapse precipitants and coping behavior between alcohol relapsers and survivors. *Behavior Research and Therapy*, **17**, 89–94.

Litman, G. K., Stapleton, J., Oppenheim, A. N., Pelig, M., and Jackson, P. (1983). Situations related to alcoholism relapse. *British Journal of Addiction*, **78**, 381–9.

Longabaugh, R. and Morgenstern, J. (1999). Cognitive-behavioral coping-skills therapy for alcohol dependence: current status and future directions. *Alcohol Research and Health*, **23**, 78–85.

Marlatt, G. A. and Gordon, J. R. (eds) (1985). *Relapse Prevention: Maintenance Strategies in the Treatment of Addictive Behaviors*. New York: Guilford Press.

Marlatt, G. A., Larimar, M. E., Baer, J. S., and Quigley, L. A. (1993). Harm reduction for alcohol problems: moving beyond the controlled drinking controversy. *Behavior Therapy*, **24**, 461–504.

Mattson, M. E. and Allen, J. P. (1991). Research on matching alcoholic patients to treatments: findings, issues, and implications. *Journal of Addictive Diseases*, **11**(2), 33–49.

McCrady, B. S. and Epstein, E. E. (1996). Theoretical bases of family approaches to substance abuse treatment. In *Treating Substance Abuse: Theory and Technique*, ed. F. Rotgers, D. S. Keller, and J. Morgenstern, pp. 117–42. New York: Guilford Press.

McKay, J. R., Maisto, S. A., and O'Farrell, T. J. (1993). End-of-treatment self-efficacy, aftercare, and drinking outcomes of alcoholic men. *Alcoholism: Clinical and Experimental Research*, **17**, 1078–83.

Miller, W. R. and Brown, J. M. (1991). Self-regulation as a conceptual basis for the prevention and treatment of addictive behaviours. In *Self-control and the Addictive Behaviours*, ed. N. Heather, W. R. Miller, and J. Greeley, pp. 3–79. Sydney, Australia: Maxwell Macmillan.

Miller, W. R. and Page, A. C. (1991). Warm turkey: other routes to abstinence. *Journal of Substance Abuse Treatment*, **8**, 227–32.

Miller, W. R. and Rollnick, S. (1991). *Motivational Interviewing: Preparing People to Change Addictive Behavior*. New York: Guilford Press.

Miller, W. R., Benefield, R. G., and Tonigan, J. S. (1993). Enhancing motivation for change in problem drinking: a controlled comparison of two therapist styles. *Journal of Consulting and Clinical Psychology*, **61**, 455–61.

Miller, W. R., Brown, J. M., Simpson, T. L., et al. (1995). What works? A methodological analysis of the alcohol treatment outcome literature. In *Handbook of Alcoholism Treatment Approaches: Effective Alternatives*, 2nd edn, ed. R. K. Hester and W. R. Miller, pp. 12–44. Boston: Allyn and Bacon.

Miller, W. R., Westerberg, V. S., Harris, R. J., and Tonigan, J. S. (1996). What predicts relapse? Prospective testing of antecedent models. *Addiction*, **91** (suppl.), 155–72.

Moak, D. H. and Anton, R. F. (1999). Alcohol. In *Addictions: A Comprehensive Guidebook*, ed. B. S. McCrady and E. E. Epstein, pp. 75–94. New York: Oxford University Press.

Monti, P. M., Abrams, D. B., Kadden, R. M., and Cooney, N. L. (1989). *Treating Alcohol Dependence: A Coping Skills Training Guide*. New York: Guilford Press.

Monti, P. M., Abrams, D. B., Binkoff, J. A., et al. (1990). Communications skills training with family and cognitive behavioral mood management training for alcoholics. *Journal of Studies on Alcohol*, **51**, 263–70.

Moos, R. H. (1993). Coping responses inventory professional manual. Odessa, Florida: Psychological Assessment Resources.

Moos, R. H., Finney, J. W., and Cronkite, R. C. (1990). *Alcoholism Treatment: Context, Process, and Outcome*. New York: Oxford University Press.

Morgenstern, J., Frey, R. M., McCrady, B. S., Labouvie, E., and Neighbors, C. J. (1996). Examining mediators of change in traditional chemical dependency treatment. *Journal of Studies on Alcohol*, **57**, 53–64.

Moser, A. E. and Annis, H. M. (1996). The role of coping in relapse crisis outcome: a prospective study of treated alcoholics. *Addiction*, **91**, 1101–13.

Oei, T. P. S. and Jackson, P. R. (1980). Long-term effects of group and individual social skills training with alcoholics. *Addictive Behaviors*, **5**, 129–36.

Oei, T. P. S. and Jackson, P. R. (1982). Social skills and cognitive behavioral approaches to the treatment of problem drinking. *Journal of Studies on Alcohol*, **43**, 532–47.

O'Malley, S. S., Jaffe, A. J., Chang, G., et al. (1992). Naltrexone and coping skills therapy for alcohol dependence: a controlled study. *Archives of General Psychiatry*, **49**, 881–7.

Pavlov, I. P. (1927). *Lectures on Conditioned Reflexes*. New York: International Publishers.

Prochaska, J. O., DiClemente, C. C., and Norcross, J. C. (1992). In search of how people change: applications to addictive behaviors. *American Psychologist*, **47**, 1102–14.

Project MATCH Research Group. (1997). Matching alcoholism treatment to client heterogeneity: project MATCH posttreatment drinking outcomes. *Journal of Studies on Alcohol*, **58**, 7–29.

Rimmele, C. T., Miller, W. R., and Dougher, M. G. (1989). Aversion therapies. In *Handbook of Alcoholism Treatment Approaches: Effective Alternatives*, ed. R. K. Hester and W. R. Miller, pp. 128–40. New York: Pergamon Press.

Rosenberg, H. and Brian, T. (1986). Cognitive-behavioral group therapy for multiple-DUI offenders. *Alcoholism Treatment Quarterly*, **3**, 47–65.

Rotgers, F. (1996). Behavioral theory of substance abuse treatment: bringing science to bear on practice. In *Treating Substance Abuse: Theory and Technique*, ed. F. Rotgers, D. S. Keller, and J. Morgenstern, pp. 174–201. New York: Guilford Press.

Rua, J. (1990). *Treatment Works: The Tragic Cost of Undervaluing Treatment in the "Drug War."* Washington, DC: National Association of State Alcohol and Drug Abuse Directors.

Schuckit, M. A. and Monteiro, M. G. (1988). Alcoholism, anxiety and depression. *British Journal of Addictions*, **83**, 1373–80.

Skinner, B. F. (1953). *Science and Human Behavior*. New York: Macmillan.

Soloman, K. E. and Annis, H. M. (1990). Outcome and efficacy expectancy in the prediction of post-treatment drinking behaviour. *British Journal of Addiction*, **85**, 659–65.

Watson, J. B. (1919). *Psychology from the Standpoint of a Behaviorist*. Philadelphia: Lippincott.

15

Cognitive approaches to understanding, preventing, and treating child and adolescent depression

Susan H. Spence[1] and Mark A. Reinecke[2]

[1] University of Queensland, Brisbane, Australia
[2] Northwestern University Medical School, Chicago, IL, USA

Depression is a significant problem among children and adolescents, with 2–5% of the population meeting diagnostic criteria for this disorder at any point in time (Fleming and Offord, 1990; Lewinsohn et al., 1993; Boyd et al., 2000). The percentage of young people affected by disorders of mood is even higher if one includes dysthymia and bipolar spectrum disorder or if we consider those who report symptoms of dysphoria but who do not meet criteria for the full clinical syndrome. The prevalence of clinical depression increases with age, being less common in preschool and primary (elementary) schoolchildren, and increasing in midadolescence. Community prevalence rates for affective disorders among schoolchildren are relatively low, ranging from 0.4% to 2.5% (Anderson et al., 1897; Kashani and Ray, 1983; Costello et al., 1988; Kashani et al., 1989). Depression is more common, however, among adolescents, with community prevalence rates ranging from 2.9% to 8% (Kashani et al., 1987; Lewinsohn et al., 1993). By the age of 18 years approximately 20% of young people will have experienced at least one episode of a depressive disorder. Moreover, 1–6% of adolescents manifest a depressive disorder at any given time (Fleming and Offord, 1990; McCracken, 1992).

In addition to the relatively high prevalence of clinical depression in young people, there are several reasons we need to take this problem seriously. First, there are a range of short-term negative consequences associated with depression, including disruption to personal relationships and school performance (Kellam et al., 1991; Petersen et al., 1993). There are also long-term negative outcomes, such as increased risk of substance abuse and impaired functioning in work, social, and family life (Harrington et al., 1990; Poznanski and Mokros, 1994; Weissman et al., 1999; Geller et al., 2001). Second, depression in young people is not a transient problem that will remit if left untreated. Studies suggest that clinical levels of child and adolescent depression frequently persist if left untreated and many cases of adult depression have their onset during adolescence (Kovacs and Gatsonis, 1989). The experience of depression during childhood and adolescence is associated with increased risk of developing depression in the future (Kovacs et al., 1984; Harrington et al., 1990; Holson et al., 2000; Kessler et al., 2001). Third, there is a strong link between depression and suicidal behavior in adolescents (Reynolds and Mazza, 1994). In 1998, the last year for which comprehensive government data are available, suicide was the third most common cause of death for youth in the USA, with a rate of 13.7 per 100 000. More adolescents committed suicide than died from the next seven causes of death combined. Adolescent depression, in short, is a problem to be taken seriously. Given that major depression is predicted to produce one of the greatest levels of global burden of disease within the next 30 years (Murray and Lopez, 1996) there is a strong case for early intervention and prevention of depression in young people.

Etiology of child and adolescent depression

It has been recognized for some time that depression is a complex disorder that is influenced by a range of biological, psychological, social, and environmental factors (Rehm and Sharp, 1996; Asarnow et al., 2001). No one variable can account for all cases of depression. Rather, it appears that a complex interplay exists between causal factors. Although much of the data is correlational, several variables have been identified as being associated with depression among youth. To date, it is not clear whether these variables are risk, vulnerability or protective factors, causes or consequences, concurrent reflections of common causal variables, or form part of the depressive syndrome. Risk factors refer to those variables that, when present, increase the probability that a problem will develop. These may include biological, environmental, or developmental factors associated with an increased likelihood of an individual becoming depressed, but are neither necessary nor sufficient for this to occur. Vulnerability factors, in contrast, represent stable or enduring factors or characteristics of individuals that predispose them to develop a specific disorder. Vulnerability factors, as such, are typically viewed as playing a causal role in the emergence of the disorder. They are mechanisms or mediating variables in the development of a clinical condition. In contrast, protective factors are variables that, when present, reduce the probability that the problem will develop. They are moderator variables that reduce the influence of risk or vulnerability factors.

It appears that some risk and vulnerability factors may be both causes and consequences of depression, having a reciprocal relationship in exacerbating and maintaining the depressive episode. These considerations are important for at least two reasons. First, it is important for scholars, in developing models of depression, to articulate clearly causal relationships between variables being examined and to note whether these variables are associated with the onset of the depressive episode, symptom severity, maintenance of the episode, treatment response, or risk of relapse and recurrence. Second, it is important to place these variables within a developmental context. Maladaptive schema or tacit beliefs, for example, are often viewed in cognitive diathesis-stress models as serving as a distal vulnerability factor for the development of clinical depression. Proximal risk factors would include maladaptive thoughts and biases in information processing that are byproducts of activated schema. The question arises, however, can schema be viewed as "stable and enduring factors" during childhood? Might they be better conceptualized as reflecting transient phenomena during a period of cognitive and emotional development? Similar considerations apply with regard to our understanding of social and biological markers of risk for depression. In as much as psychopathology during childhood may be viewed as reflecting a failure to negotiate developmental issues or tasks, or to acquire specific adaptive skills (Cicchetti and Cohen, 1995; Brooks-Gunn and Attie, 1996; Sroufe, 1997; Garber and Flynn, 2001), it becomes important to attend to the tasks of each stage of development, as well as internal and external risks and resources as they influence the child's development and adaptation. Simple, linear models for understanding mood and adaptation during childhood will likely prove inadequate. Longitudinal research with both clinical populations and at-risk, asymptomatic samples is needed to clarify the relationship between depression and indicators of vulnerability, risk, and resilience. To date, the major correlates that have been identified for child and adolescent depression include:

- family history of affective disorder;
- genetic/heritability factors;
- growth hormone and hypothalamic–pituitary axis dysregulation;
- exposure to negative life events and daily hassles;
- parental discord and family conflict;
- high levels of expressed emotion and criticism at home;
- relationship difficulties with peers, parents, and family members;
- social skills deficits;
- lack of family, peer, and social support;
- insecure attachment;
- loss of response-contingent reinforcement;
- cognitive distortions;
- pessimistic attributional style;
  - negative interpretation and expectations of events relating to the self, the world, and the future;
  - hopelessness; and helplessness;

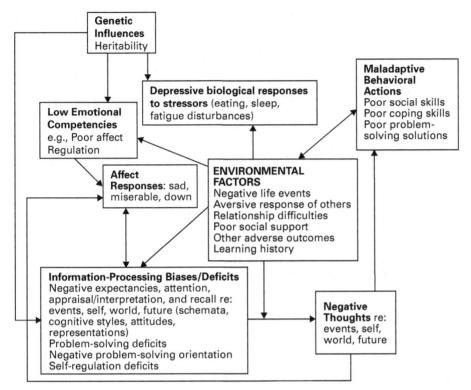

Figure 15.1   Cognitive factors within a biopsychosocial model of depression in children and adolescents.

- ruminative style;
- self-focused attention;
- self-control skills deficits; poor affect regulation;
- deficits in interpersonal and life problem-solving skills;
- negative problem-solving orientation/motivation;
- low self-esteem and low self-efficacy;
- poor coping skills;
- conduct disorder problems; substance abuse and other internalizing difficulties.

One of the challenges for researchers is to work out the ways in which risk, vulnerability, and protective factors interact to influence the likelihood that a person will experience depression. Several authors have proposed integrative cognitive models to explain the development of depression (Gotlib and Hammen, 1992; Harrington et al., 1998a). The present chapter will emphasize the role of cognitive factors in the onset and maintenance of depression in young people, within a biopsychosocial model, as outlined in Figure 15.1. This model draws on the research and theoretical contributions of many authors in the area of depression, as described below.

Before we examine the various cognitive models of the etiology of depression, it is helpful to have a framework regarding the terminology to be used. It is important to distinguish between cognitive operations, products, and schemata. *Cognitive operations* may be defined as the processes involved in the transformation of information into cognitive products, and include attention, reception, perception, encoding, storage and retrieval of memories, decision-making, and problem solving. *Cognitive products* are the thoughts, images, words, and concepts that occur within the individual's stream of consciousness. These events are the products of the interaction of environmental information, cognitive operations, and schemata. *Schemata* are tacit, higher-order cognitive constructs that account for the consistency in each person's thoughts, behavior, and emotions. They influence the way in which information is stored, organized, and linked. Schemata are proposed to influence what the individual attends to, perceives, stores into memory, recalls, and views as important (Ingram and Kendall, 1986) and are reflected in attitudes and belief systems. Cognitive schemata are seen as influencing the ways in which cognitive operations process information and thereby the cognitive products that they generate. Inaccurate, distorted, or maladaptive cognitive schemata can therefore have a marked impact upon how information is processed and, in turn, upon how the individual thinks, feels, and behaves. Most contemporary cognitive models of depression stress the interaction between cognitive operations, products, and schemata.

The evolution of cognitive models of childhood depression

As we shall see, there is not one cognitive therapy of depression, but many. Several cognitive models of depression have been proposed, each emphasizing a different cognitive component of the disorder. They share a number of philosophical assumptions and, in practice, share a number of technical similarities (Freeman and Reinecke, 1995; Dobson and Dozois, 2001).

Cognitive distortion models

Work by Aaron Beck (1967) and Albert Ellis (1958) has profoundly influenced contemporary models of adult depression. These models are founded upon the assumption that our emotions and behaviors are determined not so much by events per se, but by our interpretations, thoughts, expectancies, and beliefs about the events. They are moderation models (Clark and Beck, 1999) and typically take the form of diathesis-stress formulations, proposing that certain styles of thinking and information processing represent a diathesis which, in the presence of negative life stress, increases vulnerability to the development of depression (Abramson et al., 1999). Beck's early work (1963, 1964, 1967) focused on the role of maladaptive thoughts relating to the "cognitive triad" – negative views of the self, the world, and the future – in the maintenance of depression. He observed that the thoughts of depressed individuals were characterized by a variety of systematic distortions and proposed that these processes served to generate negative affect. These distortions or biases included catastrophizing, overgeneralization, magnification, and selective abstraction, to mention just a few. Depressed persons tend, for example, to manifest negative expectancies about their futures and about their ability to achieve desired outcomes. They manifest reduced perceptions of personal efficacy and hold excessively pessimistic expectancies about life outcomes. Beck (1983) subsequently proposed that individuals are particularly likely to experience depression if there is a congruence or match between the type of negative life events and that person's depressogenic schemata. Schemata relating to the constructs of sociotropy (placing excessive value on personal relationships) and autonomy (excessive investment in preserving independence and freedom of choice) were considered to be distal contributors to the development of depression. Individuals who adhere strongly to sociotropic values are more likely to develop depression in response to life events that threaten social relationships. In contrast, highly autonomous individuals are more susceptible to depression in situations that involve a threat to independence and freedom of choice.

Depressed children and adolescents have been observed to show a similar pattern of cognitive errors to depressed adults, including high levels of catastrophizing, overgeneralizing, personalizing, and selective abstraction (Haley et al., 1985; Leitenberg et al., 1986; McGee et al., 1986; Asarnow and Bates, 1988; Robins and Hinckley, 1989; Kazdin, 1990; Kendall et al., 1990). For example, Leitenberg et al. (1986) found that depressed children tended to endorse four types of cognitive error more often than their nondepressed peers. These errors included: (1) overgeneralized predictions of negative outcomes; (2) catastrophizing the consequences of negative events; (3) incorrectly taking personal responsibility for negative outcomes; and (4) selectively attending to negative features of an event. Interestingly, youngsters with high evaluation anxiety also endorsed a high level of all four cognitive errors. It does not appear that cognitive distortions, such as these, are specific to clinical depression. Rather, cognitive distortions appear to be associated with several forms of psychopathology during childhood (Kendall and MacDonald, 1993). There is, however, some evidence to suggest that a tendency towards cognitive distortion represents a cognitive diathesis that increases the likelihood of future development of depressive symptoms in adolescents who experience adverse life events (Lewinsohn et al., 2001), indicating a causal role in the development of depression. Interestingly, Lewinsohn et al. found that depressive outcomes were related to cognitive vulnerability only when dysfunctional attitudes exceeded a certain level, suggesting a threshold view of vulnerability.

Based on the cognitive models of Beck and Ellis, cognitive restructuring approaches were developed as a means of teaching people to identify and change their maladaptive thoughts and to reduce cognitive distortions. Such interventions have been found to be relatively effective in the treatment of adult depression (Dobson, 1989; Lambert and Davis, 2002; see Chapter 2). As a result, attempts have been made to develop similar treatments for children (Emery et al., 1983; Reinecke, 1992; Carey, 1993; Vostanis and Harrington, 1994; Rehm and Sharp, 1996; Stark et al., 2000) and adolescents (Rotheram-Borus et al., 1994; Wilkes et al., 1994; Wood et al., 1996). The effectiveness and efficacy of such approaches are discussed later in this chapter.

Self-regulation deficits

Work completed during the early 1970s suggested that deficits in the ability to regulate one's own behavior in order to attain adaptive goals may play a role in the development of depression (Rehm, 1977). Rehm, drawing upon the self-regulation theory of Kanfer (Kanfer and Phillips, 1970; Kanfer, 1975), proposed that the behavior of depressed individuals emerges as the result of deficits in self-monitoring, self-evaluation, and self-reinforcement. Depressed persons, or persons predisposed to develop depression, tend to: (1) attend selectively to negative events to the exclusion of positive events; (2) attend selectively to the immediate, as opposed to the delayed, consequences of behavior; (3) set excessively high self-evaluation standards for their behavior; (4) make negative attributions for the causes of events; (5) provide themselves with insufficient reinforcement to motivate effective behavior; and (6) administer excessive punishment to themselves, thus further decreasing effective behavior. It is interesting to note the similarity in constructs in self-control theory and attributional-style models (below) of depression, despite their emergence from very different literatures.

In keeping with the adult literature, there is also some evidence to support the role of self-control deficits in childhood depression. Depressed youngsters tend to show deficits in self-control strategies compared to nondepressed children, and set higher standards for themselves, evaluate themselves more negatively, and punish themselves more (Kaslow et al., 1984).

Self-control therapy was developed in an attempt to rectify observed self-control deficits (Rehm, 1981). This program teaches individuals to: (1) self-monitor their moods, thoughts, and activities; (2) recognize immediate versus delayed consequences of their behavior; (3) make appropriate attributions for success and failure; (4) set realistic goals, with appropriate self-evaluation and activity scheduling; and (5) increase the use of overt and covert self-reinforcement. Following positive results in the treatment of depressed adults, self-control training has been adapted for use with children (Stark et al., 1987; Stark, 1990) and adolescents (Reynolds and Coats, 1986).

Although training in self-monitoring and self-reinforcement plays a central role in self-control treatment programs, they are also regularly incorporated into other cognitive-behavioral programs. Many cognitive-behavioral treatment protocols begin by training children to monitor their thoughts, emotions, and behaviors, encouraging them to engage in more adaptive actions (such as enjoyable, social, and mastery activities), and teaching them to acknowledge their success and to reward themselves for their gains.

Helplessness, hopelessness, and attributional style

The learned helplessness theory of depression was based on observations made during animal learning experiments that dogs exposed to repeated, uncontrollable aversive events demonstrated motivational, learning, and emotional deficits. As these symptoms paralleled those observed among depressed adults, Seligman (1975) proposed that depression may stem from a perceived lack of contingency between adverse life events and an individual's actions. That is to say, persons who believe that they are helpless to control important negative outcomes subsequently become depressed.

Although this model received some empirical support, it was soon criticized as conceptually incomplete. With this in mind, Abramson et al. (1978) reformulated the model. The reformulation incorporated the concept of attribution of responsibility. They proposed that when individuals are faced with an uncontrollable event, they make attributions about its cause along three explanatory dimensions: internal or external (i.e., causes within the person versus outside the person), stable or unstable (i.e., causes that persist versus transient ones), and global or specific (i.e., causes that affect many domains versus those that are more limited). Individuals who become depressed are viewed as having tendencies to attribute negative, uncontrollable outcomes to internal, stable, and global causes. The reformulated model generated a considerable amount of research, with results generally suggesting that internal, stable, and global attributions for negative events are associated with feelings of depression (Brewin, 1985; Sweeney et al., 1986).

Subsequently, Abramson et al. (1988a, 1988b, 1989) revised the reformulated helplessness model of depression into the "hopelessness theory" of depression. They proposed the existence of a subtype of depression, "hopelessness depression," and suggested that hopelessness may serve as a proximal and sufficient (though not a necessary) cause of clinical depression. They defined hopelessness as the expectation that desired outcomes will not occur or that aversive outcomes will occur but that one cannot control them. Hopelessness is seen as stemming from tendencies to make stable, global causal attributions about negative events, infer that negative life events will have negative consequences, and draw negative inferences about the self. A depressogenic attributional style is regarded as a cognitive diathesis that in the presence but not absence of negative life events will increase the risk of hopelessness depression. Furthermore, the theory suggests that a depressogenic attributional style related to a particular content domain (e.g., for personal events) provides a specific vulnerability (in keeping with Beck, 1963, 1967) to hopelessness depression when an individual is confronted with negative life events in that same content domain (e.g. loss of a relationship). This specific vulnerability theory predicts that the cognitive diathesis only comes into operation when there is a match between content areas of the negative life event and the individual's depressogenic attributional style. It is worth noting that negativistic attributional style may be viewed as representing either a form of cognitive distortion or bias that accompanies depressed mood, or as a stable, enduring trait that serves as a vulnerability factor for depression. This model for understanding depression has recently been studied among adolescents (Hankin et al., 2001). We should also consider the possibility that it is not the presence of a negative attributional style per se that places individuals at risk for depression so much as the absence of a positive attributional style. Positive events, in this circumstance, are not attributed to oneself, but to chance or other explanations, and are expected to be one-off occurrences.

Research has provided some support for the role of hopelessness depression and attributional style in the development of depression in young people. Children who report high levels of depressive symptomatology are more likely to attribute negative events to internal, global, and stable causes, and positive events to external, unstable, and specific factors (Kaslow et al., 1984; Seligman et al., 1984; Asarnow and Bates, 1988; Bodiford et al., 1988; Curry and Craighead, 1990; Hops et al., 1990; Nolen-Hoeksema and Girgus, 1995; Gladstone et al., 1997) in comparison to nondepressed peers. Furthermore, there is some evidence to suggest that a tendency towards pessimistic thinking styles and cognitive distortion increases the likelihood of future development of depressive symptoms in adolescents (Nolen-Hoeksema et al., 1992; Garber et al., 1993), providing support for a causal role of attributional style in the development of depression. Joiner (2000) found support for the hopelessness theory in the development of depression among young psychiatric inpatients. Pessimistic attributional style in the presence but not absence of negative life events predicted future increases in depression. This relationship was mediated by changes in hopelessness. In contrast, a recent study by Spence et al. (2002) found that, although pessimistic attributional style predicted future increases in depressive symptoms among adolescents, this effect was evident irrespective of the occurrence of negative life events. These findings suggest a direct effect for attributional style rather than a cognitive-diathesis. In a further twist, Lewinsohn et al. (2001) failed to find a direct effect for attributional style in the development of adolescent depression and, in opposition to the cognitive diathesis model, found that attributional style had little effect on depression onset at high levels of stress whereas at low levels of negative life events the probability of future depression increased as a function of increasingly negative attributional style. Clearly the role of attributional style in the development of depression is complex and is not yet fully understood.

Problem-solving deficits

Several theorists have proposed that deficits in the development and use of rational problem-solving skills predispose individuals to become depressed (Marx et al., 1992; Haaga et al., 1993). D'Zurilla and Goldfried (1971) defined problem solving as a process by which an individual identifies a variety of potentially effective response alternatives for dealing with the problematic situation and increases the probability of selecting the most effective response from among these various alternatives (1971, p. 108). D'Zurilla (1986) proposed that social problem solving can be viewed as comprised of two processes, namely problem orientation and rational problem-solving skills. Problem orientation is a motivational construct incorporating an individual's awareness of problems, an assessment of his or her ability to manage these problems, and expectations about the effectiveness of problem-solving attempts. Rational problem-solving skills, in contrast, refer to the individual's ability rationally to identify and define problems, generate solutions, evaluate and select the most reasonable alternative, implement this solution, and monitor his or her effectiveness.

Research suggests that both of these aspects of problem solving – motivation and rational problem solving – may be relevant for understanding risk for depression and suicidality among adolescents (Asarnow et al., 1987; Spirito et al., 1989; Rotheram-Borus et al., 1990; Fremouw et al., 1993; Sadowski and Kelley, 1993; Reinecke et al., 2001; Spence et al., 2002). Rotheram-Borus et al. (1990), for example, observed that suicidal female adolescents developed fewer alternative solutions for problems and were more focused upon problems than were their nondistressed peers. They appear to demonstrate deficits in the use of rational problem-solving skills. A problem-solving style that results in attempts to use self-destructive or passive/avoidant solutions to life problems is also found to predict future depression in response to negative life events among adolescents (Adams and Adams, 1991). The relationship between depression and interpersonal problem solving has been found to hold even when level intellectual functioning is controlled (Sacco and Graves, 1984).

The motivational aspect of problem solving (negative problem orientation), as well as avoidant and impulsive problem-solving style, has also been shown to be associated with increased levels of depression and suicidality among clinically referred adolescents (Reinecke et al., 2001). There is also some suggestion that negative problem orientation represents a cognitive diathesis for the development of depression. Spence et al. (2002) reported that negative problem orientation in the presence but not absence of high negative life events predicted future increases in depressive symptoms among adolescents. A negative problem orientation is proposed to increase the likelihood that the young person will attempt to handle difficult life situations in an ineffective or self-destructive manner. The concept of negative problem-solving orientation, as such, is similar in many ways to the concepts of negativistic attributional style, hopelessness, and decreased self-efficacy, as outlined above.

How might problem-solving deficits contribute to an increased risk of depression among youth? One possibility is that difficulties managing interpersonal and life problems increase the chance of negative outcomes and reduce the probability of positively reinforcing experiences. It is possible, as such, that problem-solving deficits on their own do not account for the development of depression. Rather, their impact may be mediated by increased negative life events and low levels of reinforcement, two factors that have been found to be associated with an increased risk of depression (Nezu, 1986; Adams and Adams, 1991; Goodman et al., 1995).

Problem-solving training has been widely used in treating depressed adults (Nezu and Perri, 1989; D'Zurilla and Nezu, 1999). Recently, a problem-solving intervention has been developed for use with children and adolescents (Spence et al., in press). Problem-solving approaches have also been incorporated into several multi-component interventions for child and adolescent depression (Wilkes et al., 1994; Lewinsohn and Clarke, 1999). The problem-solving steps outlined by D'Zurilla and Goldfried (1971) continue to form the basis of problem-solving therapy approaches. Therapy involves teaching the child to identify and define problems, generate a range of alternative solutions (brainstorming), evaluate these alternatives with regard to their short-and long-term consequences, select the optimal solution, implement it, and assess its impact on the problem. Recent developments in problem-solving training include an increased emphasis on problem-solving motivation and on teaching an adaptive orientation towards problems and problem solving (Spence et al., in press). This phase of problem-solving training makes use of techniques based on cognitive restructuring and positive attribution training.

Schema-based models

The concept of schema – organized, tacit representations of features of stimuli and events which serve to guide the selection, encoding, retrieval, and processing of information – plays a central role in both experimental cognitive psychology and cognitive therapy. The concept of schema has been incorporated into the practice of cognitive therapy during recent years, and received its fullest elaboration in schema-focused psychotherapy (Young, 1994) and in cognitive-constructivist formulations (Guidano, 1995). These models explicitly attempt to alleviate depression by modifying tacit beliefs and expectations. Although cognitive therapists have become attentive to the role of early experiences and current social interactions in the development and maintenance of schema, relatively little work has been done in applying these models with children and adolescents.

As noted, schemata contain representations of the self and others that are abstracted from one's experiences. They stand as "general rules" for understanding oneself, the future, and one's world. Schemata can be viewed as having a number of characteristics. They vary, for example, with regard to their availability or accessibility (i.e., the ease with which they may be activated by events in the person's life) and complexity (i.e., the degree to which cognitive elements of the schema are related to other memories and beliefs). Broad schemata, such as an individual's self-concept, incorporate a relatively large number of elements (e.g., appearance, likeability, intelligence, athletic ability) and are, as a consequence, more easily activated by a range of events in a person's life. They are also, as a result, more likely to influence a person's mood. Schema may vary, as well, with regard to their flexibility, permeability, and level of abstraction. These considerations are important in our understanding of depression among youth in that their views of themselves tend to be more malleable and are tied to their performance in specific settings. Children's cognitive representations of themselves are narrower, more flexible, and more responsive to new information, and are less abstract than are those of adolescents and adults. Children's ability to reflect on their own motivations, and to identify abstract characteristics of themselves and others, develops with age. The structure and functioning of schema may change as children move from preoperational to concrete operational to formal operational thought. Developmental variations, such as these, affect both how we think about vulnerability for depression and the course of cognitive therapy. The ability to reflect on one's thoughts, to engage in hypotheticodeductive reasoning, and to form higher-order abstract views of the self develop over the course of childhood and adolescence. In as much as these are requisite skills for benefiting from standard forms of cognitive therapy, we will need to modify both our models and techniques to meet the needs of depressed youth. Cognitive therapy should not, in short, be applied in an unmodified form with children.

Integrative models

Recognizing the limitations of standard cognitive models of depression, researchers have, during recent years, attempted to integrate cognitive, social, and developmental models of depression. Attachment theory, parenting style, and research on the development of affect regulation skills during childhood have emerged as central components of these models (Baldwin, 1992; Gotlib and Hammen, 1992; Stark et al., 1996, 2000; Rudolph et al., 1997; Harrington et al., 1998a). These models provide a framework for understanding the development of depressogenic beliefs, attitudes, schema, and attributional styles, and the ways in which interpersonal and cognitive vulnerability factors interact in placing individuals at risk for depression. The University of Manchester Depression Treatment Programme (DTP), for example, explicitly acknowledges the interacting effects of genetic factors, early experience, cognitive style, social competence, life events, and mood in contributing to the development of a depressive syndrome (Harrington et al., 1998a). Recent studies with adults are consistent with these models. It has been observed, for example, that dysfunctional attitudes or schema may mediate the relationships observed between attachment style and severity of depression (Roberts et al., 1996; Reinecke and Rogers, 2001).

Unresolved conceptual issues

Studies completed to date, for the most part, support cognitive models of depression. What, then, are the difficulties with this literature? First, although research with children and adolescents is consistent with the descriptive aspects of cognitive-behavioral models of depression, it is not clear that these factors stand as vulnerability factors for depression. The possibility exists that they may be concomitants of depressed mood rather than risk or vulnerability factors. Measures of depressive thinking often normalize after the conclusion of the depressive episode. It is also possible that maladaptive schemata, problem-solving deficits, and cognitive distortions are *both* causes and consequences of the depressive episode. We cannot conclude, at this point, that these factors represent a cognitive vulnerability for depression. The possibility exists, as well, that there may be age-related differences in relationships between cognitive markers of risk or vulnerability and mood. In early childhood, for example, depression may be more closely related to the occurrence of negative life events (such as losses and separations) than to maladaptive attitudes and beliefs. During later childhood and adolescence, however, attributional style and life events may come to make independent contributions to negative mood (Peterson and Seligman, 1984). After a depressive episode has occurred, children tend to demonstrate a more negativistic attributional style, suggesting that the experience of depression may alter their cognitive style, placing them at risk for further depressive episodes.

As the thoughtful reader may have noted, many of the central constructs in the alternative cognitive models we have reviewed are, at least at first glance, conceptually similar to one another. There appear, for example, to be essential similarities between the concepts of negative problem orientation and hopelessness, helplessness and self-efficacy, and self-concept and self-schema. Research will be needed to determine the relationships between these markers of risk and vulnerability and to evaluate the discriminant validity of measures for assessing them. It also is not clear which of these cognitive concomitants of depression are core features of the disorder, and how their relationships with one another change over the course of development.

As noted, it does not appear that measures of cognitive risk and vulnerability are specific to depression. Rather, they appear to be associated with various forms of psychopathology. Although cognitive specificity – the hypothesis that specific cognitive markers of risk will be associated with specific forms of psychopathology – has not been demonstrated with depressed youth, this may stem from methodological limitations of research to date. These methodological issues include high levels of comorbidity of depression with other disorders in this age group (Kashani et al., 1987) and the fact that few studies have used appropriate mood induction or priming techniques to test cognitive diathesis-stress models.

As we have noted, research is yet to demonstrate conclusively that cognitive variables associated with adolescent depression are causally related to the emergence of clinical depression. Furthermore, it is necessary, in developing our models, to state explicitly how these variables are related to the onset, severity, and maintenance of the disorder (Reinecke and DuBois, 2001). We must clarify whether they are proximal or distal causes, whether moderator variables affect their relationship to mood, and whether we view them as necessary and/or sufficient causes of the disorder.

The cognitive models we have discussed attend to different cognitive operations, products, and schemata as if they are independent constructs. More recently, several cognitive theorists have attempted to develop integrated models capable of addressing the observed interrelationships between different aspects of cognition (Gotlib and Hammen, 1992; Harrington et al., 1998a; Stark et al., 2000). We also need to explore how individuals acquire particular cognitive styles and how these interact with other psychosocial factors that influence the development and maintenance of depression in youth. A proposed sociocognitive model for the development of depression during childhood is presented in Figure 15.1.

Clinical applications

Assessment

As we have seen, research suggests that cognitive deficits, distortions, and schema may play a role in the development and maintenance of depression. It may, as such, be important to assess these factors objectively in order to design effective and efficient interventions. Over the past decade, there has been an increasing emphasis on the use of prescriptive, manualized treatment approaches that are applied to different disorders based upon diagnosis. Although this approach has facilitated the development of empirically supported treatments for depression, it has proven to be quite controversial. Persons (1989) emphasized the importance of functional assessment as a foundation for formulation-based cognitive therapy, and Lewinsohn et al. (1994) noted the importance of functional assessment in treating depression among young people given the heterogeneous symptom presentation. We would concur. A range of cognitive and social factors appears to play a role in the presentation of depression for young people. The specific type of cognitive and social deficits, however, can vary between individuals. A detailed assessment of cognitive strengths and weaknesses, therefore, is important if we are fully to understand factors contributing to an individual's feelings of depression. Given the significant contribution of biological, environmental, and behavioral factors in the development and maintenance of depression, the assessment of the full range of cognitive factors will form an important aspect of the assessment process. We are, in short, advocating the use of formulation-based, multicomponent cognitive-behavioral therapy (CBT) approaches. Information about thoughts, attitudes, and cognitive skills needs to be integrated with data relating to affect, behavior, family situation, relationships, parenting practices, and environmental stressors in order to develop a parsimonious understanding of factors influencing the child's psychosocial functioning, as outlined in Figure 15.1.

Although it makes intuitive sense to propose that effective treatment requires an individual clinical formulation, it is important to acknowledge that we do not yet have evidence supporting the efficacy of individually tailored, formulation-driven cognitive therapy for depression. The practical implications of the model outlined in Figure 15.1 are that practitioners need to assess and intervene with children at various levels. We will want to assess objectively and address: (1) cognitive biases; (2) maladaptive beliefs and schema; (3) social skills and problem-solving deficits; (4) stressful life events; and (5) social supports. Evaluation needs to examine the content of thoughts, images, and other cognitive products. Our goal is to identify systematic distortions or errors in cognitive processing that may be modified during intervention. Recurrent patterns of cognitive distortion may be indicative of maladaptive schemata, assumptions, attitudes, and beliefs. In addition, assessment needs to investigate deficits in cognitive operations, such as problem solving, interpersonal perception, or self-control skills. These cognitive skill deficits may then be targeted for training. This is augmented by an assessment of stressful life events and social supports available to the child.

Assessment of cognitive products (thoughts and images)

There are a variety of ways to assess the content of children's thoughts and images. Hughes (1988) suggested that an interview with the child can yield useful information about the youngster's automatic thoughts about him- or herself, the world and their future. With very young children, concrete props, such as toys and puppets, may be used in conjunction with simple, nonthreatening, and specific questions to elicit thoughts about events. Self-monitoring, questionnaires, diaries, thought listing and videotape-cued recall can be used to obtain cognitive information from children, as can projective techniques such as drawings, mutual story telling, and sentence completion tasks (Reinecke, 1992). Stark (1990) described the use of cartoon sequences to teach children the basic principles of thought monitoring.

A variety of questionnaires have been developed to assess children's thoughts. Leitenberg et al. (1986), for example, developed the Children's Cognitive Error Questionnaire to assess cognitive distortions among youth. Thought listing is another method that can be used to identify cognitive events in children. The procedure involves exposing the child to some relevant event and then asking him or her to state exactly what he or she was thinking immediately before, during, or after the event. These responses are then recorded verbatim and later categorized according to set criteria, such as positive and negative expectation or coping style. This approach has been used in the assessment of anxiety in children during exposure to feared events (Prins, 1986; Kendall and Chansky, 1991). Videotaped cued recall is another method that can be used to identify specific thoughts that occur during a particular task or event. Although this method has primarily been used with anxious children, it offers promise as an assessment tool in depression. Initially children are videotaped while they take part in a relevant task or situation. They are then asked to watch a replay of their videotaped performance and to describe, at set intervals, the thoughts that they were experiencing during the actual task (Spence et al., 1999).

In summary, there are various methods that can be used to assess cognitive products with children. With careful consideration of developmental issues, reliable and valid information can be obtained.

Assessment of schema (attitudes, assumptions, attributions, and beliefs)

Assessing maladaptive assumptions, attributions, and tacit beliefs can be helpful in developing an individualized treatment plan. Various methods have been developed to assess attributional style in children. N. J. Kaslow et al. (unpublished data), for example, developed the Children's Attributional Style Questionnaire (CASQ) and a shorter revision (CASQ-R; N. J. Kaslow and S. Nolen-Hoeksema, unpublished data). This questionnaire assesses internal/external, specific/global, and stable/unstable attributions for positive and negative events. The psychometric properties are barely acceptable, however, particularly for the shorter version. Fielstein et al. (1985) also developed an Attributional Style Questionnaire consisting of 12 vignettes, each describing a social, athletic, or academic event and an outcome of that event (success or failure). Children rate the degree to which they attribute the outcome to skill/lack of skill; effort/lack of effort; good luck/bad luck; and task ease/difficulty. This measure is reported to have good psychometric properties and discriminates between children with high and low self-esteem.

The Hopelessness Scale for Children (Kazdin et al., 1986) is a widely used measure of pessimism among depressed youth. This scale includes 17 items relating to beliefs about the likelihood of future events (e. g., "All I can see ahead of me are bad things, not good things" or "I don't think I will have any real fun when I grow up"). As might be expected, scores on this scale correlate significantly with severity of depression. This scale may therefore be helpful in the assessment of depressive thinking styles related to negative expectations about the future.

Assessment of cognitive operations

Cognitive operations, such as attention, reception, perception, encoding, storage, retrieval, decision-making, planning, and self-regulation of behavior, should also be considered as possible contributors to the development and maintenance of depression. Measures of interpersonal problem-solving ability may be useful. For example, the Means–Ends Problem Solving (MEPS) inventory was designed for use with elementary schoolchildren and requires the child to complete the middle part of a problem situation when presented with the beginning and the end (Spivack et al., 1976). Performance is determined by the number of alternative means that the child suggests, elaboration of specific means, potential obstacles identified, and use of a time sequence. The Open Middle Interview (OMI; Polifka et al., 1981) is an adaptation of the MEPS and has the advantage of being scored according to the effectiveness of each solution, whereas the original MEPS considers quantity rather than quality of solutions.

A more detailed method of assessing problem-solving skills is the Purdue Elementary Problem-Solving Inventory (PEPSI; Feldhusen et al., 1972). The PEPSI involves 49 cartoon slides, each of which portrays the child in a specific, real-life problem situation. Audiotaped directions are presented, along with a choice of alternative solutions. Children mark on a record sheet their preferred solution. The PEPSI provides an indication of children's abilities to sense problems, to define problems, to analyze critical details, to see implications, and to make unusual associations. To date, this measure does not seem to have been widely used in clinical practice.

The Social Problem-Solving Inventory–Revised (SPSI-R; D'Zurilla and Nezu, 1990; D'Zurilla and Maydeu-Olivares, 1995; D'Zurilla et al., 1997) was developed as an objective self-report measure of rational problem solving and problem-solving motivation. The SPSI-R assesses cognitive, affective, and behavioral processes by which individuals attempt to identify and implement adaptive coping responses for problem situations. The measure comprises five scales, two of which pertain to general problem orientation – Negative Problem Orientation and Positive Problem

Orientation – and the remaining three assess rational problem solving, impulsivity-carelessness style and avoidant style. Research provides support for use of the SPSI-R with adolescents (Sadowski et al., 1994; Reinecke et al., 2001). A short form has also been developed (D'Zurilla et al., 1997) that is suitable for adolescents (Spence et al., 2002).

Although studies suggest that relationships may exist between social problem solving and mood, a caveat is in order. The external validity of these scales has not been demonstrated. It is not clear to what extent self-report instruments, such as these, are related to children's ability to solve problems in real-life settings. Moreover, there are few data regarding the clinical use of these measures in guiding the treatment of depressed youth, or whether observed improvements in mood over the course of treatment are mediated by the acquisition and use of rational problem-solving skills.

Effectiveness of therapies with depressed youth

Research into the efficacy and effectiveness of cognitive therapy and CBT for depression among young people lags behind that with adults. None the less, initial findings have been encouraging. Recent clinical practice guidelines for treatment of depression in young people have emphasized cognitive-behavioral methods as the treatment of choice, with drug treatment being reserved for severe cases of depression or where CBT has not been effective (National Health and Medical Research Council, 1997). Research suggests that antidepressant medication for depressed children and adolescents is only modestly effective. A recent review by Wagner and Ambrosini (2001) concluded that, for this population, tricyclic antidepressants are not superior to placebo, although the early evidence from trials with the selective serotonin reuptake inhibitors has been encouraging.

Cognitive restructuring approaches

Despite the wide acceptance of cognitive restructuring approaches, such as rational emotive therapy (Ellis, 1962) and Beck's (1976) cognitive therapy for depression, few controlled-outcome studies with children and adolescents have been completed using these approaches. Belsher et al. (1995) reported an uncontrolled, multisite trial of cognitive therapy with 18 depressed adolescent outpatients. A structured treatment program (Wilkes et al., 1994), based upon Beck's (1976) cognitive therapy for depression, was used. Following treatment, participants showed significant decreases in depressive symptoms and depressogenic cognitions. These benefits were maintained at 5-month follow-up. However, there were no control groups to permit us to determine the degree to which changes associated with cognitive therapy were greater than the passage of time or placebo effects. Furthermore, some of the sample continued with antidepressant medication, making interpretation of the results difficult. Nevertheless, the Belsher et al. (1995) results were encouraging and justified progression to controlled-outcome studies.

Butler et al. (1980) conducted one of the few controlled studies that specifically examined the effectiveness of cognitive therapy as an isolated component. This study compared cognitive restructuring with role play, an attention placebo, and a classroom control with fifth- and sixth-grade children who were selected on the basis of high depression scores or teacher referral. Cognitive restructuring involved teaching children to recognize irrational, self-deprecating automatic thoughts, and to encourage them to adopt more logical, adaptive alternatives. They were taught to monitor their thoughts and to recognize the relationship between thoughts and feelings. The role-play treatment group used role play of specific problems associated with feelings of depression to discuss personal thoughts and feelings, develop empathy for others, teach social skills, and teach a problem-solving approach to handling threatening or stressful situations. The attention-placebo students were taught a cooperative problem-solving process for resolving academic questions. Significant reductions in depression scores were found for cognitive restructuring and role-play conditions, and the no-intervention classroom control. However, the attention placebo group showed minimal change on any measures. Overall, role play and cognitive restructuring produced the most improvement across the spectrum of depression, self-esteem, and locus-of-control measures. Interestingly, more children reached nondepressed status after the role-play intervention compared to the other conditions, suggesting that cognitive restructuring may be less developmentally appropriate for this age group than the role-play approach.

Self-control training

Self-control techniques have been used in several controlled-outcome investigations. Reynolds and Coats (1986), for example, randomly assigned 30 high-school students selected on the basis of elevated depression scores to self-control training, relaxation training, or a waitlist control. The self-control intervention involved monitoring of pleasant events and mood as a means of increasing awareness of pleasant events and decreasing focus on unpleasant events, decreasing emphasis on short-term rather than long-term consequences, and increasing accurate self-evaluation, attributions, realistic goal setting, and self-reinforcement. Both self-control and relaxation training conditions showed significantly greater reductions in depressive symptoms than a waitlist, but there was minimal difference in efficacy between treatments.

Stark et al. (1987) reported a controlled-outcome study comparing self-control therapy with a behavioral problem-solving therapy for moderately to severely depressed children. Significant reductions in depressive symptoms were found for children in both treatments from pre- to posttreatment, while those in the waitlist showed minimal change. Results were maintained at 8-week follow-up. Rehm and Sharp (1996) also found reductions in depression scores among mild to moderately depressed children in a noncontrolled evaluation of self-control training.

Integrative treatment approaches

The majority of controlled evaluations of psychotherapy with depressed youth have involved integrated cognitive-behavioral interventions, rather than cognitive therapy components in isolation. Cognitive-behavioral treatment components typically include presentation of a treatment rationale and socialization to the cognitive model, mood monitoring, cognitive restructuring, increasing pleasant events, training in social skills, relaxation training, development of social problem-solving skills, and the use of adaptive self-statements. Several studies have demonstrated the positive effects of combined CBT programs in treating child and adolescent depression (Reynolds and Coats, 1986; Kahn et al., 1990; Lewinsohn et al., 1990; Vostanis and Harrington, 1994; Brent et al., 1997, 1999; Harrington et al., 1998a; Clarke et al., 1999). Lewinsohn and Clarke (1999) have reviewed psychological treatments of depression, including integrative cognitive therapies (e.g., cognitive restructuring, attributional retraining, rational emotive therapy, self-control training, problem-solving skills training), behavioral approaches (e.g., social skills and assertiveness training, increasing pleasant events), family therapies (e.g., conflict resolution, communication skills, and parenting skills), and treatments focusing on affective education and management (e.g., relaxation training, affective education, and anger management). They concluded that treatment outcome studies involving CBT (which included cognitive therapies as major components) consistently showed positive results in the treatment of depressed adolescents.

In a metaanalysis of CBT for depression and depressive symptoms during adolescence, Reinecke et al. (1998) reported moderate to large effect sizes for six treatment outcome studies. The treatment effects were substantial, although not as large as those found for cognitive therapy with adults. One possible explanation is that most studies to date have used mild to moderately depressed or nonclinical adolescent samples, among which there may be less room for improvement. It was not possible to draw conclusions about the efficacy of CBT for treating depression among prepubertal children, however, given the small number of studies in this area. We await the findings of larger controlled trials that are now underway with clinical populations.

It is important to note, however, that not all studies have reported positive findings for the use of CBT with depressed young people. Liddle and Spence (1990) found significant reductions in depression scores for children in CBT, attention placebo, and waitlist conditions, but no difference in outcome across conditions at 2-month follow-up.

The relatively transient nature of depression among many prepubertal children, particularly those selected from school screening programs, is an issue for researchers conducting treatment outcome evaluations. It is important that students are selected based on a relatively stable presentation of depression, and that elevated mood scores are not reflecting a short-term mood reaction. This requires repeat assessments of depression over at least a 4-week period. The Liddle and Spence (1990) study selected students who showed elevated depression scores on two occasions across a 2-week period. Nevertheless, after 4 months the majority of children in the waitlist group showed scores within the normal range, making it difficult to determine any superior benefits for the CBT condition.

Methodological issues and future directions for treatment research

Although studies suggest that cognitive techniques offer promise for treating depressed youth, this research suffers from numerous methodological limitations (Reinecke et al., 1998). In addition to the relatively small number of controlled clinical trials, the sample sizes have typically been small and the majority of studies have used dysphoric, rather than clinically depressed populations. Participants were generally recruited through schools, rather than clinical settings, thus it is unclear whether the findings can be generalized to clinically referred children and adolescents. The outcome measures used in most studies have emphasized dysphoria rather than clinical depression, typically using self-report of depressive symptoms rather than a clinical diagnostic evaluation. There has also been little attempt to determine whether treatments influence broader aspects of psychosocial functioning, deficits in which frequently accompany depression. Furthermore, assessment has rarely included reports from other informants, such as parents and teachers, and evaluations have generally failed to consider the clinical in addition to the statistical significance of improvements.

A further limitation is the failure of most studies to include an attention placebo control condition in order to demonstrate the treatment specific effect of cognitive therapies. In addition, long-term follow-up periods are typically inadequate, rarely exceeding 6 months. This limitation restricts the conclusions that can be drawn about the durability of treatment effects – a true concern given the high risk of recurrence and relapse of depression in young people (Wood et al., 1996; Harrington et al., 1998b; Vostanis et al., 1998). For example, Wood et al. found that more than 40% of adolescent patients who had responded to CBT had relapsed within 6 months of remission. Vostanis et al. (1998) reported that 20% of adolescents who had received CBT reported feeling depressed at the 2-year follow-up and 38.9% had experienced significant depressive symptoms during the previous year. It would be useful to investigate the benefits of booster/maintenance/continuation sessions over follow-up periods. A pilot study along these lines was conducted by Kroll et al. (1996) who found a significantly lower cumulative relapse risk for adolescents who received continued CBT sessions for 6 months following remission, compared to a historical control group who received no further intervention. Similarly, Clarke and colleagues (1999) recently demonstrated that depressed youths who had not fully recovered at the end of an 8-week treatment program benefited from additional monthly booster sessions.

In addition to the problem of relapse, a significant percentage of young people discontinue treatment prematurely, are not able to comply with the CBT treatment protocol, or remain depressed at the end of treatment. Clarke et al. (1999), for example, reported that 33% of depressed adolescents remained depressed at the end of their CBT treatment, a finding that is in line with the results of a recent metaanalysis (Lewinsohn and Clarke, 1999). Research is required into the impact of varying parameters of therapy delivery, such as number and length of sessions, and fixed versus open-ended number of sessions. We also need to examine therapeutic techniques that may enhance treatment effects, reduce dropout, and increase resistance to relapse, such as incorporating family members into the treatment process, placing a greater emphasis on the modification of depressogenic schema, or augmenting CBT with prophylactic medications.

To date, cognitive therapy has not been compared with other frequently used treatments, such as antidepressant medications, interpersonal psychotherapy, or combined CBT approaches. There is also minimal research to determine the benefits of combining cognitive therapy with other treatments. The relative benefit of combined drug plus cognitive therapy treatments warrants exploration. With adults, there is some evidence that combined drug plus cognitive therapy may reduce rate of relapse and provide more "all-round" improvements across both depressive symptoms and psychosocial adjustment, compared to either treatment alone (Manning et al., 1992). It would also be valuable to examine the efficacy of a combined interpersonal psychotherapy–cognitive therapy approach given recent evidence suggesting the important role of interpersonal problems in the development and maintenance of depression and the benefits of interpersonal psychotherapy in the treatment of this condition in adolescents (Mufson and Fairbanks, 1996; Santor and Kusamakar, 2001).

To date we have minimal information about which young people are most likely to benefit from CBT or cognitive therapy and for whom it would be therefore a treatment of choice. For example, Jayson et al. (1998) examined predictors of remission in a sample of 10–17-year-olds who had completed a program of CBT. Contrary to their predictions, younger children were more likely to be diagnosis-free at the end of treatment than their older peers. The authors had initially hypothesized that younger children would have more difficulty understanding the concepts with the cognitive therapy component of the program. It is possible, however, that this age effect could reflect factors such as the duration of depressive disorder, rather than developmental stage. Jayson et al. (1998) also found that patients with less severe deficits in adaptive functioning were more likely to remit following treatment. Interestingly, severity of depressive symptoms and recent exposure to stressful life events were not found to be significant predictors of outcome following CBT once age and adaptive functioning were controlled. CBT has also been found to be particularly effective (relative to behavioral family therapy and supportive therapy) in assisting depressed adolescents with comorbid anxiety disorders, but its relative effectiveness is reduced for teenagers whose mothers are also depressed (Brent et al., 1998, 1999). The effects of other patient variables – including general level of intelligence, level of cognitive development, cognitive flexibility, executive function, verbal abstraction capacity, comorbid psychopathology, and patient motivation and compliance – on treatment response have received relatively little study. Similarly, there is a need to examine the impact of social factors such as level of social support, negative life events, and parent–child relationship quality as potential moderators or mediators of treatment outcome.

There is a pressing need for change process studies to clarify the mechanisms of therapeutic improvement in CBT with youth. It is not at all clear, for example, that clinical improvement is predicted by, or associated with, changes in cognitive variables targeted in treatment. It would be troubling to find that cognitive variables, which are addressed in CBT, are not related to therapeutic improvement. Kolko et al. (2000) reported one of the few studies to examine this issue. After acute treatment, CBT exerted specific effects on cognitive distortion relative to either systemic-behavioral family therapy or nondirective supportive therapy. At 2-year follow-up systemic-behavioral family therapy showed a specific influence upon family conflict and parent–child relationships compared to CBT or nondirective supportive therapy. However, no measures of cognitive distortion or family functioning mediated or moderated treatment outcome.

In a similar manner, it may be helpful to begin interdisciplinary research examining the biological changes associated with psychological treatments of depression in youth. Studies with adults suggest, for example, that CBT is associated with normalization of brain metabolism among patients with OCD (Baxter et al., 1992; Schwartz et al., 1996). Research on relationships between biological and cognitive concomitants of depression among youth, however, have not been explored. Research of this nature would inform our understanding of both neurobiological substrates of mood and biobehavioral mechanisms of change.

The suggestion has been made that therapeutic progress is related not to the efficient use of strategic interventions, but to the nature of the therapeutic relationship itself. The role of the therapeutic relationship in CBT with depressed children and adolescents, however, has received little systematic examination, and this is also true for the relationships of therapeutic allegiance and outcome expectancies to treatment outcome. A recent study by Kolko et al. (2000) failed to find any link between nonspecific therapist variables and outcome for CBT with adolescents.

Although outcome studies suggest that CBT may be efficacious in treating depressed youth, evidence of the effectiveness of these approaches in community settings and with diagnostically heterogeneous populations is limited. It will be useful to examine effectiveness of CBT with different depressive subtypes and with youth with a range of comorbid conditions. The ways in which CBT approaches may be adapted to meet the specific needs of different ethnic or cultural groups is also worthy of exploration. Our goal should be one of developing interventions that are not only efficacious, but portable, useful, economical, efficient, and (for lack of a better term) "desirable for our end-user"–children and their families.

Finally, additional work is needed on the dissemination of clinical research findings. Although evidence indicates that cognitive therapy and CBT can assist depressed youth, it is not clear that these findings have had a significant effect on services that children receive. Although recent data are not available on trends in treatment utilization for depressed youth, one suspects that, by and large, children and families are not able to avail themselves of treatments, like cognitive therapy or CBT, which can be effective and which have a relatively low risk of adverse side-effects. Further research is needed, as such, on systems of care and on mental health policies that influence the dissemination and availability of cognitive therapy for youth and families. Cognitive therapy, particularly when integrated with behavioral strategies, is a promising treatment for depressed youth. For many children and families, however, it is not an available option.

Preventing depression in young people

In recent years there have been a number of empirical investigations of the prevention of adolescent depression (Harrington and Clark, 1998; Gillham et al., 2000). These can be classified into three approaches – universal, selective, and indicated prevention (Mrazek and Haggerty, 1994). Universal prevention programs focus on all individuals in a population, irrespective of the presence or absence of risk factors. Selective prevention programs focus on those youngsters who are judged to be "at risk" for the development of depression, given the presence of certain factors that have been shown to be correlates or predictors of depression. Finally, indicated interventions target those individuals who show minimal but detectable symptoms of a disorder or who show biological markers suggestive of a predisposition to that disorder.

Universal prevention

There have been few empirical investigations of universal or primary preventive interventions for preventing depression. Clarke et al. (1993) described two brief psychoeducational interventions that aimed to prevent adolescent depression, neither of which produced significant benefits. Clarke et al. (1993) criticized these programs for failing to include a skills training component to rectify those skills deficits (e.g., social or problem-solving skills deficits) associated with depression in young people. More recently, Shochet et al. (2001) reported more positive findings from a small-group, school-based program conducted by psychologists and incorporating elements of CBT and interpersonal psychotherapy. A total of 240 students, aged 12–15 years, were assigned to either a monitoring control condition or the preventive intervention (with and without parent involvement). Students who participated in the intervention reported small but significant decreases in depressive symptoms on one of two measures of depression and on a hopelessness scale. Parental involvement did not influence outcome and the positive effects were not evident for the monitoring-only group.

Spence et al. (in press) also evaluated the impact of a school-based intervention, but using a whole-class approach with the sessions being conducted by teachers. The intervention integrated cognitive restructuring/interpersonal problem-solving approaches to the management of challenging life situations. In addition to the teaching of problem-solving strategies, the program emphasized the importance of problem-solving orientation, in line with cognitive restructuring approaches. Participants were 1500 students aged 12–14 years attending one of 16 participating schools. Schools were matched in pairs on indices of size, state/private, and socioeconomic status and were then randomly assigned from within each pair to either the Problem Solving for Life program or to the monitoring control condition. Short-term results indicated that participants with initially high levels of depressive symptoms who received the intervention showed a significantly greater reduction in depression and increase in life problem-solving skills compared to their counterparts in the control group. Those with nonelevated levels of depression and who received the intervention showed a stable level of depressive symptoms whereas the control group showed a small but significant increase in depressive symptoms over time. The low-depression, intervention students also showed a significantly greater improvement in problem-solving skills over time compared to the control group. However, at 12-month follow-up there were no significant differences in depression scores between groups, although the intervention group continued to show lower use of avoidant problem-solving strategies and lower negative problem-solving orientation.

This study demonstrates the feasibility of producing short-term changes in depressive symptoms and problem-solving skills, but emphasizes the difficulty in producing lasting preventive benefits. It is likely that students at risk will require a more prolonged, intensive intervention that tackles a broader range of risk factors. As in the teaching of any skill, the acquisition of cognitive and life problem-solving skills is likely to require repeated training opportunities throughout the teenage years. One-off interventions are not effective in the teaching of skills such as arithmetic and this may well be true for psychosocial skills. Most importantly, the results of Spence et al. (in press) suggest that teachers are indeed able to teach social-cognitive skills of this type within a classroom setting.

Selective and indicated prevention

Selective and indicated preventive interventions have also produced some encouraging results. For example, Beardslee et al. (1997) evaluated two selective prevention approaches for prevention of depression among children with a depressed parent. Their results showed better adaptive functioning at 1.5-year follow-up for children who attended a clinician-facilitated psychoeducational program compared to those who were enrolled in a lecture discussion group. Programs to enhance psychological functioning have also been implemented successfully with children of substance abusers (Gross and Mccaul, 1992) and children following parents' divorce (Zubernis et al., 1999).

Indicated preventive interventions with adolescents who show subclinical symptoms of depression have also produced encouraging results. Clarke et al. (1995) reported the results of a preventive program with high-school adolescents who demonstrated depressive symptoms. These youngsters were randomly assigned to a 15-session CBT group intervention or a "usual care" control condition. Survival analyses indicated a significant 12-month advantage for the prevention program. Similarly, Jaycox et al. (1994) reported positive findings in the prevention of depression with primary schoolchildren who reported mild symptoms of depression and parental conflict in the home. At 6-month follow-up, the preventive CBT intervention group reported fewer symptoms of depression compared to a nonintervention control group, an effect that was still evident at 2-year but not 3-year follow-up (Gillham et al., 1995; Gillham and Reivich, 1999). Two other pilot studies have reported small but significant benefits for CBT approaches to prevention of children at risk (Hannan et al., 2000; Muris et al., 2001).

At first sight it is tempting to conclude that preventive efforts may be best focused upon selective or indicated populations, rather than a universal or primary prevention approach. This conclusion, however, may be premature. Universal approaches have a number of important advantages that justify continued efforts to develop effective universal prevention protocols. The advantages of universal prevention over selective or indicated programs include: (1) avoidance of labeling effects as the result of the selection process; (2) better participation rates; (3) ability to target a wide range of risk factors simultaneously; and (4) the potential for impact upon other disorders that share common etiological factors with depression. Future research should examine the cost–benefits of universal versus indicated or selective approaches to prevention of depression in young people. Furthermore, studies to date have not examined whether the effects are maintained over several years. It seems unlikely that relatively brief interventions will be able to counteract the influence of the many risk factors that influence the development of depression. It would therefore be valuable to determine the benefits of booster programs, and longer-term or maintenance interventions. A further area worthy of examination is the value of adding parent or family interventions to those focused upon the young person. To date, most preventive interventions have concentrated upon the adolescent, aiming to enhance protective skills and to reduce risk factors relating to the individual (e. g., depressogenic thinking styles). There has been little attempt to modify risk factors within the environment, such as maladaptive parenting style or lack of social support within the home. Future studies should examine the benefits of combined individual–environmental change programs compared to individually focused preventive interventions.

Prevention research offers an important opportunity for understanding the ways in which cognitive, social, biological, and environmental factors interact in contributing to risk for depression. Attempts should be made, then, to examine simultaneously a broad range of vulnerability and risk factors in normative and at-risk groups. It may be useful, as well, to develop approaches for treating early-onset depression, including mood and anxiety disorders among preschool and early school-age children. These may be viewed as gateway conditions for the development of major depression during later childhood and adolescence. Prevention efforts should focus on specific developmental periods and should attend to specific, age-related developmental tasks. Although we accept a cognitive diathesis-stress paradigm for understanding human adaptation, we cannot presume that relationships between cognitive, social, and environmental factors are similar at different ages. Rather, we should attempt to understand the ways in which individuals and families respond to stressors at different points in the lifespan and should develop prevention strategies accordingly. It is possible, as well, that social and cultural differences in coping exist. With this in mind, a focus might be placed on understanding the ways in which individuals and families from diverse backgrounds understand and cope with stressful life events.

Summary and conclusions

Cognitive approaches offer promise in the understanding, prevention, and treatment of depression among youth. In this chapter we have reviewed the development of cognitive models of child and adolescent depression, and have noted their short-comings. We have discussed interventions that have been developed based on these models, and the evidence in support of them. As we have seen, research completed to date is, in many ways, supportive of the descriptive aspects of cognitive models of depression. Depressed children and adolescents do, as predicted, appear to demonstrate a range of cognitive deficits and maladaptive beliefs. Moreover, cognitive and behavioral treatment programs based upon these models have proven to be effective, at least in the short term, for alleviating depression among youth.

As we have also seen, however, there are many unanswered questions. Existing models do not effectively attend to the full range of cognitive, biological, social, and environmental factors that have been found to be associated with risk for depression. Moreover, existing models do not specify causal relationships between variables or the ways in which identified risk factors influence one another over time in contributing to vulnerability for depression. We need to consider why some young people develop cognitive styles and cognitive skill deficits that increase the chance that they will develop depression. We also need to understand why some young people who show these cognitive features do not develop depressive disorders, whereas others do. We have only a basic understanding of the developmental antecedents of cognitive risk factors for depression. There is a pressing need for cognitive models of depression among children and adolescents to be integrated with research from the developmental psychopathology and developmental neuroscience literatures. We may wish to begin by exploring the social context in which maladaptive beliefs, attitudes, attributions, and problem-solving deficits are acquired, as well as factors that inhibit the development of affect regulation skills and adaptive coping capacities. This may be augmented by research into the relationships between cognitive risk factors for depression and biological markers – such as neurotransmitter binding and endocrine function – associated with clinical depression. The relationships between biological, genetic, cognitive, and environmental factors associated with depression among youth are almost entirely unexplored, and offer exciting opportunities for further study. We know, for example, that gene expression can be influenced by environmental events (Gottlieb, 2000) and that psychosocial interventions (such as CBT) can influence brain metabolism. It is not implausible, then, to propose that functional relationships may exist between biological and cognitive adaptive systems (Kandel, 1998).

Research completed over the past 20 years indicates that cognitive therapy offers promise in, and forms a significant component of CBT approaches to, the treatment of depressed and dysphoric youth. The treatment effects are strong and, at least for adolescents, appear to be comparable to those observed in cognitive therapy with depressed adults. The volume and methodological quality of efficacy studies have improved over the years, and controlled comparative outcome studies examining the relative effectiveness of CBT and medications for treating clinically depressed adolescents are under way. Although cognitive therapy can be effective for treating depression among youth, the mechanisms of change are not well understood. From a practical perspective, work is needed to identify techniques to enhance the outcome of therapy, reduce relapse, and prevent the development of depression.

In sum, cognitive therapy has emerged during recent years as a promising treatment for depressed youth. It is not, however, a panacea. Our models of mood, adaptation, and development are, in many ways, rudimentary. Our therapeutic techniques, though promising, are insufficient. Much work remains to be done.

REFERENCES

Abramson, L., Seligman, M. E. P., and Teasdale, J. (1978). Learned helplessness in humans: critique and reformulation. *Journal of Abnormal Psychology*, **87**, 102–9.

Abramson, L., Metalsky, G., and Alloy, L. (1988a). The hopelessness theory of depression. Does the research test the theory? In *Social Cognition and Clinical Psychology: A Synthesis*, ed. L. Y. Abramson, pp. 33–65. New York: Guilford.

Abramson, L., Metalsky, G., and Alloy, L. (1988b). The hopeless theory of depression: atributional aspects. *British Journal of Clinical Psychology*, **27**, 5–12.

Abramson, L., Metalsky, G., and Alloy, L. (1989). Hopelessness depression: a theory-based subtype of depression. *Psychological Review*, **96**, 358–72.

Abramson, L., Alloy, L., Hogan, M. E., et al. (1999). Cognitive vulnerability to depression: theory and evidence. *Journal of Cognitive Psychotherapy*, **13**, 5–20.

Adams, M. and Adams, J. (1991). Life events, depression, and perceived problem-solving alternatives in adolescents. *Journal of Child Psychology and Psychiatry*, **32**, 811–20.

Anderson, J., Williams, S., McGee, R., and Silva, P. (1897). DSM-III disorders in pre-adolescnt children. *Archives of General Psychiatry*, **44**, 69–76.

Asarnow, J. and Bates, S. (1988). Depression in child psychiatric inpatients: cognitive and attributional patterns. *Journal of Abnormal Child Psychology*, **16**, 601–15.

Asarnow, J., Carlson, G., and Guthrie, D. (1987). Coping strategies, self perceptions, hopelessness, and perceived family environments in depressed and suicidal children. *Journal of Consulting and Clinical Psychology*, **55**, 361–6.

Asarnow, J. R., Jaycox, L. H., and Tompson, M. C. (2001). Depression in youth: psychosocial interventions. *Journal of Clinical Child Psychology*, **30**, 33–47.

Baldwin, M. (1992). Relational schemas and the processing of social information. *Psychological Bulletin*, **112**, 461–84.

Baxter, L., Schwartz, J., Bergman, K., et al. (1992). Caudate glucose metabolic rate changes with both drug and behavior therapy for obsessive-compulsive disorder. *Archives of General Psychiatry*, **49**(9), 681–9.

Beardslee, W. R., Wright, E. J., Salt, P., and Drezner, K. (1997). Examination of children's response to two preventive intervention strategies over time. *Journal of American Academy of Child and Adolescent Psychiatry*, **36**, 196–204.

Beck, A. T. (1963). Thinking and depression: 1. Idiosyncratic content and cognitive distortions. *Archives of General Psychiatry*, **9**, 324–33.

Beck, A. T. (1964). Thinking and depression: 2. Theory and therapy. *Archives of General Psychiatry*, **10**, 561–71.

Beck, A. T. (1967). *Depression: Clinical, Experimental, and Theoretical Aspects.* New York: Guilford Press.

Beck, A. T. (1976). *Cognitive Therapy and the Emotional Disorders.* New York: International Universities Press.

Beck, A. T. (1983). Cognitive therapy of depression: new perspectives. In *Treatment of Depression: Old Controversies and New Approaches*, ed. P. J. Clayton and J. E., Barrett, pp. 265–90. New York: Raven Press.

Belsher, G., Wilkes, T. C. R., and Rush, A. J. (1995). An open, multi-site pilot study of cognitive-therapy for depressed adolescents. *Journal of Psychotherapy Practice and Research*, **4**, 52–66.

Bodiford, C. A., Eisenstadt, R. H., Johnson, J. H., and Bradlyn, A. S. (1988). Comparison of learned helpless cognitions and behaviour in children with high and low scores on the Children's Depression Inventory. *Journal of Clinical Child Psychology*, **17**, 152–8.

Boyd, C. P., Kostanski, M., Gullone, E., Ollendick, T., H., and Shek, D., T. L. (2000). Prevalence of anxiety and depression in Australian adolescents: comparisons with worldwide data. *Journal of Genetic Psychology*, **161**, 479–92.

Brent, D., Holder, D., Kolko, D., et al. (1997). A clinical psychotherapy trial for adolescent depression comparing cognitive, family, and supportive treatments. *Archives of General Psychiatry*, **54**, 877–85.

Brent, D., Kolko, D., Birmaher, B., et al. (1998). Predictors of treatment efficacy in a clinical trial of three psychosocial treatments for adolescent depression. *Journal of the American Academy of Child and Adolescent Psychiatry*, **37**, 906–14.

Brent, D., Kolko, D., Birmaher, B., Baugher, D., and Bridge, J. (1999). A clinical trial for adolescent depression: predictors of additional treatment in the acute and follow-up phases of the trial. *Journal of the American Academy of Child and Adolescent Psychiatry*, **38**, 263–71.

Brewin, C. (1985). Depression and causal attributions: what is their relation? *Psychological Bulletin*, **98**, 297–309.

Brooks-Gunn, J. and Attie, I. (1996). Developmental psychopathology in the context of adolescence. In *Frontiers of Developmental Psychopathology*, ed. M. Lenzenweger and J. Haugaard, pp. 148–89. New York: Oxford University Press.

Butler, L., Mietzitis, S., Friedman, R., and Cole, E. (1980). The effect of two school-based intervention programs on depressive symptoms in preadolescents. *American Educational Research Journal*, **17**, 111–19.

Carey, M. (1993). Child and adolescent depression: cognitive-behavioral strategies and interventions. In *Cognitive-behavioral Procedures with Children and Adolescents: A Practical Guide*, ed. A. Finch, W. Nelson, and E. Ott, pp. 289–314. Boston: Allyn & Bacon.

Cicchetti, D. and Cohen, D. (1995). Perspectives on developmental psychopathology. In *Developmental Psychopathology: Theory and Methods*, vol. 1, ed. D. Cicchetti and D. Cohen, pp. 3–20. New York: Wiley.

Clark, D. and Beck, A. (1999). *Scientific Foundations of Cognitive Theory and Therapy of Depression*. New York: John Wiley.

Clarke, G. N., Hawkins, W., Murphy, M., and Sheeber, L. (1993). School-based primary prevention of depressive symptomatology in adolescents: findings from two studies. *Journal of Adolescent Research*, **8**, 183–204.

Clarke, G. N., Hawkins, W., Murphy, M., et al. (1995). Targeted prevention of unipolar depressive disorder in an at-risk sample of high school adolescents: a randomized trial of group cognitive intervention. *Journal of the American Academy of Child and Adolescent Psychiatry*, **34**, 312–21.

Clarke, G. N., Rohde, P., Lewinsohn, P. M., Hops, H., and Seeley, J. R. (1999). Efficacy of acute group treatment and booster sessions. *Journal of the American Academy of Child and Adolescent Psychiatry*, **38**(3), 272–9.

Costello, E., Costello, A., Edelbrock, C., et al. (1988). Psychiatric disorders in pediatric primary care. *Archives of General Psychiatry*, **45**, 1107–16.

Curry, J. and Craighead, W. (1990). Attributional style in clinically depressed and conduct disordered adolescents. *Journal of Consulting and Clinical Psychology*, **58**, 109–16.

Dobson, K. (1989). A meta-analysis of the efficacy of cognitive therapy for depression. *Journal of Consulting and Clinical Psychology*, **57**, 414–19.

Dobson, K. and Dozois, D. (2001). Historical and philosophical bases of the cognitive-behavioral therapies. In *Handbook of Cognitive-Behavioral Therapies*, 2nd edn, ed. K. Dobson, pp. 3–39. New York: Guilford.

D'Zurilla, T. J. (1986). *Problem-solving Therapy: A Social Competence Approach to Clinical Intervention*. New York: Springer.

D'Zurilla, T. J. and Goldfried, M. R. (1971). Problem solving and behaviour modification. *Journal of Abnormal Psychology*, **78**, 107–26.

D'Zurilla, T. and Maydeu-Olivares, A. (1995). Conceptual and methodological issues in social problem solving assessment. *Behavior Therapy*, **26**, 409–32.

D'Zurilla, T. and Nezu, A. (1990). Development and preliminary evaluation of the Social Problem Solving Inventory. *Psychological Assessment*, **2**, 156–63.

D'Zurilla, T. J. and Nezu, A. M. (1999). *Problem-solving Therapy: A Social Competence Approach to Clinical Intervention*, 2nd edn. New York: Springer.

D'Zurilla, T. J., Nezu, A. M., and Maydeu-Olivares, A. (1997). *Manual for the Social Problem-Solving Inventory-Revised (SPSI-R)*. North Tonawanda, NY: Multi-Health Systems.

Ellis, A. (1958). Rational psychotherapy. *Journal of General Psychology*, **59**, 35–49.

Ellis, A. (1962). *Reason and Emotion in Psychotherapy*. New York: Lyle Stuart.

Emery, G., Bedrosian, R., and Garber, J. (1983). Cognitive therapy with depressed children and adolescents. In *Affective Disorders in Childhood and Adolescence*, ed. D. P. Cantwell and G. A. Carlson, pp. 445–71. New York: Spectrum.

Feldhusen, J., Houtz, J., and Ringenbach, S. (1972). The Purdue Elementary Problem-solving Inventory. *Psychological Reports*, **31**, 891–901.

Fielstein, E., Klein, M. S., Fischer, M., et al. (1985). Self-esteem and causal attributions for success and failure in children. *Cognitive Therapy and Research*, **9**, 381–98.

Fleming, J. and Offord, D. (1990). Epidemiology of childhood depressive disorders: a critical review. *Journal of the American Academy of Child and Adolescent Psychiatry*, **29**(4), 571–80.

Freeman, A. and Reinecke, M. (1995). Cognitive therapy. In *Essential Psychotherapies: Theory and Practice*, ed. A. Gurman and S. Messer, pp. 182–225. New York: Guilford.

Fremouw, W., Callahan, T., and Kashden, J. (1993). Adolescent suicidal risk: psychological, problem-solving, and environmental factors. *Suicide and Life-Threatening Behavior*, **23**, 46–54.

Garber, J. and Flynn, C. (2001). Vulnerability to depression in childhood and adolescence. In *Vulnerability to Psychopathology: Risk Across the Lifespan*, ed. R. Ingram and J. Price, pp. 175–225. New York: Guilford.

Garber, J., Weiss, B., and Shanley, N. (1993). Cognitions, depressive symptoms and development in adolescents. *Journal of Abnormal Psychology*, **102**, 47–57.

Geller, B., Zimerman, B., Williams, M., Bohhofner, K., and Craney, J. L. (2001). Adult psychosocial outcomes of prepubertal major depressive disorder. *Journal of the American Academy of Child and Adolescent Psychiatry*, **40**, 673–7.

Gillham, J. E. and Reivich, K. J. (1999). Prevention of depressive symptoms in school children: a research update. *Psychological Science*, **10**, 461–2.

Gillham, J., Reivich, K. J., Jaycox, L. H., and Seligman, M. E. P. (1995). Prevention of depressive symptoms in school children: two year follow-up. *Psychological Science*, **6**, 343–51.

Gillham, J., Shatte, A., and Freres, D. (2000). Preventing depression: a review of cognitive-behavioral and family interventions. *Applied and Preventive Psychology*, **9**(2), 63–88.

Gladstone, T., Kaslow, N., Seeley, J., and Lewinsohn, P. (1997). Sex differences, attributional style, and depressive symptoms among adolescents. *Journal of Abnormal Child Psychology*, **25**, 297–305.

Goodman, S. H., Gravitt, G. W., and Kaslow, N. J. (1995). Social problem solving: a moderator of the relation between negative life stress and depression symptoms in children. *Journal of Abnormal Child Psychology*, **23**, 473–85.

Gotlib, I. and Hammen, C. (1992). *Psychological Aspects of Depression: Toward a Cognitive–interpersonal Integration*. Chichester, UK: Wiley.

Gottlieb, G. (2000). Environmental and behavioral influences on gene activity. *Current Directions in Psychological Science*, **9**(3), 93–7.

Gross, J. and McCaul, E. (1992). An evaluation of a psychoeducational and substance abuse risk reduction intervention for children of substance abusers. *Journal of Community Psychology*, **20**, 75–87.

Guidano, V. (1995). Constructivist psychotherapy: a theoretical framework. In *Constructivism in Psychotherapy*, ed. R. Neimeyer and M. Mahoney, pp. 93–108. Washington, DC: American Psychological Association.

Haaga, D., Fine, J., Terrill, D., Stewart, B., and Beck, A. (1993). Social problem-solving deficits, dependency, and depressive symptoms. *Cognitive Therapy and Research*, **19**, 147–58.

Haley, G., Fine, S., Marriage, K., Moretti, M., and Freeman, R. (1985). Cognitive bias and depression in psychiatrically disturbed children and adolescents. *Journal of Consulting and Clinical Psychology*, **53**, 535–7.

Hankin, B., Abramson, L., and Siler, M. (2001). A prospective test of the hopelessness theory of depression in adolescence. *Cognitive Therapy and Research*, **25**(5), 607–32.

Hannan, A. P., Rapee, R. M., and Hudson, J. L. (2000). The prevention of depression in children: a pilot study. *Behaviour Change*, **17**, 78–83.

Harrington, R. and Clark, A. (1998). Prevention and early intervention for depression in adolescence and early adult life. *European Archives of Psychiatry and Clinical Neuroscience*, **248**(1), 32–45.

Harrington, R., Fudge, H., Rutter, M., Pickles, A., and Hill, J. (1990). Adult outcomes of childhood and adolescent depression. *Archives of General Psychiatry*, **47**, 465–73.

Harrington, R., Wood, A., and Verduyn, C. (1998a). Clinically depressed adolescents. In *Cognitive-behaviour Therapy for Children and Families*, ed. P. Graham, pp. 156–93. Cambridge, UK: Cambridge University Press.

Harrington, R., Whittaker, J., and Shoebridge, P. (1998b). Psychological treatment of depression in children and adolescents. *British Journal of Psychiatry*, **173**, 291–8.

Holson, I., Kraft, P., and Vitterso, J. (2000). Stability in depressed mood in adolescence: results from a 6-year longitudinal panel study. *Journal of Youth and Adolescence*, **29**(1), 61–78.

Hops, H., Lewinsohn, P., Andrews, J., and Roberts, R. (1990). Psychosocial correlates of depressive symptomatology among high school students. *Journal of Clinical Child Psychology*, **19**, 211–20.

Hughes, J. N. (1988). *Cognitive Behaviour Therapy with Children in Schools*. New York: Pergamon.

Ingram, R. E. and Kendall, P. C. (1986). Cognitive clinical psychology: implications of an information processing perspective. In *Information Processing Approaches to Clinical Psychology*, ed. R. E. Ingram, pp. 3–21. New York: Academic Press.

Jaycox, L. H., Reivich, K. J., Gillham, J., and Seligman, M. E. P. (1994). Prevention of depressive symptoms in school children. *Behaviour Research and Therapy*, **32**, 801–16.

Jayson, D., Wood, A., Kroll, L., Fraser, J., and Harrington, R. (1998). Which depressed patients respond to cognitive-behavioural treatment? *Journal of the American Academy of Child and Adolescent Psychiatry*, **37**, 35–9.

Joiner, T. E. (2000). A test of the hopelessness theory of depression in youth psychiatric inpatients. *Journal of Clinical Child Psychology*, **29**, 167–76.

Kahn, J. S., Kehle, T. J., Jenson, W. R., and Clark, E. (1990). Comparison of cognitive-behavioural, relaxation and self-monitoring interventions amongst middle-school students. *School Psychology Review*, **19**, 196–211.

Kandel, E. (1998). A new intellectual framework for psychiatry. *American Journal of Psychiatry*, **155**, 457–69.

Kanfer, F. H. (1975). Self management methods. In *Helping People Change*, ed. F. H. Kanfer and A. P. Goldstein, pp. 309–55. New York: Pergamon.

Kanfer, F. H. and Phillips, J. S. (1970). *Learning Foundations of Behavior Therapy*. New York: John Wiley.

Kashani, J. H. and Ray, J. S. (1983). Depressive-related symptoms among preschool-age children. *Child Psychiatry and Human Development*, **13**, 233–8.

Kashani, J. H., Carlson, G. A., Beck, N. C., et al. (1987). Depression, depressive symptoms, and depressed mood among a community sample of adolescents. *American Journal of Psychiatry*, **144**(7), 931–4.

Kashani, J. H., Orvaschel, H., Rosenberg, T., and Reid, J. (1989). Psychopathology in a community sample of children and adolescents: a developmental perspective. *Journal of the American Academy of Child and Adolescent Psychiatry*, **28**, 701–6.

Kaslow, N., Rehm, L., and Siegel, A. (1984). Social-cognitive and cognitive correlates of depression in children. *Journal of Abnormal Child Psychology*, **12**, 605–20.

Kazdin, A. E. (1990). Evaluation of the Automatic Thoughts Questionnaire: negative cognitive processes and depression among children. *Psychological Assessment*, **2**, 73–9.

Kazdin, A. E., Rodgers, A., and Colbus, D. (1986). The Hopelessness Scale for Children: psychometric characteristics and concurrent validity. *Journal of Consulting and Clinical Psychology*, **54**, 241–5.

Kellam, S. G., Werthamer-Larsson, L., Dolan, L. J., et al. (1991). Developmental epidemiologically based preventive trials: baseline modelling of early target behaviours and depressive symptoms. *American Journal of Community Psychology*, **19**, 563–84.

Kendall, P. C. and Chansky, T. E. (1991). Considering cognition in anxiety disordered youth. *Journal of Anxiety Disorders*, **5**, 167–85.

Kendall, P. C. and MacDonald, J. (1993). Cognition in the psychopathology of youth and implications for treatment. In *Psychopathology and Cognition*, ed. K. Dobson and P. Kendall, pp. 387–427. San Diego: Academic Press.

Kendall, P. C., Stark, K. D., and Adam, T. (1990). Cognitive deficit or cognitive distortion in childhood depression. *Journal of Abnormal Child Psychology*, **18**, 255–70.

Kessler, R. C., Avenevoli, S., and Merikangas, K. R. (2001). Mood disorders in children and adolescents: an epidemiologic perspective. *Biological Psychiatry*, **49**(12), 1002–14.

Kolko, D. J., Brent, D. A., Baugher, M., Bridge, J., and Birmaher, B. (2000). Cognitive and family therapies for adolescent depression: treatment specificity, mediation, and moderation. *Journal of Consulting and Clinical Psychology*, **68**, 603–14.

Kovacs, M. and Gatsonis, C. (1989). Stability and changes in childhood-onset depressive disorders: longitudinal course as a diagnositc validator. In *The Validation of Psychiatric Disorders*, ed. L. Robins, J. L. Fleiss, and J. Barrett (eds), pp. 57–75. New York: Raven Press.

Kovacs, M., Feinberg, T., Crouse-Novak, M., et al. (1984). Depressive disorders in childhood. II. A longitudinal study of the risk for a subsequent major depression. *Archives of General Psychiatry*, **41**, 643–9.

Kroll, L., Harrington, R., Jayson, D., Fraser, J., and Gowers, S. (1996). Pilot study of continuation cognitive-behavioral therapy for major depression in adolescent psychiatric patients. *Journal of the American Academy of Child and Adolescent Psychiatry*, **35**, 1156–61.

Lambert, M. and Davis, M. (2002). Treatment for depression: what the current research says. In *Comparative Treatments of Depression*, ed. M. Reinecke and M. Davison, pp. 21–46. New York: Springer.

Leitenberg, H., Yost, L.W., and Carroll-Wilson, M. (1986). Negative cognitive errors in children: questionnaire development, normative data and comparisons between children with and without self-reported symptoms of depression, low self-esteem, and evaluation anxiety. *Journal of Consulting and Clinical Psychology*, **54**, 528–36.

Lewinsohn, P. M. and Clarke, G. N. (1999). Psychosocial treatments for adolescent depression. *Clinical Psychology Review*, **19**, 329–42.

Lewinsohn, P. M., Clarke, G. N., Hops, H., and Andrews, J. (1990). Cognitive-behavioral group treatment of adolescent depression. *Behavior Therapy*, **21**, 385–401.

Lewinsohn, P., Hops, H., Roberts, R., Seeley, J., and Andrews, J. (1993). Adolescent psychopathology: I. Prevalence and incidence of depression and other DSM-III-R disorders in high school students. *Journal of Abnormal Psychology*, **102**, 133–44.

Lewinsohn, P. M., Clarke, G. N., and Rohde, P. (1994). Psychological approaches to the treatment of depression in adolescents. In *Handbook of Depression in Children and Adolescents*, ed. W. M. Reynolds and H. E. Johnston, pp. 309–44. New York: Plenum Press.

Lewinsohn, P. M., Joiner, T. E., and Rohde, P. (2001). Evaluation of cognitive diathesis-stress models in predicting major depressive disorder in adolescents. *Journal of Abnormal Psychology*, **110**, 203–15.

Liddle, B., and Spence, S. H. (1990). Cognitive-behaviour therapy with depressed primary school children: a cautionary note. *Behavioural Psychotherapy*, **18**, 85–102.

Manning, D. W., Markowitz, J. C., and Frances, A. J. (1992). A review of combined psychotherapy and pharmacotherapy in the treatment of depression. *Journal of Psychotherapy Practice and Research*, **1**, 103–16.

Marx, E., Williams, J., and Claridge, G. (1992). Depression and social problem solving. *Journal of Abnormal Psychology*, **101**, 78–86.

McCracken, J. (1992). The epidemiology of child and adolescent mood disorders. *Child and Adolescent Psychiatric Clinics of North America*, **1**, 53–72.

McGee, R., Anderson, J., Williams, S., and Silva, P. (1986). Cognitive correlates of depressive symptoms in eleven year old children. *Journal of Abnormal Child Psychology*, **14**, 517–24.

Mrazek, P. J. and Haggarty, R. J. (eds) (1994). *Reducing the Risks for Mental Disorders: Frontiers for Preventive Intervention Research*. Washington, DC: National Academy Press.

Mufson, L. and Fairbanks, J. (1996). Interpersonal psychotherapy for depressed adolescents: a one-year naturalistic follow-up study. *Journal of the American Academy of Child and Adolescent Psychiatry*, **35**, 1145–55.

Muris, P., Bogie, N., and Hoogsteder, A. (2001). Effects of an early intervention group program for anxious and depressed adolescents: a pilot study. *Psychological Reports*, **88**, 481–2.

Murray, C. J. C. and Lopez, A. D. (eds) (1996). *The Global Burden of Disease*. Harvard: WHO, World Bank, and Harvard School of Public Health.

National Health and Medical Research Council. (1997). *Clinical Practice Guidelines: Depression in Young People*. Canberra: Looking Glass Press.

Nezu, A. M. (1986). Negative life stress and anxiety: problem solving as a moderator variable. *Psychological Reports*, **58**, 279–83.

Nezu, A. and Perri, M. (1989). Social problem-solving therapy for unipolar depression: an initial dismantling investigation. *Journal of Consulting and Clinical Psychology*, **57**, 408–13.

Nolen-Hoeksema, S. and Girgus, J. S. (1995). Explanatory style, achievement, depression, and gender differences in childhood and early adolescence. In *Explanatory Style*, ed. G. Buchanan and M. E. P. Seligman, pp. 57–70. Hillsdale, NJ: Erlbaum.

Nolen-Hoeksema, S., Girgus, J. S. and Seligman, M. E. P. (1992). Predictors and consequences of childhood depressive symptoms: a 5 year longitudinal study. *Journal of Abnormal Psychology*, **101**, 405–22.

Persons, J. (1989). *Cognitive Therapy: A Case Formulation Approach*. New York: Norton.

Petersen, A. C., Compas, B. E., Brooks-Gunn, J., et al. (1993). Depression in adolescence. *American Psychologist*, **48**, 155–68.

Peterson, C. and Seligman, M. E. (1984). Causal explanations as a risk factor for depression: theory and evidence. *Psychological Review*, **91**, 347–74.

Polifka, J. A., Weissberg, R. P., Gesten, E. L., de Apodaca, R. F., and Picoli, L. (1981) *The Open Middle Interview Manual*. Available from R. P. Weissberg, Department of Psychology, Yale University, New Haven, CT.

Poznanski, E. O. and Mokros, H. B. (1994). Phenomenology and epidemiology of mood disorders in children and adolescents. In *Handbook of Depression in Children and Adolescents*, ed. W. M. Reynolds and H. E. Johnston, pp. 19–39. New York: Plenum Press.

Prins, P. J. M. (1986). Children's self-speech and self-regulation during a fear provoking behavioural test. *Behaviour Research and Therapy*, **24**, 181–91.

Rehm, L. P. (1977). A self-control model of depression. *Behavior Therapy*, **8**, 787–804.

Rehm, L. P. (1981). A self-control therapy program for treatment of depression. In *Depression: Behavioral and Directive Intervention Strategies*, ed. J. Clarkin and H. Glazer, pp. 68–110. New York: Garland Press.

Rehm, L. P. and Sharp, R. N. (1996). Strategies for childhood depression. In *Cognitive Therapy with Children and Adolescents: A Casebook for Clinical Practice*, ed. M. A. Reinecke, F. M. Dattilio, and A. Freeman, pp. 103–23. New York: Guilford Press.

Reinecke, M. (1992). Childhood depression. In *Comprehensive Casebook of Cognitive Therapy*, ed. A. Freeman and F. Dattilio, pp. 147–58. New York: Plenum.

Reinecke, M. and DuBois, D. (2001). Socio-environmental and cognitive risk and resources: relations to mood and suicidality among inpatient adolescents. *Journal of Cognitive Psychotherapy*, **15**(3), 195–222.

Reinecke, M. and Rogers, G. (2001). Dysfunctional attitudes and attachment style among clinically depressed adults. *Behavioural and Cognitive Psychotherapy*, **29**, 129–41.

Reinecke, M., Ryan, N., and DuBois, D. (1998). Cognitive-behavioral therapy of depression and depressive symptoms during adolescence: a review and meta-analysis. *Journal of American Academy of Child and Adolescent Psychiatry*, **37**(1), 26–34.

Reinecke, M., DuBois, D., and Schultz, T. (2001). Social problem solving, mood, and suicidality among inpatient adolescents. *Cognitive Therapy and Research*, **25**(6), 743–56.

Reynolds, W. R. and Coats, K. I. (1986). A comparison of cognitive-behavioural therapy and relaxation training for the treatment of depression in adolescents. *Journal of Consulting and Clinical Psychology*, **54**, 653–60.

Reynolds. W. R. and Mazza, J. J. (1994). Suicide and suicidal behaviors in children and adolescents. In *Handbook of Depression in Children and Adolescents*, ed. W. M. Reynolds and H. E. Johnston, pp. 525–80. New York: Plenum Press.

Roberts, J., Gotlib, I., and Kassel, J. (1996). Adult attachment security and symptoms of depression: the mediating roles of dysfunctional attitudes and low self-esteem. *Journal of Personality and Social Psychology*, **70**, 310–20.

Robins, C. J. and Hinckley, K. (1989). Social-cognitive processing and depressive symptoms in children: a comparison of measures. *Journal of Abnormal Child Psychology*, **17**, 29–36.

Rotheram-Borus, M., Trautman, P., Dopkins, S., and Shrout, P. (1990). Cognitive style and pleasant activities among female adolescent suicide attempters. *Journal of Consulting and Clinical Psychology*, **58**, 554–61.

Rotheram-Borus, M., Piacentini, J., Miller, S., Graae, F., and Castro-Blanco, D. (1994). Brief cognitive behavioural treatment for adolescent suicide attempters and their families. *Journal of American Academy of Child and Adolescent Psychiatry*, **33**, 508–17.

Rudolph, K., Hammen, C., and Burge, D. (1997). A cognitive-interpersonal approach to depressive symptoms in preadolescent children. *Journal of Abnormal Child Psychology*, **25**, 33–45.

Sacco, W. P. and Graves, D. J. (1984). Childhood depression, interpersonal problem-solving and self-ratings of performance. *Journal of Clinical Child Psychology*, **13**, 10–15.

Sadowski, C. and Kelley, M. L. (1993). Social problem solving in suicidal adolescents. *Journal of Consulting and Clinical Psychology*, **61**, 121–7.

Sadowski, C., Moore, L., and Kelly, M. L. (1994). Psychometric properties of the Social Problem Solving Inventory (SPSI) with normal and emotionally disturbed adolescents. *Journal of Abnormal Child Psychology*, **22**, 487–500.

Santor, D. A. and Kusamakar, V. (2001). Open trial of interpersonal therapy in adolescents with moderate to severe major depression: effectiveness of novice IPT therapists. *Journal of American Academy of Child and Adolescent Psychiatry*, **40**, 236–40.

Schwartz, J., Stoessel, P., Baxter, L., Martin, K., and Phelps, M. (1996). Systematic changes in cerebral glucose metabolic rate after successful behavior modification treatment of obsessive-compulsive disorder. *Archives of General Psychiatry*, **53**(2), 109–13.

Seligman, M. E. P. (1975). *Helplessness: On Depression, Development and Death*. San Francisco: W. H. Freeman.

Seligman, M. E. P., Kaslow, N. J., Allow, L. B., et al. (1984). Attributional style and depressive symptoms in children. *Journal of Abnormal Psychology*, **93**, 235–8.

Shochet, I. M., Dadds, M. R., Holland, D., et al. (2001). The efficacy of a universal school-based program to prevent adolescent depression. *Journal of Clinical Child Psychology*, **30**, 303–15.

Spence, S. H., Donovan, C., and Brechman-Toussaint, M. (1999). Social skills, social outcomes and cognitive features of childhood social phobia. *Journal of Abnormal Psychology*, **108**, 211–21.

Spence, S. H., Sheffield, J., and Donovan, C. L. (2002). Problem-solving orientation and attributional style: moderators of the impact of negative life events on the development of depressive symptoms in adolescence. *Journal of Clinical Child and Adolescent Psychology*, **31**, 219–29.

Spence, S. H., Sheffield, J., and Donovan, C. L. (in press). Preventing adolescent depression: an evaluation of the Problem Solving for Life program. *Journal of Consulting and Clinical Psychology*.

Spirito, A., Overholser, J., and Stark, L. (1989). Common problems and coping strategies: II. Findings with adolescent suicide attempters. *Journal of Abnormal Child Psychology*, **17**, 213–21.

Spivack, G., Platt, J. J., and Shure, M. B. (1976). *The Problem Solving Approach to Adjustment*. San Francisco: Jossey Bass.

Sroufe, L. A. (1997). Psychopathology as an outcome of development. *Development and Psychopathology*, **9**, 251–68.

Stark, K. D. (1990). *Childhood Depression: School-based Intervention*. New York: Guilford.

Stark, K. D., Reynolds, W. M., and Kaslow, N. J. (1987). A comparison of the relative efficacy of self-control therapy and a behavioural problem-solving therapy for depression in children. *Journal of Abnormal Child Psychology*, **15**, 91–113.

Stark, K. D., Schmidt, K., and Joiner, T. (1996). Depressive cognitive triad: relationship to severity of depressive symptoms in children, parents' cognitive triad, and perceived parental messages about the child him or herself, the world, and the future. *Journal of Abnormal Child Psychology*, **24**, 615–25.

Stark, K. D., Sander, J., Yancy, M., Bronick, M., and Hoke, J. (2000). Treatment of depression in childhood and adolescence: cognitive-behavioural procedures for the individual and family. In *Child and Adolescent Therapy: Cognitive-behavioural Procedures*, 2nd edn ed. P. C. Kendall, pp. 173–234. New York: Guilford Press.

Sweeney, P. D., Anderson, K., and Bailey, S. (1986). Attributional style in depression: a meta-analytic review. *Journal of Personality and Social Psychology*, **50**, 974–91.

Vostanis, P. and Harrington, R. (1994). Cognitive-behavioural treatment of depressive disorder in child psychiatric patients: rationale and description of a treatment package. *European Child and Adolescent Psychiatry*, **3**, 111–23.

Vostanis, P., Feehan, C., and Grattan, E. (1998). Two-year outcome of children treated for depression. *European Child and Adolescent Psychiatry*, **7**, 12–18.

Wagner, K. D. and Ambrosini, P. J. (2001). Childhood depression: pharmacological therapy/treatment (pharmacotherapy of childhood depression). *Journal of Clinical Child Psychology*, **30**, 88–97.

Weissman, M. M., Wolk, S., Goldstein, R. B., et al. (1999). Depressed adolescents grow up. *Journal of the American Medical Association*, **281**, 1707–13.

Wilkes, T. C. R., Belsher, G., Rush, A. J., and Frank, E. (1994). *Cognitive Therapy for Depressed Adolescents*. New York: Guilford Press.

Wood, A., Harrington, R., and Moore, A. (1996). Controlled trial of a brief cognitive-behavioural intervention in adolescent patients with depressive disorders. *Journal of Child Psychology and Psychiatry*, **37**, 737–46.

Young, J. (1994). *Cognitive Therapy for Personality Disorders: A Schema-focused Approach*. Sarasota, FL: Professional Resource Exchange.

Zubernis, L. S., Cassidy, K. W., Gillham, J. E., Reivich, K. J., and Jaycox, L. H. (1999). Prevention of depressive symptoms in preadolescent children of divorce. *Journal of Divorce and Remarriage*, **30**, 11–36.

16

Cognitive-behavioral interventions in childhood anxiety disorders

John Piacentini,[1] R. Lindsey Bergman,[1] and Julie Wargo Aikins[2]

[1]University of California at Los Angeles, CA, USA
[2]Yale University, New Haven, CT, USA

Anxiety disorders are among the most common conditions affecting children and adolescents (Costello and Angold, 1995) with most modern epidemiological reports estimating the prevalence of significant anxiety disorders at greater than 10% worldwide (Pine, 1994) and from 12% to 20% in the USA (Kessler et al., 1994; Achenbach et al., 1995; Shaffer et al., 1996). Nevertheless, and in spite of the high prevalence, anxiety in childhood has not been as well studied as many other less common childhood disorders, possibly due to the incorrect perception that this problem is typically transient and innocuous (Benjamin et al., 1990). Over the last decade, however, our understanding of the phenomenology, prevalence, and treatment of childhood anxiety has increased dramatically. Although cognitive factors are presumed to play an important role in the expression and maintenance of childhood anxiety and most treatments contain at least some cognitive techniques specifically addressing these factors, only a handful of studies have been published investigating cognitive aspects of anxiety in children and adolescents.

In addition to the epidemiological findings, recent studies suggest that anxiety disorders in childhood are highly comorbid, relatively stable over time, and associated with significant impairment both acutely and over the long term. Clinic and community studies suggest that 50–75% of anxious children demonstrate two or more anxiety diagnoses (Costello and Angold, 1995; Last et al.,1987), and that comorbidity with both mood and externalizing disorders is also common (Bernstein and Borchardt, 1991; Ollendick and King, 1994). Childhood anxiety has been found to impact negatively on school, social, and family functioning (Ialongo et al., 1994; Klein, 1995), and children with anxiety disorders have been shown to be as severely impaired as other psychiatrically disturbed youngsters on multiple functional measures, including global perceptions of competence (Benjamin et al., 1990). Prospective studies confirm that anxiety disorders often are first apparent early in childhood and often run a chronic, although fluctuating course into adulthood (Achenbach et al., 1995; Costello and Angold, 1995; Pine et al., 1998). Although methodologically limited, retrospective studies indicate that a majority of adults with anxiety disorders recall developing their condition, or a similar condition, in childhood (Kessler et al., 1994; Klein, 1995). Anxiety in childhood has also been shown to predict prospectively major depression, suicidality, and psychiatric hospitalization in adults (Ferdinand and Verhulst, 1995; Klein, 1995; Pine et al., 1998).

When taken together, the high prevalence and significant morbidity associated with childhood anxiety suggest that these disorders constitute a significant public health problem. Unfortunately, children and adolescents with anxiety disorders are less likely to receive mental health services than children with many other disorders (Benjamin et al., 1990; Klein, 1995). Nevertheless, several recent and rigorously controlled trials have documented the efficacy of cognitive-behavioral interventions for the treatment of childhood anxiety disorders. Typically delivered in a multicomponent package, the primary components of cognitive-behavioral therapy (CBT) include cognitive restructuring which seeks to identify maladaptive thoughts and teach realistic, coping-focused thinking and graduated, systematic, and controlled behavioral exposure to feared situations and stimuli (Kendall, 1994). The initial CBT packages have proven to be both portable and adaptable, and the treatment appears to be robustly effective across a variety of delivery formats, including individual, group, and family treatment (Turner and Heiser, 1999; Piacentini and Bergman, 2001). In addition to CBT, a small but growing body of evidence suggests that pharmacologic intervention, especially with the selective serotonin reuptake inhibitors (SSRIs), may also be an effective tool in the treatment of childhood anxiety disorders (March, 1999; RUPP Anxiety Study Group, 2001).

The prevailing practice in anxiety treatment research has been to group and study youngsters with social phobia, separation anxiety disorder, and generalized anxiety disorder together and separately from other *Diagnostic and Statistical Manual of Mental Disorders,* 4th edition (DSM-IV American Psychiatric Association, 1994) anxiety disorders such as obsessive-compulsive disorder (OCD), posttraumatic stress disorder (PTSD), simple phobia, and panic disorder (Birmaher et al., 1994; Pine, 1994; Kendall et al., 1997; Pine et al., 1998). The primary reason for this grouping is that these three disorders respond to treatment (both CBT and pharmacological) in roughly similar degree and fashion regardless of which of the other diagnoses are present and/or primary. Other factors responsible for this grouping derive from research documenting that these three "core" disorders share a common underlying etiological construct, are highly comorbid with each other, infrequently occur in isolation, and show similar familial associations with adult anxiety and depression (Breslau et al., 1987; Last et al., 1991; Fyer et al., 1995; Kendall and Brady, 1995). Although CBT interventions for the broad range of childhood anxiety disorders typically include exposure and cognitive restructuring, CBT for other anxiety disorders such as OCD (March and Mulle, 1998; Piacentini, 1999), panic disorder (Ollendick, 1995), and PTSD (March et al., 1998) is usually administered in somewhat different fashion from that for the three core disorders. Given that most CBT trials have targeted social phobia, separation anxiety disorder, and generalized anxiety disorder collectively (Kendall, 1994; Barrett et al., 1996a; Kendall et al., 1997), treatments addressing these conditions will be the primary focus of this chapter.

Etiological models of anxiety in children

Generally speaking, the development of most behavioral and cognitive-behavioral treatment approaches for childhood anxiety has been guided by an understanding of presumed etiological theories underlying these disorders. Although a comprehensive review of the etiology of childhood anxiety is beyond the scope of this chapter, the most prominent theories on which CBT for childhood anxiety is based are briefly reviewed below. In all likelihood, the development of anxiety is a highly complex and iterative process involving multiple individual, familial (including genetic), and environmental risk factors (Rapee, 2001).

Ethological model

The ethological model of anxiety emphasizes the concept that fear and anxiety are not only normal and expected emotional states, but that they serve an adaptive function by increasing preparedness in the face of danger and thus aiding in the avoidance of harm to the individual (Barlow, 1988). Anxiety is seen as a natural response to a perceived danger or threat that serves to prepare the organism to either fight or flee (the "fight-or-flight" response). The autonomic components of the anxiety response (increased heart rate, sweating, etc.) are understood best in terms of the function those physiological adaptations play in helping the organism survive. According to the theory, anxiety disorders result when danger is perceived (and anxiety "activated") in the absence of an actual threat or when the anxiety response is in excess of what is reasonable for a given danger or threat. In these cases, anxiety ceases to be adaptive and can instead lead to deleterious changes in behavior that can become disruptive to normal functioning.

Most CBT interventions for childhood anxiety have used the ethological model as the basis for the psychoeducational component of treatment. Understanding the adaptive function of anxiety and reconceptualizing it as a normal and expected phenomenon serves as a key basis for cognitive restructuring in CBT treatment and provides anxious youngsters with an important and effective tool for coping with heightened levels of anxiety and distress elicited during exposure exercises.

Tripartite model

The tripartite model includes many of the assumptions of the ethological model of anxiety but expands upon it considerably. Perhaps the most influential model with regard to etiology and phenomenological expression, the tripartite model views anxiety as involving cognitive, physiological, and behavioral components (Lang, 1971; Rachman and Hodgson, 1974). These components, or response systems, are considered partially independent but interactive with one another. The cognitive component involves thoughts, worry, or self-statements about danger. The physiological component involves the physical feelings or symptoms of anxiety such as muscular tension, rapid pulse, difficulty breathing, frequent or excessive sweating, and headaches. The behavioral component involves both disruption of performance, such as the inability to perform in public or complete assigned tasks, and anxiety-related escape and avoidance behaviors. According to the tripartite model, excessive or unrealistic levels of anxiety result from distortions in one or more of these response systems, which can be triggered by either external events or interoceptive stimuli. Anxiety is then further heightened and/or maintained through the unique interactions among these systems. The exact mechanisms by which distortions in the three response channels are initially triggered have yet to be elucidated. Nevertheless, the tripartite model has served as the impetus for the development of multicomponent interventions that address each of the relevant anxiety components.

Temperament

Kagan and colleagues (1989) have focused on an enduring behaviorally inhibited temperament in childhood as a vulnerability factor for the development of anxiety disorders. Behavioral inhibition includes a spectrum of behaviors exhibited in the presence of unfamiliar or novel stimuli. These behaviors, which include withdrawal, cessation of speech, comfort seeking, suppression of ongoing behavior, as well as elevated autonomic arousal, have been identified in approximately 10–15% of Caucasian children in the USA (Kagan et al., 1987). Several studies have indicated an increased risk of anxiety disorders among behaviorally inhibited children (Biederman et al., 1990, 1993; Rosenbaum et al., 1993), especially if the behavioral inhibition persists over time (Hirshfeld et al., 1992). However, it should be noted that, although behaviorally inhibited children are more likely to develop anxiety disorders than are noninhibited children, only a minority of behaviorally inhibited children develop anxiety disorders (Biederman et al.,1990; Hayward et al., 1998).

Familial determinants

Familial aggregation of anxiety disorders has been well demonstrated (Fyer et al., 1993; Beidel and Turner, 1997). Children of parents with an anxiety disorder are seven times more likely than children of nonanxious parents to develop an anxiety disorder (Turner et al., 1987) while, conversely, parents of anxious children are more likely than parents of nonanxious children to meet criteria for an anxiety disorder themselves (Last et al., 1991). Although a significant proportion of familial transmission of anxiety disorders is accounted for by genetics (Torgersen, 1983; Kendler et al., 1992a, 1992b), family environment has been shown to play an important role as well. Families of anxious youngsters have been characterized as more controlling, conflictual, and promoting less independence than families of nonanxious children (Silverman et al., 1988; Messer and Beidel, 1994; Ginsburg et al., 1995).

Barrett et al. (1996b) provided direct evidence of familial enhancement of anxious avoidance in a study examining child interpretation bias among clinically anxious, oppositional, and nonclinical 7–14-year-old children. These authors found anxious children were more likely to interpret ambiguous scenarios in a threatening manner than were nonclinical and oppositional children. However, after study youngsters had initially and individually interpreted the ambiguous situations and formulated a plan of action, these situations were then rediscussed with the entire family, after which the child provided a second (re-)interpretation of the situation. Following the parent–child discussions, anxious children's endorsement of avoidant strategies increased significantly, even compared to the previously high baseline levels. Whaley et al. (1999) found anxious mothers to be less warm and positive and more controlling, catastrophizing, and critical of their children than nonanxious mothers, with the presence of anxiety in the child exacerbating certain of these maternal behaviors even further (control, catastrophizing, criticism). Further, lower levels of maternal autonomy granting and warmth were both shown to predict increased anxiety symptomatology in their children. Collectively, these findings suggest that parental expectations and coping approaches play an important role in the development, expression, and maintenance of childhood anxiety. As a result, many cognitive-behavioral treatment researchers have begun emphasizing greater parental involvement in the child's treatment (Barrett et al., 1996a; Silverman et al., 1999b) and some have gone so far as to include intervention modules aimed at treating coexisting parental anxiety disorder as part of their overall treatment package (Barrett et al., 1996a).

Cognitive constructs

In spite of the presumed importance of cognition in the etiology and maintenance of childhood anxiety, relatively little empirical investigation has focused on this area. In an effort to extend previous findings with anxious adults (Mogg et al., 1989; Martin et al., 1992; Chen et al., 1996), it was demonstrated that anxious children as young as 6 years of age exhibit biased attention to threatening stimuli as detected with the use of a Stroop task. Vasey and colleagues (1995, 1996) replicated these findings by using developmentally appropriate probe detection tasks. In the latter studies, anxious children responded more quickly to a dot probe if it was preceded by a threatening word (e.g., death, teased, danger) than if it was preceded by a neutral word. In contrast, nonanxious children's probe detection was unaffected by the content of the preceding word.

Anxious adults have consistently been shown to display cognitive biases regarding the interpretation of ambiguous stimuli (Butler and Mathews, 1983; Mathews et al., 1989). In an effort to examine the presence of such biases among anxious children, Barrett et al. (1996b), as discussed previously, found anxious youngsters to be more likely to interpret ambiguous scenarios in a threatening manner than both clinic and control youngsters.

The adult literature also supports the notion that anxiety is linked to a tendency to exaggerate the likelihood of occurrence of negative events and to attribute negative outcomes to stable, and often internal causes (Bell-Dolan and Wessler, 1994). Examining this issue among youngsters, Boegels and Zigterman (2000) revealed that, in addition to judging situations as being more dangerous than control children and externalizing children, anxious children rated themselves as less competent at dealing with threatening situations. King et al. (1995) found that high test-anxious high-school students tended to make more negative self-evaluations than their nonanxious peers. Socially anxious children also appear to have lower expectancies of their performance during a stressful task than do their nonanxious peers (Spence et al., 1999). Similarly, when confronted with a fear-eliciting task, younger anxious children (aged 8–12 years) also reported more negative self-statements than nonanxious or moderately anxious children (Prins, 1986).

Several studies have demonstrated cognitive content-specificity for anxiety and depression in adults with thoughts of personal loss and failure associated with depression and thoughts of harm and danger associated with anxiety (for review, see Clark and Steer, 1996). In contrast, evidence for content-specificity in children and adolescents has been much less consistent. Laurent and Stark (1993) found no difference in the level of anxious self-talk among children with anxiety, depression, or both conditions. In contrast, Ronan et al. (1994) reported that endorsement of certain statements related to negative self-evaluation discriminated anxious from both depressed and nonclinical children. Moreover, these investigators (Ronan and Kendall, 1997) found some support for content-specificity (anxiety versus depression) using rationally derived item sets but only mixed support for specificity when empirically derived item sets were employed.

Distorted cognitive operations are suspected to underlie many cognitive biases, including the tendency to make fearful interpretations of ambiguous stimuli and to evaluate negatively situations and self. These distorted cognitive operations are often referred to as cognitive distortions or cognitive errors (Beck et al., 1979; Weems et al., 2001) and are meaningfully distinct from "cognitive deficits" (Kendall, 1993). Various cognitive distortions that are presumably associated with anxiety include catastrophizing (expecting the worst possible outcome of a situation and overestimating the probability that it will occur), overgeneralization (believing that a negative outcome of an isolated situation is likely to occur in a wide range of situations), personalizing (attributing control over negative outcomes to internal causes when there is no reason to do so), and selective abstraction (focusing only on the negative aspects of an event or situation while ignoring other potentially important features). There is some evidence that children with high levels of anxiety endorse more cognitive errors than do children with low levels of anxiety (Leitenberg et al., 1986; Mazur, et al., 1992). While an increase in cognitive errors has been observed among both anxious and depressed youth, both personalizing and overgeneralization seem to have stronger associations with anxiety than with depression (Epkins, 1996; Weems et al., 2001).

Although cognitive biases appear to be associated with anxiety in children and adults, the nature of this association is not completely clear. Specifically, cognitive biases may represent a vulnerability or basis for the development of anxiety or they could be a consequence of having an anxiety disorder (Vasey et al., 1995; Craske, 1999). This relationship is likely a complicated one in which tendencies toward bias may constitute an anxiety vulnerability that becomes entrenched after the onset of a specific anxiety disorder (Craske, 1999). However, regardless of whether cognitive biases are a cause or consequence of anxiety disorder, these factors almost certainly contribute to the maintenance and/or intensification of anxious response patterns.

Treatment of childhood anxiety disorders

Behavioral treatments

Although the most widely used treatment approaches for childhood anxiety now include a range of intervention strategies, including psychoeducation, and cognitive and behavioral techniques, earlier treatments for anxiety and fears in children utilized behavioral interventions almost exclusively. The most commonly used behavioral techniques included systematic desensitization, modeling, and contingency management (Ollendick and King, 1998).

Systematic desensitization

The use of systematic desensitization as a treatment approach is based on the assumption that fears and phobias are learned as a result of classical conditioning, and must be paired with incompatible stimuli or responses in order to extinguish the fear response (Wolpe, 1958). Therefore desensitization requires exposure to the feared stimulus while blocking or replacing the fear response with a pleasant or neutral one. A number of studies have found both imaginal (Kondas, 1967; Mann and Rosenthal, 1969; Miller et al., 1972; Barabasz, 1973) and in-vivo (Kuroda, 1969; Ultee et al., 1982) desensitization to be more effective than no treatment for childhood fears and phobias. However, not all of the results have been positive. Ultee et al. (1982) failed to find an advantage for imaginal desensitization compared to no treatment, while Miller et al. (1972) found imaginal desensitization equivalent to psychotherapy, although both interventions included instruction in parent training and contingency management procedures. Ultee et al.'s (1982) results suggest that in-vivo desensitization may be more effective than imaginal approaches. Ollendick and King (1998) conclude that, although systematic desensitization procedures are typically considered as effective treatments, the evidence base for this treatment is relatively thin. Moreover, most of the research in this area is relatively old, with some studies characterized by methodological flaws (Miller et al., 1972).

Modeling

Modeling is based on the theoretical assumption that observational learning may play a role in both the acquisition and amelioration of fear and anxiety (Rachman, 1977). As applied to the treatment of anxiety, observation of a model's approach to a feared situation or stimulus along with the lack of any negative repercussions befalling the model leads to a reformulation or correction of the child's fear response. Further, the positive coping approaches utilized by the model in approaching the feared stimulus may be learned as adaptive approaches for addressing this fear. Several modalities of the modeling technique have been shown to reduce child anxiety and fear effectively including live, filmed, and participant modeling (where the child is guided through anxiety-eliciting situations by the therapist) (Bandura et al., 1967; Hill et al., 1968; Ritter, 1968; Lewis, 1974). Participant modeling and modeling by peers (as opposed to adults) appear to be the most effective variations of this technique (Ollendick, 1979).

Contingency management

While systematic desensitization and modeling both focus upon the extinction of fear as a primary treatment goal, contingency management strategies differ in that they do not target anxiety reduction as the primary mechanism for addressing avoidance behaviors and other anxiety-related impairments. Instead, contingency management, which is based on operant conditioning theory, assumes that fear behaviors may be altered solely through the manipulation of their consequences (King and Ollendick, 1997). Shaping, positive reinforcement, and extinction are among the most commonly used contingency management strategies for childhood fears and anxiety (Ollendick and King, 1998). Reinforced practice (graduated exposure plus reinforcement) has been well established as an effective treatment for the amelioration of specific fears and phobias (Obler and Terwilliger, 1970; Leitenberg and Callahan, 1973; Sheslow et al., 1983; Menzies and Clarke, 1993).

Although multiple controlled trials have demonstrated the efficacy of behavioral techniques, most notably reinforced practice, for the treatment of childhood fears and phobias, empirical investigation of behavioral treatments for other childhood anxiety disorders such as separation anxiety, generalized anxiety, and school refusal are lacking (Ollendick and King, 1998). This may be due to the fact that these latter anxiety disorders involve a particularly complex set of cognitive and physiological influences that call for the application of additional nonbehavioral interventions. Indeed, as outlined in the tripartite model, since cognitions, behaviors, and physiology are believed to contribute to the development and maintenance of anxiety in a highly interrelated fashion, it follows that therapy should address each of these three components to be optimally effective (Ollendick and King, 1998).

Cognitive treatments

Either by design or result, cognitive strategies have rarely been employed as the sole treatment intervention for the treatment of childhood anxiety and fears. Instead, cognitive techniques tend to be used in combination with other, most commonly behavioral techniques. In one of the first cognitive therapy studies, Graziano and Mooney (1980) randomized 33 children with nighttime fears to either cognitive self-control training or to a waitlist control group. Children in the cognitive self-control groups were taught to relax, imagine a pleasant scene, and recite coping statements to themselves, such as "I am brave," "I can take care of myself when I'm alone," and "I can take care of myself when I'm in the dark." Parents were taught to monitor symptoms and provide immediate reinforcement for brave behavior in the form of "bravery" tokens. Although treatment response was significantly better among the youngsters in the active treatment group, it is difficult to assess the unique efficacy of the cognitive intervention given that a behavioral technique (the reward system) was also employed.

Eisen and Silverman (1993) examined the efficacy of cognitive therapy, relaxation therapy, and their combination in four youngsters with overanxious disorder using a multiple baseline design across subjects. All three interventions also contained an identical behavioral component, namely exposure to the feared stimulus. According to the authors, this methodology was employed to examine the unique benefit of the cognitive and relaxation techniques beyond that of the exposure component. All three treatment conditions led to decreased anxiety. However, the interventions tended to be most effective when matched to the individual symptom profile of the child. That is, cognitive therapy worked best for youngsters with primarily cognitive symptoms, relaxation therapy was best for youngsters with primarily somatic symptoms, and the combination treatment was most helpful for subjects with both cognitive and somatic symptoms. A similar pattern of results was found by these authors in a second case series also involving four youngsters, albeit with generalized anxiety disorder (Eisen and Silverman, 1998). While intriguing, these results require replication in larger samples and under controlled conditions. Nevertheless, the development of prescriptive intervention strategies, or treatments that are matched to specific symptom patterns, is an important goal for the focus of research efforts in the coming years.

Combined cognitive-behavioral interventions

Multicomponent cognitive-behavioral interventions for childhood anxiety were initially derived from the adult treatment literature (Barlow, 1988; Chambless and Gillis, 1993). The adult treatments were modified to address the unique developmental characteristics of children and adolescents. These developmental characteristics include less well-developed and typically more concrete cognitive abilities, poorer affect recognition and regulation skills, greater present versus future orientation, more variable motivation, and increased reliance on family, academic, and other social systems (Piacentini and Bergman, 2001). Methods to address these constraints are described more fully below.

Individual CBT

While early case studies suggested the efficacy of multicomponent cognitive-behavioral interventions with anxious children, the first controlled trials were only completed in 1994 (Kendall, 1994). In the first such trial, Kendall (1994) treated children with generalized anxiety disorder, separation anxiety disorder, and social phobia using a 16–20-session program (Coping Cat), in which the first eight sessions are utilized for skills training and the second eight sessions focus on exposure-based practice. Skill building in the Coping Cat program targets four areas: (1) the identification of anxious feelings and physiological reactions; (2) the recognition and evaluation of anxious cognitions; (3) the creation of a plan for coping with this anxiety; and (4) the evaluation of coping responses and self-reinforcement or reward strategies. Working together, the therapist and child create a FEAR plan for coping with anxiety-eliciting situations. The FEAR acronym stands for feeling frightened, expecting bad things to happen, attitudes and actions, and results and rewards. Specific techniques in this phase of treatment include the identification and evaluation of cognitive distortions such as negative self-talk, catastrophizing, and striving for perfection, cognitive restructuring to address cognitive distortions and facilitate more adaptive (i.e., nonanxious) reality-based cognitions, relaxation techniques to address somatic symptoms, and rewards for positive attempts to cope with and confront feared situations (Kendall et al., 1992).

During the latter half of the Coping Cat program, the FEAR plan is used to help children learn to cope with relevant anxious situations presented in graded fashion with easiest situations attempted first and increasingly difficult situations afterwards. Behavioral strategies such as modeling and reinforced practice are used to facilitate the in-vivo exposures characterizing this phase of treatment. Through in-session exposures and home-based "Show that I Can" tasks, children gradually learn to overcome their fears in a hierarchical fashion and to gain mastery over their anxiety.

Kendall and colleagues have examined the efficacy of the Coping Cat program in two controlled trials, both of which employed an 8-week waitlist control condition. In the first trial (Kendall, 1994), CBT led to marked improvement in symptomatology as compared to waitlist across self-and parent ratings of symptoms and distress as well as child observations. Overall, 64% of the CBT group did not meet criteria for an anxiety diagnosis at posttreatment compared to only 5% in the waitlist condition. Impressive evidence attests to the durability of this treatment as gains (assessed by child and parent ratings and diagnostic interviews) were maintained over a 2–5-year follow-up (Kendall and Southam-Gerow, 1996). A second larger randomized trial utilizing the same design as the first study yielded similar results as 71% of youth in the CBT condition no longer met criteria for anxiety at posttreatment compared to only 5.8% of waitlist children (Kendall et al., 1997). Treatment gains were maintained over a 1-year follow-up, with many youths demonstrating increasing gains over time. Taken together, findings from Kendall's studies provide strong support for the use of CBT in the treatment of childhood anxiety disorders.

Family CBT

Given the role that family appears to play in the development and maintenance of childhood anxiety, Barrett et al. (1996a) recommended the inclusion of a family component in the cognitive-behavioral treatment of anxiety for children. Family involvement in treatment recognizes the high frequency of anxiety disorders among parents of anxious children, and introduces strategies that are directed at helping parents to identify, manage, and cope with their own anxiety. Additionally, this approach attempts to promote more positive parental communication and problem-solving skills to bolster parents' ability to facilitate their child's positive coping efforts and to deal with family difficulties that could exacerbate their child's anxiety. Parents' use of contingency management techniques in response to their child's anxiety and coping approaches is emphasized as well.

Barrett et al. (1996a) compared the treatment gains associated with CBT, CBT plus family anxiety management, and a waitlist control. The cognitive-behavioral approach was based on the Coping Cat program (Kendall, 1994). Although outcome assessments were based on parental report only, the findings from this study suggest that the adjunctive family component provided significant benefits to outcome beyond the cognitive-behavioral approach alone. More specifically, while 57% of the children in the cognitive-behavioral condition no longer met anxiety disorder criteria following treatment, 84% of the CBT plus family anxiety management no longer met diagnostic criteria at the posttreatment assessment. Additionally, these treatment gains were maintained over time, with even greater decreases in anxiety diagnoses at 6 and 12 months. Notably, treatment condition interacted significantly with gender and age, such that females and younger children appeared to benefit most from the added family component.

Silverman and colleagues (Silverman et al., 1995; Silverman and Kurtines, 1996) similarly emphasized the inclusion of parents in the treatment of child anxiety. These investigators developed a treatment that focuses less upon parental anxiety, but emphasizes other ways that parents may affect their child's treatment success. For example, as a complement to exposure exercises for the children, parents learn contingency management strategies in which they support their child's approach to feared stimuli and engagement in exposures, while being careful not to respond to avoidance behaviors with positive reinforcement. Other elements of their treatment program, such as identification of anxious cognitions and somatic symptoms, cognitive restructuring, exposure to feared stimuli, relaxation strategies, and self-evaluation and reward are similar to those emphasized in the Coping Cat program (Kendall, 1994). Silverman and Kurtines (1996) suggest that control over treatment should gradually be transferred from the therapist to the parent and then to the child, positing that this type of guardianship over treatment facilitates long-term therapeutic change. Thus, as children develop skills they begin to take on more responsibility for their own treatment, allowing parental control and involvement to diminish. Through the development of greater self-management and regulation, children are able to become the central mediator of their own anxiety. Although multicomponent CBT protoocols for childhood anxiety typically include elements relevant to this notion (e.g., contingency management training and child self-control training), the specific contribution of "transfer of control" to outcome has not been explicitly tested.

Group CBT

Silverman et al. (1999a) also hypothesized that CBT, with concurrent parent sessions, might be enhanced when delivered in a group format because the group would provide an additional pathway for the transfer of control which would enhance the efficacy of the treatment and allow the group to provide valuable feedback and skill facilitation. In a controlled clinical trial in which group CBT was compared to a waitlist control condition, children in the group CBT condition demonstrated marked improvement both immediately following treatment and at 3-, 6-, and 12-month follow-up. That is, 64% of the children in the group CBT condition no longer met criteria for anxiety following the treatment, while only 13% of the waitlisted children demonstrated this same improvement. Similar patterns of improvement were demonstrated for child and parent ratings of distress.

CBT versus education support

Taken together, the findings of the clinical trials presented above provide strong support for the efficacy of child-focused CBT for the treatment of childhood anxiety and suggest that treatment may be enhanced by the inclusion of family treatment components. However, with the exception of Barrett et al. (1996a), none of the above studies included an active comparison condition or utilized a dismantling approach to identify the active components of the treatment packages employed. More recent studies have begun to address these issues. Silverman et al. (1999b) utilized a dismantling approach to compare the efficacy of contingency management or self-control paired with exposure to that associated with an education support condition. Findings suggested that exposure with either contingency management or self-control was equally effective across child, parent, and clinician ratings. In contrast to prediction, however, the education condition appeared to be an effective treatment intervention as well, with children in this group demonstrating significant treatment response. These findings are notable given the exclusion of an exposure component (usually assumed to be an important active ingredient in the treatment of anxiety) in the education-based condition.

Last et al. (1998) examined the treatment of school phobia using a standard cognitive-behavioral approach versus an education support condition. Similar to Silverman et al. (1999b), both CBT and education support conditions were found to be equally effective in the reduction of anxiety. Although these findings are clearly intriguing as well as surprising, it is possible that the education support conditions in these studies actually contained many cognitive-behavioral components, thereby blurring the distinction between the "active" and education conditions, and making the results difficult to interpret in a meaningful way. Conversely, Silverman et al. (1999b) speculate that undetermined nonspecific factors or positive expectations for treatment may have been responsible for the effectiveness of the education support condition.

Summary and future directions

Although treatment research for anxiety disorders in children still lags considerably behind that for many other childhood disorders (Anxiety Disorders Association of

America (ADAA), 1999), significant gains have been made in this area over the last decade. Childhood anxiety research has demonstrated growing sophistication in the use of etiological models as a springboard for treatment development and has begun to take the next steps in research design, moving from waitlist control and placebo comparisons to clinical trials involving active treatment conditions. Collectively, these investigations have begun to provide valuable information regarding effective treatments for childhood anxiety. However, a number of critical issues and questions remain to be addressed.

The ADAA National Institute of Mental Health (NIMH)-sponsored conference on treating anxiety disorders in youth (ADAA, 1999) identified several critical research needs pertaining to the treatment of childhood anxiety disorders. These include: (1) the need for research designs other than waitlist controls, including comparisons with specific and nonspecific placebo controls and comparisons of CBT and medication along with their combination; (2) the need for more studies investigating mechanisms of action and the process of treatment delivery; (3) the need to address the high placebo response rates characteristic of many extant treatment studies; (4) the need to broaden the definition of "treatment effectiveness" by moving away from reliance on strict, singular indicators and including other measures of improvement, including behavioral observation, physiological and psychological measures, and assessments conducted blind to treatment condition; (5) the need to evaluate the clinical significance of treatment effectiveness through the greater use of comparisons to nonclinic reference groups; (6) the need to expand intervention targets (away from the sole focus on the individual child) to include more contextually valid arenas such as the family, school, and community systems; (7) the need to identify and evaluate potential predictors and inhibitors of treatment outcome such as demographic status, comorbidity, severity, and family and school environments; and (8) the need to address long-term follow-up with special emphasis on relapse rates, continued treatment gains, and factors that attenuate or enhance treatment outcome with respect to both acute symptomatology and individual and familial functioning.

Only within the last 5–10 years have clinical trials for child anxiety disorders replaced case-study designs, and of these controlled trials most have employed waitlist control groups (Kendall, 1994; Barrett et al., 1996a; Kendall et al., 1997). Clearly, these waitlist controlled trials were an important step forward and characteristic of the development of a relatively young field of study. More recent efforts to compare CBT to nonspecific treatments such as psychoeducation have yielded mixed results, with both groups showing similar, albeit significant, improvement (Last et al., 1998; Silverman et al., 1999b). Whether or not these results reflect the instability of anxiety symptoms over time, the inadvertent inclusion of cognitive and/or behavioral techniques in the comparison treatments, or the possibility that the efficacy of

CBT is actually due to nonspecific elements of the intervention remains unclear. Studies involving active contrasts have been primarily limited to comparisons of CBT delivered in different formats, yet these studies provide evidence for the flexibility and exportability of this treatment (Barrett et al., 1996a; Mendlowitz et al., 1999).

As the efficacy of CBT for childhood anxiety becomes more firmly established, dismantling, constructive, and parametric studies will be needed to establish which features of this treatment package are critical to the creation of therapeutic change. While etiologic theories (such as the tripartite model) suggest the importance of both cognitive and behavioral components (and perhaps family components as well), only limited evidence exists addressing the incremental contribution of each of these components to treatment outcome (Barrett et al., 1996a; Silverman et al., 1999b). It is unclear whether the various treatment components employed in CBT for childhood anxiety work together in an additive or interactional manner (Borkovec, 1994).

The identification of treatment moderators and of differentially effective treatment components will play an important role in the development of prescriptive treatment approaches (i.e., approaches that seek to match specific treatment techniques to specific symptoms or symptom clusters). Pertinent to cognitive researchers, the relationship between specific cognitive variables and treatment selection and outcome has yet to be examined. Aside from Barrett et al. (1996a), who reported that younger children and females responded better to family involvement in CBT, the search for moderators and mediators of treatment outcome has not yielded significant findings (Treadwell et al., 1995; Silverman et al., 1999a). Nevertheless, initial efforts at treatment matching, such as that by Eisen and Silverman (1993, 1998), which sought to link treatment techniques to symptoms based on hypothesized etiologic processes, have yielded promising results.

For this promise to be fully realized, however, additional work is needed to elucidate further the etiologic mechanisms underlying the expression and maintenance of anxiety symptoms in children. This includes efforts to identify better and clarify both maladaptive and protective cognitive processes, studies examining behavioral parameters related to fear acquisition and conditioning, and the investigation of the biological, physiological, and neurocognitive processes underlying these domains. Finally, an enhanced understanding of the interplay among these components (à la tripartite model) will play a key role in the development of more efficiently targeted and effective interventions.

Recent and ongoing studies have begun to establish the efficacy of psychopharmacologic interventions, primarily the serotonin reuptake inhibitors, for the treatment of child anxiety disorders (March, 1999; Research Units in Pediatric Psychopharmacology (RUPP) Anxiety Study Group, 2001). As a result, research is needed to examine the efficacy of CBT as compared to that for psychopharmacologic treatment and to identify optimal strategies for selecting CBT versus medication and for sequencing and combining these two treatments. A large NIMH-funded multisite study conducted by a multidisciplinary group of CBT and psychopharmacologic treatment researchers, the Child and Adolescent Anxiety Multisite Study (CAMS) is just now getting under way to address some of these issues.

Finally, further research is needed to establish the exportability of manualized CBT treatment approaches from largely university-based settings to community, school, and hospital-based populations and to enhance efforts aimed at preventing the development of anxiety disturbance in at-risk children and adolescents. Along these latter lines, recent work by Dadds and colleagues (Dadds et al., 1999; Lowry-Webster et al., 2001) has demonstrated that universal school-based CBT programs can be effective in both preventing the onset of anxiety disorders in high-risk (e.g., subthreshold) youngsters and in reducing the level of disturbance in youngsters with preexisting anxiety disorder. Significantly larger sample sizes than those utilized to date as well as more representative community samples will be needed to achieve the research agenda outlined above. To meet this need, future studies will likely require multisite and multidisciplinary collaborative research teams rather than the single-site approach now commonplace in most childhood anxiety research.

The treatment research literature to date has yielded a number of highly promising and effective interventions for childhood anxiety disorders. The results from even more sophisticated treatment designs and continued efforts investigating the etiological underpinnings of child anxiety and their relationship to treatment outcome should greatly enhance our ability to address this important mental health problem. Eventually it may be that these research efforts will provide clinicians with the necessary knowledge to develop prescriptive interventions in which specific treatment techniques are individually packaged for a given child based on the unique pattern of the underlying behavioral, cognitive, and familial determinants of his or her anxiety symptomatology.

REFERENCES

Achenbach, T., Howell, C., McConaughy, S., and Stanger, C. (1995). Six-year predictors of problems in a national sample of children and youth: I. Cross-informant syndromes. *Journal of the American Academy of Child and Adolescent Psychiatry*, **34**, 336–47.

American Psychiatric Association. (1994). *Diagnostic and Statistical Manual of Mental Disorders*, 4th edn. Washington, DC: APA.

Anxiety Disorders Association of America (ADAA). (1999). *Treating Anxiety Disorders in Youth: Current Problems and Future Solutions*, pp. 63–76. Washington, DC: Anxiety Disorder Association of America.

Bandura, A., Grusec, J., and Menlove, F. (1967). Vicarious extinction of avoidance behavior. *Journal of Personality and Social Psychology*, **5**, 16–23.

Barabasz, A. F. (1973). Group desensitization of test anxiety in elementary school. *Journal of Psychology*, **83**, 295–301.

Barlow, D. H. (1988). *Anxiety and its Disorders: The Nature and Treatment of Anxiety and Panic.* New York: Guilford Press.

Barrett, P., Dadds, M., and Rapee, R. (1996a). Family treatment of childhood anxiety: a controlled trial. *Journal of Consulting and Clinical Psychology*, **64**, 333–42.

Barrett, P., Rapee, R., Dadds, M., and Ryan, S. (1996b). Family enhancement of cognitive styles in anxious and aggressive children. *Journal of Abnormal Child Psychology*, **24**, 187–203.

Beck, A., Rush, A., Shaw, B., and Emery, G. (1979). *Cognitive Therapy of Depression.* New York: Guilford Press.

Beidel, D. and Turner, S. (1997). At risk for anxiety: I. Psychopathology in the offspring of anxious parents. *Journal of the American Academy of Child and Adolescent Psychiatry*, **36**, 918–24.

Bell-Dolan, D. and Wessler, A. (1994). Attributional style of anxious children: extensions from cognitive theory and research on adult anxiety. *Journal of Anxiety Disorders*, **8**, 79–96.

Benjamin, R., Costello, E., and Warren, M. (1990). Anxiety disorders in a pediatric sample. *Journal of Anxiety Disorders*, **4**, 293–316.

Bernstein, G. and Borchardt, C. (1991). Anxiety disorders of childhood and adolescence: a critical review. *Journal of the American Academy of Child and Adolescent Psychiatry*, **30**, 519–32.

Biederman, J., Rosenbaum, J., Hirshfeld, D., et al. (1990). Psychiatric correlates of behavioral inhibition in young children of parents with and without psychiatric disorders. *Archives of General Psychiatry*, **47**, 21–6.

Biederman, J., Rosenbaum, J., Bolduc-Murphy, E., et al. (1993). A 3-year follow-up of children with and without behavioral inhibition. *Journal of the American Academy of Child and Adolescent Psychiatry*, **32**, 814–21.

Birmaher, B., Waterman, G. S., Ryan, N., et al. (1994). Fluoxetine for childhood anxiety disorders. *Journal of the American Academy of Child and Adolescent Psychiatry*, **33**, 993–9.

Boegels, S. and Zigterman, D. (2000). Dysfunctional cognitions in children with social phobia, separation anxiety disorder, and generalized anxiety disorder. *Journal of Abnormal Child Psychology*, **28**, 205–11.

Borkovec, T. D. (1994). Between-group therapy outcome research: design and methodology. In *Behavioral Treatments for Drug Abuse and Dependence*, ed. L. S. Onken and J. D. Blaine, pp. 249–89. NIDA Research Monograph no. 137. Rockville, MD: National Institute of Drug Abuse.

Breslau, N., Davis, G., and Prabucki, K. (1987). Searching for evidence on the validity of generalized anxiety disorder: psychopathology in children of anxious mothers. *Psychiatry Research*, **20**, 285–97.

Butler, G. and Mathews, A. (1983). Cognitive processes in anxiety. *Advances in Behaviour Research and Therapy*, **5**, 51–62.

Chambless, D. and Gillis, M. (1993). Cognitive therapy of anxiety disorders. *Journal of Consulting and Clinical Psychology*, **61**, 248–60.

Chen, E., Lewin, M., and Craske, M. (1996). Effects of state anxiety on selective processing of threatening information. *Cognition and Emotion*, **10**, 225–40.

Clark, D. and Steer, R. (1996). Empirical status of the cognitive model. In *Frontiers of Cognitive Therapy*, ed. P. Salkovkis pp. 75–96. New York: Guilford Press.

Costello, E. and Angold, A. (1995). Epidemiology. In *Anxiety Disorders in Children and Adolescents*, ed. J. S. March, pp. 109–24. New York: Guilford.

Craske, M. (1999). *Anxiety Disorders: Psychological Approaches to Theory and Treatment*. Colorado: Westview Press.

Dadds, M., Holland, D., Laurens, K., et al. (1999). Early intervention and prevention of anxiety disorders in children: results at 2-year follow-up. *Journal of Consulting and Clinical Psychology*, **67**, 145–50.

Eisen, A. and Silverman, W. (1993). Should I relax or change my thoughts? A preliminary examination of cognitive therapy, relaxation training, and their combination with overanxious children. *Journal of Cognitive Psychotherapy: An International Quarterly*, **7**, 265–79.

Eisen, A. and Silverman, W. (1998). Prescriptive treatment for generalized anxiety disorder in children. *Behavior Therapy*, **29**, 105–21.

Epkins, C. (1996). Cognitive specificity and affective confounding in social anxiety and dysphoria in children. *Journal of Psychopathology and Behavioral Assessment*, **18**, 83–101.

Ferdinand, R. and Verhulst, F. (1995). Psychopathology from adolescence into young adulthood: an 8-year follow-up study. *American Journal of Psychiatry*, **152**, 586–94.

Fyer, A., Mannuzza, S., Chapman, T., Liebowitz, M., and Klein, D. (1993). A direct interview family study of social phobia. *Archives of General Psychiatry*, **50**, 286–93.

Fyer, A., Mannuzza, S., Chapman, T., Martin, L., and Klein, D. (1995). Specificity in familial aggregation of phobic disorders. *Archives of General Psychiatry*, **52**, 564–73.

Ginsburg, G., Silverman, W., and Kurtines, W. (1995). Family involvement in treating children with phobic and anxiety disorders: a look ahead. *Clinical Psychology Review*, **15**, 457–73.

Graziano, A. and Mooney, K. (1980). Family self-control instruction for children's nighttime fear reduction. *Journal of Consulting and Clinical Psychology*, **48**, 206–13.

Hayward, C., Killen, J., Kraemer, H., and Taylor, C. (1998). Linking self-reported childhood behavioral inhibition to adolescent social phobia. *Journal of the American Academy of Child and Adolescent Psychiatry*, **37**, 1–9.

Hill, J., Liebert, R., and Mott, D. (1968). Vicarious extinction of avoidance behavior through films: an initial test. *Psychological Reports*, **22**, 192.

Hirshfeld, D., Rosenbaum, J., Biederman, J., et al. (1992). Stable behavioral inhibition and its association with anxiety disorders. *Journal of the American Academy of Child and Adolescent Psychiatry*, **31**, 103–11.

Ialongo, N., Edelsohn, G., Werthamer-Larsson, L., and Kellam, S. (1994). The significance of self-reported anxious symptoms in first-grade children. *Journal of Abnormal Child Psychiatry*, **22**, 441–55.

Kagan, J., Reznick, J., and Snidman, N. (1987). The physiology and psychology of behavioral inhibition in children. *Child Development*, **58**, 59–73.

Kagan, J., Reznick, J., and Gibbons, J. (1989). Inhibited and uninhibited types of children. *Child Development*, **60**, 838–45.

Kendall, P. (1993). Cognitive-behavioral therapies with youth: guiding theory, current status, and emerging developments. *Journal of Consulting and Clinical Psychology*, **61**, 235–47.

Kendall, P. (1994). Treating anxiety disorders in children: results of a randomized clinical trial. *Journal of Consulting and Clinical Psychology*, **62**, 100–10.

Kendall, P. and Brady, E. (1995). Comorbidity in the anxiety disorders of childhood. In *Anxiety and Depression in Adults and Children*, ed. K. Craig and K. Dobson, pp. 3–36. Newbury Park, CA: Sage Publications.

Kendall, P. and Southam-Gerow, M. (1996). Long-term follow-up of a cognitive behavioral therapy for anxiety disordered youth. *Journal of Consulting and Clinical Psychology*, **64**, 724–30.

Kendall, P., Chansky, T., Kane, M., et al. (1992). *Anxiety Disorders in Youth: Cognitive-behavioral Interventions*. Needham Heights, MA: Allyn and Bacon.

Kendall, P., Flannery-Schroeder, E., Panicelli-Mindel, S., et al. (1997). Therapy for youths with anxiety disorders: a second randomized clinical trial. *Journal of Consulting and Clinical Psychology*, **65**, 366–80.

Kendler, K., Neale, M., Kessler, R., Heath, A., and Eaves, L. (1992a). Generalized anxiety disorder in women: a population based twin study. *Archives of General Psychiatry*, **49**, 267–72.

Kendler, K., Neale, M., Kessler, R., Heath, A., and Eaves, L. (1992b). The genetic epidemiology of phobias in women. *Archives of General Psychiatry*, **49**, 273–81.

Kessler, R., McGonagle, K., Zhao, S., et al. (1994). Lifetime and 12-month prevalence of DSM-III-R psychiatric disorders in the United States. *Archives of General Psychiatry*, **51**, 8–19.

King, N. and Ollendick, T. (1997). Annotation: treatment of childhood phobias. *Journal of Child Psychology and Psychiatry*, **38**, 389–400.

King, N., Mietz, A., Tinney, L., and Ollendick, T. (1995). Psychopathology and cognition in adolescents experiencing severe test anxiety. *Journal of Clinical Child Psychology*, **24**, 49–54.

Klein, R. G. (1995). Anxiety disorders. In *Child and Adolescent Psychiatry: Modern Approaches*, ed. M. Rutter, E. Taylor, and L. Hersov, pp. 351–74. London: Blackwell Scientific.

Kondas, O. (1967). Reduction of examination anxiety and "stage fright" by group desensitization and relaxation. *Behaviour Research and Therapy*, **5**, 275–81.

Kuroda, J. (1969). Elimination of children's fears of animals by the method of experimental desensitization: an application of learning theory to child psychology. *Psychologia*, **12**, 161–5.

Lang, P. J. (1971). The application of psychophysiological methods to the study of psychotherapy and behavior modification. In *Handbook of Psychotherapy and Behavior Change: An Empirical Analysis*, ed. A. E. Bergin and S. L. Garfield, pp. 75–125. New York: Wiley.

Last, C., Strauss, C., and Francis, G. (1987). Comorbidity among childhood anxiety disorders. *Journal of Nervous and Mental Disease*, **175**, 726–30.

Last, C., Hersen, M., Kazdin, A., Orvaschel, H., and Perrin, S. (1991). Anxiety disorders in children and their families. *Archives of General Psychiatry*, **48**, 928–34.

Last, C., Hansen, C., and Franco, N. (1998). Cognitive-behavioral treatment of school phobia. *Journal of the American Academy of Child and Adolescent Psychiatry*, **37**, 404–11.

Laurent, J. and Stark, K. (1993). Testing the cognitive content-specificity hypothesis with anxious and depressed youngsters. *Journal of Abnormal Psychology*, **102**, 226–37.

Leitenberg, H. and Callahan, E. (1973). Reinforced practice and reduction of different kinds of fears in adults and children. *Behaviour Research and Therapy*, **11**, 19–30.

Leitenberg, H., Yost, L., and Carroll-Wilson, M. (1986). Negative cognitive errors in children. *Journal of Consulting and Clinical Psychology*, **54**, 528–36.

Lewis, S. (1974). A comparison of behavior therapy techniques in the reduction of fearful avoidance behavior. *Behavior Therapy*, **5**, 648–55.

Lowry-Webster, H., Barrett, P., and Dadds, M. (2001). A universal prevention trial of anxiety and depressive symptomatology in childhood: preliminary data from an Australian study. *Behaviour Change*, **18**, 36–50.

Mann, J. and Rosenthal, T. (1969). Vicarious and direct counter-conditioning of test anxiety through individual and group desensitization. *Behaviour Research and Therapy*, **7**, 359–67.

March, J. (1999). Pharmacotherapy of pediatric anxiety disorders: a critical review. In *Treating Anxiety Disorders in Youth: Current Problems and Future Solutions*, ed. D. Beidel, pp. 42–62. Washington, DC: Anxiety Disorders Association of America.

March, J. and Mulle, K. (1998). *OCD in Children and Adolescents: A Cognitive-Behavioral Treatment Manual*. New York: Guilford Press.

March, J., Amaya-Jackson, L., Murry, M., and Schulte, A. (1998). Cognitive-behavioral psychotherapy for children and adolescents with post-traumatic stress disorder following a single incident stressor. *Journal of the American Academy of Child and Adolescent Psychiatry*, **37**, 585–93.

Martin, M., Horder, P., and Jones, G. (1992). Integral bias in naming of phobia-related words. *Cognition and Emotion*, **6**, 479–86.

Mathews, A., Richards, A., and Eyesenck, M. (1989). The interpretation of homophones related to threat cues in anxiety states. *Journal of Abnormal Psychology*, **98**, 31–4.

Mazur, E., Wolchik, S., and Sandler, I. (1992). Negative cognitive errors and positive illusions for negative divorce events: predictors of children's psychological adjustment. *Journal of Abnormal Child Psychology*, **20**, 523–42.

Mendlowitz, S., Manassis, K., Bradley, S., et al. (1999). Cognitive-behavioral group treatments in childhood anxiety disorders. *Journal of the American Academy of Child and Adolescent Psychiatry*, **38**, 1233–9.

Menzies, R. and Clarke, J. (1993). A comparison of in vivo and vicarious exposure in the treatment of childhood water phobia. *Behaviour Research and Therapy*, **31**, 9–15.

Messer, S. and Beidel, D. (1994). Psychosocial correlates of childhood anxiety disorders. *Journal of the American Academy of Child and Adolescent Psychiatry*, **33**, 975–83.

Miller, L., Barrett, C., Hampe, E., and Noble, H. (1972). Comparison of reciprocal inhibition, psychotherapy, and waiting list control for phobic children. *Journal of Abnormal Psychology*, **79**, 269–79.

Mogg, K., Mathews, A., and Weinman, J. (1989). Selective processing of threat cues in anxiety states: a replication. *Behaviour Research and Therapy*, **27**, 317–23.

Obler, M. and Terwilliger, R. (1970). Pilot study on the effectiveness of systematic desensitization with neurologically impaired children with phobic disorders. *Journal of Consulting and Clinical Psychology*, **34**, 314–18.

Ollendick, T. H. (1979). Fear reduction techniques with children. In *Progress in Behavior Modification*, vol. 8, ed. M. Hersen, R. Eisler, and P. Miller, pp. 127–68. New York: Academic.

Ollendick, T. H. (1995). Cognitive behavioral treatment of panic disorder with agoraphobia in adolescents: a multiple baseline design analysis. *Behavior Therapy*, **26**, 517–31.

Ollendick, T. H. and King, N. (1994). Diagnosis, assessment, and treatment of internalizing problems in children: the role of longitudinal data. *Journal of Consulting and Clinical Psychology*, **62**, 918–27.

Ollendick, T. H. and King, N. (1998). Empirically supported treatments for children with phobic and anxiety disorders. *Journal of Clinical Child Psychology*, **27**, 156–67.

Piacentini, J. (1999). Cognitive behavior therapy for child and adolescent OCD. *Child and Adolescent Clinics of North America*, **8**, 599–618.

Piacentini, J. and Bergman, R. L. (2001). Developmental issues in cognitive therapy for childhood anxiety disorders. *Journal of Cognitive Psychotherapy*, **15**, 165–82.

Pine, D. (1994). Child–adult anxiety disorders. *Journal of the American Academy of Child and Adolescent Psychiatry*, **33**, 280.

Pine, D., Cohen, P., Gurley, D., Brook, J., and Ma, Y. (1998). The risk for early-adulthood anxiety and depressive disorders in adolescents with anxiety and depressive disorders. *Archives of General Psychiatry*, **55**, 56–64.

Prins, P. (1986). Children's self-speech and self-regulation during a fear-provoking behavioral test. *Behavior Research and Therapy*, **35**, 159–63.

Rachman, S. (1977). The conditioning theory of fear acquisition: a critical examination. *Behaviour Research and Therapy*, **15**, 375–87.

Rachman, S. and Hodgson, R. (1974). Synchrony and desynchrony in fear and avoidance. *Behaviour Research and Therapy*, **12**, 311–18.

Rapee, R. (2001). The development of generalized anxiety. In *The Developmental Psychopathology of Anxiety*, ed. M. W. Vasey and M. R. Dadds, pp. 481–503. New York: Oxford Press.

Research Units in Pediatric Psychopharmacology (RUPP) Anxiety Study Group. (2001). An eight week placebo-controlled trial of fluvoxamine for anxiety disorders in children and adolescents. *New England Journal of Medicine*, **344**, 1279–85.

Ritter, B. (1968). The group desensitization of children's snake phobias using vicarious and contact desensitization procedures. *Behaviour Research and Therapy*, **6**, 1–6.

Ronan, K. and Kendall, P. (1997). Self-talk in distressed youth: states-of-mind and content specificity. *Journal of Clinical Child Psychology*, **26**, 330–7.

Ronan, K., Kendall, P., and Rowe, M. (1994). Negative affectivity in children: development and validation of a questionnaire. *Cognitive Therapy and Research*, **18**, 509–28.

Rosenbaum, J., Biederman, J., Bolduc-Murphy, E., et al. (1993). Behavioral inhibition in childhood: a risk factor for anxiety disorders. *Harvard Review of Psychiatry*, **1**, 2–16.

Shaffer, D., Fisher, P., Dulcan, M., et al. (1996). The NIMH Diagnostic Interview Schedule for Children. Version 2.3 (DISC 2.3): description, acceptability, prevalence rates, and performance in the MECA study. *Journal of the American Academy of Child and Adolescent Psychiatry*, **49**, 865–77.

Sheslow, D., Bondy, A., and Nelson, R. O. (1983). A comparison of graduated exposure, verbal coping skills, and their combination in the treatment of children's fear of the dark. *Child and Family Behavior Therapy*, **4**, 33–45.

Silverman, W. and Kurtines, W. (1996). *Anxiety and Phobic Disorders: A Pragmatic Approach.* New York, NY: Plenum Press.

Silverman, W., Cerny, J., and Nelles, W. (1988). The familial influence in anxiety disorders: studies on the offspring of patients with anxiety disorders. In *Advances in Clinical Child Psychology*, ed. B. B. Lahey and A. E. Kazdin, pp. 223–47. New York: Plenum Press.

Silverman, W., Ginsburg, G., and Kurtines, W. (1995). Clinical issues in treating children with anxiety and phobic disorders. *Cognitive and Behavioral Practice*, **2**, 93–117.

Silverman, W., Kurtines, W., Ginsburg, G., et al. (1999a). Treating anxiety disorders in children with group cognitive-behavioral therapy: a randomized clinical trial. *Journal of Consulting and Clinical Psychology*, **67**, 995–1003.

Silverman, W., Kurtines, W., Ginsburg, G., et al. (1999b). Contingency management, self-control, and education support in the treatment of childhood phobic disorders: a randomized clinical trial. *Journal of Consulting and Clinical Psychology*, **67**, 675–87.

Spence, S., Donovan, C., and Brechman-Toussaint, M. (1999). Social skills, social outcomes, and cognitive features of childhood social phobia. *Journal of Abnormal Psychology*, **108**, 211–21.

Torgersen, S. (1983). Genetic factors in anxiety disorders. *Archives of General Psychiatry*, **40**, 1085–9.

Treadwell, K., Flannery, E., and Kendall, P. (1995). Ethnicity and gender in relation to adaptive functioning, diagnostic status, and treatment outcome in children from an anxiety clinic. *Journal of Anxiety Disorders*, **9**, 373–84.

Turner, S. and Heiser, N. (1999). Current status of psychological interventions for childhood anxiety disorders. In *Treating Anxiety Disorders in Youth: Current Problems and Future Solutions*, ed. D. Beidel, pp. 63–76. Washington, DC: Anxiety Disorders Association of America.

Turner, S., Beidel, D., and Costello, A. (1987). Psychopathology in the offspring of anxiety disorders patients. *Journal of Consulting and Clinical Psychology*, **55**, 229–35.

Ultee, C., Griffioen, D., and Schellekens, J. (1982). The reduction of anxiety in children: a comparison of the effects of "systematic desensitization in vitro" and "systematic desensitization in vivo." *Behaviour Research and Therapy*, **20**, 61–7.

Vasey, M., Daleiden, E., Williams, L., and Brown, L. (1995). Biased attention in childhood anxiety disorders: a preliminary study. *Journal of Abnormal Child Psychology*, **23**, 267–79.

Vasey, M., El-Hag, N., and Daleiden, E. (1996). Anxiety and the processing of emotionally threatening stimuli: distinctive patterns of selective attention among high- and low-test-anxious children. *Child Development*, **67**, 1173–85.

Weems, C., Berman, S., Silverman, W., and Saavedra, L. (2001). Cognitive errors in youth with anxiety disorders: the linkages between negative cognitive errors and anxious symptoms. *Cognitive Therapy and Research*, **25**, 559–75.

Whaley, S., Pinto, A., and Sigman, M. (1999). Characterizing interactions between anxious mothers and their children. *Journal of Consulting and Clinical Psychology*, **67**, 826–36.

Wolpe, J. (1958). *Psychotherapy by Reciprocal Inhibition*. Stanford, CA: Stanford University Press.

17

Attention deficit/hyperactivity disorder

Arthur D. Anastopoulos,[1] E. Paige Temple,[2] and Stephanie D. Shaffer[1]

[1] University of North Carolina at Greensboro, NC, USA
[2] Department of Psychology, Chapel Hill, NC, USA

Attention deficit/hyperactivity disorder (AD/HD; American Psychiatric Association, 1994) is the most recent in a long line of diagnostic labels used to describe individuals who display developmentally inappropriate levels of inattention, impulsivity, and/or hyperactivity. Prior to 1994, children displaying many of these same behavioral features might have been identified as having attention deficit disorder (ADD), hyperkinetic reaction of childhood, or minimal brain dysfunction. Although confusing to some, such changes in diagnostic terminology have not been without purpose. On the contrary, each labeling change has reflected important changes in the conceptualization of this disorder.

As recently as 15 years ago, it was not unusual to find people – lay individuals and healthcare professionals alike – who believed that AD/HD was a condition limited to childhood. Hence, the advice often given to parents was: "Hang in there, once children reach the teen years, they outgrow their AD/HD." We now know that nothing could be further from the truth. Not only does AD/HD occur during adolescence, it can also be found among a significant number of adults. In light of this finding, most experts in the field today view AD/HD to be a chronic condition that persists across the lifespan (Weiss and Hechtman, 1993; Barkley, 1998).

Of what relevance is cognitive therapy to the clinical management of AD/HD? To answer this question, it is first necessary to have a better understanding of what AD/HD is, and how it presents itself across the lifespan. To this end, this chapter will begin with a brief overview of this disorder. Against this background, it will then review some of the major etiological conceptualizations of AD/HD that have been put forth, including cognitive theories. The empirical support that exists for these cognitive perspectives will be considered next. This will be followed by a discussion of the various ways in which cognitive interventions may be employed with this population.

Clinical presentation

Diagnostic criteria

The diagnostic criteria for AD/HD appear in the fourth edition of the *Diagnostic and Statistical Manual* (DSM-IV; American Psychiatric Association, 1994). To receive a diagnosis of AD/HD, an individual must first display a high enough frequency of its primary symptoms. In keeping with the results of factor-analytic studies, DSM-IV presents these primary symptoms in two lists – one pertaining to inattention symptoms (e.g., often fails to give close attention to details, often has difficulty sustaining attention to task, often does not seem to listen when spoken to directly, often does not follow through on instructions, often has difficulty organizing tasks, often is easily distracted), the other related to hyperactivity-impulsivity concerns (e.g., often fidgets, often leaves seat, often is on the go, often talks excessively, often blurts out answers, often has difficulty awaiting turn, often interrupts). To meet the frequency requirement, DSM-IV stipulates that at least six of nine inattention symptoms and/or six of nine hyperactive-impulsive symptoms must be present. If so, there must also be evidence that these symptoms occur in two or more settings and that they are associated with some degree of functional impairment in an individual's daily life. Moreover, these symptoms must be developmentally deviant, have a duration of 6 months, arise prior to 7 years, and not be due to other medical and mental health conditions that better account for their existence.

According to these guidelines, *all* AD/HD diagnoses must now be accompanied by one of several possible subtyping distinctions. What mainly distinguishes one major subtype from another is whether or not the criteria for one or both primary symptom lists are met. For example, if six or more symptoms from both lists are present, and if all other AD/HD criteria are met, AD/HD, combined type (code 314.01) is the appropriate diagnosis. When there are six or more inattention symptoms, but fewer than six hyperactivity-impulsivity symptoms present, and all other AD/HD criteria are met, a diagnosis of AD/HD, predominantly inattentive type (314.00) is in order. The other possible scenario that might unfold is when there are six or more hyperactivity-impulsivity symptoms, but fewer than six inattention symptoms present. Assuming that all other AD/HD criteria are met, the proper diagnosis for this situation is AD/HD, predominantly hyperactive-impulsive type (314.01).

Many individuals incorrectly regard the predominantly inattentive and the predominantly hyperactive-impulsive classifications as pure or exclusive subtyping categories. For example, if a child has the predominantly inattentive subtype of AD/HD, many parents, teachers, and child healthcare professionals automatically assume that the child *only* displays inattentive features. Although these subtyping categories certainly can be exclusive at times, the manner in which they are defined would suggest that this was not DSM-IV's intent. A useful way to understand this situation more fully is to consider how these subtyping categories might apply to two children with very similar behavioral features. One child, for example, might display six inattention symptoms but only five hyperactive-impulsive symptoms, and therefore carry a diagnosis of AD/HD, predominantly inattentive type. The other child might have a combination of five inattention symptoms and six hyperactive-impulsive symptoms, for which AD/HD, predominantly hyperactive-impulsive type is the appropriate diagnosis. To think of the former child as having *only* inattention difficulties and the latter as having *only* hyperactive-impulsive concerns would obviously be inaccurate. In view of this possibility, clinicians and researchers must bear in mind that both subtyping categories can include symptoms that go beyond what is suggested in their labeling. Thus, a child with the predominantly inattentive type can have subclinical hyperactive-impulsive features that require therapeutic attention. Conversely, the same is true for the predominantly hyperactive-impulsive classification.

Although educators and child healthcare professionals in Europe and in many other parts of the world would certainly agree that symptoms of inattention and/or hyperactivity-impulsivity constitute a diagnostic condition, they would not refer to it as AD/HD nor would they follow DSM-IV guidelines in deciding whether or not a diagnosis was present. If any diagnosis were to be made at all, it would be hyperkinetic disorder, the criteria for which appear in the 10th edition of the *International Classification of Diseases* (ICD-10; World Health Organization, 1993). Somewhat akin to DSM-IV, ICD-10 uses separate symptom listings, encompassing a total of 18 symptoms. Unlike DSM-IV, however, ICD-10 utilizes a nine-item inattention list, a five-item hyperactivity list, and a four-item list of impulsivity symptoms, each of which also differs in the symptom cut-off points that they employ. For example, at least six inattention symptoms, three hyperactivity symptoms, and one impulsivity symptom must be present before considering a hyperkinetic disorder diagnosis. ICD-10 further requires that these symptoms: (1) have an early childhood onset no later than 7 years of age; (2) have a duration of at least 6 months; (3) be developmentally deviant; and (4) not be due to pervasive developmental disorder or certain other psychiatric conditions (e.g., mood disorder).

What should be apparent is that the DSM-IV and ICD-10 diagnostic guidelines are similar in a number of ways. This is not a chance occurrence, as systematic efforts were made during the development of DSM-IV to create a classification system that would allow for direct comparison with equivalent ICD-10 disorders. Thus, the content of the symptom lists overlaps across the two systems. Their criteria for onset and duration, as well as a portion of their exclusionary criteria, are similar as well. Both systems also require clear evidence of cross-situational pervasiveness.

Amidst these many similarities, significant differences exist. Perhaps the most important of these is that ICD-10 does not allow for any diagnostic subtyping involving the primary features of hyperkinetic disorder. Thus, any comparisons between DSM-IV and ICD-10 must necessarily be limited to a consideration of AD/HD, combined type, and hyperkinetic disorder, respectively. A related concern is that, with only one form of hyperkinetic disorder available for consideration, fewer individuals would be expected to receive this type of clinical diagnosis. To the extent that this is a valid assumption, it would have tremendous clinical and research implications. Another important difference between ICD-10 and DSM-IV may be found among their exclusionary criteria. In ICD-10, the co-occurring presence of a depressive episode or an anxiety disorder automatically precludes making a diagnosis of hyperkinetic disorder. Although DSM-IV recognizes that such conditions can preclude an AD/HD diagnosis, it also allows for the possibility that they might instead be comorbid with AD/HD.

Situational variability

Contrary to the belief of many individuals, AD/HD is not an all-or-none phenomenon, either always present or never present. Instead, it is a condition whose primary symptoms show significant fluctuations in response to different situational demands (Zentall, 1985). One of the most important factors determining this variation is the degree to which children with AD/HD are interested in what they are doing. AD/HD symptoms are much more likely to occur in situations that are highly repetitive, boring, or familiar, versus those that are novel or stimulating (Barkley, 1977). Another determinant of situational variation is the amount of imposed structure. In many free-play or low-demand settings, where children with AD/HD have the freedom to do as they please, their behavior is often indistinguishable from that of normal children (Luk, 1985). Significant AD/HD problems may arise, however, when others place demands on them or set rules for their behavior. Presumably due to increased demands for behavioral self-regulation, group settings are far more problematic for children with AD/HD than would be the case in one-to-one situations. There is also an increased likelihood for AD/HD symptoms to arise in situations where feedback is dispensed infrequently and/or on a delayed basis (Douglas, 1983).

In view of this tendency for AD/HD symptoms to be subject to situational variability, it should come as no great surprise that children with AD/HD often display tremendous inconsistency in their task performance, both in terms of their productivity and accuracy (Douglas, 1972). Such variability may be evident with respect to their in-class performance or test scores (e.g., getting a grade of 90 one day, 60 the next), or it may involve fluctuations in their completion of homework or routine home chores. Although it may be argued that all children display a certain amount of variability in their daily activities, it is clear from clinical experience and research that children with AD/HD exhibit this to a much greater degree. Thus, instead of reflecting "laziness," as some might infer from their behavior, the inconsistent performance of children with AD/HD may represent yet another manifestation of this disorder.

Prevalence

According to DSM-IV, the overall prevalence of AD/HD among children – that is, the sum total of all subtyping categories – is 3–5% (APA, 1994). Community-based estimates of the overall prevalence have ranged from 7.5% to 21.6% for both parent- and teacher-generated samples (Wolraich, et al., 1996; Gaub and Carlson, 1997; DuPaul et al., 1998). That these would be higher than the 3–5% prevalence described in DSM-IV is not at all surprising, given that the community rates were derived primarily on the basis of the AD/HD symptom frequency requirement alone. Having been determined in this way, such figures very likely include many children for whom AD/HD would not be diagnosed, due to the fact that they would not meet all of the necessary DSM-IV criteria.

Among clinic samples (Lahey et al., 1994), the combined type would appear to be the most commonly encountered subtype category, whereas the inattentive type occurs most often in community samples (Wolraich et al., 1996; Gaub and Carlson, 1997; DuPaul et al., 1998). According to teachers, younger children display the combined subtype most often, whereas older children and adolescents are much more likely to be identified with the inattentive classification (DuPaul et al., 1997). Similar findings have emerged from parent ratings of older children and adolescents, but parents are much more likely to identify very young children as having the hyperactive-impulsive subtype (DuPaul et al., 1998). Of additional interest is that the overall prevalence of DSM-IV-defined AD/HD – that is, the total for all three major subtypes – seems to decline with age. In terms of gender issues, boys outnumber girls across all subtypes, with ratios ranging from 6:1 to 9:1 in clinic samples and 1.3:1 to 3.3:1 in community samples, depending on the informant and subtype under consideration (Arnold, 1996). Although there have been some indications that AD/HD appears more often among those from lower socio-economic (Szatmari, 1992) and minority (DuPaul et al., 1998) backgrounds, the exact distribution of this disorder across the socioeconomic spectrum and across different cultures is not well established.

Developmental course

Most individuals with AD/HD begin to display their symptoms in early childhood, with hyperactive-impulsive difficulties typically preceding inattention. Most often such symptoms appear around 3–4 years, but they can also surface during infancy or upon school entrance. Upon reaching late childhood and early adolescence, many children with AD/HD begin to display significantly fewer hyperactive-impulsive symptoms. Some may also show a reduction in their overall level of inattention, but to a much lesser degree. This change in symptom presentation may help to explain why only 50–80% of the children identified as AD/HD will continue to meet full diagnostic criteria for this condition as adolescents (Barkley et al., 1990). Only 30% will continue to meet diagnostic criteria for this condition as adults (Gittelman et al., 1985; Mannuzza et al., 1993), but as many as 50% will continue to exhibit subclinical levels of these symptoms, which interfere with daily functioning (Weiss and Hechtman, 1993). The overall frequency of AD/HD symptoms seems to decline gradually across adulthood (Murphy and Barkley, 1996a). Unlike what has been observed for children and adolescents, such declines are evident for both hyperactive-impulsive and inattention symptoms.

Psychosocial impact

Having AD/HD places individuals at risk for a multitude of psychosocial difficulties across the lifespan. The exact nature of these complications is determined in large part by a consideration of what is considered typical or normal at any given stage of development. Preschoolers with AD/HD place enormous caretaking demands on their parents (Shelton et al., 1998) and frequently display aggressive behavior when interacting with siblings or peers (Campbell, 1990). Difficulties acquiring academic readiness skills may be evident as well, but these tend to be of less clinical concern than the family or peer problems that preschoolers present. As children with AD/HD move into the elementary school years, academic problems take on increasing importance (DuPaul and Stoner, 1994). Together with their ongoing family (Johnston, 1996) and peer relationship problems (Lahey et al., 1997), such school-based difficulties set the stage for the development of low self-esteem and other emotional concerns (August et al., 1996). Similar problems persist into adolescence, but on a much more intense level. New problems may develop as well (e.g., traffic violations, experimentation with alcohol and drugs), stemming from the increased demands for independence, self-regulation, and self-control that teenagers with AD/HD face (Klein and Mannuzza, 1991; Barkley et al., 1992). AD/HD can also make the transition into adulthood very difficult.

Particularly noteworthy in this regard are the obstacles that AD/HD imposes on adults in their efforts to establish and maintain a family or career (Murphy and Barkley, 1996b).

Comorbidity

In addition to being affected by its primary symptoms, individuals with AD/HD are at increased risk for having secondary or comorbid diagnoses. Preschoolers and children with AD/HD frequently display oppositional defiant disorder (ODD; Jensen et al., 1997). Among adolescents with AD/HD, conduct disorder is quite common (Barkley et al., 1991). When AD/HD is accompanied by either ODD or CD, there is also an increased risk for depression and anxiety disorders to be present (August et al., 1996). Antisocial personality disorder, major depression, and substance abuse are just a few of the many comorbid problems that may be found among adults with AD/HD (Klein and Mannuzza, 1991). In combination with AD/HD, such comorbid conditions increase the severity of an individual's overall psychosocial impairment, thereby making the prognosis for such individuals less favorable.

Etiology

Biological accounts

Among the studies that have examined the etiology of AD/HD, inconsistent findings have emerged, presumably due to cross-study differences in defining AD/HD samples, small sample sizes, and other methodological limitations. As a result of such circumstances, what we know about the etiology of AD/HD might best be described as theoretical rather than factual.

Bearing this limitation in mind, several lines of evidence point towards biological factors being involved in the etiology of AD/HD. Research has suggested that abnormalities in brain chemistry (Arnsten et al., 1996), brain structure (Castellanos et al., 1996), and brain function (Zametkin et al., 1990) may play an important role. Multiple pathways presumably lead to these abnormalities. Among these, genetic mechanisms (Biederman et al., 1992; Levy et al., 1997) and certain pregnancy complications, such as excessive maternal consumption of alcohol and/or nicotine (Streissguth et al., 1995), very likely account for a significant percentage of children who have AD/HD. For some children, AD/HD may be acquired after birth, resulting from head injury, elevated lead levels, and other biological complications.

Although the exact manner in which these biological pieces fit together is far from clear, recent findings have offered some interesting leads. Particularly promising is the possibility that recently identified dopamine gene defects (Cook et al., 1995; Lahoste et al., 1996) may be a precursor to the dopamine deficiencies that have been reported in the neurochemical literature (Raskin et al., 1984; Pliszka et al., 1996). These deficiencies in turn may be linked to some of the structural and functional abnormalities that have been observed, particularly in the frontostriatal region (Castellanos et al., 1996), where dopamine systems are known to be at work. These in turn set the stage for AD/HD to occur.

With further advances in medical technology, especially neuroimaging procedures, our understanding of these biological mechanisms should increase dramatically. In the meantime, it will remain important to continue integrating biological theories with psychological conceptualizations in order to arrive at a more complete understanding of this disorder.

Psychosocial conceptualizations

Although a few environmental theories have been proposed to explain AD/HD (Block, 1977; Willis and Lovaas, 1977; Jacobvitz and Sroufe, 1987), there is little empirical justification for claiming that poor parenting, chaotic home environments, or poverty *cause* AD/HD. The results of twin studies in particular have highlighted this limited role, by showing that less than 5% of the variance in AD/HD symptomatology can be accounted for by environmental factors (Levy et al., 1997). When AD/HD is found among children who come from such family circumstances, one might reasonably speculate that the parents of such children may themselves be individuals with childhood and adult histories of AD/HD. If so, this would help to explain why their homes might be so chaotic and, at the same time, provide support for a genetic explanation for the child's AD/HD condition. Under this same scenario, the resulting chaos in the home might then be viewed as a factor exacerbating, rather than causing, the child's preexisting, inborn AD/HD condition.

Psychological conceptualizations

Over the years numerous psychological theories have also been put forth to explain the manner in which AD/HD affects psychosocial functioning. Many of the early accounts, which did not have the benefit of the above-noted neurobiological findings, focused almost exclusively on attentional processes that were believed to be at the core of AD/HD difficulties. Although these attentional hypotheses were intuitively appealing and compatible with the diagnostic criteria that were in use at that time (i.e., DSM-III; APA, 1980), investigators soon began to question whether attentional deficits were truly core problems. The impetus for this challenge stemmed in part from the failure of such conceptualizations to account for why children with AD/HD displayed appropriate levels of attention in some situations and not others. In an effort to address this concern, investigators began to put forth alternative explanations, implicating core deficiencies in the regulation of behavior to situational demands (Routh, 1978), self-directed instruction (Kendall and Braswell, 1985), the self-regulation of arousal to environmental demands (Douglas, 1983), and rule-governed behavior (Barkley, 1981). Though differing somewhat, each of these alternative views shared the belief that poor executive functioning was a central problem.

Building on what is now known about the biology of AD/HD, more recent theories have taken on a distinctive neuropsychological flavor, emphasizing the impulsivity features of this disorder. For example, Quay (1997) has proposed that AD/HD stems from an impairment in a neurologically based behavioral inhibition system. In an extensive elaboration of this same theme, Barkley (1998) has contended that a deficit in behavioral inhibition leads to impairment in four major areas of executive functioning: working memory, emotion regulation, internalization of language, and reconstitution. Such deficits in executive functioning lead directly to the various academic, behavioral, and social deficits that are observed within AD/HD populations.

Cognitive models

Cognitive models of AD/HD and its associated features have periodically appeared in the literature over the past 30 years. Most of these models were inspired by the seminal work of Meichenbaum and Goodman (1971), who observed significant reductions in impulsivity among children participating in their cognitive self-instructional training (CSIT) program. Borrowing from the Russian psychologists, Vygotsky and Luria, Meichenbaum and Goodman (1971) constructed a theoretically driven treatment program that assumed that the behavioral difficulties of impulsive children stemmed from deficiencies in their verbal mediation skills. Mimicking the developmental progression that presumably led to the verbal control of behavior, CSIT began with an adult verbally coaching the child through the steps necessary to complete a task. Next, the adult encouraged the child to use overt language to guide his or her own behavior. Thereafter, the child would whisper self-instructions to guide his or her behavior. In the final step of the program, the child would "think" the self-instructions to guide him- or herself through an assigned task. In this way, CSIT achieved two important therapeutic goals that paralleled normal development – namely, shifting control of the child's behavior from other to self, and shifting control of the child's behavior from overt to covert (internalized) language.

The success of Meichenbaum and Goodman's (1971) study and the theoretical appeal of their treatment approach spawned a tremendous amount of interest in the use of CSIT and related treatments that emphasized verbal self-regulation training (Bornstein and Quevillon, 1976; Kendall and Braswell, 1985). Included among these were various self-monitoring, self-reinforcement, and self-instructional techniques. Much of the appeal for their clinical application stemmed from their apparent focus on some of the primary deficits of AD/HD, including impulsivity, poor organizational skills, and difficulties with rules and instructions. Also contributing to their popularity was their presumed potential for enhancing treatment generalization, above and beyond that achieved through more traditional contingency management programs.

Research on self-monitoring has shown that it can improve on-task behavior and academic productivity in some children with AD/HD (Shapiro and Cole, 1994). The combination of self-monitoring and self-reinforcement can also lead to improvements in on-task behavior and academic accuracy (Hinshaw et al., 1984), as well as in peer relations (Hinshaw, 2000). Behavioral improvements have also been reported for aggressive AD/HD children who received a combination of self-control and anger management training (Miranda and Presentacion, 2000). As for self-instructional training, the picture is less clear, with many studies (Abikoff and Gittelman, 1985) failing to replicate earlier reported successes (Meichenbaum and Goodman, 1971; Bornstein and Quevillon, 1976).

Readily apparent in these studies are several limitations. For example, in order to achieve desired treatment effects in the classroom, children with AD/HD must be reinforced for utilizing self-instructional strategies. Hence, contrary to initial expectations, this form of treatment apparently does not free children from control by the social environment. Instead, what it seems to accomplish is to shift such external control to a slightly less direct form. Another limitation is that treatment effects seldom generalize to settings where self-instructional training is not in effect, or to academic tasks that are not specifically part of the training process (Barkley et al., 1980). In this regard, self-instructional training does not, as had been hoped, circumvent the problem of situation-specificity of treatment effects, which has plagued the use of contingency management methods for many years.

In sum, verbal self-regulation treatment approaches began with much promise but have not received strong empirical support over the years. Although they can be helpful for some children with this AD/HD (Kendall, 2000), they often do not produce the kinds of behavioral improvements that would be considered therapeutically meaningful. Thus, there is little justification for their routine inclusion in treatment plans for children with AD/HD.

Cognitive models in a different light

Given their theoretical appeal, why haven't these cognitive models of AD/HD received the strong empirical support so many expected? Part of the answer to this question may come from a consideration of recent conceptualizations of AD/HD. As noted above, many contemporary researchers now view AD/HD to be the result

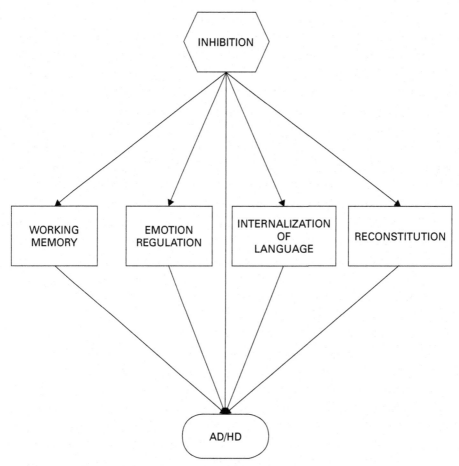

Figure 17.1   Barkley model of attention deficit/hyperactivity disorder (AD/HD).

of a core deficit in behavioral inhibition (Quay, 1997; Barkley, 1998). In an extensive elaboration of this theme, Barkley (1998) has postulated that a deficit in the behavioral inhibition center of the brain interferes with the development and subsequent performance of four major executive functions, which in turn leads to the clinical presentation of AD/HD (Figure 17.1). As conceptualized by Barkley, an underaroused cortical inhibition center makes it difficult for individuals with AD/HD to: (1) stop before initiating a response; (2) stop a response that has already been initiated; and/or (3) block out mental interference. This failure to inhibit properly interferes with the development and subsequent functioning of an individual's nonverbal working memory, internalization of speech, self-regulation of affect, and capacity for reconstitution. Of particular relevance for the present discussion is the executive function that Barkley (1998) terms internalization of speech. This executive function is nothing more than the same verbal self-regulation process that captured the attention and interest of Meichenbaum and Goodman (1971) and others (Bornstein and Quevillon, 1976; Kendall and Braswell, 1985). What makes Barkley's reference to this process different is where he places it in his model. Rather than being the starting point for AD/HD, verbal self-regulation deficits are thought to play a mediating role, linking deficits in behavioral inhibition to the expression of AD/HD. More to the point, if an individual can't block out mental interference, he/she will not be able to utilize internal language to guide behavior, at least not effectively. Thus, for internal speech and the other executive functions to be maximally effective, the cortical inhibition center must be functioning normally. Presumably, such is not the case for individuals with AD/HD.

With this in mind it becomes easier to understand why CSIT and other verbal self-control training programs do not work particularly well as a treatment for AD/HD. To the extent that they address an executive function (i.e., internalization of speech) and not the core deficit (i.e., behavioral inhibition) that precedes this, the likelihood for success is quite slim. Stated another way, verbal self-regulation training is too far downstream in the process that leads to AD/HD. To be successful, therefore, the focus of treatment needs to be more upstream, targeting the behavioral inhibition deficit, which is the presumed starting point of the process leading to AD/HD.

Although intuitively appealing, it is important to remember that Barkley's (1998) conceptualization of AD/HD is a relatively new theory and is only in the beginning stages of being examined empirically. In its present form it does not explain all that is known about AD/HD. Missing, for example, are corollaries that might help explain the developmental pathways from AD/HD to its various comorbid conditions, such as ODD or depression. At a more basic level, the theory also lacks empirical validation for the presumed links between behavioral inhibition and the executive functions. Some studies have shown that groups of children with AD/HD do not have the same capacity for behavioral inhibition as do normal controls. Other studies have found executive function deficits among children with AD/HD. What has yet to be explored is the extent to which these deficits in behavioral inhibition and executive functioning occur together within the same sample, not only in group comparisons but also within the same individuals. For the theory to have merit, this type of connection will need to be established.

If this type of research were to show that deficits in behavioral inhibition are associated with deficiencies in verbal self-regulation, such a finding would have enormous clinical implications. For example, it would be reasonable to predict that verbal self-regulation training could become more effective if combined with treatments that address the behavioral inhibition deficit more directly, thereby setting the stage for improvements in verbal self-regulation to occur. Stimulant medication therapy is one such treatment that can improve an individual's capacity for behavioral inhibition. Unfortunately, only a small number of studies have tested stimulant medication and verbal self-regulation training in combination. Results from these studies have been mixed at best (Hinshaw et al., 1984; Abikoff and Gittelman, 1985; Horn et al., 1991; Wilens et al., 1999), thus leaving unanswered this important clinical and theoretical question.

Opportunities for using cognitive interventions

In light of Barkley's (1998) conceptualization of AD/HD and the absence of strong empirical support, CSIT and other types of verbal self-regulation training programs do not appear to be well suited to addressing AD/HD, at least in terms of its primary symptoms. This does not necessarily mean that there is no room for cognitive interventions in the clinical management of AD/HD. Based upon a consideration of how AD/HD presents itself clinically across the lifespan, there would seem to be numerous ways in which cognitive therapy strategies could be employed both in the assessment and in the treatment of individuals who have this condition.

Misperceptions of clinical presentation

At the beginning of an evaluation a clinician might ask a child's parents, "What does your child do that makes you think he/she might have AD/HD?" Not uncommonly, parents might answer, "Well, he/she definitely has problems paying attention, but he/she is not hyperactive." More often than not, implicit in this response is the faulty belief that motor restlessness has to be in its extreme form before it can be labeled hyperactivity. Moreover, there is an underlying assumption that hyperactivity can only be expressed through physical actions. Due to such misconceptions, parents might later have difficulty accepting diagnostic feedback, if indeed the clinician concludes that AD/HD is present. To help correct such thinking and thereby facilitate parental acceptance of the diagnosis, clinicians must clarify why they believe a hyperactivity component is present. For example, they might need to call attention to the fact that hyperactivity can be displayed motorically or vocally. They should also acknowledge that, in extreme cases, children who are hyperactive can indeed be "in constant motion," "bouncing off the walls," and so forth. At the same time, however, they must point out that while most people think of hyperactivity in this way, it can also present itself in less severe forms, such as "fidgeting when seated," or "talking excessively."

For many parents and teachers, the fact that AD/HD symptoms are subject to situational variability can be very confusing. It can also at times be a source of great tension and conflict, especially when one person (e.g., mother) believes that AD/HD is present and another (e.g., father) does not. At the root of disagreements like these is dichotomous, all-or-none thinking. After all, the reasoning goes, if

AD/HD really is present, it would be there all the time and everyone would see it … if it's not always there, then it can't be AD/HD. Such disagreements, whether they exist between mothers and fathers or between parents and teachers, need to be defused. To this end, clinicians can utilize cognitive restructuring techniques that first point out the all-or-none nature of the thinking that fuels the disagreement. Thereafter, clinicians can cite research findings that provide the data necessary for adapting a more realistic view of how AD/HD varies in accordance with situational demands. Similar restructuring strategies can be employed in the treatment of adults with AD/HD. Such an opportunity might arise when one person in a relationship needs to gain a better understanding of why his or her partner displays variability in behavior and performance from day to day.

Clarifying the rationale for multimethod assessment

Clinical evaluations of children with AD/HD must be comprehensive and multi-modal in nature, so as to capture its situational variability, its comorbid features, and its impact on home, school, and social functioning (Anastopoulos and Shelton, 2001). This may include not only the traditional methods of parent and child interviews, but also standardized child behavior rating scales, parent self-report measures, direct behavioral observations of AD/HD symptoms in natural or ana-log settings, and clinic-based psychological tests. All sources of information about the child are of clinical value, but input obtained from parents and teachers is generally more reliable and valid than that obtained from the child via interview or psychological testing. For this reason, parent and teacher input typically carries greater weight in the overall interpretation of obtained results.

Many parents find the above approach to assessment incompatible with what they thought might be done to determine the presence or absence of AD/HD. "After all," they might reason, "if you're trying to find out whether my child has AD/HD, why are you spending so much time interviewing me and having me fill out questionnaires … why aren't you spending more time testing my child?" Left unanswered, such matters can cause parents to feel threatened or to question the competence of the evaluating clinician. This in turn can interfere with their acceptance of any diagnostic feedback, as well as their willingness to implement treatment recommendations.

In anticipation of such problems, clinicians must explain the rationale for their assessment approach. In particular, they need to mention that directly testing their child involves relatively novel and interesting psychological test materials that are administered under closely supervised, high-feedback, one-to-one conditions. Such circumstances decrease the likelihood that AD/HD symptoms will surface. For this reason, the most accurate sampling of a child's behavior stems from parent and teacher input, based on observations of the child in situational contexts (e.g., large group setting) that are more likely to elicit AD/HD symptomatology. This type of explanation often serves to alleviate any parental concerns or doubts that might interfere with their receptivity to diagnostic and treatment feedback.

Past and future perspectives

Cognitive restructuring techniques can also be used to address the confusion and emotional distress so often surrounding the developmental course of AD/HD. Upon learning for the first time that their child has AD/HD, many parents become quite distraught. For one thing, they feel as if they've lost something. The child for whom they had so many hopes and aspirations no longer exists in their minds. Replacing this idealized child is one whom they fear is destined to a life of failure and frustration. Although it is certainly the case that children with AD/HD are at increased risk for such outcomes, not all experience them. Protective factors, such as beginning treatment early and living in a stable home environment, can greatly reduce such risks. Calling this to the attention of parents often serves to address the negative fortune-telling aspects of their thinking. This is turn can provide them with much needed relief, as well as hope that serves to motivate them to pursue whatever treatment options are recommended.

From a somewhat different perspective, the developmental course of AD/HD can also be addressed when working with adults. Not uncommonly, many adults with AD/HD do not learn of this diagnosis until late in life. Although AD/HD is by no means an answer to every life problem an individual might have, it can certainly help explain why someone might have had difficulties in school, frequent job changes, or relationship problems. Thus, once informed of their diagnostic status, adults with AD/HD can begin working with a clinician in looking back over their lives, often reframing past failures. For many such individuals this can be tremendously therapeutic.

Distress over diagnostic feedback

Another clinical concern that can arise at times is parental guilt over a child's AD/HD diagnosis. Many parents often wonder whether they did something wrong. Some friends and relatives may have even gone so far as to tell them that they had. Hearing the diagnosis, therefore, sometimes serves to confirm parents' worst fears – that they had done something wrong and were bad parents, all of which serves to increase their sense of guilt, frustration, and despair. To address this situation, clinicians need to point out that research has shown that faulty parenting is *not* a cause of AD/HD. On the contrary, most of the current research findings point towards biological causes, including genetic transmission and prenatal complications. Emphasizing the biological nature of this disorder very often serves to help parents see their child's problems in a different light. Although this information may not fully eliminate a parent's negative self-perception and feelings, it can begin a process of reframing parental views of their contribution to their child's problems. This in turn sets the stage for them to let go of any faulty beliefs that they may have (e.g., "I must be a bad parent"), thereby reducing any associated guilt feelings or other types of personal distress.

Addressing comorbid concerns

Earlier in this chapter attention was called to the fact that children and adults with AD/HD are at increased risk for secondary complications, including various types of emotional difficulties. Because children with AD/HD frequently experience a great deal of failure or chronic feelings of underachievement, they may begin to experience diminished self-esteem or other symptoms of depression. Although there certainly can be a reality base for such feelings, many children with AD/HD begin to view themselves in ways that go beyond what is a realistic appraisal, and therefore engage in distorted thinking patterns that exacerbate their emotional distress. For example, they may conclude that "I can't do anything right" or that "Nobody likes me." Here again, cognitive restructuring techniques can be immensely helpful in altering such distorted thinking, thereby reducing such mild depressive symptomatology. When secondary depressive disorders or anxiety conditions accompany AD/HD, they too need to be addressed clinically. To this end, empirically validated cognitive treatments can be used. Similar strategies can be employed to address secondary emotional and personality disorders that are so often found in adults with AD/HD (Wilens et al., 1999).

Preparing children for medication trials

Cognitive therapy procedures can also be used in alleviating the anxiety that a child with AD/HD might feel in anticipation of an upcoming stimulant medication trial. How? One way to do so is to create visual imagery related to the child's life experience. For example, one can ask the child, "Are you a fast runner?" Just about every child says yes. The clinician then asks, "What are the names of some kids that don't run as fast as you?" After getting a name or two, the clinician then poses, "Let's suppose that you and this friend are about to run a race . . . but in this race, you have heavy weights attached to your ankles . . . if that were to happen, who would win the race?" Invariably the child admits that the friend would, at which point the clinician says, "Having those weights on is a lot like having AD/HD . . . it keeps you from doing what you can do and know how to do . . . what would happen if we took off those weights?" After the child responds that he or she would run faster and win once again, the clinician offers the rationale for the medication trial by saying, "Well, that's why we sometimes give special medication to children . . . it helps remove some of the 'weight' from you, and that makes it possible for you to be all that you can be." This type of visual imagery helps the child see the benefits of medication without making it sound like it's magic. Similarly, by highlighting that the medication enables the child to "be all that you can be," it reinforces the notion that any therapeutic gains are in part due to the child's skills. This point is particularly important as one wants to avoid having the child attribute any difficulties to not taking the medication, and similarly giving credit for all improvements to the medication. In short, the goal of this discussion is to help the child understand the basics of medication in a developmentally appropriate fashion and to appraise the benefits of medication in a realistic and balanced way. Doing so goes a long way toward enhancing the child's self-esteem and self-efficacy.

Facilitating home- and school-based interventions

Due to the increased incidence of various psychosocial difficulties among the parents of children with AD/HD, clinicians must sometimes recommend that they too receive therapy services, such as individual or marital counseling. Again, cognitive therapy is often well suited to addressing these parental concerns. In addition to providing therapeutic benefits for the parents themselves, these adjunctive procedures can produce indirect benefits for their children. This is because, when parental distress is reduced, parents very often become better able to implement recommended treatment strategies, such as parent training, on behalf of their child.

Even when parents are not troubled by psychological distress, they can still engage in cognitive distortions that interfere with their implementation of their child's home-based treatment. Such distortions often arise during parent training. For example, when presented with the idea of learning specialized parenting techniques, many parents inform therapists, "I've tried that already, nothing works." Upon hearing such overgeneralizations, therapists must first ask the parents to provide a detailed description of the techniques they have used. Against this background, therapists must then provide the details of the parenting techniques that they plan to teach, making sure to highlight any and all important differences. Although this information may not convince parents that the new techniques will work, more often than not they become receptive to the idea that alternatives do exist and, consequently, also become more willing to give recommended techniques a try.

Clinicians working with AD/HD populations might also find it useful to incorporate cognitive restructuring techniques in their dealings with teachers and other school personnel. Some teachers are highly resistant to recommendations that special modifications be made in the classroom. After all, the reasoning goes, "If I change things for one child, then I'll have to change things for everyone else." Pointing out the overgeneralization in this statement and reminding them that the other students in the classroom do not have AD/HD often serves to alter teacher perceptions of this situation, thereby increasing their willingness to implement modifications that will facilitate the overall classroom behavior and performance of a child with AD/HD.

Summary and conclusions

AD/HD is a chronic and pervasive condition characterized by developmentally inappropriate levels of inattention and/or hyperactivity-impulsivity. Contrary to popular belief, AD/HD symptoms are highly subject to situational variability, occurring most often under low- and delayed-feedback conditions that are boring, repetitive, or familiar. Although the details of what causes AD/HD are not well understood, there has been a recent convergence of theory and empirical findings, pointing towards a combination of genetic, neurochemical, and other neurobiological factors being involved. Due to the highly variable manner in which epidemiological research has been conducted, the exact prevalence of AD/HD has been difficult to determine. What is clear is that AD/HD occurs more often among boys and among younger children. AD/HD symptoms typically arise in early childhood and persist across the lifespan, with hyperactivity-impulsivity symptoms diminishing somewhat over time. At least in clinic-referred populations, AD/HD is often accompanied by secondary behavioral, academic, social, emotional, and family complications, which increase the severity of psychosocial impairment, thereby making the prognosis for such individuals less favorable.

Early applications of cognitive therapy to AD/HD populations emphasized the use of verbal self-regulation training. Such an approach was based on the assumption that verbal mediation deficits were central to understanding this disorder. Contrary to the expectations of many, research findings have not provided strong support for using this type of treatment routinely in the clinical management of AD/HD. One possible explanation for the limited success of these cognitively based treatment strategies is that they do not target neurologically based deficits in behavioral inhibition, which presumably precede verbal self-regulation in the chain of events leading to the AD/HD.

Although verbal self-control training may not be well suited to addressing its primary symptoms, the manner in which AD/HD presents itself affords clinicians many opportunities for using restructuring, visual imagery, and other cognitive techniques. Such strategies can be used at many points in the clinical management of individuals with AD/HD, including both the assessment and treatment phases.

Future directions

There are few boundaries on how clinicians might employ cognitive therapy in their ongoing assessment and treatment of children and adults with AD/HD. At present, very little information of this sort is available. Clearly, there is a need for

AD/HD experts and cognitive therapy experts to join forces for the purpose of developing assessment and treatment procedures that address the clinical needs of this population.

In the child domain, consideration could be given to developing an assessment procedure that taps into parental assumptions about AD/HD as a disorder, including parental attributions about its causes and beliefs about the efficacy of various treatments. Similar assessment devices might also be developed for use with affected children and their teachers. Once developed, such measures can then be used to examine what role cognitive therapy variables might play in predicting treatment outcome or in mediating previously reported treatment-induced changes in parenting functioning, such as decreased parenting stress following participation in cognitive-behavioral parent-training programs (Anastopoulos et al., 1993).

In the adult domain, similar assessment endeavors could be undertaken. To the extent that AD/HD is a disorder characterized primarily by behavioral inhibition deficits, this has implications for the type of cognitive distortions that adults with AD/HD might make. More specifically, one could predict that adults with AD/HD would be especially prone to cognitive distortions that highlight their deficit in behavioral inhibition, such as jumping to conclusion errors. Although intuitively appealing, there is currently no empirical support for this contention. None the less, it would seem to be an area fruitful for future research and clinical applications.

To the extent that parent and teacher cognitions interfere with the success of home and school-based interventions, it may also be useful for future researchers to begin examining how cognitive therapy, directed systematically at these important adults in the child's life, can improve their implementation of and adherence to treatments that they deliver on behalf of the child. Although cognitive interventions have met with limited success in the treatment of children with AD/HD, the verdict is still out on their efficacy with adolescents and adults with this same condition. Why should cognitive interventions work with these teens and adults when they haven't worked particularly well for children? One could speculate that, as their brains mature, teens and adults acquire an increased capacity for behavioral inhibition. If so, this increased capacity may set the stage for them to benefit from cognitive therapy and other verbal self-control techniques.

For both children and adults, there is also a need for examining the efficacy of cognitive interventions when used as adjunctive procedures in the treatment of depression and other comorbid conditions. Further research examining the efficacy of cognitive interventions when combined with pharmacotherapy would also seem to be in order.

These are but a few of the many possible directions that future research and clinical practice might take. Hopefully those who read this chapter will be inspired to think of other ways in which cognitive therapy can be used when working with AD/HD populations.

REFERENCES

Abikoff, M. and Gittelman, R. (1985). Hyperactive children treated with stimulants: is cognitive training a useful adjunct? *Archives of General Psychiatry*, **42**, 953–61.

American Psychiatric Association. (1980). *Diagnostic and Statistical Manual of Mental Disorders*, 3rd edn. Washington, DC: American Psychiatric Association.

American Psychiatric Association. (1994). *Diagnostic and Statistical Manual of Mental Disorders*, 4th edn. Washington, DC: American Psychiatric Association.

Anastopoulos, A. D. and Shelton, T. L. (2001). *Assessing Attention-Deficit/Hyperactivity Disorder*. New York: Kluwer Academic/Plenum.

Anastopoulos, A. D., Shelton, T. L., DuPaul, G. J., and Guevremont, D. C. (1993). Parent training for attention-deficit hyperactivity disorder: its impact on parent functioning. *Journal of Abnormal Child Psychology*, **21**, 581–96.

Arnold, L. E. (1996). Sex differences in ADHD: conference summary. *Journal of Abnormal Child Psychology*, **24**, 555–70.

Arnsten, A. F. T., Steere, J. C., and Hunt, R. D. (1996). The contribution of alpha$_2$ noradrenergic mechanism to prefrontal cortical cognitive function. *Archives of General Psychiatry*, **53**, 448–55.

August, G. J., Realmuto, G. M., MacDonald, A. W., Nugent, S. M., and Crosby, R. (1996). Prevalence of ADHD and comorbid disorders among elementary school children screened for disruptive behavior. *Journal of Abnormal Child Psychology*, **24**, 571–95.

Barkley, R. A. (1977). The effects of methylphenidate on various measures of activity level and attention in hyperkinetic children. *Journal of Abnormal Child Psychology*, **5**, 351–69.

Barkley, R. A. (1981). *Hyperactive Children: A Handbook for Diagnosis and Treatment*. New York: Guilford.

Barkley, R. A. (1998). *Attention-Deficit Hyperactivity Disorder – A Handbook for Diagnosis and Treatment*, 2nd edn. New York: Guilford.

Barkley, R. A., Copeland, A. P., and Sivage, C. (1980). A self-control classroom for hyperactive children. *Journal of Autism and Developmental Disorders*, **10**, 75–89.

Barkley, R. A., Fischer, M., Edelbrock, C. S., and Smallish, L. (1990). The adolescent outcome of hyperactive children diagnosed by research criteria: I. An 8 year prospective follow-up study. *Journal of the American Academy of Child and Adolescent Psychiatry*, **29**, 546–57.

Barkley, R. A., Anastopoulos, A. D., Guevremont, D. C., and Fletcher, K. E. (1991). Adolescents with attention deficit hyperactivity disorder: patterns of behavioral adjustment, academic functioning, and treatment utilization. *Journal of the American Academy of Child and Adolescent Psychiatry*, **30**, 752–61.

Barkley, R. A., Anastopoulos, A. D., Guevremont, D. C., and Fletcher, K. E. (1992). Adolescents with attention deficit hyperactivity disorder: mother–adolescent interactions, family beliefs and conflicts, and maternal psychopathology. *Journal of Abnormal Child Psychology*, **20**, 263–88.

Biederman, J., Faraone, S. V., Keenan, K., et al. (1992). Further evidence for family-genetic risk factors in attention deficit hyperactivity disorder: patterns of comorbidity in probands and relatives in psychiatrically and pediatrically referred samples. *Archives of General Psychiatry*, **49**, 728–38.

Block, G. H. (1977). Hyperactivity: a cultural perspective. *Journal of Learning Disabilities*, **110**, 236–40.

Bornstein, P. H. and Quevillon, R. P. (1976). The effects of a self-instructional package on over-active preschool boys. *Journal of Applied Behavior Analysis*, **9**, 179–88.

Campbell, S. B. (1990). *Behavior Problems in Preschoolers: Clinical and Developmental Issues.* New York: Guilford.

Castellanos, F. X., Giedd, J. N., Marsh, W. L., et al. (1996). Quantitative brain magnetic resonance imaging in attention-deficit hyperactivity disorder. *Archives of General Psychiatry*, **53**, 607–16.

Cook, E. H., Stein, M. A., Krasowski, M. D., et al. (1995). Association of attention deficit disorder and the dopamine transporter gene. *American Journal of Human Genetics*, **56**, 993–8.

Douglas, V. I. (1972). Stop, look, and listen: the problem of sustained attention and impulse control in hyperactive and normal children. *Canadian Journal of Behavioral Science*, **4**, 259–82.

Douglas, V. I. (1983). Attention and cognitive problems. In *Developmental Neuropsychiatry*, ed. M. Rutter, pp. 280–329. New York: Guilford.

DuPaul, G. J. and Stoner, G. (1994). *ADHD in the Schools: Assessment and Intervention Strategies.* New York: Guilford Press.

DuPaul, G. J., Power, T. J., Anastopoulos, A. D., et al. (1997). Teacher ratings of attention-deficit/hyperactivity disorder symptoms: factor structure and normative data. *Psychological Assessment*, **9**, 436–44.

DuPaul, G. J., Anastopoulos, A. D., Power, T. J., et al. (1998). Parent ratings of attention-deficit/hyperactivity disorder symptoms: factor structure and normative data. *Journal of Psychopathology and Behavioral Assessment*, **20**, 83–102.

Gaub, M. and Carlson, C. (1997). Behavioral characteristics of DSM IV AD/HD subtypes in a school-based population. *Journal of Abnormal Child Psychology*, **25**, 103–11.

Gittelman, R., Mannuzza, S., Shenker, R., and Bonagura, N. (1985). Hyperactive boys almost grown up: I. Psychiatric status. *Archives of General Psychiatry*, **42**, 937–47.

Hinshaw, S. P. (2000). Attention-deficit/hyperactivity disorder: the search for viable treatments. In *Child and Adolescent Therapy: Cognitive-behavioral Procedures*, ed. P. C. Kendall, pp. 88–128. New York: Guilford Press.

Hinshaw, S. P., Henker, B., and Whalen, C. K. (1984). Self-control in hyperactive boys in anger-inducing situations: effects of cognitive-behavioral training and of methylphenidate. *Journal of Abnormal Child Psychology*, **12**, 55–77.

Horn, W. F., Ialongo, N., Pacoe, J. M., et al. (1991). Additive effects of psychostimulants, parent training, and self-control therapy with ADHD children: a 9-month follow-up. *Journal of the American Academy of Child and Adolescent Psychiatry*, **32**, 182–9.

Jacobvitz, D. and Sroufe, L. A. (1987). The early caregiver–child relationship and attention-deficit disorder with hyperactivity in kindergarten: a prospective study. *Child Development*, **58**, 1488–95.

Jensen, P. S., Martin, D., and Cantwell, D. P. (1997). Comorbidity of ADHD: implications for research, practice, and DSM-V. *Journal of the American Academy of Child and Adolescent Psychiatry*, **36**, 1065–79.

Johnston, C. (1996). Parent characteristics and parent–child interactions in families of non-problem children and ADHD children with higher and lower levels of oppositional-defiant behavior. *Journal of Abnormal Child Psychology*, **24**, 85–104.

Kendall, P. C. (2000). *Child and Adolescent Therapy: Cognitive-behavioral Procedures*. New York: Guilford Press.

Kendall, P. C. and Braswell, L. (1985). *Cognitive-behavioral Therapy for Impulsive Children*. New York: Guilford.

Klein, R. G. and Mannuzza, S. (1991). Long-term outcome of hyperactive children: a review. *Journal of American Academy of Child and Adolescent Psychiatry*, **30**, 383–7.

Lahey, B. B., Applegate, B., McBurnett, K., et al. (1994). DSM-IV field trials for attention deficit/hyperactivity disorder in children and adolescents. *American Journal of Psychiatry*, **151**, 1673–85.

Lahey, B. B., Carlson, C. L., and Frick, P. J. (1997). Attention deficit disorder without hyperactivity: a review of research relevant to DSM IV. In *DSM IV Sourcebook*, vol. 3, ed. T. A. Wideger, A. J. Frances, H. A. Pincus et al., pp. 189–209. Washington, DC: American Psychiatric Association.

Lahoste, G. J., Swanson, J. M., Wigal, S. B., et al. (1996). Dopamine D_4 receptor gene polymorphism is associated with attention deficit hyperactivity disorder. *Molecular Psychiatry*, **1**, 121–4.

Levy, F., Hay, D. A., McStephen, M., Wood, C., and Waldman, I. (1997). Attention-deficit hyperactivity disorder: a category or a continuum? Genetic analysis of a large-scale twin study. *Journal of the American Academy of Child and Adolescent Psychiatry*, **36**, 737–44.

Luk, S. (1985). Direct observation studies of hyperactive behaviors. *Journal of the American Academy of Child Psychiatry*, **24**, 338–44.

Mannuzza, S., Klein, R. G., Bessler, A., Malloy, P., and LaPadula, M. (1993). Adult outcome of hyperactive boys: educational achievement, occupational rank, and psychiatric status. *Archives of General Psychiatry*, **45**, 13–18.

Meichenbaum, D. and Goodman, J. (1971). Training impulsive children to talk to themselves: a means of developing self-control. *Journal of Abnormal Psychology*, **77**, 115–26.

Miranda, A. and Presentacion, M. J. (2000). Efficacy of cognitive-behavioral therapy in the treatment of children with ADHD, with and without aggressiveness. *Psychology in the Schools*, **37**, 169–82.

Murphy, K. and Barkley, R. A. (1996a). Prevalence of DSM-IV symptoms of ADHD in adult licensed drivers: implication for clinical diagnosis. *Journal of Attention Disorders*, **1**, 147–61.

Murphy, K. and Barkley, R. A. (1996b). Attention deficit hyperactivity disorder in adults. *Comprehensive Psychiatry*, **37**, 393–401.

Pliszka, S. R., McCracken, J. T., and Maas, J. W. (1996). Catecholamines in attention-deficit hyperactivity disorder: current perspectives. *Journal of the American Academy of Child and Adolescent Psychiatry*, **35**, 264–72.

Quay, H. C. (1997). Inhibition and attention deficit hyperactivity disorder. *Journal of Abnormal Child Psychology*, **25**, 7–13.

Raskin, L. A., Shaywitz, S. E., Shaywitz, B. A., Anderson, G. M., and Cohen, D. J. (1984). Neuro-chemical correlates of attention deficit disorder. *Pediatric Clinics of North America*, **31**, 387–96.

Routh, D. K. (1978). Hyperactivity. In *Psychological Management of Pediatric Problems*, ed. P. Magrab, pp. 3–48. Baltimore, MD: University Park Press.

Shapiro, E. S. and Cole, C. L. (1994). *Behavior Change in the Classroom: Self-Management Interventions*. New York: Guilford Press.

Shelton, T., Barkley, R., Crosswait, C., et al. (1998). Psychiatric and psychological morbidity as a function of adaptive disability in preschool children with aggressive and hyperactive-impulsive-inattentive behavior. *Journal of Abnormal Child Psychology*, **26**, 475–94.

Streissguth, A. P., Booksetin, F. L., Sampson, P. D., and Barr, H. M. (1995). Attention: prenatal alcohol and continuities of vigilance and attentional problems from 4 through 14 years. *Development and Psychopathology*, **7**, 419–46.

Szatmari, P. (1992). The epidemiology of attention-deficit hyperactivity disorders. In *Child and Adolescent Psychiatric Clinics of North America: Attention-deficit Hyperactivity Disorder*, ed. G. Weiss, pp. 361–72. Philadelphia: Saunders.

Weiss, G. and Hechtman, L. (1993). *Hyperactive Children Grown Up*, 2nd edn. New York: Guilford Press.

Wilens, T. E., McDermott, S. P., Biederman, J., et al. (1999). Cognitive therapy in the treatment of adults with ADHD: a systematic chart review of 26 cases. *Journal of Cognitive Psychotherapy*, **13**, 215–26.

Willis, T. J. and Lovaas, I. (1977). A behavioral approach to treating hyperactive children: the parent's role. In *Learning Disabilities and Related Disorders*, ed. J. B. Millichap, pp. 119–40. Chicago: Yearbook.

Wolraich, M. L., Hannah, J. N., Pinnock, T. Y., Baumgaertel, A., and Brown, J. (1996). Comparison of diagnostic criteria for attention-deficit hyperactivity disorder in a county-wide sample. *Journal of the American Academy of Child and Adolescent Psychiatry*, **35**, 319–24.

World Health Organization. (1993). *The ICD-10 Classification of Mental and Behavioral Disorders: Diagnostic Criteria for Research*. Geneva, Switzerland: World Health Organization.

Zametkin, A. J., Nordahl, T. E., Gross, M., et al. (1990). Cerebral glucose metabolism in adults with hyperactivity of childhood onset. *New England Journal of Medicine*, **323**, 1361–6.

Zentall, S. (1985). A context for hyperactivity. In *Advances in Learning and Behavioral Disabilities*, vol. 4, ed. K. D. Gadox and I. Bialer, pp. 273–343. Greenwich, CT: JAI Press.

18

Cognitive-behavioral interventions for children with conduct problems

John E. Lochman, Thomas N. Magee, and Dustin A. Pardini

University of Alabama, Tuscaloosa, AL, USA

In this chapter we will provide an overview of cognitive-behavioral therapy for children with symptoms of conduct disorder (CD) and oppositional defiant disorder (ODD). After examining the characteristics of children with these aggressive, disruptive behaviors, the chapter will present a history of cognitive-behavioral therapy with conduct problem children, and then will present a contemporary model of social-cognitive processing difficulties among aggressive children. An intervention model that is derived from this conceptual model, and which served as the basis for an Anger Coping Program and a Coping Power Program, will then be described. Outcome research which has examined the efficacy of several forms of cognitive-behavioral interventions for conduct problem children will be reviewed, and the chapter will end with a discussion of the clinical and research implications of the intervention research in this area.

Conduct disorder and oppositional defiant disorder

CD, aggression, and delinquency, are all terms that refer to antisocial behaviors that indicate an inability or failure of an individual to conform to his or her societal norms, authority figures, or to respect the rights of others (Frick, 1998a; Lochman, in press a). These behaviors can range from chronic annoying of others and argumentativeness with adults to stealing, vandalism, and physical harm to others. While these behaviors cover a broad spectrum of problems, they are highly correlated, with few children showing one type of behavior in the absence of others (Frick et al., 1993). This relatedness of behaviors is considered to be indicative of a single psychological dimension, generally referred to as antisocial behaviors or conduct problems.

Antisocial behaviors of children and adolescents have long been a major concern of society. This attention seems justified given the increased attention society has given to juvenile correction facilities, early intervention programs such as Fast Track, developed by the Conduct Problems Prevention Research Group (1992, 1999a, 1999b), and the enormous financial costs of youth crime. In addition, conduct problems in children represent the childhood behavioral problems most referred to mental health professionals, especially for boys (Frick, 1998b). Aggressive and disruptive behavior is one of the most enduring dysfunctions in children, and, if left untreated, frequently results in high personal and emotional cost to the child, the family, and to society in general. As a direct result, much research has investigated the causes, treatment, and prevention of conduct problems.

As a clinical syndrome with a broad list of symptoms, it is logical to expect much heterogeneity within the group that falls under the umbrella term of conduct problems. In addition to heterogeneity in the type of conduct problems manifested, children with conduct problems also can differ in the causal factors involved, the developmental course of the problems, the response to treatment, and the interaction between any of these.

While there is a strong agreement that children with conduct problems are a very heterogeneous group, there is significantly less consensus about the most appropriate method of classifying conduct problems into meaningful subtypes. One of the most widely used and accepted classifications of disruptive behavior disorders is the criteria in the *Diagnostic and Statistical Manual of Mental Disorders*, fourth edition (DSM-IV; American Psychiatric Association (APA), 1994). The criteria employ a two-dimensional approach with an explicit symptom list for making a diagnosis. This system divides conduct problems into two syndromes: conduct disorders (CD) and oppositional defiant disorder (ODD). CD is defined as symptoms consisting of aggressive conduct that threatens physical harm to other people or animals, nonaggressive conduct that causes property loss or damage, deceitfulness and theft, and serious violations of rules. ODD is defined as a recurrent pattern of negativistic, defiant, disobedient, and hostile behavior toward authority figures.

The DSM-IV also distinguishes between children who begin showing conduct problems in early childhood from those who begin conduct problems closer to adolescence. If any symptoms are present prior to age 10, with the child meeting criteria for CD, he or she is classified as childhood-onset type. However, if criteria are met for CD and no symptoms are present prior to age 10, the child is classified as adolescent-onset type.

Conceptually there seems to be an important relationship between CD and ODD. Research indicates that CD is a developmentally advanced form of ODD, and that there are similar correlates for both ODD and CD. Both children with ODD and children with CD come from lower socioeconomic status (Frick et al., 1992; Keenan et al., 1995), are more likely to have a parent with a history of antisocial personality disorder (Faraone et al., 1991; Frick et al., 1992), and have parents who use ineffective discipline practices (Frick et al., 1993).

Undoubtedly, the frequency with which children or adolescents manifest clinically significant and impairing levels of conduct problems is greatly determined by the definition used for such conduct when surveying populations. The DSM-IV notes a prevalence ranging between 2% and 16% for ODD (APA, 1994). For CD, rates of 6–16% for males and 2–9% for females have been cited (APA, 1994). Sex ratios in research studies have been approximately 3–4:1 (males to females) for both ODD and CD. Both disorders, therefore, occur more commonly in males than in females, but ratios vary widely as a function of both the age of the child and the definition of the disorder (APA, 1994; Hinshaw and Anderson, 1996). The higher rate for boys is associated primarily with childhood onset; male to female ratio evens out in adolescence. Characteristic symptom patterns tend to differ as well. Child-onset conduct problems tend to reflect aggressive behavior, whereas adolescent onset tends to reflect more delinquent behavior (vandalism, theft; Zoccolillo, 1993).

Children who meet criteria for ODD or CD are likely to meet criteria for other disorders as well. This coexistence of more than one disorder is referred to as comorbidity. Comorbidity with ODD and CD is the rule rather than the exception, especially with regard to attention deficit/hyperactivity disorder (AD/HD). In clinic samples, of children with CD, 75–90% had co-occurring AD/HD (Abikoff and Klein, 1992). Comorbidity with AD/HD seems to affect the manifestation and course of CD. The presence of AD/HD in CD/ODD children produces more severe, chronic, and aggressive conduct problems and increased peer rejection (Abikoff and Klein, 1992). CD and ODD can also be comorbid with anxiety (60–75% of clinic-referred CD children) and depression (15–31% of CD children) (Zoccolillo, 1993; Hinshaw et al., 1993). For these comorbid children, affect regulation difficulties may lead to their co-occurring problems with the display of anger, anxiety, and depression.

One of the most distressing qualities of CD is the enduring stability over time of these disorders over the course of childhood and adolescence and even potentially into adulthood. Aggression may be one of the most enduring forms of psychopathology in children (Frick, 1998b). Longitudinal research has indicated that CD is often a precursor of antisocial personality disorder (APD) in adulthood (Frick, 1998b). It is estimated that approximately half of children with CD develop significant APD symptomatology. Two factors that predict the development of APD are the number of CD symptoms the child exhibits and early age of onset of symptoms (APA, 1994). In addition, ODD and CD children who show pervasive symptoms in a variety of settings (e.g., home, school, community) are at risk for a wide range of negative outcomes in adolescence, including truancy, substance use, early teenage parenthood, and delinquency (Lochman and Wayland, 1994; Lochman and The Conduct Problems Prevention Research Group, 1995).

There is a strong consensus among researchers that conduct disorders are the result of a complex interaction of causal factors (Frick, 1994; Lochman, in press a). Distal and proximal causes of conduct problems appear to cluster into four categories: biological factors, family context, social ecology and peer relationships, and social cognition. Due to the state of research on biological correlates coupled with stronger, more consistent research in other areas, the biological correlates of conduct problems are not discussed in this chapter.

Three dimensions of the family are consistently related to the development of conduct problems: poor psychiatric adjustment, poor parental socialization, and marital instability/divorce (Frick, 1994). Second, from a social ecological perspective, one of the most consistently documented predictors of conduct problems has been low socioeconomic status. Closely related to low socioeconomic status, other ecological factors, such as poor schools, disadvantaged neighborhood, and the environmental stressors associated, have also been shown to result in conduct problems. Third, early peer rejection is associated with later development of conduct problems (Coie et al., 1992; Miller-Johnson et al., 1998). Preadolescent peer rejection is predictive of adolescent association with a deviant peer group, which has shown to increase the risk of substance abuse, school truancy, and violence (Lochman and Wayland, 1994). Fourth, children with conduct problems have deficits in social cognition and information processing. This pattern of cognitive distortions and deficiencies will be examined within the social-cognitive model which serves as the basis for our form of cognitive-behavioral intervention. Before examining contemporary social-cognitive models, we will next explore the development of cognitive models in earlier decades.

History of early cognitive intervention models

Current conceptualizations of cognitive-behavioral and social-cognitive theory, as well as their application in the treatment of disruptive behavior disorders in children, are deeply rooted in social learning theories that were initially developed and tested about 50 years ago. Some of the groundbreaking work in this field began with Rotter's model of how social environments influence early child development and psychological disorders (Rotter, 1954). Many of the general principles used in his theory were derived from studies examining learning in animals (Hull, 1943) and conceptualizations of personality development as a dynamic process in childhood (Jones and Burks, 1936). As a result, human behavior was viewed not only as reaction to basic human drives and specific reinforcement contingencies, but as a malleable process that fluctuates with the subjective value that individuals place on reinforcers and their expectation that reward(s) could be obtained in a given social situation. For example, if a child who wants maternal attention (outcome value) believes that an emotional outburst would elicit this response (high outcome expectancy), and a prosocial verbal request would not (low outcome expectancy), then the child would tend to utilize emotional outbursts as a way to have his or her needs met. These expectancies could be either situation-specific or they could become generalized across various settings in the form of social schemata (Jessor, 1954).

Walter Mischel, a protégé of Rotter, may have been the first researcher to publish an article proposing the cognitive social learning conceptualization of human behavior most closely related to current conceptualizations of social-cognitive theory (Mischel, 1973). At the time, Mischel's theoretical work was an attempt to combine the most recent developments in social learning theory (Bandura, 1969) with an extensive research literature in cognitive processing and symbolic mental representations (Neisser, 1967). The result was a comprehensive theory of personality development that described the complex and dynamic interactions between individuals and their environment in terms of cognitive processing and behavioral abilities. Processes and abilities such as cognitive and behavioral construction competencies, encoding strategies and construct development, subjective outcome expectancies and values, self-imposed behavioral regulation systems, and behavioral planning, were viewed as personal variables that mediated the relation between environmental stimulation and overt behavior in humans. According to this model, situational variables were said to influence behaviors in so far as they changed or otherwise impacted an individual's cognitive schema at these various stages or levels, while simultaneously conceding that an individual's overt behavior could also modify and change the amount and type of situations experienced.

Early social-cognitive treatments

Many of the early treatments for childhood disruptive behavior disorders that were based on principles of cognitive social learning theory focused primarily on teaching behavioral self-control. The methodology for many of these treatment protocols came from investigations examining how self-control normally develops in children. Specifically, developmental theorists Luria (1961) and Vygotsky (1962) proposed that children learn to master their own behavior in a predictable pattern that is contingent upon early cognitive development. Their model of self-mastery asserts that the behavior of preverbal children is initially directed and controlled by the verbalizations of adults, but as children develop the ability to speak, they begin using overt self-verbalizations, and later internalized self-talk, to master their own behavior. According to this view, the behavior problems of hyperactive and impulsive children are seen as deficiencies in their ability to use internal verbalizations to control or regulate their overt behavior (Meichenbaum and Goodman, 1969).

Armed with theoretical and scientific knowledge pertaining to the nature and development of self-control in children, Meichenbaum developed a cognitive self-guidance treatment program for impulsive children. The program taught children to control their own behavior by modeling self-control verbalizations and teaching them to engage in their own private-self speech when performing various tasks (Meichenbaum and Goodman, 1971). Impulsive children who underwent treatment showed improvement in their ability to use private self-speech to orient their attention and think carefully when making important decisions. A more comprehensive strategy developed by Kendall included teaching impulsive children general steps to problem solving and how to use internalized coping statements to deal with frustration and failures (Kendall and Braswell, 1982). These early therapy studies with impulsive children demonstrated that disruptive behavioral symptoms could be treated using techniques based on cognitive social learning theory.

Current social-cognitive models

Many of the most recent interventions for disruptive behavior disorder are based on cognitive-behavioral theories of antisocial and delinquent behavior. The premise behind many of these approaches is that cognitions or thoughts influence the behavior that an individual displays in various situations, and thus aims to alter both an individual's general response (behavioral) patterns and the cognitions that accompany or precede the behaviors. Cognitive-behavioral interventions with aggressive children are thus designed to have an impact on social behavior and related cognitive processes. This form of intervention is based on a social-cognitive theoretical model, which describes social behavior as a function of perceptions of the social environment and ideas regarding how best to resolve perceived social conflicts.

Anger arousal model

An early form (the Anger Control Program) of our current cognitive behavior intervention program was based on an anger arousal model (Lochman et al., 1981) which was primarily derived from Novaco's (1978) work with aggressive adults. In this conceptualization of anger arousal, which stressed sequential cognitive processing, the child responded to problems such as interpersonal conflicts or frustrations with environmental obstacles (i.e., difficult schoolwork). However, it was not the stimulus event itself that provoked the child's response, but rather the child's cognitive processing of and about that event. This first stage of cognitive processing was similar to Lazarus's (Smith and Lazarus, 1990) primary appraisal stage, and consisted of labeling, attributions, and perceptions of the problem event. The second state of processing, similar to Lazarus's (Smith and Lazarus, 1990) secondary appraisal, consisted of the child's cognitive plan for his/her response to the perceived threat or provocation. This level of cognitive processing was accompanied by anger-related physiological arousal. The anger arousal model indicated that the child's cognitive processing of the problem event and of his/her planned response led to the child's actual behavioral response (ranging from aggression to assertion, passive acceptance or withdrawal) and to the positive or negative consequences that the child experienced as a result.

Serving as the basis for the social cognitive model in our revised Anger Coping Program (Lochman et al., 1991, 2000a), this social-cognitive model stressed the reciprocal interactive relationships between the initial cognitive appraisal of the problem situation, the cognitive appraisal of the problem solutions, the child's physiological arousal, and the behavioral response. The Anger Coping Program introduced the role that affect labeling, cognitive operations, and schematic propositions can have on the child's social-cognitive processes. In this model, there is greater emphasis on the recursive nature of the different elements in the model, with all processing steps/components having some influence in all other elements. There is greater emphasis placed on the ongoing nature of interpersonal interaction. The level of physiological arousal will depend on the individual's biological predisposition to become aroused, and will vary depending on the interpretation of the event. The level of arousal will further influence the social problem solving, operating either to intensify the fight-or-flight response, or interfering with the generation of solutions. This model helps to explain the chronic nature of aggressive children's difficulties, as there is emphasis on the ongoing and reciprocal nature of interactions, which suggests that there will be a cyclical element to aggressive children's difficulties, and it may be difficult for them to extricate themselves from the aggressive behavior pattern.

Social information-processing model

The social information-processing model developed by Dodge (1993; Dodge et al., 1986) explicitly expands on substeps in the child's cognitive processing of social problems and serves as an important heuristic for research with aggressive children. In this model, there are five sequential steps involved in the processing of social information, which include encoding relevant social cues, interpreting these cues, generating possible solutions, evaluating these solutions, and enacting the chosen response. The first two steps involve cognitive processing of the problem event, and the next two steps involve cognitive processing about responses. Aggressive children have been found to have difficulties at each of these stages.

Aggressive children have cognitive distortions when: (1) encoding incoming social information; and (2) interpreting social events and others' intentions; cognitive deficiencies in (3) generating alternative adaptive solutions for perceived problems; and (4) evaluating the consequences for different solutions; and behavioral deficiencies enacting (5) the solution believed to be most appropriate.

Considerable research has indicated that aggressive children do have the deficiencies hypothesized above. In terms of the initial state, or the encoding of information, aggressive children have been found to recall fewer relevant cues about events (Lochman and Dodge, 1994), to base interpretations of events on fewer cues (Dodge and Newman, 1981; Dodge et al., 1986), to attend selectively to hostile rather than neutral cues (Milich and Dodge, 1984; Gouze, 1987), and to recall the most recent cues in a sequence, with selective inattention to earlier presented cues (Milich and Dodge, 1984). MacKinnon et al. (1990) have suggested that these biases at the encoding phase, which involves selective attention to particular cues in the environment, are a direct result of prior social interactions and in fact are a logical outcome of the aggressive child's early relationships which are affectively toned. Accordingly, the child learns to pay attention to interaction patterns and social cues that are effectively similar to cues he or she has previously experienced; if a child has experienced primarily negative or aggressive interactions with the parent, he or she will more likely attend to, and process, aggressively toned cues.

At the next stage, or the interpretation stage, aggressive children have been shown to have a hostile attributional bias, as they tend to infer excessively that others are acting towards them in a provocative and hostile manner (Dodge et al., 1986; Katsurada and Sugawara, 1998). Both aggressive girls (Feldman and Dodge, 1987) and aggressive boys (Waas, 1988; Guerra and Slaby, 1989; Sancilio et al., 1989; Lochman and Dodge, 1994) have been found to have this attributional bias. Lochman and Dodge (1998) found that aggressive boys have underperceptions of their own aggressive behavior, as well as distorted overperceptions of others' aggression. As a result, aggressive boys develop attributions that their peers have relative responsibility for conflict rather than assuming responsibility themselves. These attributional biases tend to be more prominent in reactively aggressive children than in proactively aggressive children (Dodge et al., 1997), which offers support for the need for a subclassification of aggressive children, as the particular social-cognitive deficits may be different in differentially aggressive children (Crick and Dodge, 1996).

The third information-processing stage involves a generative process whereby potential solutions for coping with a perceived problem are recalled from memory. At this stage, aggressive children demonstrate deficiencies in both the quality and the quantity of their problem-solving solutions (Lochman et al., 1991). These differences are most pronounced for the quality of the solutions offered, with aggressive children offering fewer verbal assertion solutions (Asarnow and Callan, 1985; Lochman and Lampron, 1986; Joffe et al., 1990), fewer compromise solutions (Lochman and Dodge, 1994), more direct action solutions (Lochman and Lampron, 1986), a greater number of help-seeking or adult intervention responses (Asher and Renshaw, 1981; Dodge et al., 1984; Lochman et al., 1989; Rabiner et al., 1990), and more physically aggressive responses (Slaby and Guerra, 1988; Waas, 1988; Waas and French, 1989; Pepler et al., 1998) to hypothetical vignettes describing interpersonal conflicts. In terms of the quantity of solutions offered by aggressive children, there is little evidence in general that they offer a fewer number of responses (Rubin et al., 1991; Bloomquist et al., 1997), although the most severely aggressive and violent youth do have a deficiency in the number of solutions they can generate to resolve social problems (Lochman and Dodge, 1994). The nature of the social problem-solving deficits for aggressive children can vary depending on their diagnostic classification. Boys with CD diagnoses produce more aggressive/antisocial solutions in vignettes about conflicts with parents and teachers, and fewer verbal/nonaggressive solutions in peer conflicts, in comparison to boys with ODD (Dunn et al., 1997). Thus, children with CD have broader problem-solving deficits in multiple interpersonal contexts, in comparison to ODD children.

The fourth processing step involves a two-step process: first, identifying the consequences for each of the solutions generated; and second, evaluating each solution and consequence in terms of the individual's desired outcome. In general, aggressive children evaluate aggressive behavior as less negative (Deluty, 1983) and more positive (Crick and Werner, 1998) than children without aggressive behavior difficulties. Children's beliefs about the utility of aggression and about their ability to enact an aggressive response successfully can operate to increase the likelihood of aggression being displayed, as children who hold these beliefs will be more likely also to believe that this type of behavior will help them to achieve the desired goals, which then influences response evaluation (Perry et al., 1986; Lochman and Dodge, 1994). Recent research has found that these beliefs about the acceptability of aggressive behavior lead to deviant processing of social cues, which in turn then leads to children's aggressive behavior (Zelli, et al., 1999), indicating that these information-processing steps have recursive effects, rather than strictly linear effects on each other.

The final processing stage enumerated by Dodge et al. (1986) involves behavioral enactment, or displaying the response that was chosen in the above steps. Aggressive children have been found to be less adept at enacting positive or prosocial interpersonal behaviors (Dodge et al., 1986). This interpretation would suggest that improving the ability to enact positive behaviors may influence aggressive children's belief about their ability to engage in these more prosocial behaviors and thus functions to change the response evaluation.

Crick and Dodge (1994) proposed a more recent modification of the original model. They indicated this revised model describes more of the online processing that actually occurs when individuals are engaged in social interactions, and also contains an explicit reference to the idea that the consequences of one's behavior will feed back into the system and function as the stimulus for the subsequent interaction. Additionally, a sixth step was included in the information-processing model; this involves a clarification of goals that the individual wishes to attain. This stage in the process involves selecting the desired goal from different possible goals (i.e., to avoid punishment, to get even with another individual, to affiliate), or determining which goal predominates during the particular interaction. The goal that the individual chooses to pursue will then affect the responses generated for resolving the conflict, which occurs in the next processing stage. Within this model, the database can be accessed at any of the processing stages, and can be influenced by stored knowledge related to similar situations; furthermore, each stage will provide information for the database, which will then have an impact on future interactions.

Despite these advances, there is still a need for research examining how deficits at earlier stages of social information processing influence those processes that occur at later stages. There are also relatively few longitudinal studies that have investigated what types of social-cognitive problems are the most powerful predictors of antisocial behavior and at what age these problems have the greatest impact on the later development of conduct problems. Future studies examining these issues will provide a greater understanding of the recursive nature of contemporary social information-processing models and help pinpoint the specific processing problems that should be addressed by social-cognitive interventions at different developmental periods.

Research has begun to examine whether subtypes of children with specific types of aggressive behavior patterns may have different patterns of social-cognitive deficiencies. Dodge and Coie (1987) differentiated proactive aggressive children, who engage in aggressive behavior in a relatively planful, unemotional way, from reactive aggressive children, who become impulsively aggressive when they are anger-aroused following perceived provocations. Reactive aggressive children have been found to be more likely to have social-cognitive difficulties throughout the full array of information-processing steps, particularly being overly sensitive to hostile cues and having higher rates of hostile attributional biases, and proactive aggressive children have been primarily characterized by their higher expectations that aggressive behavior will work for them (Dodge et al., 1997). Harsh parenting and neighborhood violence appear to be factors contributing to the development of reactive aggression, and to reactive aggressive children's hostile attributional biases

(J. E. Lochman and K. C. Wells, unpublished data; J. E. Lochman et al., unpublished data). While these findings on subtypes of aggression, along with the previously noted research comparing the social problem-solving skills of outpatient children with CD versus ODD (Dunn et al., 1997), have important implications for designing targeted interventions aimed at treating specific subtypes of aggressive children, future research should continue to explore the nature of the social-cognitive difficulties in other subgroups of antisocial children (e.g., overt versus covert delinquents, childhood versus adolescent-onset CD) to increase our understanding of how these deficits influence the development of specific types of antisocial behavior over time.

Role of schemata

Recent revisions of social-cognitive models have more explicitly introduced the role that children's cognitive schemata have on their information processing (Crick and Dodge, 1994; Lochman et al., 1991, 1993, 2000). Schemata account for how organisms actively construct their perceptions and experiences, rather than merely being passive receivers and processors of social information (Ingram and Kendall, 1986). Schemata have been defined in somewhat different ways by various theoreticians and researchers, but they are commonly regarded as consistent core beliefs and patterns of thinking (Lochman and Lenhart, 1995). These underlying cognitive structures form the basis for individuals' specific perceptions of current events (De Rubeis and Beck, 1988). Similar to Adler's concept of "style of life" (Freeman and Leaf, 1989), schemata are cognitive blueprints or master plans which construe, organize, and transform people's interpretations and predictions about events in their lives (Kelly, 1955; Mischel, 1990). Schemata have certain basic attributes. First, a distinction can be made between *active* schemata, which are often conscious and govern everyday behavior, and *dormant* schemata, which are typically out of individuals' awareness and emerge only when the individuals are faced with specific events or stressors (Lochman and Lenhart, 1995). The dormant schemata are in a state of "chronic accessibility" (Higgins et al., 1982; Mischel, 1990) or state of potential activation, ready to be primed by minimal cues. Thus, individuals' beliefs and expectations, which emerge when they are intensely stressed or aroused, may not be at all apparent when they are calm and nonaroused. Second, existing schemata can be either compelling or noncompelling (Freeman and Leaf, 1989).

Noncompelling schemata are not strongly held by a person, and can be given up easily. In contrast, compelling schemata are strongly entrenched in the person's way of thinking. They promote more filtering and potential distortions of the person's perceptions of self and others (Fiske and Taylor, 1984). The compelling schemata lead to more rapid judgments about the presence of these schema-related traits in self and others, and they often operate outside conscious awareness (C. A. Erdley, unpublished data). Third, schemata can be more or less permeable. Permeable schemata permit a person to alter his or her interpretation of events through successive approximations, a process identified as "constructive alternativism" by Kelly (1955). A person with relatively permeable schemata can readily adapt his or her schemata to the specific situations and conditions he or she encounters, thereby adding new elements and complexity to the schema. Schemata are typically more permeable and situational as individuals develop and have experiences in a number of situations (Rotter et al., 1972; Mischel, 1990). Relatively nonpermeable schemata are preemptive, and promote rigid black–white thinking (Kelly, 1955).

The process of altering schemata is essentially conservative (Lochman and Dodge, 1998), as preexisting beliefs are accepted over new ones, and self-centered, because one's own personal preexisting beliefs are held more strongly than new information provided by others (Fiske and Taylor, 1984). Nonpermeable schemata are self-maintaining because they lead the individual to seek and recall information that is consistent with his or her conceptions of others and self. Fourth, schemata permit individuals to predict the outcomes of events (Adler, 1964). Schemata allow people to operate efficiently in their social worlds by providing expectations for how others will react and how they will be able to meet their own goals and needs (Lochman and Dodge, 1998).

Schemata within the social cognitive model

Schemata have been proposed to have a significant impact on the information-processing steps within the social cognition model underlying cognitive-behavioral interventions with aggressive children (Lochman et al., 1991, 2000). Ingram and Kendall (1986; Kendall, 1991) have organized individuals' cognitive processing of events into four categories in their Cognitive Taxonomic System. Cognitive products refer to the actual cognitions that individuals have in the present when dealing with events (e.g., attributions, decisions, beliefs, thoughts, recognition of stimuli), and cognitive operations represent the procedures which process information (e.g., attention, encoding, retrieval). Cognitive operations operate on the immediate stimuli and on schemata to produce cognitive products. Schemata have two forms within the Cognitive Taxonomic System: cognitive structures and cognitive propositions. Cognitive structures are the architecture of the cognitions in memory, representing the structure in which information is organized and stored. These functional psychological mechanisms store information in both short- and long-term memory, placing information in interconnecting categories and nodes. Cognitive propositions are the content within the cognitive structures, and are the information that is actually stored. Cognitive propositions include information in both semantic memory (general knowledge that has been acquired and learned) and in episodic memory (personal information gleaned through one's experiences in the world). Within the social-cognitive model, social-cognitive products include elements within the social information-processing steps such as encoded cues, attributions, problem solutions, goals, and anticipated consequences which individuals experience during moment-to-moment processing.

Schematic propositions are those beliefs, ideas, and expectations, which can have direct and indirect effects on the social-cognitive products. Schematic propositions include information stored in memory about individuals' beliefs, general social goals, generalized expectations, and their understanding of their competence and self-worth (Lochman and Lenhart, 1995).

Direct effects of schemata on social information processing
Schemata can influence the sequential steps of information processing in different ways. Early in the information-processing sequence, when the individual is perceiving and interpreting new social cues, schemata can have a clear direct effect by narrowing the child's attention to certain aspects of the social cue array (Lochman et al., 1981). A child who believes it is essential to be in control of others and who expects that others try to dominate him or her, often in aversive ways, will attend particularly to verbal and nonverbal signals about someone else's control efforts, easily missing accompanying signs of the other person's friendliness, or attempts to negotiate. Children's schema about control and aggression will also heavily influence the second stage of processing, as the child interprets the malevolent meaning and intentions in others' behavior (Lochman and Lenhart, 1995).

Schemata can also play a significant role in the fourth stage of information processing, as the child anticipates consequences for different problem solutions available to him or her, and as the child decides which strategy will be enacted. Social goals and outcome expectations are schemata, which, from a Social Learning Theory view (Rotter et al., 1972; Mischel, 1990), combine to produce children's potential for behaving in specific ways. When the child places a higher value on certain goals or reinforcements, the child will then engage in behaviors that he or she expects will have a high probability of meeting this goal. Aggressive adolescent boys have been found to place higher value on social goals for dominance and revenge, and lower value on social goals for affiliation, than do nonaggressive boys (Lochman et al., 1993). In this study, there was a clear relation between social goal choice and problem solving, indicating a direct effect of cognitive schemata on information processing. Aggressive boys proposed using fewer bargaining solutions and more aggressive and verbal assertion solutions, in comparison to nonaggressive boys, but this problem-solving difference was only evident when the boys' main social goals were taken into account. Thus children's schemata about social goals and outcome expectations can affect their response decisions in the fourth stage of information processing.

Indirect effects of schemata on information processing

Schemata can also have indirect or mediated effects on information processing through the influence of schemata on children's expectations for their own behavior and for other's behavior in specific situations, through the associated affect and arousal when schemata are activated, and through schemata influence on the style and speed of processing (Lochman and Lenhart, 1995). Schemata about attributes of self and of others, such as aggressiveness or dominance, produce expectations about the anticipated presence or absence of these attributes as individuals prepare to interact with people in specific situations. Research by Lochman and Dodge (1998) indicated that aggressive boys' perceptions of their own aggressive behavior was primarily affected by their prior expectations, while nonaggressive boys relied more on their actual behavior to form their perceptions. These results indicate that the schemata of aggressive boys about their aggressive behavior are strong and compelling, leading the aggressive boys to display cognitive rigidity between their expectations and perceptions. The aggressive boys' perceptions of their behavior, driven by their schemata, were relatively impermeable to actual behavior, and instead were heavily governed by the boys' preconceptions.

Schemata are complex blends of cognition and associated emotion, and as schemata are activated during interactions, they can contribute to the intense levels of affect and arousal that a person can experience in response to a provocative event. Thus, while provocative events produce some emotional and physiological arousal in most children, the intense reactive anger and rage of some individuals can be due to the activation of their schemata about the general hostility of others, and of their schemata that others are responsible for initiating unjust and unfair conflicts. Emotions have been hypothesized to be the glue between attributions and behavior (Weiner, 1990) and the adaptational systems which motivate individuals to solve their perceived problems (Smith and Lazarus, 1990). For example, when a child attributes blame for a conflict to another person, the child experiences anger, but when the child has perceived self-responsibility for the problem, the child experiences guilt (Weiner, 1990). These attribution–emotion linkages can then produce quite different decisions about behavioral responses (e.g., aggression versus apology, help-seeking, nonconfrontation, or compromise). Schemata about accountability and responsibility, with their implications for who receives blame or credit for events, are closely linked to the experience of anger. Accountability appraisals generate "hot" emotional reactions when a provocative person is perceived to act intentionally, unjustly, and in a controllable manner (Smith and Lazarus, 1990). The arousal and emotional reactions in early stages of interactions then serve to flood the information-processing system (Lochman, 1984), and to maintain the hostile attributions and aggressive response style over time during an interaction. This makes it more difficult for the aggressive individual to avoid escalating cycles of aggression and violence. Aggressive children and adolescents are further hampered by schemata and appraisal styles which make them relatively unaware of emotional states associated with vulnerability (e.g., fear, sadness), leading them to overlabel their arousal during frustration or conflict as anger (Lochman and Dodge, 1994).

Assessment issues with schemata

Because schemata are often activated by specific environmental situations and may operate outside conscious awareness, the assessment of these complex cognitive structures using traditional paper-and-pencil measures is fairly controversial. In order to address this issue, some researchers have begun using primed experimental tasks to assess clinically important cognitive processes in children with conduct problems (for review, see Frick and Loney, 2000), and others have assessed the operation of schemata in direct laboratory situations. Many of the primed experimental techniques make inferences about the nature of children's schemata by observing their reactions to various computer tasks. One computer-based measure that has received considerable clinical attention is based upon Newman and colleagues, work with antisocial adults and is designed to assess children's sensitivity to cues of punishment when engaged in goal-directed behavior (Shapiro et al., 1988; Daughtery and Quay, 1991; O'Brien and Frick, 1996). Although there are several permutations of this paradigm, each involves a computerized game where children initially have a high probability of obtaining a reward (e.g., money, points used to buy prizes) by performing a simple behavioral response. As the game continues there is a gradual increase in the probability that the child will lose his or her previously obtained reward if he or she continues to respond. Although the children have no control over the contingencies operating in the game, they are allowed to stop playing at any time. Across several studies children with conduct problems have been shown to play consistently more trials in comparison to normal children (Daughtery & Quay, 1991) and children with other adjustment problems (O'Brien and Frick, 1996). These results have been used to support the notion that children with conduct problems have a goal-directed schema that is activated by cues of reward, making them relatively insensitive to cues of punishment. Even more interesting are findings by O'Brien and Frick (1996), suggesting that this response style may be unique to a subgroup of conduct-disordered children who also exhibit high levels of callous and unemotional traits (e.g., lacking empathy, lacking guilt, showing little emotion).

Alternatively, in research assessing children's schematic expectations in laboratory settings, children's expectations for the behavior of self and of an unknown peer during an upcoming interaction task have been assessed prior to a brief competitive interaction (Lochman, 1987; Lochman and Dodge, 1998). Using this paradigm, Lochman and Dodge (1998) had found that aggressive children's schematic expectations were relatively rigid and impermeable to behavioral experience because aggressive children's perceptions' of self and others' behavior, collected after the interactions, were primarily predicted by their prior expectations rather than the direct observations of their actual behavior during the interaction. In contrast, the perception ratings made by nonaggressive children after the interactions were primarily predicted by the participants' actual observed behaviors rather than their prior expectations. This research suggests that attributes of schemata, such as expectations and goals, can be directly assessed in laboratory settings without attempting to resort to children's self-reports of these often unconscious processes.

Contemporary cognitive-behavioral interventions: the Anger Coping and Coping Power Programs

The social-cognitive model that we have discussed serves as the foundation for our cognitive-behavioral intervention programs for aggressive children. The intervention model needs to be closely linked to the conceptual model, which characterizes the development and maintenance of the aggressive, disruptive behavior which is the focus of this chapter. Thus, the intervention should clearly target the specific social-cognitive distortions and deficiencies which are evident for aggressive children. The conceptual social-cognitive model provides a template (or a schema for intervention) for identifying the relevant intervention goals for aggressive children in general, and these intervention goals can then guide the development of a structured intervention manual. In addition, the social-cognitive model can be very useful during clinical assessment, and can be used to identify the specific types of cognitive distortions and deficits that are evident for specific aggressive children (Lochman and Lenhart, 1995; Lochman et al., 2000a). As noted previously, aggressive children vary widely in the particular social-cognitive difficulties they display, with some conduct problem children having the full array of social-cognitive deficiencies and others having deficits only at certain steps in the information-processing stages. In this section we will provide an example of contemporary cognitive-behavioral interventions for aggressive children by describing the Anger Coping Program, and its extension, the Coping Power Program.

Anger Coping Program

The Anger Coping Program is a structured 18-session group intervention for aggressive children which has been refined over a period of 20 years, and evolved from an earlier 12-session Anger Control Program (Lochman et al., 1981). The Anger Coping Program has been used in school settings for prevention and early intervention purposes, and in specialty programs for ODD and CD children in outpatient mental health clinics. Sessions typically last 45–60 min in school-based groups, and 60–90 min in outpatient groups. Sessions are moderately structured, with specific goals, objectives, and planned exercises for each session. This model was designed for use with elementary-school and middle-school-age children, and has been used primarily with children in the fourth to sixth grades, although the program can be adapted for children several years older and younger than that age range. The groups typically have four to six children, and although all have aggressive and disruptive behavior, we recommend that the each group contains a range of social-cognitive strengths and weaknesses evident in the children.

A detailed session-by-session outline of the Anger Coping Program can be found elsewhere (Lochman et al., 1987a,b, 1999). The goals for group sessions include: (1) introduction and establishment of the group rules and reinforcement systems (session 1); (2) goal-setting (session 2); (3) anger management training (sessions 3 and 4); (4) perspective-taking (sessions 5 and 6); (5) awareness of physiological arousal and anger (session 7); and (6) social problem solving (sessions 8–18). The two overarching goals for this cognitive-behavioral program are, first, to assist children in finding ways to cope with the intense surge of physiological arousal and anger which they experience immediately after a provocation or frustration, and, second, to assist children in retrieving from memory an array of possible competent strategies that they could use to resolve adaptively to the frustrating problem or conflict that they are experiencing.

Anger management training is addressed by assisting children in recognizing the level of arousal and anger they experience in difficult interpersonal situations, the triggers that lead to these high arousal reactions, and then in assisting children to use several coping techniques to manage the arousal, and to avoid an impulsive rage-filled response. The coping techniques to which children are introduced include distraction, relaxation, and self-talk. The use of self-talk is a central focus of this part of the program, and is meant to disrupt children's reflexive aggressive responses, and to facilitate a more adaptive problem-solving process. Children practice using coping self-instructions and distraction techniques while other group members are teasing them, first using puppets, and then directly role-playing the responses to teasing. Children are reinforced for creating a repertoire of coping self-statements that are relevant and useful for them.

The longest section of the Anger Coping Program focuses on social problem solving, which also includes integrating work from other sections of the program on anger management and perspective-taking. Children practice brainstorming multiple possible solutions to social problems, and then evaluate the long-term and short-term consequences of each solution. A brief video is used to illustrate the problem-solving process, and then group members plan and make their own problem-solving videotape about one or more problem situations that are common to them.

Coping Power Program

The Coping Power Program (Lochman and Wells, 1996; Lochman, in press a) is a lengthier, multicomponent version of the Anger Coping Program, designed to enhance outcome effects, and to provide for better maintenance of gains over time. The Coping Power Program has added sessions to the basic Anger Coping framework, creating a Coping Power Program Child Component (for a total of 33 group sessions), addressing additional substantive areas such as emotional awareness, relaxation training, social skills enhancement, positive social and personal goals, and dealing with peer pressure. Other elements of the Coping Power Program Child Component include regular individual sessions which take place every 4–6 weeks, and which are designed to increase individualized generalization of the program content to the children's actual social situations. Periodic consultation is provided to the teachers of children who are making some progress in group sessions but who are still having recurrent behavior problems at school. The Coping Power Program also has a Coping Power Program Parent Component which is designed to be integrated with the Coping Power Program Child Component, and to cover the same 15–18-month period of time. The 16 parent group sessions address parents' use of social reinforcement and positive attention, their establishment of clear house rules, behavioral expectations, and monitoring procedures, their use of a range of appropriate and effective discipline strategies, their family communication, their positive connection to school, and their stress management. Parents are informed of the skills their children are working on in their sessions, and are encouraged to facilitate and reinforce children for their use of these new skills. The Coping Power Program Parent Component also includes periodic individual contacts with the parents through home visits and telephone contacts to promote generalization of skills.

Outcome effects of cognitive-behavioral interventions

Recent efforts have been made to identify empirically supported treatments for a variety of types of developmental psychopathology, including externalizing conduct problems in children. Kazdin and Weisz (1998) have identified three groups of promising treatments for children with externalizing behavior problems. In addition to parent training (Patterson et al., 1992) and multisystemic therapy (Henggeler et al., 1992), cognitive problem-solving skills training approaches have been found to produce significant reductions in aggressive and antisocial behavior. As part of a task force on effective psychosocial interventions, Brestan and Eyberg (1998) reviewed the intervention research on children with conduct problems and concluded that two parent training interventions had well-established empirical support, and 10 other programs were probably efficacious based on their outcome research reports. These probably efficacious treatments included four which had prominent cognitive-behavioral components, and which will be reviewed below (Anger Coping Program, the Montreal Delinquency Prevention Program, Problem-Solving Skills Training (PSST), and Anger Control Training). In addition, several other recently researched cognitive-behavioral intervention programs are also reviewed (Adolescent Transition Program; Dinosaur School).

Anger Coping Program

Although the specifics of this intervention have been previously discussed, the effectiveness of these programs will now be analyzed. A preliminary uncontrolled study of the Anger Coping Program for aggressive children in the second and third grades showed significant posttreatment reductions in teacher-reported aggressive and off-task behavior (Lochman et al., 1981). This finding spurred subsequent studies comparing the Anger Coping Program to alternative interventions and untreated control conditions. One such investigation found that aggressive boys randomly assigned to the Anger Coping Program displayed less parent-reported aggressive behavior, fewer problems associated with disruptive and aggressive behavior in the classroom, and higher levels of self-esteem at posttreatment in comparison to children randomly assigned to minimal treatment and no treatment conditions (Lochman et al., 1984). The addition of a goal-setting component tended to enhance treatment effectiveness, and children who exhibited poorer problem-solving skills, higher levels of peer rejection, and greater internalizing symptoms at baseline tended to show the greatest behavioral improvements at follow-up (Lochman et al., 1984, 1985). Although follow-up studies have shown that an extended 18-session Coping Power Program produced greater reductions in off-task classroom behavior (Lochman, 1985), the addition of teacher consultation and impulse-control training (Lochman and Curry, 1986) did not tend to enhance intervention effects. In addition to the consistent findings from this series of studies that indicate the Anger Coping Program can produce reductions in children's aggression in the home and school settings at the end of intervention, Lochman and Lampron (1988) found that the Anger Coping Program had improved levels of on-task behavior at school at a 7-month follow-up. Furthermore, at a 3-year follow-up when boys were 15 years old on average, boys who received the Anger Coping Program training exhibited lower levels of substance use and maintained increases in self-esteem and problem-solving skills (Lochman, 1992), indicating the presence of long-term maintenance of social-cognitive gains and prevention effects in the area of on-set of substance use. The Anger Coping boys functioning in these domains was within the range of a nonaggressive comparison group, indicating the clinical significance of these positive effects. However, the Anger Coping boys did not have significant reductions in delinquent behavior at follow-up, and their reductions in independently observed off-task behavior were maintained only for a subset of Anger Coping boys who had received a brief booster intervention for themselves and their parents in the school year following their initial Anger Coping group. Thus, this child-centered cognitive-behavioral intervention reduced children's disruptive behaviors immediately after treatment, but evidence suggests that some of these treatment effects may dissipate over time, especially in the absence of booster intervention.

These findings led the investigators to expand the child component and add a parenting module in a new Coping Power Program (Lochman and Wells, 1996). Two grant-funded studies are currently in process to examine the efficacy of the Coping Power Program. In the first of these studies (J. E. Lochman and K. C. Wells, unpublished data; Lochman, in press b), 183 boys who had high rates of teacher-rated aggression in fourth or fifth grades were randomly assigned to either a school-based Coping Power child component, to a combination Coping Power Program including both child and parent components, or to an untreated control condition. The 33-session child component was based on the Anger Coping program, and provided for more intensive and sustained treatment of the social-cognitive deficits and distortions of aggressive children. The 16-session parent component was provided in community and school settings over the same 15-month period of time. Initial outcome analyses indicate that the Coping Power intervention has had broad effects at postintervention on boys' social competence, social information processing, locus of control, temperament, and aggressive behavior, and on parents' parenting practices, anger, and their marital relationship. In analyses of the 1-year follow-up assessment for the first of the two cohorts, most of these effects were maintained. Most intervention effects, especially in the arena of children's social competence, social information processing, and school behavior, were apparent in both intervention cells, indicating the influence of the child intervention, but certain effects, such as parents' sense of efficacy and satisfaction with their parenting, aspects of their marital relationship, and reductions in children's aggressive behavior in the home at follow-up, were only evident in the combined intervention cell, indicating the importance of multicomponent interventions impacting both children's social-cognitive processes and parents' parenting practices.

In the second ongoing study of the Coping Power Program we are examining whether the effects of the Coping Power Program, offered as an indicated prevention intervention for targeted high-risk aggressive children, can be enhanced by combining the indicated intervention with a universal prevention intervention randomly offered to half of the fifth-grade teachers and the parents of the students in these classrooms. Initial midintervention analyses with 245 aggressive children indicate that both the universal and indicated interventions produce significant effects on children's social competence and behavior and on parents' positive involvement with their children (J. E. Lochman and K. C. Wells, unpublished data). Early findings from these two studies indicate the effects of this form of cognitive-behavioral intervention can be enhanced by including both child and parent intervention components, and that the intervention effects are evident as early as midintervention and are maintained at 1-year follow-up.

Dinosaur School – child training

This program was initially developed as part of a larger preventive intervention designed to examine the relative and additive effectiveness of parent training and child training for 4–7 year-olds with early-onset conduct problems (Webster-Stratton and Hammond, 1997). The child component, which was referred to as Dinosaur School, addresses issues that young children with conduct problems frequently face: social skills problems, an inability to empathize emotionally or engage in perspective-taking, effective conflict resolution, and dealing with feelings of loneliness, stress, and anger. The parenting component consisted of videotaped programs on parenting and interpersonal skills that have previously proven to be effective in reducing noncompliant behaviors (Webster-Stratton, 1990). Analysis of treatment groups revealed that the child training led to a significant reduction in the amount of conduct problems reported in the home and increases in social problem-solving skills in comparison to controls. Moreover, at 1-year follow-up nearly two-thirds of children in the child treatment group had parent ratings of behavioral problems in the normal rather than clinically significant range. Although the combination of child and parent training proved superior to each of the component pieces, this finding indicates that cognitive-behavioral treatments directed at young children can be effective in reducing disruptive behavior problems and could potentially be used when parents are unwilling or unable to participate in treatment.

The Montreal Delinquency Prevention Program

This intervention took place over the course of 2 years and consisted of a parent training component based on the strategy developed by the Oregon Social Learning

Center (Patterson, 1982) and a child component consisting of social skills and self-control trainings that took place in the second and third grades (Tremblay et al., 1996). Investigations have revealed that, by age 12, boys who received the intervention were less likely to have serious adjustment problems in school (Tremblay et al., 1992) and antisocial friends (Vitaro and Tremblay, 1994) and they reported fewer instances of trespassing and stealing (McCord et al., 1994) than untreated boys. Moreover, during adolescence individuals who received the treatment were less likely to be involved in gangs (Tremblay et al., 1996) and reported lower levels of delinquency and substance use (Tremblay et al., 1995) than the untreated controls. Since many of these treatment effects emerged at age 12 and remained stable up until the age of 15, the results of this preventive intervention provide substantial evidence that early cognitive-behavioral interventions in the elementary school years can produce effects that last throughout adolescence. It should be noted that these effects are for the parent and child training combined, making it difficult to interpret the unique effect that the child-centered cognitive-behavioral component had on treatment gains.

Problem-Solving Skills Training

PSST is probably one of the most extensively researched cognitive-behavioral treatments for antisocial behavior in childhood. The program itself focuses on teaching and reinforcing prosocial problem-solving skills among children with disruptive behavior disorders in order to promote their ability to manage effectively potentially volatile interpersonal situations. Research examining the PSST program has indicated that it is superior to nondirective relationship therapy and control conditions in reducing global measures of externalizing and internalizing problems, including aggression, and increasing social activities and overall school adjustment among psychiatric inpatient children (Kazdin et al., 1987). A subsequent study revealed that the addition of an in-vivo practice component to PSST can improve children's social and behavioral functioning at school. This effect, however, was found only at posttreatment, not 1-year follow-up. Both the original and modified PSST were more effective in reducing disruptive behaviors and increasing prosocial activities at both home and school in comparison to nondirective behavior therapy, and these effects remained at 1-year follow-up (Kazdin et al., 1989). Interestingly, another study indicated that PSST could be better than parent management training at increasing children's social competence at school and reducing self-reports of aggression and delinquency, although a combination of both treatments seems to be optimal (Kazdin et al., 1992). An accumulated body of evidence suggests, then, that PSST is an effective and long-lasting treatment for antisocial behavior in children. It also indicates that cognitive-behavioral treatments for disruptive behavior disorders may be superior to other active forms of treatment.

Anger Control Training

This program is an emotional arousal control training for aggressive adolescents which utilizes techniques like stress inoculation and relation training, cognitive restructuring, behavioral self-management, and imagery (Fiendler et al., 1984). An initial study with delinquent junior-high-school students indicated that self-control training increased problem-solving ability and self-control and reduced the amount of disruptive classroom behavior (Feindler et al., 1984). Moreover, research with adolescents at a residential treatment facility indicated that this treatment improved participants' ability to cope effectively with anger-provoking stimuli and reduced their defiant and aggressive behavior within the treatment facility, but this study failed to assign subjects randomly to experimental conditions (Feindler et al., 1986). Whereas these results provide support for the use of cognitively oriented self-control therapy as a means of treating aggressive behavior during adolescence, further studies using sound experimental designs and examining long-term effects are needed before firm conclusions regarding firm clinical utility may be drawn.

Adolescent transition program

The Adolescent Transition Program, which was designed as a preventive intervention for high-risk adolescents and their families, uses both parent-directed and child-directed group interventions to curb maladaptive developmental processes (Dishion and Andrews, 1995). The parent component is designed to teach family management skills (Patterson, 1982) and the teen component uses social modeling and cognitive-behavioral techniques to teach goal setting, assertiveness, limit setting, and interpersonal skills during the sixth grade. Pioneering work by Dishion and Andrews (1995) examined the effectiveness of the parent and child components separately as well as the effectiveness of both components combined. Interestingly, participants who attended the teen-focused group as part of treatment exhibited higher levels of teacher-rated disruptive behavior and tobacco use at the end of treatment, in contrast to controls, while families assigned exclusively to the parent-training condition showed improvements in ratings of disruptive behavior in comparison to controls. This seemingly detrimental effect of the peer group training on participants' drug use and ratings of disruptive behavior remained at 1-year follow-up. This finding seems to indicate that, whereas some cognitive-behavioral interventions may be beneficial in reducing antisocial behavior, certain risk factors for delinquency, such as affiliation with a deviant peer group, may be artificially facilitated by the intervention itself, thereby escalating the development of problematic behaviors.

Implications and issues

This review of effects of cognitive-behavioral interventions with children who have symptoms of ODD and CD supports the conclusions of Kazdin and Weisz (1998) and of Brestan and Eyberg (1998) that this family of interventions is indeed promising. Based on this review of cognitive-behavioral conceptual and intervention models, on the intervention research in this area, and on our own experience using these methods, certain implications and issues are evident for clinical practice and for the next phases of research. To optimize the efficacy and effectiveness of cognitive-behavioral interventions, greater attention needs to be directed toward using multicomponent interventions, at individualizing programs to meet the needs of specific children, at clarifying the cultural and developmental appropriateness of the interventions, at clarifying whether interventions are equally applicable for use in school, outpatient, inpatient and residential settings, and at clarifying the importance of group process and group composition in group-based cognitive-behavioral interventions. Future intervention research in this area should examine the role of mediator and moderator variables, the maintenance of intervention-induced change over time, and factors which influence the successful dissemination of empirically supported programs (Brestan and Eyberg, 1998; Kazdin and Weisz, 1998; J. E. Lochman et al., unpublished data).

Clinical issues
Multicomponent interventions

Intervention research with aggressive children indicates that cognitive-behavioral strategies that address both children's social-cognitive processes and parents' parenting practices produce broader positive effects and better maintenance of behavioral improvements over time than do interventions that focus on children or parents alone (Kazdin et al., 1992; Webster-Stratton and Hammond, 1997; Lochman, in press b). Thus, optimal intervention planning would include structured, empirically supported interventions for children and for parents. Interventions that have both child and parent components can address a wider set of risk and protective factors than can an intervention with single components. Other intervention components, including teacher consultation, teacher training to implement programs directly in the classroom, and academic tutoring, can also augment and reinforce the effects of comprehensive interventions for children with early-onset conduct problems (Conduct Problems Prevention Research Group, 1999a).

Individualizing intervention

Cognitive-behavioral interventions should be individualized in at least two ways. First, even though there is a guiding social-cognitive model indicating the targeted goals for structured interventions, the interventions need to be adapted to meet the specific deficits and strengths of specific aggressive children. As we learn more about meaningful subtypes of children with aggressive, disruptive disorders (Dodge et al., 1997; Frick, 1998b), and we determine how different subtypes of children have different patterns of social-cognitive difficulties, we can develop individualized treatment plans that emphasize certain aspects of cognitive-behavioral treatments more than others for particular children. Second, the delivery of cognitive-behavioral protocols can be adjusted to meet emerging clinical issues. For example, when children begin discussing an event which has recently occurred, clinicians should respond by shifting their agenda for the session, and modeling and reinforcing problem-solving skills, rather than rigidly focusing on the planned activities for the day. It is critical that clinicians keep in mind the overall objectives of the program, as well as the objectives of each session, so that the clinicians' flexible responses to children's problems and to group process problems can still have a direct impact on the targeted social-cognitive difficulties of aggressive children.

Ethnic and community context

Interventions must be delivered in ways that make them relevant and appropriate for the varying types of populations that can be found in urban, suburban, and rural settings. Lochman et al. (2000a) note that the effects of a cognitive-behavioral intervention like the Anger Coping Program could be limited by certain cultural constraints. Within African-American, low-income populations, children's abilities to accept and use nonaggressive strategies to solve problems may be limited by their parents' modeling of physical aggression through their greater use of corporal punishment, and by their parents' direct advice to retaliate when confronted by certain types of threatening situations. These parental responses often stem from the parents' desire to protect their children within a threatening, violent environment. Intervention may need explicitly to advocate the use of "code switching" among these youth (Lochman et al., 2000a), so that children can acquire a different code of behavior depending on the environment they are in (e.g., a violent, crime-ridden neighborhood versus a relatively orderly school).

Developmental appropriateness

Children's cognitive, social, and emotional developmental level should be carefully considered before using cognitive-behavioral interventions. Many of these interventions were originally developed for children or adolescents within certain age ranges, and the supportive intervention research may have been limited to those age ranges. Thus, the use of the structured intervention program with children outside that age range may be ineffective, because the targeted skills and program activities are not developmentally appropriate. To make the Anger Coping Program relevant for children in the early years of elementary school, activities have to be more concrete, highly engaging, briefly presented, and make frequent use of stimulating books, puppets, and arts-and-crafts activities. Interventions have to be highly structured because children at this age typically are less able to engage in constructive group behavior such as turn-taking, sitting in one's seat, and making relevant comments. Moreover, normative levels of perspective-taking and sequential problem solving are much lower at this age range (Lochman et al., 1999, 2000a in press). In a similar vein, the Anger Coping Program can be adapted for use by older adolescents. This requires a greater emphasis on discussion and the risks posed by peer pressure and deviant peer groups. Lochman et al. (1999) discuss the types of content and structural changes that should be made with both young children and older adolescents.

Applications to school-based, outpatient, and residential settings

The Anger Coping Program was originally developed for use in school-based settings, and this method of intervention delivery has certain advantages. These advantages include: (1) an opportunity for early screening, early intervention, and prevention with children with emerging disruptive behavior disorders; (2) an opportunity to work on children's interpersonal behavior problems within one of the settings where many of these problems occur; (3) a ready and easy opportunity to consult with children's teachers on a regular basis, thus extending the "reach" of the intervention by directly establishing contingencies for children's behavior in the classrooms and by reinforcing teachers' skills in facilitating the development of children's social-cognitive skills; (4) inclusion of school personnel such as school counselors and school psychologists as co-leaders, thus increasing the likelihood that the intervention will be accepted by other staff within the school setting and that the intervention will be maintained over time; and (5) often higher attendance rates for children in their groups than would be the case if children were being seen in an outpatient setting. We have found that the Anger Coping Program can also be used in outpatient settings. This has certain other advantages, including: (1) the inclusion of parents into parent groups that meet at the same time as the child groups; (2) an extension of group meeting time, often to 90 min, permitting more intensive work within the group sessions; and (3) opportunities to provide the Anger Coping Program as part of an integrated treatment plan, which can include medication and other psychosocial treatments for comorbid conditions such as AD/HD and anxiety disorders. Similar advantages occur when children are in residential or inpatient settings, and the Anger Coping Program appears to be an appropriate component treatment in these settings (Lochman et al., 1992, unpublished data). In all of these settings, we have found that many of the Anger Coping Program activities can be adapted for use in individual therapy, and we believe that periodic adjunctive individual therapy sessions are useful with ongoing group treatment as well. Research on other social problem-solving interventions have demonstrated the efficacy of these cognitive-behavioral interventions with inpatient and outpatient children (Kazdin et al., 1987, 1992).

Group process issues

When these cognitive-behavioral interventions are delivered within the context of group therapy, the therapists have to be attentive to the development of negative group process of possible iatrogenic effects which can occur when group members reinforce each other's deviant beliefs (Dishion and Andrews, 1995). At the stage of composing a group, we have found that the likelihood of creating a productive group increases when the children selected have the kinds of problem-solving deficits that are the focus of the Anger Coping Program, when some group members can serve as solid peer models for how to enact more competent, verbal assertion, and negotiation strategies, and when group members have at least a minimal level of motivation to work on their anger management difficulties. During the course of group sessions, we attempt to facilitate a positive group process by including positive feedback from all group members at the end of group sessions, including group-wide contingencies for earning group reinforcements which thus promote cooperative behavior among group members, and encouraging the group to plan prosocial group activities which can positively impact others outside the group (e.g., creating drug prevention posters which focus on handling peer pressure and which can be mounted in their school). When disagreements and conflicts develop between group members during sessions, these can be opportunities directly to model and reinforce the social-cognitive skills. These become the focus of cognitive-behavioral interventions, including finding ways to cool down, listening to the other person's point of view, getting a better understanding of the perspective of their peers, and using verbal assertion and negotiation skills.

Research issues

Future intervention research with conduct problem children should focus on multicomponent interventions, methods for individualizing interventions, culturally and developmentally relevant interventions, efficacy of these interventions in different settings, and the identification and management of group process problems. Other research issues include the following (Lochman, 2000).

Mediational processes

A clear strength of cognitive-behavioral interventions for conduct problem children is that the intervention model is based on a clear conceptual model of what the mutable mediating processes should be. However, little research has attempted to confirm the mediational effects of changes in social-cognitive processes on change in behavior, as a result of cognitive-behavioral interventions. Thus, research needs to examine if the interventions have had an immediate proximal effect on children's social-cognitive processes and on parenting practices, and then whether these proximal effects lead to distal reductions in CD, delinquency, and substance abuse. These mediational analyses not only further understanding of how interventions actually work, but they can also provide critical tests for the theory underlying the intervention.

Moderator effects

In an effort to determine which children may benefit from an intervention, and which may not respond as well, research needs to examine moderator variables. These moderator variables can include characteristics of the children, as well as characteristics of the children's family and neighborhood. Prior research on risk factors leading to adolescent antisocial behavior can be a useful source for identifying possible moderating factors. Children who have low levels of fear and high levels of psychopathy, for example, have been found to be less responsive to positive parenting practices (Colder et al., 1997; Wooton et al., 1997).

Maintenance of change

Recognizing that aggressive, disruptive behavior in children and adolescents is highly stable over time and can represent a chronic disorder, intervention research needs to identify factors which serve to maintain children's behavioral gains beyond the end of intervention. The effects of booster interventions and intervention components which are specifically designed to promote relapse prevention can be empirically investigated.

Dissemination research

Even though cognitive-behavioral interventions have been found to be efficacious in controlled trials, these empirically supported treatments may not be as effective in some real-life settings and they have had relatively little impact on clinical and prevention work in communities. Intervention research needs to examine factors in the training process and in the host systems (community agencies; schools) which affect dissemination. There is a critical need to understand what are the key factors within communities and within agencies which can lead that community or agency to be more or less accepting of a new intervention. Agency acceptance may be affected by such factors as the level of support for the program by key administrators, and by staff's ability freely and critically to review the program before its acceptance. Variations in how training is provided may also have effects on the effectiveness of the implementation of empirically supported cognitive-behavioral programs.

REFERENCES

Abikoff, H. and Klein, G. (1992). Attention-deficit hyperactivity and conduct disorder: co-morbidity and implications for treatment. *Journal of Consulting and Clinical Psychology*, **60**, 881–92.

Adler, A. (1964). *Social Interest: A Challenge to Mankind*. New York: Capricorn.

American Psychiatric Association. (1994). *The Diagnostic and Statistical Manual of Mental Disorders*, 4th edn. Washington, DC: American Psychiatric Association.

Asarnow, J. R. and Callan, J. W. (1985). Boys with peer adjustment problems: social cognitive processes. *Journal of Consulting and Clinical Psychology*, **53**, 80–87.

Bandura, A. (1969). *Principles of Behavior Modification*. New York: Holt, Rinehart & Winston.

Bloomquist, M. L., August, G. J., Cohen, C., et al. (1997). Social problem solving in hyperactive-aggressive children: how and what they think in conditions of automatic and controlled processing. *Journal of Clinical Psychology*, **26**(2), 172–80.

Brestan, E. V. and Eyberg, S. M. (1998). Effective psychosocial treatments of conduct-disordered children and adolescents: 29 years, 82 studies, and 5272 kids. *Journal of Clinical Child Psychology*, **27**, 180–9.

Coie, J. D., Lochman, J. E., Terry, R., and Hyman, C. (1992). Predicting early adolescent disorder from childhood aggression and peer rejection. *Journal of Consulting and Clinical Psychology*, **60**, 787–92.

Colder, C. R., Lochman, J. E., and Wells, K. C. (1997). The moderating effects of children's fear and activity level on relations between parenting practices and childhood symptomatology. *Journal of Abnormal Child Psychology*, **25**, 251–63.

Conduct Problems Prevention Research Group. (1992). A developmental and clinical model for the prevention of conduct disorder: the fast track program. *Development and Psychopathology*, **4**, 509–27.

Conduct Problems Prevention Research Group. (1999a). Initial impact of the fast track prevention trial for conduct problems: I. The high-risk sample. *Journal of Consulting and Clinical Psychology*, **67**, 631–47.

Conduct Problems Prevention Research Group. (1999b). Initial impact of the fast track prevention trial for conduct problems: II. Classroom effects. *Journal of Consulting and Clinical Psychology*, **67**, 648–57.

Crick, N. R. and Dodge, K. A. (1994). A review and reformulation of social-information processing mechanisms in children's social adjustment. *Psychological Bulletin*, **115**, 74–101.

Crick, N. R. and Dodge, K. A. (1996). Social information-processing mechanisms on reactive and proactive aggression. *Child Development*, **67**(3), 993–1002.

Crick, N. R. and Werner, N. E. (1998). Response decision processes in relational and overt aggression. *Child Development*, **69**(6), 1630–9.

Daugherty, T. K. and Quay, H. C. (1991). Response perseveration and delayed responding in childhood behavior disorders. *Journal of Child Psychology and Psychiatry*, **32**, 453–61.

Deluty, R. H. (1983). Children's evaluation of aggressive, assertive, and submissive responses. *Journal of Consulting and Clinical Psychology*, **51**, 124–9.

DeRubeis, R. J. and Beck, A. T. (1988). Cognitive therapy. In *Handbook of Cognitive-behavioral Therapies*, ed. K. S. Dobson, pp. 85–135. New York: Guilford Press.

Dishion, T. J. and Andrews, D. W. (1995). Preventing escalation in problem behaviors with high-risk young adolescents: immediate and 1-year outcomes. *Journal of Consulting and Clinical Psychology*, **63**, 538–48.

Dodge, K. A. (1993). The future of research on the treatment of conduct disorder. *Development and Psychopathology*, **5**, 311–19.

Dodge, K. A. and Coie, J. D. (1987). Social information processing factors in reactive and proactive aggression in children's peer group. *Journal of Personality and Social Psychology*, **53**, 1146–78.

Dodge, K. A. and Newman, J. P. (1981). Biased decision making processes in aggressive boys. *Journal of Abnormal Psychology*, **90**, 375–90.

Dodge, K. A., Murphy, R. R., and Buchsbaum, K. (1984). The assessment of intention-cue detection skills in children: implications for developmental psychopathology. *Child Development*, **55**, 163–73.

Dodge, K. A., Petit, G. S., McClaskey, C. L., and Brown, M. M. (1986). Social competence in children. *Monographs of the Society for Research in Child Development*, **51**.

Dodge, K. A., Lochman, J. E., Harnish, J. D., Bates, J. E., and Pettit, G. (1997). Reactive and proactive aggression in school children and psychiatrically impaired chronically assaultive youth. *Journal of Abnormal Psychology*, **106**(1), 37–51.

Dunn, S. E., Lochman, J. E., and Colder, C. R. (1997). Social problem-solving skills in boys with conduct and oppositional defiant disorders. *Aggressive Behavior*, **23**, 457–69.

Faraone, S. V., Biederman, J., Keenan, K., and Tsuang, M. T. (1991). Separation of DSM-III attention deficit disorder and conduct disorder: evidence from a family genetic study of American child psychiatry patients. *Psychological Medicine*, **21**, 109–21.

Feindler, E. A., Marriott, S. A., and Iwata, M. (1984). Group anger control training for junior high school delinquents. *Cognitive Therapy and Research*, **8**, 299–311.

Feindler, E. A., Ecton, R. B., Kingsley, D., and Dubey, D. R. (1986). Group anger-control training for institutionalized psychiatric male adults. *Behavior Therapy*, **17**, 109–23.

Feldman, E. and Dodge, K. A. (1987). Social information processing and sociometric status: sex, age, and situational effects. *Journal of Abnormal Child Psychology*, **15**, 211–27.

Fiske, S. T. and Taylor, S. E. (1984). *Social Cognition*. Reading, MA: Addison-Wesley.

Freeman, A. and Leak, R. C. (1989). Cognitive therapy applied to personality disorders. In *Comprehensive Handbook of Cognitive Therapy*, ed. A. Freeman, K. M. Simm, L. E. Beutler, and H. Arkowitz, pp. 403–33. New York: Plenum.

Frick, P. J. (1994). Family dysfunction and the disruptive behavior disorders: a review of recent empirical findings. In *Advances in Clinical Child Psychology*, vol. 16, ed. T. H. Ollendick and R. J. Prinz, pp. 203–22. New York: Plenum.

Frick, P. J. (1998a). *Conduct Disorders and Severe Antisocial Behavior*. New York: Pelnum.

Frick, P. J. (1998b). Conduct disorders. In *Handbook of Child Psychopathology*, 3rd edn, T. H. Ollendick and M. Hersen, pp. 213–34). New York: Plenum.

Frick, P. J. and Loney, B. R. (2000). The use of laboratory and performance-based measures in the assessment of children and adolescents with conduct disorders. *Journal of Clinical Child Psychology*, **29**, 540–54.

Frick, P. J., Lahey, B. B., Loeber, R., et al. (1992). Familial risk factors to oppositional defiant disorder and conduct disorder: parental psychopathology and maternal parenting. *Journal of Consulting and Clinical Psychology*, **60**, 49–55.

Frick, P. J., Lahey, B. B., Loeber, R., et al. (1993). Oppositional defiant disorder and conduct disorder: a meta-analytic review of factor analyses and cross-validation in a clinic sample. *Clinical Psychology Review*, **13**, 319–40.

Gouze, K. R. (1987). Attention and social problem solving as correlates of aggression in preschool males. *Journal of Abnormal Child Psychology*, **15**, 181–97.

Guerra, N. G. and Slaby, R. G. (1989). Evaluative factors in social problem solving by aggressive boys. *Journal of Abnormal Child Psychology*, **17**, 277–89.

Henggeler, S. W., Melton, G. B., and Smith, L. A. (1992). Family preservation using multisystemic treatment: an effective alternative to incarcerating serious juvenile offenders. *Journal of Consulting and Clinical Psychology*, **60**, 953–61.

Higgins, E. T., King, G. A., and Marvin, G. H. (1982). Individual construct accessibility and subjective impressions and recall. *Journal of Personality and Social Psychology*, **43**, 35–47.

Hinshaw, S. P. and Anderson, C. A. (1996). Conduct and oppositional defiant disorders. In *Child Psychopathology*, ed. E. J. Mash and R. A. Barkley, pp. 113–52. New York: Guilford Press.

Hinshaw, S. P., Lahey, B. B., and Hart, E. L. (1993). Issues of taxonomy and co-morbidity in the development of conduct disorder. *Development and Psychopathology*, **5**, 31–50.

Hull, C. L. (1943). *Principles of Behavior: An Introduction to Behavior Theory*. New York: Appleton-Century-Crofts.

Ingram, R. E. and Kendall P. C. (1986). Cognitive clinical psychology: implications of an informational processing perspective. In *Information Processing Approaches to Clinical Psychology*, ed. R. E. Ingram, pp. 3–21. New York: Academic.

Jessor, R. (1954). The generalization of expectancies. *Journal of Abnormal Social Psychology*, **49**, 196–200.

Joffe, R. D., Dobson, K. S., Fine, S., Marriage, K., and Haley, G. (1990). Social problem-solving in depressed, conduct-disordered, and normal adolescents. *Journal of Abnormal Child Psychology*, **18**, 565–75.

Jones, N. C. and Burks, B. S. (1936). Personality development in childhood. *Social Research in Child Development Monogram*, **1**, 1–205.

Katsurada, E. and Sugawara, A. I. (1998). The relationship between hostile attributional bias and aggressive behavior in preschoolers. *Early Childhood Research Quarterly*, **13**(4), 623–36.

Kazdin, A. E. and Weisz, J. R. (1998). Identifying and developing empirically supported child and adolescent treatments. *Journal of Consulting and Clinical Psychology*, **66**, 19–36.

Kazdin, A. E., Esveldt-Dawson, K., French, N. H., and Unis, A. S. (1987). Problem-solving skills training and relationship therapy in the treatment of antisocial child behavior. *Journal of Consulting and Clinical Psychology*, **55**, 76–85.

Kazdin, A. E., Bass, D., Siegal, T., and Christopher, T. (1989). Cognitive-behavioral therapy and relationship therapy in the treatment of children referred for antisocial behavior. *Journal of Consulting and Clinical Psychology*, **57**, 522–35.

Kazdin, A. E., Siegal, T. C., and Bass, D. (1992). Cognitive problem-solving skills training and parent management training in the treatment of antisocial behavior in children. *Journal of Consulting and Clinical Psychology*, **60**, 733–47.

Keenan, K., Loeber, R., Zhang, Q., Stouthamer-Loeber, M., and Van Kammen, W. B. (1995). The influence of deviant peers on the development of boys' disruptive and delinquent behavior: a temporal analysis. *Development and Psychopathology*, **7**, 715–26.

Kelly, G. A. (1955). *The Psychology of Personal Constructs*. New York: Norton.

Kendall, P. C. (1991). Guiding theory for therapy with children and adolescents. In *Child and Adolescent Therapy: Cognitive-behavioral Procedures*, ed. P. C. Kendall, pp. 3–22. New York: Guilford Press.

Kendall, P. C. and Braswell, L. (1982). Cognitive-behavioral self-control therapy for children: a components analysis. *Journal of Consulting and Clinical Psychology*, **5**, 672–89.

Lochman, J. E. (1984). Psychological characteristics and assessment of aggressive adolescents. In *The Aggressive Adolescent: Clinical Perspectives*, ed. C. R. Keith, pp. 17–62. New York: Free Press.

Lochman, J. E. (1985). Effects of different treatment lengths in cognitive-behavioral interventions with aggressive boys. *Child Psychiatry and Human Development*, **16**, 45–56.

Lochman, J. E. (1987). Self and peer perceptions and attributional biases of aggressive and non-aggressive boys in dyadic interactions. *Journal of Consulting and Clinical Psychology*, **55**, 404–10.

Lochman, J. E. (1992). Cognitive-behavioral interventions with aggressive boys: three-year follow-up and preventive effects. *Journal of Consulting and Clinical Psychology*, **60**, 426–32.

Lochman, J. E. (2000). Parent and family skills training in targeted prevention programs for at-risk youth. *Journal of Primary Prevention*, **21**, 253–65.

Lochman, J. E. (in press a). Conduct Disorder. In *Encyclopedia of Psychology and Neuroscence*, ed. W. E. Craighead and C. B. Nemeroff. New York: Wiley.

Lochman, J. E. (in press b). Preventive intervention with precursors to substance abuse. In *Handbook of Drug Abuse Theory, Science, and Practice*, ed. W. J. Bukoski and Z. Sloboda. New York: Plenum.

Lochman, J. E. and Curry, J. F. (1986). Effects of social problem-solving training and self-instruction training with aggressive boys. *Journal of Clinical Child Psychology*, **15**, 159–64.

Lochman, J. E. and Dodge, K. A. (1994). Social cognitive processes of severely violent, moderately aggressive, and nonaggressive boys. *Journal of Consulting and Clinical Psychology*, **62**, 366–74.

Lochman, J. E. and Dodge, K. A. (1998). Distorted perceptions in dyadic interactions of aggressive and nonaggressive boys: effects of prior expectations, context, and boys' age. *Development and Psychopathology*, **10**, 495–512.

Lochman, J. E. and Lampron, L. B. (1986). Situational social problem-solving skills and self-esteem of aggressive and nonaggressive boys. *Journal of Abnormal Child Psychology*, **14**, 605–17.

Lochman, J. E. and Lampron, L. B. (1988). Cognitive behavioral intervention for aggressive boys: seven month follow-up effects. *Journal of Child and Adolescent Psychotherapy*, **5**, 15–23.

Lochman, J. E. and Lenhart, L. (1995). Cognitive behavioral therapy of aggressive children: effects of schemas. In (Eds.), *Cognitive Behavioral Approaches for Children and Adolescents: Challenges for the Next Century*, ed. H.P.J.G. Van Bilsen, P. C. Kendall, and J. H. Slavenburg, pp. 145–66. New York: Plenum.

Lochman, J. E. and Wayland, K. K. (1994). Aggression, social acceptance, and race as predictors of negative adolescent outcomes. *Journal of the American Academy of Child and Adolescent Psychiatry*, **33**, 1026–35.

Lochman, J. E. and Wells, K. C. (1996). A social-cognitive intervention with aggressive children: prevention effects and contextual implementation issues. In *Prevention and Early Intervention: Childhood Disorders, Substance Use and Delinquency*, ed. R. D. Peters and R. J. McMahon, pp. 111–43. Thousand Oaks, CA: Sage.

Lochman, J. E., Nelson, W. M., and Sims, J. P. (1981). A cognitive behavioral program for use with aggressive children. *Journal of Clinical Child Psychology*, **13**, 146–8.

Lochman, J. E., Burch, P. P., Curry, J. F., and Lampron, L. B. (1984). Treatment and generalization effects of cognitive-behavioral and goal setting interventions with aggressive boys. *Journal of Consulting and Clinical Psychology*, **52**, 915–16.

Lochman, J. E., Lampron, L. B., Burch, P. R., and Curry, J. E. (1985). Client characteristics associated with behavior change for treated and untreated boys. *Journal of Abnormal Child Psychology*, **13**, 527–38.

Lochman, J. E., Lampron, L. B., Gemmer, T. C., and Harris, S. R. (1987). Anger-coping interventions for aggressive children: guide to implementation in school settings. In *Innovations in Clinical Practice: A Source Book*, vol. 6, ed. P. A. Keller and S. Heyman, pp. 339–56. Sarasota, FL: Professional Resource Exchange.

Lochman, J. E., Lampron, L. B., and Rabiner, D. L. (1989). Format and salience effects in the social problem-solving of aggressive and nonaggressive boys. *Journal of Clinical Child Psychology*, **18**, 230–6.

Lochman, J. E., White, K. J., and Wayland, K. K. (1991). Cognitive-behavioral assessment and treatment with aggressive children. In *Child and Adolescent Therapy*, ed. P. C. Kendall, pp. 25–65. New York: Guilford Press.

Lochman, J. E., White, K. J., Curry, J. F., and Rumer, R. (1992). Antisocial behavior. In *Inpatient Behavior Therapy for Children and Adolescents*, ed. V. B. Van Hasselt and D. J. Kolko, pp. 277–312. New York: Plenum.

Lochman, J. E., Wayland, K. K., and White, K. J. (1993). Social goals: relationship to adolescent adjustment and to social problem solving. *Journal of Abnormal Child Psychology*, **21**, 135–51.

Lochman, J. E. and the Conduct Problems Prevention Research Group. (1995). Screening of child behavior problems for prevention programs at school entry. *Journal of Consulting and Clinical Psychology*, **63**, 549–59.

Lochman, J. E., FitzGerald, D. P., and Whidby, J. M. (1999). Anger management with aggressive children. In *Short-term Psychotherapy Groups for Children*, ed. C. Schaefer, pp. 301–49. Northvale, NJ: Jason Aronson.

Lochman, J. E., Whidby, J. M., and FitzGerald, D. P. (2000a). Cognitive-behavioral assessment and treatment with aggressive children. In *Child and Adolescent Therapy*, 2nd edn, ed. P. C. Kendall, pp. 31–87. New York, NY: Guilford Press.

Lochman, J. E., Curry, J. F., Dane, H., and Ellis, M. (2000b). The anger coping power: an empirically-supported treatment for aggressive children. *Residential Treatment for Children and Youth*, **18**, 63–73.

Luria, A. R. (1961). *The Role of Speech in the Regulation of Normal and Abnormal Behavior*. New York: Live-right.

Mackinnon, C. E., Lamb, M. E., Belsky, J., and Baum, C. (1990). An affective-cognitive model of mother–child aggression. *Development and Psychopathology*, **2**, 1–13.

McCord, J., Tremblay, R. E., Vitaro, F., and Desmarais-Gervais, L. (1994). Boys' disruptive behavior, school adjustment, and delinquency: the Montreal prevention experiment. *International Journal of Behavioral Development*, **17**, 739–52.

Meichenbaum, D. H. and Goodman, J. (1969). The developmental control of operant motor responding by verbal operants. *Journal of Experimental Child Psychology*, **7**, 553–65.

Meichenbaum, D. H. and Goodman, J. (1971). Training impulsive children to talk to themselves: a means for developing self-control. *Journal of Abnormal Psychology*, **7**, 553–65.

Milich, R. and Dodge, K. A. (1984). Social information processing in child psychiatric populations. *Journal of Abnormal Child Psychology*, **12**, 471–90.

Miller-Johnson, S., Lochman, J. E., Coie, J. D., Terry, R., and Hyman, C. (1998). Co-occurrence of conduct and depressive problems at sixth grade: substance use outcomes across adolescence. *Journal of Abnormal Child Psychology*, **26**, 221–32.

Mischel, W. (1973). Toward a cognitive social learning conceptualization of personality. *Psychological Review*, **80**, 252–83.

Mischel, W. (1990). Personality disposition revisited and revised: a view after three decades. In *Handbook of Personality: Theory and Research*, ed. L. Pervin, pp. 111–34. New York: Guilford Press.

Neisser, U. (1967). *Cognitive Psychology*. New York: Wiley.

Novaco, R. W. (1978). Anger and coping with stress: cognitive behavioral interventions. In *Cognitive Behavioral Therapy: Research and Application*, ed. J. P. Foreyet and D. P. Rathjen, pp. 136-74. New York: Plenum.

O'Brien, B. S. and Frick, P. J. (1996). Reward dominance: associations with anxiety, conduct problems, and psychopathology in children. *Journal of Abnormal Child Psychology*, **24**, 223–40.

Patterson, G. R. (1982). *Coercive Family Process*. Eugene, OR: Castalia.

Patterson, G. R., Reid, J. B., and Dishion, T. J. (1992). *Antisocial Boys*. Eugene, OR: Castalia.

Pepler, D. J., Craig, W. M., and Roverts, W. I. (1998). Observations of aggressive and nonaggressive children on the school playground. *Merrill Palmer Quarterly*, **44**(1), 55–76.

Perry, D. G., Perry, L. C., and Rasmussen, P. (1986). Cognitive social learning mediators of aggression. *Child Development*, **57**, 700–11.

Rabiner, D. L., Lenhart, L., and Lochman, J. E. (1990). Automatic vs. reflective problem solving in relation to children's sociometric status. *Developmental Psychology*, **71**, 535–43.

Rotter, J. B. (1954). *Social Learning and Clinical Psychology*. New York: Prentice-Hall.

Rotter, J. B., Chance, J. E., and Phares, E. J. (1972). *Applications of a Social Learning Theory of Personality*. New York: Holt, Rinehart, and Winston.

Rubin, K. H., Bream, L. A., and Rose-Krasnor, L. (1991). Social problem solving and aggression in childhood. In *The Development and Treatment of Childhood Aggression*, ed. D. J. Pepler and K. H. Rubin, pp. 219–48. Hillsdale, NJ: Erlbaum.

Sancilio, M., Plumert, J. M., and Hartup, W. W. (1989). Friendship and aggressiveness as determinants of conflict outcomes in middle childhood. *Developmental Psychology*, **25**, 812–19.

Shapiro, S. K., Quay, H. C., Hogan, A. E., and Shwartz, K. P. (1988). Response perseveration and delayed responding in undersocialized aggressive conduct disorder. *Journal of Abnormal Psychology*, **97**, 371–3.

Slaby, R. G. and Guerra, N. G. (1998). Cognitive mediators of aggression in adolescent offenders: an assessment. *Developmental Psychology*, **24**, 580–8.

Smith, C. A. and Lazarus, R. W. (1990). Emotion and adaptation. In *Handbook of Personality: Theory and Research*, ed. L. Previn, pp. 609–37. New York: Guilford Press.

Tremblay, R. E., Vitaro, F., Bertrand, L., et al. (1992). Parent and child training to prevent early onset of delinquency: the Montreal longitudinal-experimental study. In *Preventing Antisocial Behavior: Interventions from Birth Through Adolescence*, ed. J. McCord and R. E. Tremblay, pp. 117–38. New York: Guilford Press.

Tremblay, R. E., Kurtz, L., Masse, L. C., Vitaro, F., and Pihl, R. O. (1995). A bimodal preventive intervention for disruptive kindergarten boys: its impact through mid-adolescence. *Journal of Consulting and Clinical Psychology*, **63**, 560–8.

Tremblay, R. E., Masse, L. C., Pagani, L., and Vitaro, F. (1996). From childhood physical aggression to adolescent maladjustment. In *Preventing Childhood Disorders, Substance Abuse and Delinquency*, ed. R. D. Peters and R. J. McMahon, pp. 268–89. Thousand Oaks, CA: Sage Publications.

Vitaro, F. and Tremblay, R. E. (1994). Impact of a prevention program on aggressive-disruptive children's friendships and social adjustment. *Journal of Abnormal Child Psychology*, **22**, 457–75.

Vygotsky, L. S. (1962). *Thought and Language*. New York: Wiley.

Waas, G. A. (1988). Social attributional biases of peer-rejected and aggressive children. *Child Development*, **59**, 969–75.

Waas, G. A. and French, D. C. (1989). Children's social problem solving: comparison of the open middle interview and children's assertive behavior scale. *Behavioral Assessment*, **11**, 219–30.

Webster-Stratton, C. (1990). Long-term follow-up of families with young conduct-problems children: from preschool to grade school. *Journal of Consulting and Clinical Psychology*, **19**, 1344–9.

Webster-Stratton, C. and Hammond, M. (1997). Treating children with early-onset conduct problems: a comparison of child and parent training interventions. *Journal of Consulting and Clinical Psychology*, **65**, 93–109.

Weiner, B. (1990). Attribution in personality psychology. In *Handbook of Personality: Theory and Research*, ed. L. Pervin, pp. 609–37. New York: Guilford Press.

Wooton, J. M., Frick, P. J., Shelton, K. K., and Silverthorn, P. (1997). Ineffective parenting and childhood conduct problems: the moderating role of callous-unemotional traits. *Journal of Consulting and Clinical Psychology*, **65**, 301–8.

Wyer, R. S., Jr, Lambert, J. A., Budesheim, T. L., and Greenfield, D. H. (in press). Theory and research on person impression information: a look to the future. In *The Construction of Social Judgement*, ed. L. Martin and A. Tesser, Hillsdale, NJ: Erlbaum.

Zelli, A., Dodge, K. A., Lochman, J. E., Laird, R. D., and the Conduct Problems Prevention Research Group. (1999). The distinction between beliefs legitimizing aggression and deviant processing of social cues: testing measurement validity and the hypothesis that biased processing mediates the effects of beliefs on aggression. *Journal of Personality and Social Psychology*, **77**, 150–66.

Zoccolillo, M. (1993). Gender and the development of conduct disorder. *Development and Psychopathology*, **5**, 65–78.

19

Processes of change in cognitive therapy

Sona Dimidjian[1] and Keith S. Dobson[2]

[1] University of Washington, Seattle, WA, USA
[2] University of Calgary, Alberta, Canada

Introduction

Cognitive therapy (CT) has been applied to a diverse range of clinical problems, including depression, anxiety, eating disorders, personality disorders, addictive behaviors, and marital distress (DeRubeis et al., 2001). CT is one of the most widely studied psychotherapies, as recent decades have witnessed a proliferation of research investigating its efficacy. Outcome data attest to the efficacy of CT across the broad range of clinical problems, including those noted above.

Unfortunately, while there are many studies investigating the outcome of CT, the volume of research examining the process of change in CT has been more modest. In fact, only recently have researchers systematically begun to address questions regarding the active ingredients of CT and particular mediators or moderators of change. These areas of research, however, have profound practical and theoretical implications and will likely be an increasing focus of attention in the future. Greater knowledge about particular process variables has the potential to enhance treatment development efforts, and point the way toward interventions that are more powerful and efficient than those of today. Additionally, the impact on clinician training and the treatment and service delivery and dissemination could have significant public health relevance.

This chapter focuses on the process of change in CT. Towards this end, we first propose a basic model of therapeutic change, which we use to elucidate the particular components of the cognitive theory of clinical change. Next, we present an integrative review of the empirical literature on the process of change in CT. Although we discuss research on the process of change in the treatment of a wide range of disorders, it should be noted that the majority of the extant research has focused in particular on processes of change in CT for depression. As a consequence, this area is disproportionately represented in the following discussion. Nevertheless, our review attends to the ways in which the empirical results intersect with the overall CT theory of change, which has a broad relevance to a range of clinical problems. We conclude with a discussion of theoretical and methodological issues that will be important to address in future research on processes of change in CT.

The cognitive theory of therapeutic change

CT is only one among many therapies that fall in the domain of treatments largely identified as cognitive or cognitive-behavioral (Dobson, 2001). The majority of studies reviewed in this chapter focus on the model of CT that was developed by Beck and colleagues initially for the treatment of depression (Beck et al., 1979) and later applied to a range of other clinical problems. This model has been the most widely disseminated and investigated model of CT and has, in fact, come to be considered the "standard form" of CT (Clark, 1995).

Although the specific interventions of standard CT vary depending on the target disorder, phase of treatment, and particular client, most variations are unified by shared assumptions about the processes of change in treatment. A basic model of the clinical change process was proposed by Hollon and Kris (1984) and included a consideration of clinical outcomes, mechanisms of change, active treatment components, patient prognostic indicators, and "extra-therapy factors" such as psychosocial stress. Building on this basic model, we have outlined the elements of therapeutic change in Figure 19.1 in order to facilitate a discussion of the cognitive theory of therapeutic change.

Although the various components of the change process cannot, in truth, be fully separated, the basic components of the clinical change process are depicted heuristically in Figure 19.1 to organize our following review of the process research. In addition, it is important to note that, although feedback loops exist between many of the components of the change process, these have not been depicted in the diagram for ease of representation. With these caveats in mind, thus, we begin by exploring the therapist and patient factors relevant to the study of therapeutic process, indicated on the left side of the figure. A range of important client-related factors have been identified in the literature to date, including sociodemographic variables, symptom severity, individual reasons for clinical problems, and other personal characteristics. Moreover, while the role of therapist factors has not historically received a great deal of attention, increased focus has been placed on issues of treatment adherence and competence in recent years (Waltz et al., 1993). The recent attention on credentialing in CT illustrates the increasing focus on issues of competence, in particular (Dobson and Khatri, 2000).

We next consider the central part of the figure, namely, research on active ingredients of change in CT, including theory-specific and nonspecific or common

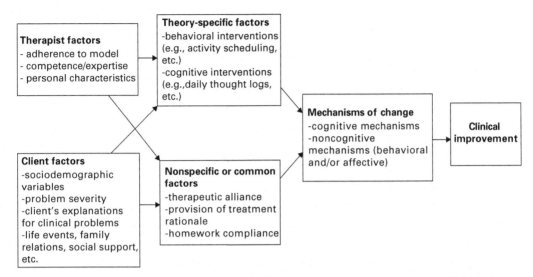

Figure 19.1   Model of therapeutic change in cognitive therapy. Adapted from Hollon and Kris (1984).

factors. We highlight, in particular, research seeking to determine the active ingredients of CT. The CT model of therapeutic change specifies that the primary active ingredients of treatment delivery are contained in the theory-specific category. In contrast, nonspecific factors, such as the therapeutic relationship and the act of providing a treatment rationale, are generally assumed to be necessary, though not sufficient ingredients (Beck et al., 1979).

In the next section of the diagram the mechanisms of change are depicted. The mechanisms of change are presumed to mediate the effect of the treatment delivery components on clinical outcomes. The cognitive theory of change is perhaps best characterized by its emphasis on cognitive mechanisms as central to clinical improvement. As Beck (1991, p. 194) summarizes: "My theory of change stipulates that symptomatic improvement in the acute disorders (e.g., depression, generalized anxiety disorder, and panic) is produced by deactivation of the hypervalent depressotypic, anxiotypic, or panicotypic schemas, respectively." This basic proposition is one of the chief unifying threads among the variety of versions of CT (see also Brewin, 1989).

How do client factors contribute to change in cognitive therapy?

The role of client factors has been evaluated most often in the context of CT for depression. A range of specific client factors have been associated with outcome. For instance, poor outcomes have been associated with a number of sociodemographic and depression-related factors, including high levels of initial severity and cognitive dysfunction (Rude and Rehm, 1991; Sotsky et al., 1991), comorbid personality disorders (Persons and Burns, 1985; Frank et al., 1987; Shea et al., 1990; Burns and Nolen-Hoeksema, 1992), presence of relationship discord or disturbance (Beach et al., 1990; Prince and Jacobson, 1995), and marital status (i.e., being separated, divorced, widowed, or never married) (Jarrett et al., 1991; Sotsky et al., 1991). The associations between these client-related factors and outcome suggest that both intrapersonal and environmental or interpersonal variables may be important in the process of change in CT.

Cognitive and personality functioning has also been related to outcome in CT. CT appears to be more effective with depressed clients who have externalizing coping styles (i.e., those who control stress poorly, are irritable and impulsive, and project blame on to others) in contrast to those with nonexternalizing coping styles (Beutler et al., 1991). Preliminary evidence also suggests that clients with well-assimilated problems do better in CT than in psychodynamic, experiential, or interpersonal therapy (Stiles et al., 1997); well-assimilated problems were identified as those that a client can clearly describe to the therapist, in contrast to problems that are presented with vague description or avoidance or of which the client indicates little or no awareness (Stiles et al., 1997).

Muran et al. (1994) examined the relationship between therapeutic alliance and client pretreatment interpersonal problems among clients treated with CT for a range of affective disorder diagnoses. They concluded that alliance was negatively related to particular types of pretreatment interpersonal problems (e.g. "hostile-dominant"), and positively related to others (e.g., "friendly-submissive"). In contrast to the above-reported findings, Whisman (1993) summarizes a range of variables that have failed to predict outcome among clients receiving CT. He notes: "intelligence, learned resourcefulness, and the presence of endogenous depression are apparently unrelated to outcome."

Some investigators have explored the role of the particular explanations that clients give for their clinical problems in the process of change. In a study with depressed clients, Addis and Jacobson (1996) found that clients who gave existential reasons for their depression experienced better outcomes in CT than in the behavioral activation component of CT. Clients who gave relationship-oriented reasons for their depression, however, consistently exhibited poor responses to the CT treatment. Similarly, Fennell and Teasdale (1987) also demonstrated that CT was more effective with clients who agreed with the CT rationale provided in CT.

Relatedly, some investigators have focused on the role of attributional style as a predictor of response and relapse following successful CT. For instance, Jacobson et al. (1996) examined the role of attributional style, as measured by the Attributional Style Questionaire, in the outcome of acute treatment for major depression.

This study found that early change in attributional style was present among clients receiving a behavioral-only intervention, but not among clients receiving a standard CT intervention. The results of Gollan et al. (in preparation), however, fail to provide support for the role of attributional style in the prediction of relapse over a 24-month follow-up period. It is possible that the lack of significant findings for attributional style reflects problems with the measurement of the construct of interest; however, these results may also point to the fact that client rationales for treatment may be distinct from more global considerations of attributional or cognitive style. The developing literature on attributional and cognitive style (Abramson et al., 1999; Alloy, 2001; Alloy et al., 1999) will continue to offer important insights into these processes.

In addition to further research on the above client variables, efforts to understand better the potentially moderating effects of sociodemographic variables on outcome and process in CT are warranted. For example, although there are descriptions of the application of cognitive-behavioral therapy in a manner that is sensitive to diversity considerations (such as the special issue of *Cognitive and Behavioral Practice*, in winter, 1996), the role of client ethnicity has rarely been considered systematically in evaluations of CT (Hays, 1995; Organista and Munoz, 1996). Future investigations also need to incorporate a focus on sexual orientation, in order to determine whether the process of CT is similar or unique with clients of color and gay and lesbian clients as compared to heterosexual clients (Purcell et al., 1996). In addition, the role of client religious beliefs may also be important to consider (Miller and Martin, 1988; Propst et al., 1992; Miller, 1999). These areas of diversity research are particularly important to increase our knowledge of processes of change for *all* CT clients, and, where necessary, to increase the sensitivity to, and competence for, effectively dealing with client diversity among cognitive therapists.

Future research is needed to determine with greater confidence the role of client factors in the process of change in CT. Future investigators can build upon the findings reported to date in order to provide additional support for particular variables. Given what is already known about patient characteristics associated with better or worse CT outcome, the possibility of client treatment matching in CT may also yield important new directions (Shoham-Salomon and Hannah, 1991; Beutler and Baker, 1998). In general, however, research on client predictors will be enhanced by greater attention to theory-specified avenues of study. As Blatt and Felsen (1993) note, "One of the contemporary challenges in psychotherapy research is the identification of theory-related patient qualities that lend themselves to systematic study" (p. 254). In addition, as noted above, research on client factor in CT for depression is significantly more advanced than such research on CT for other clinical problems; future research will need to determine whether the potential directions suggested by the research on depression are applicable to other clinical problems.

How do therapist factors contribute to change in cognitive therapy?

Although therapist factors represent an important element of the cognitive theory of therapeutic change, this area has received scant attention from CT researchers to date. In 1985, Luborsky et al. observed:

the therapist is not simply the transmitter of a standard therapeutic agent. Rather, the therapist is an important, independent agent of change with the ability to magnify or reduce the effects of the therapy. This, of course, may be obvious to clinicians who are in the position of making referrals to colleagues; however, there has been little quantitative evidence to support this clinical impression (p. 609).

Unfortunately, it is likely that the amount of research in this area has been limited by problems with restricted variability among the therapists typically employed in most efficacy studies, given the small number of research therapists in most trials, and what is often their high levels of experience and clinical training (Whisman, 1993).

The concepts of therapist adherence and competence are particularly important to the consideration of therapist factors in processes of change. Adherence is conceptualized as the degree to which therapists implement CT techniques. A related concept has been that of "purity" or "potency" of the treatment, as might be suggested by the ratio of CT interventions to interventions not specified by CT. Adherence to CT has been typically measured with the Collaborative Study Psychotherapy Rating Scale. Competence, conceptualized as the degree to which interventions are delivered skillfully, has generally been measured with the Cognitive Therapy Rating Scale (J. B. McGlinchey and K. S. Dobson, unpublished data).

It is generally assumed that positive outcome will be related to higher degrees of both adherence and competence. Unfortunately, relatively few studies have examined the role of adherence or competence in the assessment of outcome, despite the fact that outcome studies are increasingly using measures of adherence and competence to document the integrity of the investigated treatments (Waltz et al., 1993). DeRubeis and Feeley (1990) and Feeley et al. (1999) examined the relationship between outcome and therapist adherence, finding that adherence to specific types of CT interventions was associated with positive outcome. Luborsky et al. (1985) found that the relative purity with which CT was delivered was associated with outcome in the treatment of opiate addiction. Shaw et al. (1999) also provide some support for the relationship between therapist competence and outcome among patients treated for depression.

A number of investigators have also examined the role of other therapist characteristics on therapy outcome. Zlotnick et al. (1998), for instance, examined the role of therapist and patient gender in the treatment of major depression in the Treatment of Depression Collaborative Research Program (TDCRP). Contrary to expectations, they found that gender of therapist, gender match or mismatch between therapist and patient, and patient preferences regarding gender and/or match were unrelated to treatment outcome, dropout, or the patient's rating of the therapist's level of empathy.

In another analysis of TDCRP therapists, Blatt et al. (1996) found that, compared to low or moderately effective therapists, more effective therapists were more likely to be psychologically minded as opposed to biologically minded, to evidence low endorsement of biological interventions in their daily clinical practices, and to expect that outpatient treatment would take longer. Interestingly, differential outcome among therapists was not related to level of general clinical experience or specific experience treating depression. Luborsky et al. (1985) have suggested that the level of therapist personal adjustment and interest in helping are associated with positive outcome.

Given the relative paucity of research in this area, significant questions remain about which therapist factors are important to pursue in future investigations. Replication of some of the above-reported results is necessary, as are investigations of models that incorporate other therapist factors not previously addressed in CT research. Possible future directions include, for instance, an assessment of the role of therapist conviction in the CT model. Research on the effect of investigator allegiance on outcome data (Dobson and Pusch, 1993; Gaffan et al., 1995; Jacobson, 1999) may have an important corollary in therapist allegiance to the practice of CT. In addition, therapist factors that affect perceived credibility with clients (e.g., age, experience) may be important to explore further. It is possible that future work in this area may be best undertaken in the context of more naturalistic designs in which investigators can explore a wider range of therapist adherence, competence, and other personal characteristic variables.

What are the active ingredients of cognitive therapy?

CT is a multifaceted treatment, which includes attention to nonspecific factors such as a positive therapeutic alliance, and a range of behavioral and cognitive interventions. For this reason, understanding the "active ingredients" of CT is central to an examination of processes of change. Towards this end, a number of studies have identified particular components of the overall package of CT in an attempt to specify which ingredients are likely to account for therapeutic change. Research has generally focused on the relative importance of interventions common to most psychotherapeutic models, and those specified by cognitive theory. Each of these domains is discussed in turn in the sections that follow.

The empirical status of nonspecific factors in cognitive therapy

Within the large category of "nonspecific" or common factors, CT process research has tended to focus on two general areas: the quality of the therapeutic relationship and the provision of the treatment rationale. Given that such factors are often considered necessary but nonsufficient aspects of CT, research has generally sought to address the question of whether or not cognitive interventions account for change beyond that accounted for by such "nonspecific" or common factors.

The therapeutic relationship

The quality of the therapeutic relationship is generally believed to be an important factor in most psychosocial treatment models. In fact, a metaanalysis examining the relationship between therapeutic alliance and outcome (Horvath and Symonds, 1991) concluded that the alliance–outcome relationship was relatively robust across a wide range of treatment modalities. In CT, a unique type of therapeutic relationship is prescribed, which is characterized primarily by the quality of "collaborative empiricism" (Beck et al., 1979; Beck, 1995). This relationship is considered to be a critical part of the therapy, in that it sets the framework for the implementation of the primary cognitive interventions. The therapeutic relationship is, therefore, considered to be necessary, though not sufficient for therapeutic change. In line with this theory, a large number of studies has examined the relative role of theory-specified interventions and qualities of the therapeutic relationship in the prediction of positive treatment response.

In a study of CT with depressed and anxious clients, Persons and Burns (1985) concluded that patient ratings of the quality of the therapeutic relationship made an independent contribution to mood changes during a single session, over and above change accounted for by lowered belief in automatic thoughts and patient characteristics. Burns and Nolen-Hoeksema (1992) found that patients' ratings of therapist empathy were associated with outcome. Similarly, Krupnick et al. (1996) found that patients' ratings of therapeutic alliance predicted outcome of CT patients in the TDCRP. Castonguay et al. (1996) examined the predictive ability of therapeutic alliance in the context of other nonspecific factors (e.g., client emotional involvement) and CT-specific interventions. Quantitative analyses suggested that the quality of the working alliance was uniquely associated with outcome. Exploratory descriptive analyses of sessions also suggested that some cognitive interventions, when applied in the context of a poor working alliance, may have detrimental effects.

Unfortunately, despite the numerous associations between alliance and outcome, the majority of studies on therapeutic alliance to date have suffered from a number of methodological problems that limit our ability to interpret findings. As Feeley et al. (1999) describe, most studies rely on purely correlational data and fail to establish the temporal precedence of the alliance variable. Because many investigators have not sufficiently specified whether clinical improvements precede positive alliance or vice versa, it is difficult to tease apart the causal direction of the alliance–outcome relationship. A few studies have, however, attempted to account for this potential temporal confound. Gaston et al. (1991), for instance, found that treatment alliance explained considerable amounts of the variance in outcome over and above initial severity and previous change; although due to limited power, these analyses were not statistically significant. In contrast, however, Beckham (1989) found that depressed patients' ratings of therapeutic alliance did not predict later clinical improvement.

DeRubeis and Feeley (1990) also failed to find an association between alliance or "facilitative" intervention in CT and outcome; in fact, they found that therapeutic alliance was associated with *prior* but not *subsequent* symptomatic change. In a later investigation, Feeley et al. (1999) again found no relation between alliance and subsequent change. In this study, however, prior symptomatic change only predicted subsequent alliance at the level of a nonsignificant trend. Overall, they concluded that therapeutic alliance is more reasonably conceptualized as a consequence of change which has already occurred, rather than a cause of subsequent change. Therapeutic alliance also appeared to function as a consequence of clinical improvement in Tang and DeRubeis' (1999b) analysis of "critical sessions" in which alliance gains were noted following significant clinical gains. These data thus suggest that, as clients improve in treatment, they become more committed to therapy and rate the alliance more positively.

Finally, it should be noted that a number of investigators have called for a more careful examination of the ways in which the therapeutic relationship can be actively used to facilitate change in CT. Jacobson (1989) suggested that cognitive-behavioral therapies should devote increased attention to the ways in which the therapeutic relationship itself could be used "as a vehicle for change." Kohlenberg and Tsai (1991) have developed a model of treatment, entitled Functional Analytic Enhanced Cognitive Therapy (FECT), which explicitly details the ways in which an increased focus on the therapeutic relationship can enhance the CT technology. Safran and Segal (1990) have similarly emphasized the need for increased attention to the role of the therapeutic relationship in CT.

In summary, a number of important and interesting directions are highlighted by the extant research on the role of the therapeutic relationship in CT. Compelling evidence regarding the importance of the therapeutic alliance in CT has been demonstrated in a number of studies. At the same time, however, measurement issues and concerns about temporal confounds need to be considered in an evaluation of these results. Future research will need to help tease apart the direction of the relationship between alliance and symptomatic improvement. Moreover, it will be important to consider the construct of therapeutic relationship more carefully. As Jones and Pulos (1993) noted, "most psychotherapists have not found the therapeutic alliance construct sufficient for assessing the effectiveness of their techniques or for explaining how patients change; it located the common core at too high a level of abstraction" (p. 306). Finally, it will be important to evaluate whether standard CT is making the best possible use of the therapeutic relationship. Although efficacy studies attest to the power of CT, not all patients benefit from CT; future research may demonstrate that making greater use of the therapeutic relationship to promote change will significantly enhance the power of CT.

Provision of a treatment rationale

In addition to the establishment of a therapeutic relationship, most therapeutic models incorporate the use of some type of treatment rationale. Such rationales typically provide an explanatory framework for both the development of pathology and the process of change or recovery. The treatment rationale is typically an important part of the early stage of CT, and often includes the provision of written materials explaining the treatment model. A number of investigators have suggested that this rationale is a critical part of the change process in CT.

In the area of depression, for instance, Teasdale (1985) and Fennell and Teasdale (1987) have suggested that the treatment rationale helps to alleviate "depression about depression" and increase feelings of hopefulness. In these ways, the provision of a treatment rationale is hypothesized to be a core active ingredient of CT. Ilardi and Craighead (1994) have also argued that two nonspecific factors, the treatment rationale and the assignment of homework, are integral to positive outcome in CT. In support of this assertion, they report that the majority of clinical improvement in CT occurs in the first 4 weeks and that during this time period CT-specific techniques are rarely applied. Ilardi and Craighead suggest that "Although the traditional view of CBT has held that depressotypic thoughts about the future could best be modified through the use of direct cognitive restructuring techniques, it appears . . . that hopelessness is often amenable to change in response to the reassuring nonspecific aspects of the CBT therapy situation itself (i.e., hearing a credible rationale, engaging in a procedure touted as being capable of producing improvement . . .)" (p. 152).

Tang and DeRubeis (1999a) question both the methods and conclusions of Ilardi and Craighead and others who place heavy emphasis on common factors in CT. First, they argue that, in fact, 40–60% of CT sessions typically occur within the first 4 weeks, thereby providing adequate time for significant CT interventions to be applied. Second, they point to the inherent problems with using group mean time course to make inferences about active ingredients of the cognitive-behavioral therapy package. Hollon (1999) also echoed these criticisms, emphasizing the importance of cognitive change interventions as opposed to nonspecific factors. Clearly, further research is required to explicate the relationship between nonspecific and specific therapy factors in CT (Tang and DeRubeis, 1999b).

Homework compliance

The assignment of between-session homework tasks is another therapeutic factor common to most forms of standard CT. Numerous studies have found an association between client compliance with CT homework assignments and positive outcome across a wide range of samples (Fennell and Teasdale, 1987; Persons et al., 1988; Neimeyer and Feixas, 1990; Burns and Nolen-Hoeksema, 1991, 1992; Addis and Jacobson, 2000). In fact, Persons et al. (1988) found a threefold improvement among subjects who complied with homework assignments in CT for depression. Moreover, a recent study by Burns and Spangler (2000), using structural equation modeling, has provided evidence that homework compliance and positive outcome are not only associated but that homework compliance exerts a large causal effect on depressive severity. Finally, another recent metaanalytic study investigating the association of homework assignment and homework completion with outcome also provided support for the role of both (Kazantis et al., 2000).

On the whole, thus, research on homework compliance appears to support both the practical and theoretical importance of this component of CT. From a pragmatic standpoint, assigning homework and maximizing client compliance appear to be strongly associated with positive change over time. These data also provide theoretical support for the emphasis on practicing skills that is common to most cognitive theories of change.

The empirical status of theory-specific interventions

CT specifies both behavioral and cognitive interventions (Beck et al., 1979), and numerous theoretical debates have ensued over the years regarding which of these interventions are most critical to positive therapeutic outcomes. There is current debate, for instance, regarding the relative importance of teaching patients how to manage negative automatic thoughts that arise in different situations, versus those cognitive techniques designed to induce change at deeper levels. In addition, others have argued for the viability of purely behavioral explanations of CT's effects, questioning whether cognitive interventions are in fact important elements of CT at all (Beidel and Turner, 1986; Jacobson et al., 1996). The roles of behavioral and cognitive interventions in CT for depression are discussed in turn below.

Behavioral interventions in CT

In contrast to the examination of the relative efficacy of specific cognitive techniques, studies examining the relative importance of cognitive versus behavioral techniques have a long and controversial history. In the early 1980s, for instance, Beidel and Turner (1986) and Latimer and Sweet (1984) challenged the theoretical and empirical foundation for the incorporation of cognitive techniques into traditional behavior therapy models. Numerous empirical investigations on this issue have been conducted as well; in large part, these studies have relied upon dismantling designs to isolate the behavioral and the cognitive-behavioral components of CT.

In the area of depression, a series of investigators have attempted to examine whether cognitive interventions add to the efficacy of purely behavioral packages (Shaw, 1977; Wilson et al., 1983). In one of the more recent and notable studies, Jacobson and colleagues (Jacobson et al., 1996; Gortner et al., 1998) examined competing hypotheses about the basis for cognitive therapy's effects by isolating the behavioral activation component of CT in the treatment of major depression. In this study, 150 subjects were randomly assigned to one of three conditions, all of which were based on the Beck et al. (1979) manual for the treatment of depression. The first condition focused exclusively on behavioral activation interventions and included behavioral strategies common to standard CT for depression such as monitoring daily activities, assessing pleasure and mastery, graded task assignment, and so forth. The second condition included behavioral activation interventions and interventions that focused on identifying and modifying negative automatic thoughts. Finally, the full CT condition included behavioral activation interventions, automatic thoughts interventions, and core schema-focused interventions. Each condition lasted for 20 treatment sessions.

Although each condition was associated with positive treatment outcomes, this study failed to find significant differences between the treatment components at the conclusion of acute treatment (Jacobson et al., 1996) or at any point over the 2-year follow-up period (Gortner et al., 1998). These results suggested that simply activating clients produced equivalent changes to the full CT package in both the acute and long-term treatment of clients with major depressive disorder. These results challenge the cognitive assumptions about the active ingredients of change, suggesting that the behavioral interventions of CT may be, in fact, not only necessary but sufficient in the treatment of depression.

While the dictates of science prohibit acceptance of the null hypothesis, the design of this study was noteworthy in its careful attention to factors that might otherwise support rival interpretations, namely it included careful procedures for monitoring treatment adherence and competence and included investigators committed to the performance of both the behavioral and cognitive conditions to minimize possible allegiance effects. Unfortunately, however, the absence of a placebo condition prohibits the determination of whether the behavioral and cognitive conditions were equally effective or equally ineffective. Further, as all conditions included the nonspecific aspects of CT, such as a collaborative relationship, and homework, the relative contributions of these factor versus the specific interventions used in each treatment condition cannot be assessed. For these reasons, the Jacobson et al. (1996) study is currently being replicated using behavioral activation, the complete CT package, and a selective serotonin reuptake inhibitor in a large placebo-controlled trial at the University of Washington. It is noteworthy, however, that a recent meta-analysis of the efficacy of CT (Gloaguen et al., 1998) failed to find any superiority of CT over behavioral therapy for depression.

In the anxiety disorders area, other studies have paralleled the results of the Jacobson et al. (1996) study. A number of early metaanalyses failed to find significant advantages for CT when compared to behavioral methods. For instance, building upon earlier reviews by Shapiro and Shapiro (1982) and Miller and Berman (1983), Berman et al. (1985) concluded that systematic desensitization interventions produced equivalent outcomes to cognitive techniques in the treatment of a wide range of anxiety problems; moreover, no additive benefits were found for the combination of treatments. A number of subsequent studies also failed to document additive benefits of cognitive techniques specifically in the treatment of social phobia (Stravynski et al., 1982; Emmelkamp et al., 1985; Jerremalm et al., 1986; Mersch et al., 1989) and simple phobias (Biran et al., 1981; Biran and Wilson, 1981). In the treatment of generalized anxiety disorder, Borkovec and Costello (1993) concluded that relaxation and CT produced roughly equivalent outcomes at posttest to those treated with relaxation interventions, although there was evidence that CT patients showed higher end-state functioning at 1-year follow-up. Results from Kendall et al. (1997) also provide some suggestive evidence supporting the relative importance of the behavioral exposure component in cognitive-behavioral therapy for youths with anxiety disorders. In contrast to the above studies, other research has found that the cognitive components of standard cognitive-behavioral models provide clear and significant additive effects. For instance, Mattick et al. (1989) compared exposure and cognitive restructuring in the treatment of social phobia and found that patients treated with the combined package demonstrated better outcomes on a range of variables.

Although a great deal of research has been conducted on the relative importance of cognitive and behavioral interventions, considerable uncertainty persists. Moreover, even though therapist allegiance has been largely ruled out as a confound in the results of clinical trials of CT for depression (Gaffan et al., 1995), lingering questions about the impact of investigator allegiance and criticisms of the competence of study therapists have unfortunately added to the ambiguity of such findings (Jacobson and Gortner, 2000). Results from current ongoing investigations will likely help to elucidate further the relative power of behavioral and cognitive interventions. In the meantime, however, it is clear that cognitive therapists should not neglect or underrate the importance of the behavioral interventions specified by most CT models.

Cognitive interventions in CT

Interestingly, little research has examined which cognitive interventions in CT account for outcome, despite the diversity of cognitive interventions included in a typical regimen of CT, and the considerable debate regarding which of these interventions are most important for producing enduring treatment gains.

Six investigations provide evidence linking a range of specific cognitive interventions to positive clinical outcomes. In one of the first investigations of specific cognitive interventions, Teasdale and Fennell (1982) examined the treatment of five depressed patients and found that interventions that actively modified thoughts led to greater reduction in depression than did interventions that simply explored thoughts. Jarrett and Nelson (1987) focused on the cognitive interventions of self-monitoring, logical analysis, and hypothesis testing in the treatment of depressed patients. They concluded that self-monitoring was not associated with most measures of change, whereas logical analysis and hypothesis testing were equally associated with change. Focusing specifically on the assignment of homework, Persons et al. (1988) found that depressed patients who completed homework assignments improved three times as much as those who did not complete assignments.

DeRubeis and Feeley (1990) and Feeley et al. (1999) also examined the role of CT-specific techniques, focusing specifically on ratings of "concrete techniques" and "abstract techniques," which were obtained from ratings of early treatment sessions. These groups of interventions were derived from a factor analysis of the Collaborative Study Psychotherapy Rating Scale CSPRS: S. D. Hollon et al., unpublished data). "Concrete techniques" included: set and follow agenda, review homework, ask for specific examples of beliefs, ask patient to report cognitions verbatim, label cognitive errors, examine evidence concerning beliefs, practice rational responses with patient, assign homework, assign/review self-monitoring, and ask patient to record thoughts. "Abstract techniques" included: encourage independence, discuss relationship of thoughts and feelings, discuss CT rationale, explore personal meaning of thoughts, explore underlying assumptions, encourage distancing of beliefs, negotiate content of session, and explain direction in session.

The results of this study suggested that concrete techniques predicted subsequent change in depression. In contrast, "abstract" techniques bore no relation to outcome. The investigators speculated that perhaps the abstract techniques are generally less appropriate for the early parts of a typical course of CT; these techniques were not adequately measured in their design. The problem-focused, pragmatic elements of CT, however, were clearly important to implement early in the process of therapy. Of note, however, is another study conducted by Startup and Shapiro (1993), which failed to replicate DeRubeis and Feeley's factor analysis of the CSPRS into the concrete and abstract factors.

In contrast to the above studies, two studies have raised questions about the impact of the cognitive interventions prescribed by standard CT. Hayes et al. (1996) found that cognitive therapists focused on making changes in depressed clients' beliefs about their interpersonal relationships more often than on making changes in clients' actual interpersonal relationships. Moreover, therapists were less likely to implement these interventions within a developmental context (i.e., in the context of exploring past or current relationships with parents or primary caregivers). Interestingly, however, interventions that addressed cognitive change were not associated with improvements in depression. In fact, cognitive interventions that aimed to change patients' beliefs about their interpersonal relationships were associated with worse outcomes. In contrast, interventions that focused on making actual changes in interpersonal relationships and interventions that included a developmental focus were associated with clinical improvement.

Jones and Pulos (1993) reported similar results in a study of therapeutic process in CBT and psychodynamic therapy. They examined the relationship of outcome to factor-analytically derived scales of "cognitive-behavioral technique" and "psychoanalytic technique." Their CBT factor included the following interventions: therapist behaves in a didactic manner, discussion of specific activities or tasks to attempt outside session, therapist acts to strengthen defenses, discussion centers on cognitive themes, therapist explains rationale, therapist gives advice and guidance, therapist exerts control over the interaction, therapist condescends or patronizes client, therapist self-discloses, therapist is directly reassuring. Results suggested that the CT technique factor was not associated with outcome among patients treated with CT. In contrast, the "psychodynamic technique" factor, which emphasized developmental, affective, and therapeutic process factors, was associated with improvement on the majority of outcome measures.

Thus, it is clear that some important evidence has been provided for specific components of the CT package. In particular, active modification of thoughts, logical analysis and hypothesis testing, the assignment of homework, and the aggregate of "concrete" CT interventions (identified by DeRubeis and Feeley) have received some empirical validation. Nevertheless, a number of important issues require further attention.

First, it will be important for future research to determine whether the phase of treatment is an important variable to consider in the evaluation of relative importance of cognitive techniques. For instance, are some techniques more applicable, appropriate, or necessary in some phases of treatment than others? Second, research in this area will benefit from the development of greater consensus about which techniques are, in fact, "cognitive." The use of factor-analytically derived scales may be an important part of this effort; however, such techniques may also risk identifying interventions as "cognitive" that would not be theoretically prescribed by standard CT. For instance, Jones and Pulos' (1993) inclusion of "therapist condescends or patronizes client" and/or "therapist self-discloses" as CBT interventions would likely be questioned by many cognitive therapists and theorists. On a related note, however, some of the studies raise the question of whether standard cognitive techniques could be enhanced by the integration of a greater interpersonal and/or developmental focus. Third, it is important to note that the studies in this area have largely focused on treatment for depression; therefore, it will be important for future research to identify whether these results generalize to the treatment of other clinical disorders. Fourth, it is clear that only a few of the widely used cognitive techniques have been specifically evaluated; thus, further research is clearly necessary to provide a more comprehensive picture of the relative importance of the cognitive components employed in a typical regimen of CT.

On balance, although the efficacy literature supports the status of CT as an effective treatment technology, considerable discussion and data need to be developed about the specific agents of change. In this regard, recent developments of schema-focused CT (Young, 1999), bear some commentary. To our knowledge, there is no evidence that an increased emphasis on core schemata or underlying beliefs, either through the application of more interventions aimed at this level of thinking, or through prolonged length of treatment, has a positive relationship to treatment outcome or lowered relapse rates. Indeed, as noted above, the evidence appears that behavioral components may equal the outcome associated with cognitive components of the therapy (Jacobson et al., 1996; Gortner et al., 1998), that change tends to happen early in CT when the focus is typically more on behavioral aspects of depression (Ilardi and Craighead, 1994), and that the more specific aspects of CT have a stronger relationship to outcome than the more abstract aspects (DeRubeis and Feeley, 1990; Feeley et al., 1999). Given the apparent disjuncture between the mounting evidence and the conceptual model related to schema-focused CT, future efforts to examine the outcomes and processes associated with longer-term, schema-focused CT are clearly warranted.

Finally, it is important to consider what types of research designs are most conducive to an interest in linking particular interventions with outcome. Ablon and Jones (1999) note: "specific interventions do not have fixed meanings independent of context and cannot be assumed to contribute discretely and uniquely to outcome. This is one important reason why it has been difficult to identify the effects of particular kinds of interventions ... in group designs that average effects across patient–therapist pairs" (p. 73). The advantages and disadvantages of group correlational designs as opposed to alternative qualitative designs will be important to consider (Stiles and Shapiro, 1994; Ablon and Jones, 1999) in future efforts to understand the relative importance of particular cognitive interventions.

What are the mechanisms of change in CT?

Does CT work, as cognitive theory specifies, by influencing cognition? Although outcome research demonstrates that CT is an efficacious treatment for many clinical problems, one cannot simply extrapolate from such results support for the notion that CT is effective *because* it modifies cognitive phenomena. Similarly, although the studies reviewed above inform us about possible active ingredients of change in CT, they do not explicitly specify mechanisms of change. Given these facts, numerous process researchers have sought to assess directly the mechanisms of change in CT. Whereas a few studies have examined the role of noncognitive mechanisms of change (e.g., behavioral or affective processes), most research to date has focused on testing the cognitive mediation hypothesis, investigating whether cognitive phenomena are indeed primary change mechanisms in CT. Each of these areas is reviewed in turn.

Evaluating the role of noncognitive factors as mechanisms of change

Some studies have raised interesting questions about the plausibility of noncognitive mediational models of depression, focusing in particular on behavioral factors (Beidel and Turner, 1986; Jacobson et al., 1996) or affective factors (Greenberg and Safran, 1984, 1989; Castonguay et al., 1996). For instance, although the Jacobson et al. (1996) study did not provide a direct test of behavioral mediation of treatment effects, the results led the investigators to speculate about the possibility that increases in positive reinforcement in depressed patients' environments may be important mediators of change.

In regard to affective processes, a number of writers have called for an increased focus in CT on the importance of emotion in the process of change (Greenberg and Safran, 1984, 1989; Safran and Segal, 1990). In an empirical investigation of this proposition, Castonguay et al. (1996) examined, among other factors, the degree of depressed clients' emotional involvement in treatment. Results suggested that client emotional involvement was uniquely related to reductions in posttreatment Beck Depression Inventory scores. These results led Castonguay et al. to conclude that the client's affective processes may represent a largely unexplored but important potential mediator of change. In contrast, however, Borkovec and Costello (1993) found that patients with generalized anxiety disorder who received nondirective therapy performed significantly worse on outcome measures, despite receiving the highest ratings of emotional experiencing during treatment sessions. Future research is needed to explore the relative importance of cognitive factors given these other possible noncognitive mediators across the wide range of clinical problems addressed by CT.

Evaluating the role of cognition as a mechanism of change

The role of cognitive phenomena in the mediation of change has been widely addressed by CT researchers. Most studies have tackled this question by comparing the effect of CT and alternative psychosocial or pharmacological treatments on measures of cognitive processing. These studies have largely focused on the question of whether CT is either uniquely (or, at least, differentially) able to produce change in cognition. In general, studies attempting to isolate such mode-specific effects of CT have yielded mixed results.

A number of studies have provided evidence of mode-specific effects for CT in the treatment of anxiety. Mattick et al. (1989) found that CT patients treated for panic disorder showed more change on cognitive variables than did those treated with exposure interventions. In the treatment of generalized anxiety disorder, Borkovec and Costello (1993) also reported evidence of mode-specific effects. Patients treated with CT demonstrated greater change on measures of worry and depression, while behaviorally treated patients showed greater change on measures of daily anxiety.

Among depressed patients, Rush et al. (1982) found greater improvement in hopelessness and more generalized positive changes in self-concept among patients receiving CT compared to those receiving pharmacotherapy (PT).

Whisman et al. (1991) examined specificity of treatment effects among a sample of inpatients treated with pharmacotherapy (PT) alone or PT plus CT. Subjects were evaluated immediately following treatment and at 6- and 12-month follow-ups. The results suggested significant decreases in automatic thoughts (as measured by the Automatic Thoughts Questionnaire) and hopelessness (as measured by the Hopelessness Scale) in both treatment groups over the course of treatment (though not in dysfunctional attitudes, as measured by the Dysfunctional Attitudes Scale, or cognitive bias, as measured by the Cognitive Bias Questionnaire). Furthermore, both groups evidenced similar degrees of depression severity at posttreatment and follow-up. CT patients, however, reported less hopelessness and fewer cognitive biases at the end of treatment and at the 6- and 12-month follow-up points (and fewer dysfunctional attitudes at the 6-month follow-up). Whisman et al. (1991) concluded that these results support the cognitive model of change and the specificity of effects of CT.

Bowers (1990) also tested for mode-specific effects among depressed inpatients and reported some evidence that patients treated with medication and CT, or treated with medication and relaxation training, evidenced lower scores on the Automatic Thoughts Questionnaire relative to patients treated with medication alone; however, there were no group differences on measures of hopelessness or the Dysfunctional Attitudes Scale. Similarly, McKnight et al. (1992) also showed that depressed patients treated with CT evidenced greater improvements in dysfunctional thoughts (as measured by the Personal Beliefs Inventory) as compared to patients treated with medication. Finally, most recently, Segal et al. (1999) found that patients successfully treated with CT evidenced less dysfunctional attitudes following a negative mood induction than did patients successfully treated with PT. Importantly, dysfunctional attitudes at posttest also predicted relapse during a 30-month follow-up, suggesting that cognitive improvement is not only specific to successful CT, but also to the prevention of relapse.

In contrast to the above-reported findings, however, a second group of studies has failed to find any mode-specific effects. In one of the earliest studies of differential treatment mechanisms, Zeiss et al. (1979) found that patients in CT, behavior therapy, and interpersonal therapy exhibited equivalent change on measures of cognitive, behavioral, and interpersonal factors. Consistent with Zeiss et al. (1979), Blackburn and Bishop (1983) failed to find specific effects for subjects treated with CT and/or PT on the standardized measure of cognitive functioning used (i.e., the Hopelessness Scale). Similarly, Wilson et al. (1983) found that, at the end of treatment, CT and behavior therapy for depression had equivalent effects on "cognitive targets" (i.e., positive cognitions, negative cognitions, and irrational beliefs). Simons et al. (1984) also found little evidence for mode-specific effects among subjects receiving CT and those receiving PT, noting that their findings call into question the "causal" status of cognitive factors.

In an examination of the TDCRP data, Imber et al. (1990) also concluded that there was little support for mode-specific hypotheses of differential treatment effects for CT, PT, or interpersonal therapy. No significant differences between treatments in social/interpersonal functioning or biological functioning were found, and differential change for the CT treatment was found on only one of the cognitive measures examined, the need for social approval factor of the Dysfunctional Attitudes Scale. No differences were found, however, on the perfectionism factor of the Dysfunctional Attitudes Scale, the full Dysfunctional Attitudes Scale score, or two cognitive subscales derived from the Hamilton Rating Scale for Depression and the Beck Depression Inventory. Imber et al. (1990) concluded that: "Perhaps the most parsimonious interpretation of our findings is that there are core processes that operate across treatments, overriding differences among techniques" (p. 357; see also Jacobson et al., 1996).

Finally, a third group of studies has suggested that, while CT may not uniquely influence cognition, cognitive changes may nevertheless be uniquely related to clinical improvement among patients treated with CT. Rush et al. (1981) concluded that, while CT and imipramine treatment patients evidenced similar changes on cognitive measures, cross-lagged panel correlations suggested that early cognitive change predicted later change in vegetative and motivational symptoms among CT patients. In the imipramine group, however, no predictive patterns were observed. DeRubeis et al. (1990) also examined the effect of early cognitive change among a sample of patients treated with CT (either singly or in combination with PT) or with PT alone. Results suggested that both groups evidenced significant pre–post change on the cognitive measures, such that CT was not uniquely associated with change in cognition. However, early cognitive change (as measured by the Automatic Thoughts Questionnaire, the Dysfunctional Attitude Scale, and the Hopelessness Scale) predicted later depression in the CT group – but not in PT. Early change in depression, however, was not predictive of later change in cognitive processes for either group.

Echoing other investigators, DeRubeis et al. (1990) conclude that cognitive change does not play a "causally sufficient" role in the remediation of depression; however, it does appear to be an important mediator of change in CT. A metaanalysis of studies investigating cognitive mediators of change (Oei and Free, 1995) reported results consistent with Rush et al. (1981) and DeRubeis et al. (1990). Findings suggested that change in cognitive style occurred in all treatment studies (including waitlist controls); moreover, there was no differential degree of improvement in CT versus the other active treatments investigated. However, results did suggest that changes in cognition appeared to be significantly related to changes in depression, as measured by the Beck Depression Inventory, among patients treated with CT or other psychosocial treatments, though not patients in medication or waitlist control groups. Interestingly, however, this pattern of results was not confirmed when the Hamilton Rating Scale for Depression was used as the measure of depression severity.

Thus, research to date is clearly equivocal with respect to the mediational status of cognition in the process of change in CT. Although some studies support such a cognitive mediational hypothesis, numerous investigators conclude that the failure of many studies to document mode-specific effects challenges the plausibility of such a hypothesis. The lack of consensus in this area is further complicated by the cogent methodological and conceptual criticisms that some researchers have raised. Hollon et al. (1987), for instance, explain that it is erroneous to conclude that a lack of specificity de facto represents a lack of causal mediation. They present a number of alternative explanatory models that must be considered before the causal status of a potential mediator can be effectively challenged. Whisman (1993) also identified a number of methodological weaknesses of the extant research on cognitive mediation. He reports that most studies have suffered from inadequate power to detect differences between groups on measures of cognitive phenomena. In addition, he notes that some studies that report mode-specific differences (Rush et al., 1982) fail to address the relationship between symptomatic improvement and improvement in cognitive functioning. Finally, he raises questions about the measurement strategies adopted in most studies, citing concerns about the validity, sensitivity, and specificity of measures, the need for priming strategies (Miranda and Persons, 1988; Miranda et al., 1990), and obscuration of mode-specific effects that may result from combining multiple factors into single full-scale scores. Most pointedly, critics such as Coyne and Gotlib (1983, 1986) have suggested that the emphasis on cognitive phenomena has been to the exclusion of other important processes (such as in the interpersonal realm), and that cognitive phenomena in depression in particular may in fact be epiphenomenal to other emotional/interpersonal factors.

Interestingly, recent work by Tang and DeRubeis (1999b) may provide another methodology for examining the mediational status of cognitive change, which bypasses many of the methodological and conceptual problems noted above. Tang and DeRubeis analyzed individual patient time course data and assessed presence of cognitive change by rating audiotapes of sessions on the Patient Cognitive Change Scale. Tang and DeRubeis found that many patient trajectories are most accurately described by patterns of sudden and rapid change – and that evidence of cognitive change is often observed in the sessions preceding such symptomatic improvement. Based on these results, Tang and DeRubeis (1999b) conclude: "these results provide direct support for the cognitive mediation hypothesis of CBT. They revealed that in about 50% of the treatment responders, superior treatment outcome was preceded by sudden gains, which were in turn immediately preceded by substantial cognitive changes" (p. 902).

Clearly, more work is required to understand fully mediators of change in CT. Moreover, even if further research is able to document the mediational status of cognition in general, questions abound regarding the role of specific aspects of cognition. Numerous investigators have discussed varying models of cognitive mediation (Hollon et al., 1990; Barber and DeRubeis, 1989; Persons, 1993; Clark et al., 1999). These discussions have focused on the relative support for the following models: *accommodation*, in which basic cognitive processes and/or structures are modified or changed; *deactivation*, in which basic cognitive processes and/or structures are not changed but rather are deactivated, while other more adaptive processes or structures are activated; or *compensation*, in which specific skills are acquired that will allow individuals to interrupt negative cognitive patterns. Further theoretical clarification and empirical investigation of these models are clearly important in the effort to understand the central mediators of change in CT.

Methodological recommendations for future research

Although future directions have been outlined above for each specific domain addressed by process research on CT, a number of general methodological issues must also be considered if future research is to elucidate better the processes of change in CT. Unfortunately, it is important to note that such methodological problems often arise because questions about process of change are treated as secondary to questions of efficacy in larger outcome investigations, thus reflecting a more pervasive problem in psychotherapy process research. Future investigations would do well to balance concerns about outcome with the following process issues in the planning of major research endeavors.

A number of researchers, for instance, have questioned whether the measures employed in studies to date are in fact specific and sensitive to the constructs most salient to a cognitive model of therapeutic change. Barber and DeRubeis (1989) suggest that part of the ambiguity of results may be related to the fact that methods and measures have not successfully targeted "compensatory" skills, which they hypothesize to be a primary mechanism of action in CT. Whisman et al. (1991) ask whether measures should target "surface" cognitive dysfunction or "core" processes. Hollon and Kris (1984) propose the distinction between cognitive product, cognitive structure, and cognitive process, which may also be important to capture in investigations of therapeutic change.

The self-report nature of most cognitive measures used to date may also be problematic. DeRubeis et al. (2001) suggest that CT patients may respond to self-report measures by employing compensatory skills learned in treatment, thus prohibiting assessment of underlying schemata. Towards this end, mood induction procedures may prove to be particularly useful in studies of processes of change. In general, it is clear that greater specificity within cognitive theory regarding the salience of particular constructs to therapeutic process would facilitate future research, which in turn would enhance theoretical models of the process of change in CT.

A related research issue concerns the timing of assessments of process variables. Imber et al. (1990), for instance, suggest that their pattern of largely null findings may be related to the fact that they assessed patients at posttreatment. They raise the possibility that mode-specific effects may be apparent earlier in treatment, particularly for treatment responders; however, by the time such patients are assessed at posttest, these mode-specific changes have generalized to the other salient domains of functioning, thus preventing investigators from identifying mode-specific effects. Future research would benefit from both early and later assessment of cognitive processes, in attempting to assess their hypothetically causal role in CT.

Finally, it will be important for all future investigations to document carefully the integrity of treatments provided. Because CT is a multifaceted treatment, including a wide variety of cognitive and behavioral interventions, the use of standardized treatment manuals and careful tests of adherence and competence will be important in order to specify accurately the nature of the independent variable. Documenting treatment integrity in these ways will allow for greater generalizability of results and ease of comparison across studies.

Conclusion

This chapter has examined the difficult but critical area of process of change in CT. Based on a model of therapeutic change in CT, we have reviewed literature in the areas of client and therapist factors, nonspecific and treatment-specific components, as well as mechanisms of change. Within each area we have summarized the state of the extant literature, and offered suggestions for both theory and research development.

Despite the strong claim that CT works for a variety of clinical problems, it is our overall impression that the data to date offer many alternative hypotheses than the theory-consistent model that CT works because it changes cognitions. Although evidence that cognitive processes predict negative experience has existed for some time, and the primacy of cognitive change in CT has only recently been demonstrated in a convincing fashion (Tang and DeRubeis, 1999b). Further, given the number of studies that have failed to support cognitive primacy, or that question the additive beneficial effect of truly cognitive interventions in CT (Jacobson et al., 1996), it must be concluded that at present the mechanisms of change in CT are not well understood. As such, we believe that a considerable amount of energy needs to be directed towards questions of mechanisms of change in CT.

In addition to their obvious contribution to our understanding of the model of change, well-designed and controlled process investigations have the potential to contribute enormously to the delivery and practice of CT. Given today's climate of reduced resources for mental health services, questions about processes of change are increasingly important. Identifying the active ingredients of CT may help to guide us towards more parsimonious treatment models that may be more amenable to broad dissemination (Jacobson and Gortner, 2000; Hamilton and Dobson, 2001). Alternatively, such research may also spur investigators to enhance particular components of the overall CT package to increase the power of the current treatment technology. Determining critical mechanisms of change may also help to focus our intervention strategies, for as Hollon and Kris note (1984): "Once we know what active changes need to occur within the client for clinical improvement to take place, we can then devise the optimal clinical interventions for a given client or type of disorder" (p. 56). The studies conducted to date represent an important beginning. It is hoped that this review and recommendations provided herein will serve to identify new and important directions and encourage further exploration of the processes of change in CT.

REFERENCES

Ablon, J. S. and Jones, E. E. (1999). Psychotherapy process in the national institute of mental health treatment of depression collaborative research program. *Journal of Consulting and Clinical Psychology*, **67**(1), 64–75.

Abramson, L. T., Alloy, L. B., Hogan, M. E., et al. (1999). Cognitive vulnerability to depression: theory and evidence. *Journal of Cognitive Psychotherapy: An International Quarterly*, **13**, 5–20.

Addis, M. and Jacobson, N. S. (1996). Reasons for depression and the process of cognitive-behavioral psychotherapies. *Journal of Consulting and Clinical Psychology*, **64**(6), 1417–24.

Addis, M. E. and Jacobson, N. S. (2000). A closer look at the treatment rationale and homework compliance in cognitive-behavioral therapy for depression. *Cognitive Therapy and Research*, **24**, 313–26.

Alloy, L. B. (2001). The developmental origins of cognitive vulnerability to depression: negative interpersonal context leads to personal vulnerability. *Cognitive Therapy and Research*, **25**, 349–52.

Alloy, L. B., Abramson, L. Y., Whitehouse, W. G., et al. (1999). Depressogenic cognitive styles: predictive validity, information processing and personality characteristics, and developmental origins. *Behaviour Research and Therapy*, **37**, 503–31.

Barber, J. P. and DeRubeis, R. J. (1989). On second thought: where the action is in cognitive therapy for depression. *Cognitive Therapy and Research*, **13**, 441–57.

Beach, S. R. H., Sandeen, E. E., and O'Leary, K. D. (1990). *Depression in Marriage: A Model for Etiology and Treatment*. New York: Guilford Press.

Beck, A. T. (1991). Cognitive therapy as the integrative therapy. *Journal of Psychotherapy Integration*, **1**(3), 191–8.

Beck, J. (1995). *Cognitive Therapy: Basics and Beyond*. New York: Guilford Press.

Beck, A. T., Rush, A. J., Shaw, B. F., and Emery, G. (1979). *Cognitive Therapy of Depression*. New York: Guilford Press.

Beckham, E. E. (1989). Improvement after evaluation in psychotherapy of depression: evidence of a placebo effect? *Journal of Clinical Psychology*, **45**, 945–50.

Beckham, E. E. and Watkins, J. T. (1989). Process and outcome in cognitive therapy. In *Comprehensive Handbook of Cognitive Therapy*, ed. A. Freeman, K. Simon, L. Beutler, and H. Arkowitz, pp. 61–81. New York: Plenum Press.

Beidel, D. C. and Turner, S. M. (1986). A critique of the theoretical bases of cognitive-behavioral theories and therapy. *Clinical Psychology Review*, **6**, 177–97.

Berman, J. S., Miller, R. C., and Massman, P. J. (1985). Cognitive therapy versus systematic desensitization: is one treatment superior? *Psychological Bulletin*, **97**(3), 451–61.

Beutler, L. E. and Baker, M. (1998). The movement towards empirical validation: at what level should we analyze, and who are the consumers? In *Empirically Supported Therapies: Best Practice in Professional Psychology*, ed. K. S. Dobson and K. D. Craig, pp. 43–65. Thousand Oaks, CA: Sage Books.

Beutler, L. E., Engle, D., Mohr, D., et al. (1991). Predictors of differential response to cognitive, experiential, and self-directed psychotherapeutic procedures. *Journal of Consulting and Clinical Psychology*, **59**(2), 333–40.

Biran, M. and Wilson, G. T. (1981). Treatment of phobic disorders using cognitive and exposure methods: a self-efficacy analysis. *Journal of Consulting and Clinical Psychology*, **49**, 886–99.

Biran, M., Augusto, F., and Wilson, G. T. (1981). In vivo exposure vs cognitive restructuring in the treatment of scriptophobia. *Behaviour Research and Therapy*, **19**, 525–32.

Blackburn, I. M. and Bishop, S. (1983). Changes in cognition with pharmacotherapy and cognitive therapy. *British Journal of Psychiatry*, **143**, 609–17.

Blatt, S. J. and Felsen, I. (1993). Different kinds of folks may need different kinds of strokes: the effect of patients' characteristics on therapeutic process and outcome. *Psychotherapy Research*, **3**(4), 245–59.

Blatt, S. J., Zuroff, D. C., Quinlan, D. M., and Pilkonis, P. A. (1996). Interpersonal factors in brief treatment of depression: further analyses of the National Institute of Mental Health treatment of depression collaborative research program. *Journal of Consulting and Clinical Psychology*, **64**(1), 162–71.

Borkovec, T. D. and Costello, E. (1993). Efficacy of applied relaxation and cognitive-behavioral therapy in the treatment of generalized anxiety disorder. *Journal of Consulting and Clinical Psychology*, **61**(4), 611–19.

Bowers, W. A. (1990). Treatment of depressed in-patients: cognitive therapy plus medication, relaxation plus medication, and medication alone. *British Journal of Psychiatry*, **156**, 73–8.

Brewin, C. R. (1989). Cognitive change processes in psychotherapy. *Psychological Review*, **96**(3), 379–94.

Burns, D. D. and Nolen-Hoeksema, S. (1991). Coping styles, homework compliance, and the effectiveness of cognitive-behavioral therapy. *Journal of Consulting and Clinical Psychology*, **59**, 305–11.

Burns, D. D. and Nolen-Hoeksema, S. (1992). Therapeutic empathy and recovery from depression in cognitive-behavioral therapy: a structural equation model. *Journal of Consulting and Clinical Psychology*, **60**, 441–9.

Burns, D. D. and Spangler, D. L. (2000). Does psychotherapy homework lead to improvements in depression in cognitive-behavioral therapy or does improvement lead to increased homework compliance? *Journal of Consulting and Clinical Psychology*, **68**, 46–56.

Castonguay, L. G., Goldfried, M. R., Wiser, S., Raue, P. J., and Hayes, A. M. (1996). Predicting the effect of cognitive therapy for depression: a study of unique and common factors. *Journal of Consulting and Clinical Psychology*, **64**(30), 497–504.

Clark, D. (1995). Perceived limitations of standard cognitive therapy: a consideration of efforts to revise Beck's theory and therapy. *Journal of Cognitive Psychotherapy*, **9**, 153–72.

Clark, D. A., Beck, A. T., and Alford, B. A. (1999). *Scientific Foundations of Cognitive Theory and Therapy of Depression*. New York: John Wiley.

Coyne, J. C. and Gotlib, I. H. (1983). The role of cognition in depression: a critical appraisal. *Psychological Bulletin*, **94**, 472–505.

Coyne, J. C. and Gotlib, I. H. (1986). Studying the role of cognition in depression: well-trodden paths and cul-de-sacs. *Cognitive Therapy and Research*, **10**, 695–705.

DeRubeis, R. J. and Feeley, M. (1990). Determinants of change in cognitive therapy for depression. *Cognitive Therapy and Research*, **14**, 469–82.

DeRubeis, R. J., Hollon, S. D., Evans, M. D., et al. (1990). How does cognitive therapy work? Cognitive change and symptom change in cognitive therapy and phamacotherapy for depression. *Journal of Consulting and Clinical Psychology*, **58**, 862–9.

De Rubeis, R. J., Beck, A. T., and Tang, T. (2001). Cognitive therapy. In *Handbook of Cognitive-behavioral Therapies*, 2nd edn, ed. K. S. Dobson, pp. 349–92. New York: Guilford Press.

Dobson, K. S. (ed.) (2001). *Handbook of Cognitive-behavioral Therapies* 2nd edn. New York: Guilford Press.

Dobson, K. S. and Khatri, N. (2001). Cognitive therapy: looking forward, looking back. *Journal of Clinical Psychology: Science and Practice*, **56**, 907–23.

Dobson, K. S. and Pusch, D. (1993). Towards a definition of the conceptual and empirical boundaries of cognitive therapy. *Australian Psychologist*, **28**(3), 137–44.

Emmelkamp, P. M., Mersch, P. P., Vissia, E., and Van-der-Helm, M. (1985). Social phobia: a comparative evaluation of cognitive and behavioral interventions. *Behaviour Research and Therapy*, **23**, 365–9.

Feeley, M., DeRubeis, R. J., and Gelfand, L. A. (1999). The temporal relation of adherence and alliance to symptom change in cognitive therapy for depression. *Journal of Consulting and Clinical Psychology*, **67**(4), 578–82.

Fennell, M. J. and Teasdale, J. D. (1987). Cognitive therapy for depression: individual differences and the process of change. *Cognitive Therapy and Research*, **11**(2), 253–71.

Frank, E., Kupfer, D. J., Jacob, M., and Jarrett, D. (1987). Personality features and response to acute treatment in recurrent depression. *Journal of Personality Disorders*, **1**(1), 14–26.

Gaffan, E. A., Tsaousis, I., and Kemp-Wheeler, S. M. (1995). Researcher allegiance and meta-analysis: the case of cognitive therapy for depression. *Journal of Consulting and Clinical Psychology*, **63**, 966–80.

Gaston, L., Marmar, C. R., Gallagher, D., and Thompson, L. W. (1991). Alliance prediction of outcome beyond in-treatment symptomatic change as psychotherapy processes. *Psychotherapy Research*, **1**(2), 104–14.

Gloaguen, V., Cottraux, J., Cucherat, M., and Blackburn, I. M. (1998). A meta-analysis of the effects of cognitive therapy in depressed patients. *Journal of Affective Disorders*, **49**(1), 59–72.

Gollan, J. K., Jacobson, N. S., Gortner, E. T., and Dobson, K. S. (in preparation). Predictors of depression relapse following cognitive behavior therapy.

Gortner, E. T., Gollan, J. K., Dobson, K. S., and Jacobson, N. S. (1998). Cognitive-behavioral treatment for depression: relapse prevention. *Journal of Consulting and Clinical Psychology*, **66**, 377–84.

Greenberg, L. S. and Safran, J. D. (1984). Integrating affect and cognition: a perspective on the process of therapeutic change. *Cognitive Therapy and Research*, **8**(6), 559–78.

Greenberg, L. S. and Safran, J. D. (1989). Emotion in psychotherapy. *American Psychologist*, **44**(1), 19–29.

Hamilton, K. E. and Dobson, K. S. (2001). Empirically supported treatments in psychology: implications for international dissemination. *International Journal of Health and Clinical Psychology*, **1**, 35–51.

Hayes, A. M., Castonguay, L. G., and Goldfried, M. R. (1996). Effectiveness of targeting the vulnerability factors of depression in cognitive therapy. *Journal of Consulting and Clinical Psychology*, **64**(3), 623–7.

Hays, P. A. (1995). Multicultural applications of cognitive-behavior therapy. *Professional Psychology: Research and Practice*, **26**, 309–15.

Heimberg, R. G. and Barlow, D. H. (1991). New developments in cognitive-behavioral therapy for social phobia. *Journal of Clinical Psychiatry*, **52**, 21–30.

Hollon, S. D. (1999). Rapid early response in cognitive behavior therapy: a commentary. *Clinical Psychology: Science and Practice*, **6**(3), 305–9.

Hollon, S. D. and Kris, M. R. (1984). Cognitive factors in clinical research and practice. *Clinical Psychology Review*, **4**, 35–76.

Hollon, S. D., DeRubeis, R. J., and Evans, M. D. (1987). Causal mediation of change in treatment for depression: discriminating between nonspecificity and noncausality. *Psychological Bulletin*, **102**, 139–49.

Horvath, A. O. and Symonds, B. D. (1991). Relation between working alliance and outcome in psychotherapy: a meta-analysis. *Journal of Counseling Psychology*, **38**, 139–49.

Ilardi S. S. and Craighead W. E. (1994). The role of nonspecific factors on cognitive-behavior therapy for depression. *Clinical Psychology: Science and Practice*, **1**(2), 138–56.

Imber, S. D., Pilkonis, P. A., Sotsky, S. M., and Elkin, I. (1990). Mode-specific effects among three treatments for depression. *Journal of Consulting and Clinical Psychology*, **58**, 352–9.

Jacobson, N. S. (1989). The therapist–client relationship in cognitive behavior therapy: implications for treatment of depression. *Journal of Cognitive Psychotherapy*, **3**, 85–96.

Jacobson, N. S. (1999). The role of the allegiance effect in psychotherapy research: controlling and accounting for it. *Clinical Psychology: Science and Practice*, **6**(1), 116–19.

Jacobson, N. S. and Gortner, E. T. (2000). Can depression be de-medicalized in the 21st century: scientific revolutions, counter-revolutions, and the magnetic field of normal science. *Behavior Research and Therapy*, **38**, 103–17.

Jacobson, N. S., Dobson, K. S., Truax, P. A., et al. (1996). A component analysis of cognitive-behavioral treatment for depression. *Journal of Consulting and Clinical Psychology*, **64**, 295–304.

Jarrett, R. B. and Nelson, R. O. (1987). Mechanisms of change in cognitive therapy of depression. *Behavior Therapy*, **18**, 227–41.

Jarrett, R. B., Eaves, G. G., Grannemann, B. D., and Rush, A. J. (1991). Clinical, cognitive, and demographic predictors of response to cognitive therapy for depression: a preliminary report. *Psychiatry Research*, **37**(3), 245–60.

Jerremalm, A., Jansson, L., and Oest, L. G. (1986). Individual response patterns and the effects of different behavioral methods in the treatment of dental phobia. *Behaviour Research and Therapy*, **24**, 587–96.

Jones, E. E. and Pulos, S. M. (1993). Comparing the process in psychodynamic and cognitive-behavioral therapies. *Journal of Consulting and Clinical Psychology*, **61**(2), 306–16.

Kazantzis, N., Deane, F. P., and Ronan, K. R. (2000). Homework assignments in cognitive and behavioral therapy: a meta-analysis. *Clinical Psychology: Science and Practice*, **7**, 189–202.

Kendall, P. C., Flannery-Schroeder, E., Panichelli-Mindel, S. M., et al. (1997). Therapy for youths with anxiety disorders: a second randomized clincal trial. *Journal of Consulting and Clinical Psychology*, **65**(3), 366–80.

Kohlenberg, R. J. and Tsai, M. (1991). *Functional Analytic Psychotherapy: Creating Intense and Curative Therapeutic Relationships*. New York: Plenum Press.

Krupnick, J. L., Sotsky, S. M., Simmens, S., et al. (1996). The role of the therapeutic alliance in psychotherapy and pharmacotherapy outcome: Findings in the National Institute of Mental Health treatment of depression collaborative research program. *Journal of Consulting and Clinical Psychology*, **64**, 532–9.

Latimer, P. R. and Sweet, A. A. (1984). Cognitive versus behavioral procedures in cognitive-behavior therapy: a critical review of the evidence. *Journal of Behavior Therapy and Experimental Psychiatry*, **15**, 9–22.

Luborsky, L., McLellan, A. T., Woody, G. E., O'Brien, C. P., and Auerbach, A. (1985). Therapist success and its determinants. *Archives of General Psychiatry*, **41**, 602–11.

Mattick, R. P., Peters, L., and Clark, J. C. (1989). Exposure and cognitive restructuring for social phobia: a controlled study. *Behavior Therapy*, **20**, 3–23.

McKnight, D. L., Nelson-Grey, R. O., and Barnhill, J. (1992). Dexamethasone suppression test and response to cognitive therapy and antidepressant medication. *Behavior Therapy*, **23**, 99–111.

Mersch, P. P., Emmelkamp, P. M., Boegels, S. M., and Van der Sleen, J. (1989). Social phobia: individual response patterns and the effects of behavioral and cognitive interventions. *Behaviour Research and Therapy*, **27**, 421–34.

Miller, W. R. (ed.) (1999). *Integrating Spirituality into Treatment: Resources for Practitioners*. Washington, DC: American Psychological Association.

Miller, R. C. and Berman, J. S. (1983). The efficacy of cognitive behavior therapies: a quantitative review of the research evidence. *Psychological Bulletin*, **94**(1), 39–53.

Miller, W. R. and Martin, J. E. (eds) (1988). *Behavior Therapy and Religion: Integrating Spiritual and Behavioral Approaches to Change*. Thousand Oaks, CA: Sage Publications.

Miranda, J. and Persons, J. B. (1988). Dysfunctional attitudes are mood-state dependent. *Journal of Abnormal Psychology*, **97**(1), 76–9.

Miranda, J., Persons, J. B., and Byers, C. N. (1990). Endorsement of dysfunctional beliefs depends on current mood state. *Journal of Abnormal Psychology*, **99**(3), 237–41.

Muran, J. C., Segal, Z. V., Samstag, L., and Crawford, C. E. (1994). Patient pretreatment interpersonal problems and therapeutic alliance in short-term cognitive therapy. *Journal of Consulting and Clinical Psychology*, **62**(1), 185–90.

Neimeyer, R. A. and Feixas, G. (1990). The role of homework and skill acquisition in the outcome of group cognitive therapy for depression. *Behavior Therapy*, **21**, 281–92.

Oei T. P. and Free, M. L. (1995). Do cognitive behavior therapies validate cognitive models of mood disorders? A review of the empirical evidence. *International Journal of Psychology*, **30**(20), 145–80.

Organista, K. C. and Munoz, R. F. (1996). Cognitive-behavioral therapy with Latinos. *Cognitive and Behavioral Practice*, **3**, 255–70.

Persons, J. B. (1993). The process of change in cognitive therapy: schema change or acquisition of compensatory skills. *Cognitive Therapy and Research*, **17**, 123–37.

Persons, J. B. and Burns, D. D. (1985). Mechanisms of action of cognitive therapy: the relative contribution of technical and interpersonal interventions. *Cognitive Therapy and Research*, **9**, 539–51.

Persons, J. B., Burns, D. D., and Perloff, J. M. (1988). Predictors of dropout and outcome in cognitive therapy for depression in a private practice setting. *Cognitive Therapy and Research*, **12**, 557–75.

Prince, S. E. and Jacobson, N. S. (1995). A review and evaluation of marital and family therapies for affective disorders. *Journal of Marital and Family Therapy*, **21**(4), 377—401.

Propst, L. R., Ostrom, R., Watkins, P., et al. (1992). Comparative efficacy of religious and non-religious cognitive-behavioral therapy for the treatment of clinical depression in religious individuals. *Journal of Consulting and Clinical Psychology*, **60**, 94–103.

Purcell, D. W., Campos, P. E., and Perilla, J. L. (1996). Therapy with lesbians and gay men: a cognitive-behavioral perspective. *Cognitive and Behavioral Practice*, **3**, 391–416.

Rude, S. S. and Rehm, L. P. (1991). Response to treatment for depression: the role of initial status on targeted cognitive and behavioral skills. *Clinical Psychology Review*, **11**, 493–514.

Rush, A. J., Kovacs, M., Beck, A. T., Weissenburger, J., and Hollon, S. D. (1981). Differential effects of cognitive therapy and pharmacotherapy in depressive symptoms. *Journal of Affective Disorders*, **3**, 221–9.

Rush, A. S., Beck, A. T., Kovacs, M., Weissenburger, J., and Hollon, S. D. (1982). Comparison of the effects of cognitive therapy and pharmacotherapy on hopelessness and self-concept. *American Journal of Psychiatry*, **139**, 862–6.

Safran, J. D., and Segal, Z. V. (1990). *Interpersonal Process in Cognitive Therapy*. New York: Basic Books.

Segal, Z. V., Gemar, M., and Williams, S. (1999). Differential cognitive response to a mood challenge following successful cognitive therapy or pharmacotherapy for unipolar depression. *Journal of Abnormal Psychology*, **108**(1), 3–10.

Shapiro, D. A. and Shapiro, D. (1982). Meta-analysis of comparative therapy outcome studies: a replication and refinement. *Psychological Bulletin*, **92**(3), 581–604.

Shaw, B. F. (1977). Comparison of cognitive therapy and behavior therapy in the treatment of depression. *Journal of Consulting and Clinical Psychology*, **45**(4), 543–51.

Shaw, B. F., Elkin, I., Yamaguchi, J., et al. (1999). Therapist competence ratings in relation to clinical outcome in cognitive therapy of depression. *Journal of Consulting and Clinical Psychology*, **67**(6), 837–46.

Shea, M. T., Pilkonis, P. A., Beckham, E., et al. (1990). Personality disorders and treatment outcome in the NIMH treatment of depression collaborative research program. *American Journal of Psychiatry*, **147**(6), 711–18.

Shoham-Salomon, V. and Hannah, M. T. (1991). Client–treatment interaction in the study of differential change processes. *Journal of Consulting and Clinical Psychology*, **59**, 217–25.

Simons, A. D., Garfield, S. L., and Murphy, G. E. (1984). The process of change in cognitive therapy and pharmacotherapy for depression. *Archives of General Psychiatry*, **41**, 45–51.

Sotsky, S. M., Glass, D. R., Shea, T., et al. (1991). Patient predictors of response to psychotherapy and pharmacotherapy: findings from the NIMH treatment of depression collaborative research program. *American Journal of Psychiatry*, **148**, 997–1008.

Startup, M. and Shapiro, D. A. (1993). Therapist treatment fidelity in prescriptive vs. exploratory psychotherapy. *British Journal of Clinical Psychology*, **32**(4), 443–56.

Stiles, W. B. and Shapiro, D. A. (1994). Disabuse of the drug metaphor: psychotherapy process outcome correlations. *Journal of Consulting and Clinical Psychology*, **62**(5), 942–8.

Stiles, W. B., Shankland, M. C., Wright, J., and Field, S. D. (1997). Aptitude–treatment interactions based on clients' assimilation of their presenting problems. *Journal of Consulting and Clinical Psychology*, **65**(5), 889–93.

Stravynski, A., Marks, I., and Yule, W. (1982). Social skills problems in neurotic outpatients: social skills training with and without cognitive modification. *Archives of General Psychiatry*, **39**(12), 1378–85.

Tang, T. Z. and DeRubeis, R. J. (1999a). Reconsidering rapid early response in cognitive behavioral therapy for depression. *Clinical Psychology: Science and Practice*, **6**(3), 283–8.

Tang, T. Z. and DeRubeis, R. J. (1999b). Sudden gains and critical sessions in cognitive-behavioral therapy for depression. *Journal of Consulting and Clinical Psychology*, **67**(6), 894–904.

Teasdale, J. D. (1985). Psychological treatments for depression: how do they work? *Behavior Research and Therapy*, **23**, 157–65.

Teasdale, J. D. and Fennell, M. J. (1982). Immediate effects on depression of cognitive therapy interventions. *Cognitive Therapy and Research*, **6**(3), 343–52.

Waltz, J., Addis, M. E., Koerner, K., and Jacobson, N. S. (1993). Testing the integrity of a psychotherapy protocol: assessment of adherence and competence. *Journal of Consulting and Clinical Psychology*, **61**(4), 620–30.

Whisman, M. A. (1993). Mediators and moderators of change in CT of depression. *Psychological Bulletin*, **114**(2), 248–65.

Whisman, M. A., Miller, I. W., Norman, W. H., and Keitner, G. I. (1991). Cognitive therapy with depressed inpatients: specific effects on dysfunctional cognitions. *Journal of Consulting and Clinical Psychology*, **59**, 282–8.

Wilson, P. H., Goldin, J. C., and Charbonneau-Powis, M. (1983). Comparative efficacy of behavioral and cognitive treatments of depression. *Cognitive Therapy and Research*, **7**, 111–24.

Young, J. E. (1999). *Cognitive Therapy for Personality Disorders: A Schema-focused Approach*, 3rd edn. Sarasota, FL: Professional Resource Press.

Zeiss, A. M., Lewinsohn, P. M., and Munoz, R. F. (1979). Nonspecific improvement effects in depression using interpersonal skills training, pleasant activity schedules, or cognitive training. *Journal of Consulting and Clinical Psychology*, **47**, 427–39.

Zlotnick, C., Elkin, I., and Shea, M. T. (1998). Does the gender of a patient or the gender of the therapist affect the treament of patients with major depression? *Journal of Consulting and Clinical Psychology*, **66**(4), 655–9.

20

Cognitive therapy in the twenty-first century: current status and future directions

David A. Clark[1] and Mark A. Reinecke[2]

[1] University of New Brunswick, Fredericton, Canada
[2] Northwestern University, Chicago, IL, USA

Introduction

In the last two decades cognitive-clinical psychology has made impressive gains in the scope of its application to diverse clinical disorders, the complexity of its theoretical formulations, and the sophistication of its research methodology. If one were to compare current cognitive theory, research and treatment with the earliest writings of Beck (1967), Ellis (1962), Meichenbaum (1977), Rehm (1977) and Mahoney (1974), there can be little doubt that we have come a long way from those first forays into the cognitive basis of psychological disorders. If one ever questioned whether cognitive therapy (CT) represented a paradigmatic shift in clinical psychology (Wilson, 1978), a look back over the last 20 or 30 years of research and treatment advances should dispel any doubt.

As evident from the chapters in the current volume, correlational and experimental investigations into the cognitive basis of clinical disorders represents a prominent research perspective that is evident across a wide range of psychological problems. Moreover, the basic elements of CT and cognitive-behavioral therapy (CBT) have been applied to a diverse group of disorders in children, adolescents, and adults. We have a much better understanding of the cognitive concomitants of certain clinical disorders, and of the role of cognition in the etiology, persistence, and severity of disorders. The more scientific and rigorous experimental methodology of information processing has been employed to test various cognitive hypotheses. A variety of different treatment strategies have been developed under the rubric of CT or CBT, and some, such as CT for depression and panic disorder, have become established as empirically supported interventions (Chambless et al., 1998). There is also an increasing recognition that a more integrative perspective is required that acknowledges the reciprocal relations between biology, environment, development, behavior, and cognition in the pathogenesis of disorders. In many ways, then, CT and CBT have matured, becoming an established research and treatment perspective that deals with clinical problems across the lifespan.

Despite these advances, progress in cognitive research and treatment has been uneven across disorders. As evident in the preceding chapters, the cognitive approach in some disorders is 20 years behind the advances seen in other clinical domains. For example, cognitive research and treatment in schizophrenia (Chapter 13), alcohol abuse and dependence (Chapter 14), and narcissistic personality disorder (Chapter 8) are considerably behind cognitive applications to adult depression (Chapter 2), panic disorder (Chapter 6), social phobia (Chapter 11) and obsessive-compulsive disorder (Chapters 5 and 7). Moreover, cognitive research and treatment in childhood and adolescence generally lag behind the advances seen in adult psychopathology, even though some of the earliest cognitive-behavioral interventions focused on clinical problems in children (Meichenbaum and Goodman, 1971; B. N. Camp and M. A. Bash, unpublished data; Kendall and Finch, 1976; Spivack et al., 1976). There also appears to be an ever-widening gap between experimental researchers situated in academic laboratories who research the cognitive concomitants of psychopathology, and cognitively trained healthcare providers focused on the exigencies of therapeutic change and the application of effective treatments within a competitive, cost-conscious healthcare environment. The former continue to advocate a solid basis in experimental cognitive and social cognitive psychology (MacLeod, 1993; Teasdale and Barnard, 1993; Williams et al., 1997), whereas the latter are more influenced by eclecticism and integration with other schools of psychotherapy (for discussion, see Alford and Beck, 1997). This rift between research and practice could hinder further advances because it might compromise the solid basis that CT has historically maintained in cognitive theory and research on psychopathology (e.g., Beck's cognitive theory and therapy of depression; Clark and Beck, 1999). This gap is in part fueled by the perception that the findings from information-processing experiments in psychopathology have little theoretical or practical relevance (Clark and Beck, 1999; Chapter 6), and the realization that CT could be effective for reasons irrelevant to the cognitive model (Chapter 2).

Most of the major currents and crosscurrents that run through cognitive-clinical research and treatment are well discussed by the contributors to this volume. In this final chapter we highlight these issues in order to suggest directions for future development in cognitive-clinical psychology. We begin by discussing the advances that have been made over the past three decades on the cognitive basis and treatment of clinical disorders. We then discuss some of the critical questions that should be addressed for further advances in the nature and treatment of psychopathology. The chapter concludes with some final observations on the status of CT and research at the outset of the twenty-first century.

Advances in cognitive-clinical research and therapy

Cognitive perspective on clinical disorders

Diverse conceptual foundation

As can be seen from the preceding chapters, the theoretical formulations of cognitive-clinical psychology have a diverse and complex conceptual basis that spans a broad range of thought in experimental cognitive and social psychology, as well as clinical psychopathology, behavioral science, and psychiatry. It is true that some theoretical views may be particularly prominent in certain clinical domains, such as Beck's cognitive theory in adult unipolar and bipolar depression, panic disorder, social phobia, and eating disorders. However, this theoretical dominance does not signify stagnation or a narrow, unimaginative conceptual basis. Instead there is an impressive amount of vitality, breadth, and originality in cognitive-clinical models that draws from a broad knowledge base in psychology and psychiatry.

This diversity of theoretical influence can be seen in a number of chapters. Mennin et al. in Chapter 4 discuss Borkovec's avoidance theory of worry as the dominant model in generalized anxiety disorder (GAD). They then present a new emotion regulation perspective that views worry as an ineffective cognitive control strategy used to suppress emotional experiences that individuals with GAD find subjectively aversive. Hofmann (Chapter 6) argues that there are shortcomings in D. M. Clark's catastrophic misinterpretation model of panic, and so advocates taking a closer look at alternative explanations. Salkovskis and Wahl (Chapter 7) present a responsibility model of obsessive-compulsive disorder (OCD) that draws heavily from earlier behavioral accounts of the disorder. Hembree and Foa (Chapter 10) discuss an emotional processing theory of posttraumatic stress disorder (PTSD) that is based on Lang's bioinformational theory of emotion. Corrigan and Calabrese (Chapter 13) review research on information-processing deficits and social cognition as a basis for a cognitive model of schizophrenia. Raytek et al. (Chapter 14) draw on Marlett and Gordon's relapse prevention model, and Prochaska and colleagues' motivation to change, to understand alcohol dependence and its treatment.

In childhood psychopathology, the influence of a single cognitive theory, such as Beck's cognitive model of depression, is even less pronounced. In fact, as noted earlier, the development of cognitive models specific to childhood disorders has lagged behind work with adults. Piacentini et al. (Chapter 16) note that there has been little empirical research on cognition in childhood anxiety. The research that has been done tends to borrow the cognitive constructs of adult anxiety and applies them to children. There is a stronger research base for dysfunctional cognition in childhood depression. Spence and Reinecke (Chapter 15) review research on self-control deficits, negative attributional style, problem-solving deficits, and maladaptive schemata in childhood depression. Thus there appears to be a broader and more advanced cognitive theory and research of childhood depression. Lochman et al. (Chapter 18) present a social information-processing model and supporting research for conduct disorder. They note that more recent revisions of this model incorporate the notion of core dysfunctional schemata that may drive the biased and faulty processing that leads to aggression in children with conduct disorder or oppositional defiant disorder. Finally it is interesting that, despite some very early work on verbal self-regulation in impulsive children, Anastopoulos et al. (Chapter 17) note that further advances on a cognitive model of impulsivity or attention deficit/hyperactivity disorder (AD/HD) have stalled, in part because of poor empirical support for the verbal regulation approaches. In sum, we find considerable variability across disorders in the extent and sophistication of cognitive theory and research. In clinical disorders where there has been considerable research on a cognitive model, there is evidence of contributions from diverse conceptual backgrounds and research traditions.

Applied science approach

Teasdale and Barnard (1993) defined the applied science approach as starting with a concrete "real-world" problem, such as depression, and then using this real-world problem as a reference point for gauging any subsequent experimentation or theorizing. The critical question from this perspective is: how well does a theory or body of research explain the clinical phenomena under consideration? Cognitive clinical theories have a long tradition in clinical observation. Beck's cognitive model of depression, for example, began with his clinical observations of the thinking pattern of depressed patients undergoing psychoanalytic treatment (Clark and Beck, 1999). Subsequently, the validity of cognitive formulations has been judged not only in terms of how well they account for research findings, but also by their fit with what is known about a particular clinical disorder.

The applied science criterion was mentioned by a number of contributors. Hofmann (Chapter 6), for example, was critical of the catastrophic misinterpretation model of panic because it cannot explain gender differences in incidence of panic disorder, nor can it explain why panic attacks often co-occur with other disorders like schizophrenia. Scott (Chapter 3) questions the validity of the cognitive account of mania because it does not map on to the known features of this clinical phenomenon. Salkovskis and Wahl (Chapter 7) discuss the adequacy of their CBT responsibility theory in terms of how well it accounts for the persistence, severity, and subjective features of obsessions. Newman and Ratto (Chapter 8) consider the relevance of Young's schema-focused model for narcissistic personality disorder by evaluating how well the five types of early maladaptive schemata map on to the clinical presentation of narcissistic personality disorder. Hembree and Foa (Chapter 10) provide a particularly good example of an applied science critique.

They noted that early schema theories of PTSD proposed that pathological emotional responses arise when a traumatic experience is discrepant with pretrauma core beliefs that the self is worthy and the world is relatively safe. This perspective would predict that individuals with multiple traumas should recover more quickly than individuals with a first-time trauma because the trauma information matches the internal constructs of the multiple trauma victim, that the self is unworthy and the world is unsafe. However, this is not the case. Individuals with multiple traumas have a greater likelihood of suffering PTSD symptoms. This is a very nice example of a theory-derived prediction that is not confirmed by what is known about the "real-world" problem it seeks to explain. Because of the strong clinical nature of cognitive theories, a great deal of weight is placed on how well these formulations explain clinical phenomena.

There are other ways in which conceptual models can fail. As Elster (1990) notes, models can fail through indeterminacy and inadequacy. They can also fail through "conceptual entropy" – a lack of clinical momentum and utility. A theory may be seen as indeterminant to the extent that it fails to yield specific predictions, and is inadequate to the extent that its predictions are falsified or disconfirmed. Of these, the latter is the more serious concern. A theory may have a relatively narrow range of convenience, and yet have some predictive strength, explanatory power, and clinical utility. A model can, in short, be weak but not useless. It is a more serious concern if the model makes predictions that are falsified by observation. It is worse, in many ways, for a theory to predict wrongly, than to predict weakly but truthfully.

Over the course of time, there is a natural tendency for models to increase both in range and specificity. We are seeing this in cognitive models of psychopathology – they are being applied to an ever-wider range of issues, and are simultaneously becoming more sophisticated. This can, and does, create a tension. As models are applied to new domains they may lose their specificity, predictive utility, and explanatory power. It is worth noting, however, that models can retain clinical utility even as evidence accumulates that is inconsistent with them. Cartesian models, for example, remain quite useful for navigation, even though we know the world isn't flat. Similarly, Newtonian models of mechanics work perfectly well at day-to-day speeds and masses. Unless they undergo an ongoing process of refinement, however, models begin to fail as their range of convenience increases. This may or may not, however, be associated with a loss of clinical utility. Simple cognitive and behavioral interventions may continue to be quite effective even as evidence accumulates that the underlying processes of psychotherapeutic change are more complex. It is worth noting that many models in the social sciences are abandoned not as a result of empirical disputation, but because clinicians and scholars lose interest. They get stale. Conceptual entropy sets in. Without energy and momentum, models fail to work. The solution is ongoing empirical test and revision. Models, like sharks, must continually move forward or they die. Cognitive models generate continuing interest because of their openness to revision. These revisions occur in response to the model's difficulty in accounting for some aspect of a clinical disorder (i.e., clinical utility is weakened), or in accounting for relevant research findings.

Empirically based methodology

One of the legacies of the behavioral influence on cognitive-clinical psychology is the emphasis on empirical verification. As noted previously, cognitive theories are evaluated in terms of how well they account for research findings on the cognitive basis of particular disorders. In fact, Teasdale and Barnard (1993) were critical of Beck's cognitive model of depression because they claimed that it did not account for much of the laboratory findings on cognitive functioning in depression. A number of the contributors to this volume provide a critical evaluation of cognitive theories in reference to their ability to account for the results of relevant empirical research. Solomon and Haaga (Chapter 2), for example, conclude that there is fairly consistent empirical support for Beck's cognitive model of depression at the descriptive level, but the findings from diathesis-stress research show weaker and inconsistent support for cognitive vulnerability. Clark and Purdon (Chapter 5) are cautious about the validity of contemporary cognitive-behavioral theories of OCD because of the paucity of observational and experimental research on the cognitive constructs of OCD. Wilson and Rapee (Chapter 11) review a fairly advanced experimental literature on the cognitive constructs of social phobia, in order to determine whether the cognitive model of social phobia by Clark and Wells (1995), or the one proposed by Rapee and Heimberg (1997), provides a better account of the experimental findings. Spence and Reinecke (Chapter 15) also evaluate the existing cognitive models of childhood depression in reference to the extant research on depressive cognition in childhood. Unfortunately, in many disorders, such as bipolar depression, alcohol abuse and dependence, personality disorders, childhood anxiety, and AD/HD, the empirical literature is not sufficiently advanced to provide even an initial evaluation of cognitive theory.

Two conditions must be met in order to test a cognitive theory empirically. First the theory must contain constructs and hypotheses that are stated in a clear, testable form, with high informative content and high predictive value (Chapter 6). Theories that lack these characteristics will have little scientific value. A number of the theories presented by contributors appear to have good scientific value. Hofmann (Chapter 6) noted that D. M. Clark's catastrophic misinterpretation model of panic has generated a number of testable hypotheses, although recent elaborations and clarifications threaten to make the model difficult, if not impossible, to test empirically. Solomon and Haaga (Chapter 2) and Spence and Reinecke (Chapter 15) present hypotheses about the cognitive dysfunction in adult and childhood depression that have been subjected to considerable empirical research. Mennin's et al.'s theory of emotional dysregulation in GAD (Chapter 4) appears to make clear, testable predictions. Specific experimental investigations have tested Salkovskis and Wahl's (Chapter 7) theory of inflated responsibility in OCD, as well as certain constructs in social phobia such as heightened self-focused attention, biased attentional processing of external social threat stimuli, and performance–standard discrepancies (Chapter 11). The cognitive model of bulimia nervosa presented in the chapter by le Grange (Chapter 12) also has a number of testable elements.

The chapter by DuBois et al. (Chapter 9) deserves special mention in this regard. Cognitive theories of most disorders, whether in childhood/adolescence or adulthood, posit the presence of maladaptive or negative self-representation. In most of these theories the conceptualization of the self is fairly rudimentary. DuBois and colleagues make a convincing argument that cognitive theories, and ultimately CT, would benefit substantially in precision and predictive value if cognitive-clinical researchers paid closer attention to theory and research in the self literature.

The second condition that is necessary for a strong empirically based cognitive theory is a range of highly reliable and valid measures of cognitive content, process, and structure. The state of cognitive assessment and research design varies greatly across clinical domains. Some areas, such as research on depression, panic, social phobia, GAD, OCD and, to a lesser extent, PTSD and eating disorders, have a fairly large experimental and information-processing research base. In other clinical disorders, such as childhood anxiety, AD/HD, alcohol dependence, schizophrenia, and bipolar depression, the research literature is much more confined to retrospective self-report questionnaires. Although the assessment of cognitive content or appraisals is a critical part of the evaluation of cognitive theories (McNally, 2001a), experimental methodology, including research from an information-processing paradigm, is important for investigating cognitive function in clinical disorders. A number of researchers have been critical of the overreliance on retrospective, structured self-report questionnaires for the assessment of cognition and underlying schemata (Gotlib and McCabe, 1992; Clark, 1997; Glass and Arnkoff, 1997).

The cognitive nature of clinical disorders

A number of the review chapters in this volume cite research indicating that maladaptive and biased cognitive content, structures, and processes are activated during the acute phase of a clinical disorder. This has been demonstrated for depression, panic disorder, social phobia, GAD, OCD, PTSD, bulimia nervosa, and conduct disorder. Moreover this dysfunctional and biased cognition bears a close reciprocal relation with affect. It involves automatic, preconscious, and involuntary processing as well as more elaborative, effortful, and strategic processing capabilities.

The cognitive basis in clinical disorders is important because it reflects the representation of personal meaning (i.e., schemata). This provides a guide for formulating treatments at the cognitive level. It is because these meaning-making structures or schemata are so fundamental to disorders that treatment is focused on their modification. What has been demonstrated empirically, then, is that biased and dysfunctional cognition is a critical feature of anxiety and depressive disorders, in particular. Furthermore, the close affinity between cognitive dysfunction and the persistence and severity of symptoms indicates that the cognitive constructs referred to in the preceding chapters are not merely epiphenomena of the disorder, but rather they are intricately tied to the persistence and severity of the clinical state. This has been clearly shown for adult depression, and many of the anxiety disorders. Outside the anxiety/depression axis, the central role of cognitive processes and structures has yet to be firmly established. Having said this, it must also be recognized that much of the biased and dysfunctional cognitive processing does abate with recovery from the clinical state. The very fact that there is such a close tie between cognitive functioning and the course of an illness further highlights the cognitive basis of many disorders.

One aspect of the descriptive level of cognitive theory that deserves special mention is the view that a specific cognitive profile distinguishes each clinical disorder. Beck (1971) stated that the cognitive content or meaning of an event determines the type of emotional experience or psychological disturbance. Thus each psychological disorder is thought to have a distinct cognitive profile that is evident in the content and orientation of the negative cognitions and processing bias associated with the disorder (Clark and Beck, 1999). It is recognized that some cognitive constructs may be common across a variety of disorders whereas other constructs may be unique or specific to particular clinical states. Moreover, it is primarily the content or orientation of the cognitive bias that is unique to disorders, with dysfunction in cognitive structure and process more likely common across clinical domains. Solomon and Haaga (Chapter 2) concluded that cognitions of personal loss and failure might be unique to depression but that themes of threat and danger may be evident in both depression and anxiety. Spence and Reinecke (Chapter 15) arrived at a similar conclusion for childhood depression, although cognitive specificity may be more apparent in adult than childhood psychopathology (Clark and Beck, 1999). In other disorders, specific cognitive biases have been proposed, although research is lacking on whether these biases are unique to particular disorders. In a recent metaanalysis of 13 studies of cognitive content-specificity, R. Beck and Perkins (2001) reported that all effect sizes for comparisons between measures of depressive and anxious cognitions and symptoms were significant. However, when a quantitative comparison was made between the effect sizes, depressive cognitions and symptoms showed some evidence of specificity whereas anxious cognitions and symptoms lacked the same level of specificity. These findings, then, support Solomon and Haaga's (Chapter 2) contention that cognitive content-specificity may be evident in depression but not anxiety.

In the present volume specific cognitive themes have been identified for many clinical disorders. Scott (Chapter 3) suggested that causal attributions for disruption in circadian rhythm may be specific in bipolar depression. Salkovskis and Wahl (Chapter 7) identified appraisals of inflated personal responsibility as characteristic of OCD. Newman and Ratto (Chapter 8) proposed specific beliefs of entitlement in narcissistic personality disorder and Mennin et al. (Chapter 4) highlighted the use of worry to control emotional dysregulation in GAD. The catastrophic misinterpretation of bodily sensations is considered the sine qua non of panic disorder (Chapter 6), whereas cognitions and processing bias focused on the negative evaluation of others in social situations are considered core cognitive features of social phobia (Chapter 11). Clark and Purdon (Chapter 5) proposed that misinterpretation of failed thought control is a central cognitive aspect of obsessional rumination. Hembree and Foa (Chapter 10) indicated that perceptions of the world as extremely dangerous and the self as extremely incompetent were critical features of PTSD. Le Grange (Chapter 12) noted that dysfunctional beliefs and overvalued ideals about one's weight, body shape, and food are characteristic of bulimia nervosa. Raytek et al. (Chapter 14) identified certain thoughts, beliefs, and expectancies about the positive effects of alcohol and decreased self-efficacy of one's ability to abstain from alcohol. Finally, cognitive deficits in the area of behavioral inhibition were highlighted by Anastopoulos et al. (Chapter 17) for AD/HD, and Lochman et al. (Chapter 18) identified hostile attributional biases, and schemata of dominance and revenge as characteristics of children with conduct problems.

Clearly more comparative research is needed that includes other clinical disorders in order to determine whether particular cognitive constructs are distinct features of a disorder or are common across many different clinical states. This research, however, is fraught with conceptual haziness. Our ability to test these models is dependent, as well, on the capacity to identify diagnostically homogeneous comparison groups. This can be difficult given high rates of comorbidity for many disorders and the occurrence of subtypes. Cognitive specificity is founded on an assumption that discriminable and independent psychiatric disorders exist. This may not be a supportable assumption. The validity of categorically discrete diagnostic taxonomies is open to question (e.g., research on negative affectivity and of dimensional classification of disorders among youth), and diagnostic systems are continually being revised in light of new evidence. The difficulty may be with the diagnostic schemes we are using as well as the cognitive models we have developed to describe them. It's difficult to demonstrate specificity when subjects are diagnostically and symptomatically heterogeneous, or if the taxonomy lacks validity.

Cognitive vulnerability and recovery

Beck's cognitive theory of depression is the most advanced articulation of the view that certain cognitive constructs are predisposing factors that contribute to an increased risk for the onset and recurrence of depression (Beck, 1987; Clark and Beck, 1999). Beck proposes that certain exaggerated and maladaptive self-referent beliefs or schemata involving themes of helplessness (i.e., autonomy) or social acceptance (i.e., sociotropy) remain dormant until triggered by a congruent life event such as a loss of social resources for the highly sociotropic person or loss of independence or mastery for the highly autonomous individual. Once these maladaptive schemata are activated, the person is at increased risk for an onset or recurrence of depression. Beck's cognitive vulnerability perspective on depression, then, posits a diathesis-stress model for understanding the etiology of depression.

Most of the research on cognitive vulnerability has focused on onset, exacerbation, and recurrence of depressive disorders and symptoms. Some studies investigate whether maladaptive cognition is present before or after a depressive episode, whereas others examine cognitive diathesis-stress in cross-sectional and prospective research designs. As reviewed by Solomon and Haaga (Chapter 2), there is evidence that dysfunctional beliefs are present in high-risk individuals in the nondepressed state (e.g., previously depressed individuals) but only if the these schemata are activated, such as in a mood-priming experiment. There is mixed support for diathesis-stress from prospective studies, with the most consistent evidence for congruence between negative interpersonal events and maladaptive sociotropic cognitive-personality vulnerability. The strongest evidence for cognitive vulnerability comes from the Temple-Wisconsin Cognitive Vulnerability to Depression Project (Abramson et al., 1999; Alloy et al., 2000). As well, Segal and his colleagues used a mood-priming manipulation to show that dysfunctional beliefs predict relapse and recurrence of depression in recovered depressives (Segal et al., 1999). These results, then, suggest that a preexisting cognitive vulnerability may be present that increases the risk for depression. Questions, however, still remain on whether the contribution of cognitive variables to the onset or recurrence of depression is necessary, substantial, or specific to a disorder (Hammen, 2001).

Research on cognitive vulnerability in other clinical conditions is not sufficiently advanced even to draw preliminary conclusions. Scott (Chapter 3) concluded that there was no evidence for trait vulnerabilities in bipolar disorder, but there is some initial evidence that negative cognitive style might interact with negative life events to increase both depressive and manic symptoms. Garber and Flynn (2001) note that three short-term prospective studies found evidence of an interaction between negative cognition (attributions, self-worth) and negative life events for depression in children. However, very little prospective research exists on predisposing cognitive vulnerability in childhood or adult anxiety disorders (Malcarne and

Hansdottir, 2001; McNally, 2001b) or eating disorders (Chapter 12). In some cases there has been speculation on factors that predispose to disorder but very little direct research evidence. The conceptual and methodological progress on cognitive vulnerability research in depression should provide some guidance for conducting vulnerability research in other disorders.

Cognitive treatment of clinical disorders

Articulated treatment protocols

Since the first published treatment manuals for CT and cognitive-behavioral treatment (Meichenbaum, 1977; Beck et al., 1979), substantial progress has been made in elaborating, expanding, and refining cognitive intervention strategies for a wide variety of disorders. Many of these advances in treatment are described in the present volume. Chapters 7–10, 12, 14, 15, 17, 18, and 19 discuss specific elements of CT or CBT that should be included for an intervention to be effective. The current emphasis on detailed specification of cognitive treatment protocols is a historical legacy of behavior therapy. It has enhanced the dissemination of CT, enabled the provision of higher-quality therapy training, allowed the development of standards to ensure treatment integrity, and facilitated outcome and process research on cognitive psychotherapy. In sum, the development of well-articulated CT and CBT intervention packages for a variety of disorders has been the big success story for this school of psychotherapy.

Symptom reduction

In numerous outcome studies, CT produced significantly greater reductions in symptoms during the acute phase of disorders than a waitlist control condition. Moreover, CT is now considered an empirically supported treatment for major depression and panic disorder in adults (Chambless et al., 1998; DeRubeis and Crits-Christoph, 1998). The effectiveness of CT was addressed in most of the chapters. Its efficacy has been demonstrated for depression in children, adolescents and adults (Chapters 2 and 15) panic disorder (Chapter 6), social phobia (Chapter 11), bulimia nervosa (Chapter 12), alcohol abuse and dependence (Chapter 14), and childhood anxiety (Chapter 16). Cognitive intervention is effective for the treatment of conduct disorder but only when it is included in a treatment package that has a strong behavioral and problem-solving orientation (Chapter 18). CT may be slightly less effective in the treatment of GAD (Chapter 4). Its effectiveness for bipolar depression (Chapter 3) and schizophrenia (Chapter 13) is tentative, requiring more outcome research before treatment efficacy can be determined. For PTSD (Chapter 10) and OCD (Chapter 5) it is not clear if the addition of cognitive interventions improves treatment efficacy beyond what is achieved with a purely behavioral approach (e.g., exposure). The inclusion of cognitive interventions in the treatment of AD/HD has not been encouraging (Chapter 17) and its effectiveness in most of the personality disorders, such as narcissistic personality disorder, is unknown. For depression, recent evidence also indicates that CT is as effective as medication in the treatment of the severely depressed individual (DeRubeis et al., 1999). In sum, the results of numerous outcome studies indicate that CT is a versatile, highly effective psychotherapy for many different forms of childhood and adult psychopathology.

Relapse prevention

Several outcome studies include follow-up to determine whether the therapeutic gains made during the acute phase of treatment are maintained once therapy is terminated. Patients who successfully responded to CT are compared to responders from other treatment conditions, most often medication. For depression, there is evidence that CT is associated with significantly lower relapse rates than antidepressant medication (Chapter 2). Hollon et al. (1996) concluded that depressed patients treated with CT are half as likely to relapse as those treated with medication and then discontinued. In the Minnesota Cognitive-Pharmacotherapy Project, 50% of the medication-only group who had no continuation of medication over the 2-year follow-up relapsed after successful treatment, whereas only 21% of the CT and 15% of the combined CT plus medication group relapsed (Hollon et al.). DeRubeis et al. (2001) noted that only 10 sessions of CT following a successful course of pharmacotherapy are as effective in preventing relapse as continuation of active medication. The superior prophylactic effect of CT for depression has been an important finding for those who advocate the inclusion of cognitive interventions in the standard treatment protocol for major depression in adults.

With the possible exception of CT for bulimia nervosa, the follow-up research on CT for other disorders is more limited than in adult depression. Scott (Chapter 3) did report some encouraging evidence of lower relapse rates for bipolar patients treated with CT, as did Corrigan and Calabrese (Chapter 13) for CT of schizophrenia, but too few outcome studies have completed their follow-up periods to confirm these findings. Mennin et al. (Chapter 4) concluded that the majority of the 50–60% of patients with GAD who achieve high end-state functioning after CT maintain their treatment gains. Maintenance of CT treatment gains have also been reported for panic disorder (Chapter 6), social phobia (Chapter 11), PTSD (Chapter 10), and bulimia nervosa (Chapter 12). The long-term effectiveness of CT has not been as well investigated in the childhood disorders. Overall, though, the follow-up data on CT indicate that treatment gains tend to be well maintained in those who are treatment responders in the acute symptomatic phase of a disorder. In many cases treatment gains are maintained at a level that exceeds what is achieved with other types of interventions, such as medication only.

Combined treatment

Most of the CT treatment protocols utilized in comparative outcome studies employ a multicomponent treatment package that includes cognitive, behavioral, and social interventions. Below we discuss findings from dismantling studies which attempt to determine which of these components are the active therapeutic ingredients of CT or CBT. A different question is whether CT effectiveness can be improved by adding another treatment modality such as medication or behavior therapy. CT plus medication may be only slightly more effective than CT alone in the treatment of depression (Hollon et al., 1996). CT plus some form of behavior therapy (e.g., relaxation training) may be more effective than CT alone for GAD (Chapter 4), OCD (Chapter 5), PTSD (Chapter 10), conduct disorder (Chapter 18), and probably depressive and anxious disorders in childhood (Chapters 15 and 16). Le Grange (Chapter 12) concluded that the combination of CBT and medication was only slightly better than CBT alone in the treatment of bulimia nervosa. In some cases, the addition of pharmacotherapy could be contraindicated because it reduces the effectiveness of CBT. McLean and Woody (2001) note that there is some evidence that concurrent use of benzodiazepines might interfere with the effects of exposure to fear stimuli in the treatment of panic disorder and agoraphobia. Clearly, then, more is not always better in the treatment of psychological disorders.

Issues and future direction in cognitive-clinical research and therapy

Cognitive clinical research

Much progress has been made in our understanding of the cognitive basis of many clinical disorders. This has been reviewed in the preceding section and discussed by most of the contributors to this volume. However, there are a number of unresolved issues that will determine the integrity of cognitive theory. A more detailed discussion of these issues can be found in individual chapters. Here we provide an overview of areas where further theoretical and empirical work is needed.

There are many different terms and concepts derived from different theoretical models to describe the cognitive content, process, and structure of the various clinical disorders. The measures of these different concepts are often quite highly correlated, which suggests a considerable degree of commonality or overlap. In the end it is often unclear whether different cognitive constructs are really all that distinct from each other. For example, Hofmann (Chapter 6) questioned the relation between high anxiety sensitivity and catastrophic misinterpretation of bodily sensations in panic disorder. A number of items in the Anxiety Sensitivity Index deal with misinterpretation of bodily sensations. Although a number of different appraisals and beliefs have been proposed for the persistence of obsessions, recent findings indicate that these different concepts are very highly correlated (Chapter 5).

On the other hand, at times it is assumed that different concepts of similar phenomena are equivalent, when in fact they are significantly different. For example, it has been assumed that Blatt's concept of the self-critical personality is similar to Beck's personality construct of autonomy. In reality, these two constructs are quite different (Clark and Beck, 1999). As well, sociotropy and dependency may have important conceptual differences (Rude and Burnham, 1995), even though they are assumed to be practically interchangeable. Solomon and Haaga (Chapter 2) also remind us that the boundary between normal and abnormal cognitive functioning is not clear-cut because all subjective interpretation and judgment is at best an approximate representation of reality. Thus more research is needed to clarify the nature of the constructs that define our cognitive models of psychopathology. As well, further investigation is needed on the common and specific cognitive features of disorders in addition to depression and anxiety.

The interrelationships among the various cognitive constructs are still not well understood. For example, Beck's cognitive theory assumes a hierarchy of minor and major modes, core schemata, conditional and compensatory rules, and then automatic thoughts and biased cognitive processing (Beck, 1996). Young and Flanagan (1998) propose five types of early maladaptive schemata that are assumed to be a more fundamental representation of cognitive dysfunction, especially in personality disorders (Chapter 8). However, there is very little empirical evidence that would substantiate this hierarchical or "deep versus surface" conceptualization of the cognitive basis of psychopathology.

The relation between cognition and emotion was a matter of intense debate in the late 1980s. Although this debate ceased, there was no real resolution. It is evident that dysfunctional cognition can be either a cause or a consequence of emotion, and that teasing apart the one effect from the other has proven to be a most difficult task. The relationship between cognition and emotion is complex (Lazarus, 1991). Cognitive therapists and researchers often equate "emotion" with "subjectively experienced affect," which is only one component of most contemporary models of emotion. The research on emotion cited by many cognitive-behavioral theorists is neither recent nor sophisticated. We need, as a group, to integrate findings in CBT with a broader understanding of the emotion and emotional development literatures. Even in terms of clinical disorders, the role of various dysfunctional cognitive processes in the onset, maintenance, and recovery process is still unclear.

Many more questions than answers remain about cognitive vulnerability to clinical disorders. In many cases the necessary prospective studies have not been conducted. Even with disorders like depression that have seen more intense research on cognitive vulnerability, many questions remain. Numerous studies have shown that dysfunctional cognition is a concomitant of clinical disorder, but evidence for the causal status of these variables has been much more elusive. Is a particular cognitive dysfunction necessary or sufficient in the pathogenesis of a disorder? Is it a proximal or distal contributory factor to etiology? What model of vulnerability most accurately describes the interaction of cognitive diathesis and life events in the onset of disorder? How often is cognitive vulnerability an important etiological factor in onset? The relationship of cognitive factors to biological markers of vulnerability and treatment response is only beginning to be investigated. From a developmental perspective, little is known about how social and environmental risks and resources interact in contributing to cognitive vulnerability. Continuity and change over the course of development have not been given adequate attention in the cognitive-clinical perspective. Methodological limitations are also apparent. With the possible exception of the Temple-Wisconsin Cognitive Vulnerability to Depression Project (Abramson et al., 1999), few prospective studies have been sufficiently rigorous to provide a valid test of the cognitive diathesis-stress vulnerability hypothesis (Clark and Beck, 1999; Chapter 2).

An equally important but different question concerns the role of cognitive variables in risk for relapse and recurrence of a clinical episode. Solomon and Haaga (Chapter 2) noted that factors leading to recurrence of depression cannot be assumed to be causal in the initial onset of a disorder. However, determining the nature and extent of the role of maladaptive cognition in relapse and recurrence is an important clinical question that deserves considerably more research attention in its own right. Segal et al. (1996), for example, proposed that kindling and sensitization are processes that might explain the heightened risk for symptom recurrence among previously depressed individuals who also show more dysfunctional schema activation during mild dysphoric mood states.

Cognitive and cognitive-behavioral therapy

Compared to other schools of psychotherapy, CT and CBT are far ahead in the amount and the quality of psychotherapy outcome and process research it has produced. As noted above, we now know that CT is an effective treatment for a range of clinical disorders in children, adolescents, and adults, that it produces enduring treatment gains, and that a large number of clinicians have been schooled in the finer points of CT. With such progress in mind, it might be surprising to learn that there are many fundamental questions that remain about the efficacy of CT and CBT. Many of these issues have been highlighted in the preceding chapters, but no more so than in the chapter by Dimidjian and Dobson (Chapter 19). They provide a well-informed critical review of the psychotherapy process research on CT and conclude that the mechanisms of change in CT are not well understood. We consider three areas of CT that require further research; questions about the comparative efficacy of CT, the mechanisms of change in CT, and who is most likely to benefit from CT or CBT.

Comparative treatment efficacy

Although CT is effective for a wide range of clinical problems, it may not be any more effective than other clearly specified forms of psychotherapy. Solomon and Haaga (Chapter 2) concluded that CT for depression has not been shown to be superior to alternative plausible psychological treatments. Hembree and Foa (Chapter 10) reported that exposure alone was as effective for PTSD as exposure plus cognitive restructuring. Clark and Purdon (Chapter 5) noted that cognitive interventions for OCD were equivalent or slightly superior to exposure/response prevention for obsessions and compulsions. However, most of the cognitive interventions for OCD included behavioral elements such as exposure and response prevention. As noted previously, it is not known whether cognitive restructuring, for example, adds significantly to the efficacy of behavior therapy for OCD. For GAD, treatments that combine cognitive and behavioral interventions are more effective than single-component treatments (Chapter 4). Wilson and Rapee (Chapter 11) commented that cognitive interventions and exposure both lead to reductions in social phobia, but firm conclusions cannot be made on whether cognitive restructuring directly adds to the effectiveness of behavioral interventions.

Raytek at al. (Chapter 14) indicated that CBT for alcohol abuse and dependence may produce equivalent outcomes to other interventions such as relapse prevention treatment, motivational enhancement therapy, or the 12-step program. In fact, they reported somewhat inconsistent conclusions from various metaanalyses and large-scale studies which raise questions about the specific contribution that "purely" cognitive strategies make in the treatment of alcohol dependence. Interestingly, le Grange (Chapter 12) concluded that CBT was clearly superior to other credible psychotherapies in the treatment of bulimia nervosa, with the possible exception of interpersonal therapy.

With children and adolescents, Piacentini et al. (Chapter 16) reported that an education support condition was as effective in treating anxiety in children as CBT. Spence and Reinecke (Chapter 15) concluded that integrative treatment approaches were most successful in treating childhood and adolescent depression. The relative contribution of cognitive components to their effectiveness is not known. Lochman et al. (Chapter 18) concluded that CBT interventions that are multicomponent and also include instruction in parenting practices are more effective in treating aggressive children than interventions that focus on parents or children alone.

Dimidjian and Dobson (Chapter 19), in their review of the relative contribution of cognitive and behavioral interventions in CT and CBT, concluded that the behavioral interventions may be necessary and sufficient for the treatment of depression, and that cognitive interventions may not add significantly to their effectiveness. Solomon and Haaga (Chapter 2), however, were critical of the component analysis research on which this conclusion is based. They state that, by holding behavioral activation constant across treatment conditions, individuals in the behavioral activation-only condition would receive more behavioral activation than individuals in the behavioral activation plus cognitive restructuring condition. They argue that conclusions on the efficacy of cognitive restructuring are difficult to reach from such a research design.

It is evident that more research is needed that compares CT or CBT to alternative psychotherapies. In addition these studies should include an attention-placebo control condition in order to tease apart causal mediating variables in the effectiveness of treatment (Hollon et al., 1996). By comparing treatments derived from different theoretical orientations that employ different intervention strategies, researchers will learn more about which therapeutic ingredients might be most effective for inducing change within a particular disorder. It is also possible that CT or CBT may be clearly superior for one disorder, equivalent for another disorder, and a weaker treatment option for a third condition. At this point, it would appear that cognitive strategies are neither necessary nor sufficient for creating significant and lasting therapeutic change in children and adults with psychological disorders. Therapy component research might be helpful in determining the relative contribution of behavioral and cognitive interventions, but caution must be exercised in drawing conclusions from this type of research alone.

One further cautionary note should be added. It is important that the conceptual and technical bounds of what constitutes CBT be more clearly articulated. Many treatments are, in practice, fairly similar to CBT. How far can the model be pressed before it is no longer recognized as CBT (e.g., cognitive-analytic psychotherapy, eye movement desensitization reprocessing, cognitive-developmental psychotherapy)? CT has always embraced technical eclecticism (i.e., use of a diverse range of therapeutic tools in order to induce cognitive change) without necessarily endorsing theoretical eclecticism. Nevertheless, there is continuing debate over the extent to which CT is a distinct school of psychotherapy, as opposed to a broader integrative perspective on therapeutic change (Clark, 1995; Alford and Beck, 1997).

Mechanisms of change

According to CT, cognitive interventions achieve symptom reduction by targeting the maladaptive thoughts and beliefs that are thought to maintain clinical disturbance. To investigate this question, a series of studies have examined whether there are mode-specific treatment effects with CT. These studies seek to determine whether cognitive interventions produced greater change on cognitive outcome variables than other interventions that do not directly target cognitive variables. Dimidjian and Dobson (Chapter 19) reviewed this literature and concluded that there is at best conflicting evidence of mode-specific effects with CT. It appears that CT is not alone in producing change in cognition. However there is evidence that change in negative cognition may be related to symptomatic improvement, although it is difficult to draw causal inferences from this research. Evidence for cognitive mediation of CT is provided by recent research on the course of change in CT. Tang and DeRubeis (see review by DeRubeis et al., 2001) found evidence that 50% of CT treatment responders showed sudden gains in symptom reduction and these gains were preceded by cognitive change in the previous session. As noted by Dimidjian and Dobson (Chapter 19), this issue is difficult to investigate and there have been a number of methodological and conceptual criticisms of this research. Nevertheless, the question of cognitive mediation in CT is very important not only for understanding and improving the delivery of CT, but for testing specific predictions derived from cognitive theories of disorders.

Another issue related to mechanisms of change concerns the ingredients in CT that are most active in producing therapeutic effectiveness. CT and CBT are multicomponent treatment packages that employ a number of active intervention strategies. Various dismantling studies have examined the relative contribution of these facets of the treatment package. Dimidjian and Dobson (Chapter 19) concluded that there was evidence that a good therapeutic alliance characterized by "collaborative empiricism" was related to better outcome. DeRubeis at al. (2001), however, arrived at a different conclusion, stating that the positive correlation between therapeutic alliance and treatment outcome is doubtful. They noted that it is difficult to determine from correlations averaged across sessions whether good therapeutic alliance was a cause or consequence of symptom change. The provision of a treatment rationale and homework assignments have also been suggested as active ingredients of CT and CBT. Dimidjian and Dobson (Chapter 19) note a number of methodological and conceptual problems in the empirical evidence cited as support for this view. However, there is fairly convincing evidence that not only the provision of homework, but also homework compliance may be related to better outcome in CT (Chapter 19). Finally, there is evidence that therapist competence and adherence to CT treatment rationale and implementation are related to better outcome, although the paucity of research makes firm conclusions difficult to reach (Chapter 19). Clearly, we are only beginning to disentangle the active ingredients of complex treatments like CT and CBT.

Prescriptive and prognostic indicators

As with any treatment intervention, it is important to know who is most likely to benefit from CT or CBT, and what variables may be predictive of poor outcome. Some of this research has focused specifically on CT, especially cognitive interventions for depression, whereas other studies have investigated client variables for psychotherapy more generally. Dimidjian and Dobson (Chapter 19) and Solomon and Haaga (Chapter 2) review both of these research literatures and offer some suggestions on client variables that might be associated with a better response to CT. These include: (1) presentation of a well-assimilated problem; (2) tendency to adopt an externalized, self-directed coping style; (3) acceptance of the CT treatment rationale; and (4) a capacity for flexible, constructive thinking.

A variety of indicators have been implicated as a poor prognosis or outcome for CT. These include: (1) comorbid personality disorder; (2) presence of relationship or marital discord; (3) high levels of initial symptom severity and cognitive dysfunction; and (4) dispositional resistance. However, Dimidjian and Dobson (Chapter 19) and Solomon and Haaga (Chapter 2) both raise several limitations and inconsistencies with this research and so caution against drawing firm conclusions. Also, it is possible that CT or CBT prescriptive or prognostic indicators will vary depending on the clinical disorder. For example, Mennin et al. (Chapter 4) raised the possibility that presence of depressive symptoms might weaken the impact of CT or CBT for GAD, although this is based on only one study. Raytek et al. (Chapter 14) indicated that clients with higher levels of commitment to abstinence and greater intention to avoid high-risk situations might have lower risk for relapse. At this time, the research is very tentative on the prescriptive and prognostic indicators of CT. Within each clinical disorder, much more research is needed on the benefactors and detractors of CT efficacy before any practice recommendations can be issued on who will or will not benefit from a trial of CT or CBT. Another related issue raised by Dimidjian and Dobson (Chapter 19) concerns the impact of client diversity on treatment effectiveness. More research is needed on the impact of client ethnicity, sexual orientation, religious beliefs, and other sociodemographic variables on CT outcome for various clinical disorders.

Conclusion

The cognitive perspective has had a substantial impact on theory, research, and treatment of psychological and psychiatric disorders in children, adolescents, and adults. The present volume is our attempt to bring together leading researchers who deal with a range of psychopathology evident across the lifespan, and present them with the task of providing a critical review of cognitive research and treatment within a specific clinical domain. The scope and depth of cognitive research and treatment are enormous, as attested by the size of the current volume. Yet, we realize that important areas of cognitive research and therapy are missing from this volume, such as sexual dysfunctions, marital discord, and various personality disorders, to name but a few. Throughout this volume and in this concluding chapter, we have highlighted the progress that has been made in understanding the cognitive basis of disorders and in offering effective treatment interventions. Although much has been accomplished, it is also apparent that there are many important unresolved issues and inconsistent findings that provide cognitive-clinical researchers with an inexhaustible research agenda for many years to come.

REFERENCES

Abramson, L. Y., Alloy, L. B., Hogan, M. E., et al. (1999). Cognitive vulnerability to depression: theory and evidence. *Journal of Cognitive Psychotherapy: An International Quarterly*, **13**, 5–20.

Alford, B. A. and Beck, A. T. (1997). *The Integrative Power of Cognitive Therapy*. New York: Guilford Press.

Alloy, L. B., Abramson, L. Y., Hogan, M. E., et al. (2000). The Temple-Wisconsin cognitive vulnerability to depression project: lifetime history of Axis I psychopathology in individuals at high and low cognitive risk for depression. *Journal of Abnormal Psychology*, **109**, 403–18.

Beck, A. (1967). *Depression: Causes and Treatment*. Philadelphia: University of Pennsylvania Press.

Beck, A. T. (1971). Cognition, affect, and psychotherapy. *Archives of General Psychiatry*, **24**, 495–500.

Beck, A. T. (1987). Cognitive models of depression. *Journal of Cognitive Psychotherapy: An International Quarterly*, **1**, 5–37.

Beck, A. T. (1996). Beyond belief: a theory of modes, personality, and psychopathology. In *Frontiers of Cognitive Therapy*, ed. P. M. Salkovskis, pp. 1–25. New York: Guilford Press.

Beck, R. and Perkins, T. S. (2001). Cognitive content-specificity for anxiety and depression: a meta-analysis. *Cognitive Therapy and Research*, **25**, 651–63.

Beck, A. T., Rush, A. J., Shaw, B. F., and Emery, G. (1979). *Cognitive Therapy of Depression*. New York: Guilford Press.

Chambless, D. L., Baker, M. J., Baucom, D. H., et al. (1998). Update on empirically validated therapies, II. *Clinical Psychologist*, **51**, 3–16.

Clark, D. A. (1995). Perceived limitations of standard cognitive therapy: a consideration of efforts to revise Beck's theory and therapy. *Journal of Cognitive Psychotherapy: An International Quarterly*, **9**, 153–72.

Clark, D. A. (1997). Twenty years of cognitive assessment: current status and future directions. *Journal of Consulting and Clinical Psychology*, **65**, 996–1000.

Clark, D. M. and Wells, A. (1995). A cognitive model of social phobia. In *Social Phobia: Diagnosis, Assessment and Treatment*, ed. R. G. Heimberg, M. R. Liebowitz, D. A. Hope, and F. R. Schneier, pp. 69–93. New York: Guilford Press.

Clark, D. A., and Beck, A. T., with Alford, B. A. (1999). *Scientific Foundations of Cognitive Theory and Therapy of Depression*. New York: John Wiley.

DeRubeis, R. J. and Crits-Christoph, P. (1998). Empirically supported individual and group psychological treatments for adult mental disorders. *Journal of Consulting and Clinical Psychology*, **66**, 37–52.

DeRubeis, R. J., Gelfand, L. A., Tang, T. Z., and Simons, A. (1999). Medications versus cognitive behavioral therapy for severely depressed outpatients: mega-analysis of four randomized comparisons. *American Journal of Psychiatry*, **156**, 1007–13.

DeRubeis, R. J., Tang, T. Z., and Beck, A. T. (2001). Cognitive therapy. In *Handbook of Cognitive-behavioral Therapies*, 2nd edn ed. K. S. Dobson, pp. 349–92. New York: Guilford Press.

Ellis, A. (1962). *Reason and Emotion in Psychotherapy*. Secaucus, NJ: Lyle Stuart.

Elster, J. (1990). When rationality fails. In *The Limits of Rationality*, ed. K. Cook and M. Levi, pp. 19–51. Chicago, IL: University of Chicago Press.

Garber, J. and Flynn, C. (2001). Vulnerability to depression in childhood and adolescence. In *Vulnerability to Psychopathology: Risk Across the Lifespan*, ed. R. E. Ingram and J. M. Price, pp. 175–225. New York: Guilford Press.

Glass, C. R. and Arnkoff, D. B. (1997). Questionnaire methods of cognitive self-statement assessment. *Journal of Consulting and Clinical Psychology*, **65**, 911–27.

Gotlib, I. H. and McCabe, S. B. (1992). An information-processing approach to the study of cognitive functioning in depression. In *Progress in Experimental Personality and Psychopathology Research*, ed. E. F. Walker, B. A. Cornblatt, and R. H. Dworkin, vol. 15, pp. 131–61. New York: Springer.

Hammen, C. (2001). Vulnerability to depression in adulthood. In *Vulnerability to Psychopathology: Risk Across the Lifespan*, ed. R. E. Ingram and J. M. Price, pp. 226–57. New York: Guilford Press.

Hollon, S. D., DeRubeis, R. J., and Evans, M. D. (1996). Cognitive therapy in the treatment and prevention of depression. In *Frontiers of Cognitive Therapy*, ed. P. M. Salkovskis, pp. 293–317. New York: Guilford Press.

Kendall, P. C. and Finch, A. J., Jr (1976). A cognitive-behavioral treatment for impulse control: a case study. *Journal of Consulting and Clinical Psychology*, **44**, 852–7.

Lazarus, R. (1991). *Emotion and Adaptation*. New York: Oxford University Press.

MacLeod, C. (1993). Cognition in clinical psychology: measures, methods or models? *Behaviour Change*, **10**, 169–95.

Mahoney, M. J. (1974). *Cognition and Behavior Modification*. Cambridge, MA: Ballinger.

Malcarne, V. L. and Hansdottir, I. (2001). Vulnerability to anxiety disorders in childhood and adolescence. In *Vulnerability to Psychopathology: Risk Across the Lifespan*, ed. R. E. Ingram and J. M. Price, pp. 271–303. New York: Guilford Press.

McLean, P. D. and Woody, S. R. (2001). *Anxiety Disorders in Adults: An Evidence-based Approach to Psychological Treatment*. Oxford: Oxford University Press.

McNally, R. J. (2001a). On the scientific status of cognitive appraisal models of anxiety disorder. *Behaviour Research and Therapy*, **39**, 513–21.

McNally, R. J. (2001b). Vulnerability to anxiety disorders in adulthood. In *Vulnerability to Psychopathology: Risk Across the Lifespan*, ed, R. E. Ingram and J. M. Price, pp. 304–21. New York: Guilford Press.

Meichenbaum, D. H. (1977). *Cognitive-behavior Modification: An Integrative Approach*. New York: Plenum Press.

Meichenbaum, D. H. and Goodman, J. (1971). Training impulsive children to talk to themselves: a means of developing self-control. *Journal of Abnormal Psychology*, **77**, 115–26.

Rapee, R. M. and Heimberg, R. G. (1997). A cognitive-behavioral model of anxiety in social phobia. *Behaviour Research and Therapy*, **35**, 741–56.

Rehm, L. P. (1977). A self-control model of depression. *Behavior Therapy*, **8**, 787–804.

Rude, S. S. and Burnham, B. L. (1995). Connectedness and neediness: factors of the DEQ and SAS dependency scales. *Cognitive Therapy and Research*, **19**, 323–40.

Segal, Z. V., Williams, J. M., Teasdale, J. D., and Gemar, M. (1996). A cognitive science perspective on kindling and episode sensitization in recurrent affective disorder. *Psychological Medicine*, **26**, 371–80.

Segal, Z. V., Gemar, M., and Williams, S. (1999). Differential cognitive response to a mood challenge following successful cognitive therapy or pharmacotherapy for unipolar depression. *Journal of Abnormal Psychology*, **108**, 3–10.

Spivack, G., and Platt, J. J., and Shure, M. B. (1976). *The Problem- solving Approach to Adjustment*. San Francisco: Jossey-Bass.

Teasdale, J. D. and Barnard, P. J. (1993). *Affect, Cognition and Change: Remodelling Depressive Thought*. Hove, UK: Erlbaum.

Williams, J. M. G., Watts, F. N., MacLeod, C., and Mathews, A. (1997). *Cognitive Psychology and Emotional Disorders*, 2nd edn. Chichester: John Wiley.

Wilson, G. T. (1978). Cognitive behavior therapy: paradigm shift or passing phase? In *Cognitive Behavior Therapy: Research and Application*, ed. J. P. Foreyt and D. P. Rathjen, pp. 7–32. New York: Plenum Press.

Young, J. E. and Flanagan, C. (1998). Schema-focused therapy for narcissistic patients. In *Disorders of Narcissism: Diagnostic, Clinical, and Empirical Investigations*, ed. E. F. Ronningstam, pp. 239–62. Washington, DC: American Psychiatric Press.

Index

Printed in the United States
by Baker & Taylor Publisher Services